Mounting Optics
in Optical Instruments

Mounting Optics
in Optical Instruments

Paul R. Yoder, Jr.

SPIE PRESS
A Publication of SPIE—The International Society for Optical Engineering
Bellingham, Washington USA

Library of Congress Cataloging-in-Publication Data

Yoder, Paul R.
    Mounting optics in optical instruments / Paul R. Yoder, Jr.
     p. cm.
    Includes bibliographical references and index.
    ISBN 0-8194-4332-8
    1. Optical instruments--Design and construction. I. Title.

TS513 .Y62 2002
681'.25—dc21   2001049278

Published by

SPIE—The International Society for Optical Engineering
P.O. Box 10
Bellingham, Washington 98227-0010 USA
Phone: (1) 360.676.3290
Fax: (1) 360.647.1445
Email: spie@spie.org
Web: www.spie.org

Printed in the United States of America.

Dedication

I gratefully and lovingly dedicate this book to Betty, David, Marty, Carol, and Alan who have encouraged me to continue writing technical books since I really enjoy such efforts and cannot see my way clear as yet to abandon my adopted field of optomechanics to just sit on the porch or in my rocking chair and watch the rest of the world have all the fun.

Table of Contents

Preface	xiii
Terms and Symbols	xv
1. Introduction	1
1.1 Applications of Optical Components	1
1.2 Key Environmental Considerations	3
1.2.1 Temperature	4
1.2.2 Pressure	4
1.2.3 Moisture and other contamination	5
1.2.4 Vibration and shock	5
1.2.5 Radiation	7
1.2.6 Fungus	7
1.2.7 Abrasion and erosion	7
1.3 Extreme Service Environments	7
1.4 Environmental Testing	10
1.5 Key Material Properties	10
1.5.1 Optical glasses	11
1.5.2 Optical plastics	14
1.5.3 Optical crystals	14
1.5.4 Mirror materials	14
1.5.5 Materials for mechanical components	15
1.5.6 Adhesives and sealants	16
1.6 Dimensional Instability	17
References	18
2. The Optic-to-Mount Interface	21
2.1 Mechanical Constraints	21
2.1.1 General considerations	21
2.1.2 Lens interfaces	22
2.1.3 Prism interfaces	25
2.1.4 Mirror interfaces	29
2.1.5 Interfaces with other optical components	29
2.2 Consequences of Mounting Forces	29
2.3 Sealing Considerations	30
2.4 Cost and Manufacturability	31
References	32
3. Mounting Individual Lenses	33
3.1 Spring Mountings for Lenses and Filters	33
3.2 Burnished Cell Mountings	35
3.3 Snap and "Interference Fit" Rings	36
3.4 Retaining Ring Constraints	43
3.4.1 Threaded retaining ring	44
3.4.2 Clamping (flange) ring	48
3.4.3 Distributing preload uniformly	52
3.5 Constraining the Lens with Multiple Spring Clips	53
3.6 Geometry of the Lens-to-Mount Interface	56
3.6.1 The "sharp-corner" interface	56
3.6.2 The tangential (conical) interface	59

3.6.3 The toroidal interface	60
3.6.4 The spherical interface	63
3.6.5 Interfaces on bevels	65
3.7 Elastomeric Mountings	66
3.8 Advantages of a Spherical Lens Rim	75
3.9 Flexure Mountings	76
3.10 Aligning the Lens in Its Mount	81
3.11 Mounting Plastic Components	88
References	90
4. Multiple-Component Lens Assemblies	93
4.1 Spacer Design and Manufacture	93
4.2 Drop-In Assembly	101
4.3 Lathe Assembly	102
4.4 "Poker-Chip" Assembly	104
4.5 Precision Alignment of Multiple-Lens Assemblies	108
4.6 Assemblies with Plastic Housings and Lenses	116
4.7 Modular Assembly	117
4.8 Catadioptric Systems	121
4.9 Sealing and Purging Considerations	123
4.10 Internal Mechanisms	126
4.10.1 Focus mechanisms	126
4.10.2 Zoom mechanisms	130
References	131
5. Mounting Optical Windows, Filters, Shells, and Domes	135
5.1 Simple Window Mountings	135
5.2 Mounting "Special" Windows	139
5.3 Windows Subject to Pressure Differential	145
5.4 Filter Mountings	147
5.5 Mounting Shells and Domes	151
References	152
6. Prism Design	155
6.1 Geometric Considerations	155
6.1.1 Refraction and reflection	155
6.1.2 Total internal reflection	161
6.2 Aberration Contributions of Prisms	162
6.3 Typical Prism Configurations	163
6.3.1 Right-angle prism	163
6.3.2 Beamsplitter (or beamcombiner) cube prism	163
6.3.3 Amici prism	165
6.3.4 Porro prism	166
6.3.5 Abbe version of the Porro prism	167
6.3.6 Rhomboid prism	167
6.3.7 Porro erecting system	169
6.3.8 Abbe erecting system	169
6.3.9 Penta prism	170
6.3.10 Roof penta prism	170
6.3.11 Amici/penta erecting system	170
6.3.12 Dove prism	173
6.3.13 Double Dove prism	173

6.3.14 Reversion prism 175
6.3.15 Pechan prism 176
6.3.16 Delta prism 177
6.3.17 Schmidt prism 178
6.3.18 45° Bauernfeind prism 179
6.3.19 Internally reflecting axicon prism 179
6.3.20 Cube corner prism 180
6.3.21 Biocular prism system 181
6.3.22 Dispersing prisms 182
6.3.23 Thin-wedge prisms 185
6.3.24 Risley wedge system 187
6.3.25 Sliding wedge 187
6.3.26 Focus-adjusting wedge system 187
6.3.27 Anamorphic prism systems 189
References 192

7. Techniques for Mounting Prisms 193
7.1 Semikinematic Mountings 193
7.2 Mechanically Clamped Nonkinematic Mountings 208
7.3 Bonded Prism Mountings 212
7.3.1 General considerations 212
7.3.2 Cantilevered bonding techniques 216
7.3.3 Double-sided bonded support techniques 217
7.4 Flexure Mountings for Prisms 222
References 224

8. Mirror Design 227
8.1 First- and Second-Surface Mirrors 227
8.2 Determination of Mirror Aperture 233
8.3 Weight Reduction Techniques 235
8.3.1 Contoured-back configurations 237
8.3.2 Cast ribbed substrate configurations 247
8.3.3 Machined-back and built-up structural configurations 248
8.3.4 Thin facesheet configurations 257
8.4 Metallic Mirrors 260
8.5 Pellicles 264
References 267

9. Techniques for Mounting Small Mirrors 269
9.1 Mechanically Clamped Mirror Mountings 269
9.2 Bonded Mirror Mountings 277
9.3 Multiple Mirror Mountings 281
9.4 Flexure Mountings for Mirrors 287
9.5 Center Mountings for Circular-Aperture Mirrors 295
9.6 Mounting Metal Mirrors 297
9.7 Gravitational Effects on Small Mirrors 300
References 308

10. Techniques for Mounting Large Mirrors 311
10.1 Mounts for Variable-Orientation Applications 311
10.1.1 Counterweighted lever-type mountings 311
10.1.1.1 General principles 311
10.1.1.2 The 2.13-m (84-in.) Kitt Peak telescope 313

          10.1.1.3 The 5.1-m (200-in.) Hale telescope   316
       10.1.2 Hindle Mounts   319
          10.1.2.1 The 10-m (394-in.) Keck telescope   319
          10.1.2.2 A laser beam expander   323
          10.1.2.3 The SOFIA telescope   326
       10.1.3 Pneumatic and hydraulic mounts   329
          10.1.3.1 General principles   329
          10.1.3.2 A large UK telescope   333
          10.1.3.3 The converted "multiple mirror" telescope   334
          10.1.3.4 The Gemini telescopes   340
    10.2 Mounts for Fixed-Orientation Applications   343
       10.2.1 General principles   343
       10.2.2 Air bag-type axial supports   348
       10.2.3 Spring-type axial supports   350
       10.2.4 Mercury tube and strap radial supports   354
          10.2.4.1 Mercury tube supports   354
          10.2.4.2 Strap supports   354
    10.3 Supports for Large, Spaceborne Mirrors   357
       10.3.1 General considerations   357
       10.3.2 The infrared astronomical satellite telescope   357
       10.3.3 The Hubble telescope   360
       10.3.4 The Chandra telescope   364
    References   367

11. Estimation of Mounting Stresses in Optical Components   371
    11.1 General Considerations   371
    11.2 Average Compressive Stress   372
    11.3 Peak Axial Contact Stress in a Lens   373
       11.3.1 The sharp-corner interface   376
       11.3.2 The tangential interface   378
       11.3.3 The toroidal interface   380
       11.3.4 The spherical interface   381
       11.3.5 The flat-bevel interface   381
    11.4 Parametric Comparisons of Interface Types   381
    11.5 Contact Stress in a Lens Clamped with Spring Clips   386
       11.5.1 Springs with spherical pads   386
       11.5.2 Springs with cylindrical pads   390
    11.6 Contact Stress in Small Clamped Mirrors   391
    11.7 Contact Stress in Clamped Prisms   392
       11.7.1 Contact stress with curved interfaces   392
       11.7.2 Contact stress at flat prism locating pads   397
    11.8 Tensile Stress in the Single-Sided Bonded Interface   397
    11.9 Bending Stresses in Circular-Aperture Clamped Optics   398
       11.9.1 Causes of bending   398
       11.9.2 Bending stress in the optical component   399
       11.9.3 Change in surface sag of a bent optic   400
    References   402

12. Effects of Temperature Changes on Optical Component Mountings   403
    12.1 Athermalization Techniques   403
       12.1.1 Reflective systems   403

12.1.2 Refracting systems 406
12.2 Effects of Temperature Gradients 414
    12.2 1 Radial temperature gradients 415
    12.2.2 Axial temperature gradients 417
12.3 Change in Axial Preload Caused by a Temperature Change 418
12.4 Change in Lens Axial Clearance at Increased Temperature 422
12.5 Providing Residual Axial Preload on a Lens at Maximum Temperature 423
12.6 Contact Stress in a Lens at Low Temperature 424
12.7 Stress in Multiple-Lens Assemblies 425
    12.7.1 Cemented doublet lens 425
    12.7.2 Air-spaced doublet lens 428
    12.7.3 General case of the multiple-component lens 432
12.8 Radial Stresses in Rim-Mounted, Circular-Aperture Optics 432
    12.8.1 Radial stress in an optic at low temperature 433
    12.8.2 Tangential (hoop) stress in the mount wall 435
12.9 Growth of Radial Clearance at Increased Temperatures 436
12.10 Thermally Induced Stresses in Bonded Optics 437
    References 440

13. Hardware Examples 443
13.1 Lens Assembly Designed to Resist Thermal Shock 443
13.2 Infrared Sensor Lens Assembly 445
13.3 Cemented Doublet Binocular Objective Assembly 446
13.4 Modular Binocular Objective Assembly 447
13.5 Air-Spaced Triplet Telescope Objective Assembly 446
13.6 Commercial Mid-IR Lenses 449
13.7 Motorized Dual Field-of-View Lens Assembly 452
13.8 All-Plastic Projection Lens Assembly 452
13.9 Microscope Objective Assembly 456
13.10 A Simple Focusing Eyepiece Assembly 457
13.11 Collimator Assembly Designed for High Shock Loading 459
13.12 Elastomeric-Supported Camera Lens Assembly 462
13.13 Projection Lens Assembly 463
13.14 Astrographic Telescope Objective Assembly 464
13.15 Solid Catadioptric Lens Assembly 466
13.16 All-Aluminum Catadioptric Lens Assembly 469
13.17 Catadioptric Star-Mapping Objective Assembly 471
13.18 Long-Focal-Length Catadioptric Camera Objective Assembly 473
13.19 A 72-in. (1.8-m) Focal Length f/4 Aerial Camera Objective 477
13.20 Passively Stabilized 10:1 Zoom Lens Assembly 482
13.21 Camera Assembly for the DEIMOS Spectrograph 484
13.22 Nine Cameras for the Earth-Observing System, Multiangle Imaging Spectro-Radiometer 486
13.23 Bonded Porro Prism Erecting System for a Binocular 490
13.24 Large Flexure-Mounted Mirror Assembly 495
13.25 Mountings for Large Dispersing Prisms in an Echellette Spectrograph/Imager 497
13.26 Mountings for Prisms in an Articulated Telescope 502
13.27 Semikinematic Design for Constraining a Penta Prism with Springs 506

       13.27.1 Constraint perpendicular to the plane of reflection   506
       13.27.2 Constraint in the plane of reflection   509
    13.28 Mounting for the Geostationary Operational Environmental Satellite Telescope Secondary Mirror   514
    13.29 Mounting for the Far Ultraviolet Spectroscopic Explorer Spectrograph Gratings   515
    13.30 Mounting Configuration for the Very Large Telescope Secondary Mirror   519
      References   520

Appendix A Unit Conversion Factors   525

Appendix B Mechanical Properties of Materials   527
    B1 Selected mechanical properties of 68 selected Schott glasses   528
    B2 Comparison of 11 lightweight optical glasses (L) with the nearest standard glass types (S)   532
    B3 Selected optical and mechanical characteristics of commonly used optical plastics   533
    B4 Optomechanical properties of selected alkali halides and alkaline earth halides   535
    B5 Mechanical properties of selected IR-transmitting glass and other oxides   537
    B6 Mechanical properties of diamond and selected IR-transmitting semiconductor materials   540
    B7 Mechanical properties of selected IR-transmitting chalcogenide materials   542
    B8a Mechanical properties of selected nonmetallic mirror substrate materials   543
    B8b Mechanical properties of selected metallic and composite mirror substrate materials   545
    B9 Comparison of material figures of merit especially pertinent to mirror design   547
    B10a Characteristics of aluminum alloys used in mirrors   549
    B10b Characteristics of aluminum matrix composites   550
    B10c Beryllium grades and some of their properties   551
    B10d Characteristics of major silicon carbide types   552
    B11 Techniques for machining, finishing, and coating materials for optical applications   553
    B12 Mechanical properties of selected metals used for mechanical parts in optical instruments   554
    B13 Typical physical characteristics of optical cements   558
    B14 Typical characteristics of representative structural adhesives   559
    B15 Typical physical characteristics of representative elastomeric sealants   564
    B16 Typical minimum values for fracture strength S_F of infrared window materials   566
    B17 Coefficient of thermal defocus (δ) and thermo-optical coefficient (γ) for selected optical materials   567

Appendix C Torque-Preload Relationship for a Threaded Retaining Ring   573

Appendix D The Lens Temperature Sensitivity Factor K_3   575

Index   579

PREFACE

This work is intended to provide practitioners in the fields of optical engineering and optomechanical design with a comprehensive understanding of the principal ways in which optical components such as lenses, windows, filters, shells, domes, prisms, and mirrors of all sizes typically are mounted in optical instruments. It also addresses the advantages and disadvantages of various mounting arrangements and provides some analytical tools that can be used to evaluate and compare different optomechanical designs. The presentation includes the theoretical background for some of these tools and cites the sources for the most of the equations listed. Each section contains an illustrated discussion of the technology involved and, wherever feasible, one or more worked-out practical examples.

Two chapters deal with the fundamentals of design for optical components. These are Chapters 6 on prism design and Chapter 8 on mirror design. These topics are considered appropriate, and indeed necessary, as background for considering how best to mount these very important types of optics.

The book is based, in part, on short courses entitled *Precision Optical Component Mounting Techniques* and *Principles for Mounting Optical Components* offered by SPIE—The International Society for Optical Engineering— that I have had the privilege of teaching over a period of several years. Many, but not all, of the techniques for mounting optics covered here have been presented previously in the tutorial texts *Mounting Lenses in Optical Instruments*[1] and *Design and Mounting of Prisms and Small Mirrors in Optical Instruments*[2] as well as in my earlier reference book *Opto-Mechanical Systems Design*.[3] Several recent designs for mounting optics are included here to broaden the coverage and to bring the material more nearly up to date. Coverage of window-type optics and of large mirrors has been expanded over the previous works.

Wherever possible, numerical values given in this book are expressed in both the metric or Système International (SI) units and the units in customary use in the United States and Canada. The latter are abbreviated in this book as "USC" as in some recent textbooks. Examples taken directly from the literature may be expressed only in the system used by the original author. Units can be easily changed from one system to the other through use of the conversion factors given in Appendix A.

All the designs discussed here are drawn from the literature, my own experiences in optical instrument design and development, and the work of colleagues. I acknowledge with my deepest thanks the contributions of others, including the many participants in the above-mentioned SPIE short courses and the readers of my previous books, and sincerely hope that I have accurately recorded and explained the information they have given to me. I acknowledge and thank Donald O'Shea and Daniel Vukobratovich, who reviewed the manuscript for this book and suggested many improvements. I also thank Mary Haas, Rick Hermann, and Sharon Streams for their outstanding copy editing and editorial suggestions. While these people helped me to present the material clearly, correctly, and completely, I am solely responsible for and deeply regret any errors that remain.

The mounting stress theories discussed in Chapter 11 are considered to be conservative approximations. They are intended to indicate whether a given design can be judged to be adequate from a stress viewpoint or if it should be analyzed by more elaborate finite-element and/or statistical techniques. The same is true of the treatment of temperature effects on axial preload in Chapter 12. These topics would benefit greatly from further investigation, refinement, and (it is hoped) verification by other workers based on more precise computational methods, such as finite-element analysis. I would welcome comments, corrections, and suggestions for improvements in the presentations of these topics and/or in any other portion of this book.

A feature included with this book is a CD-ROM containing two Microsoft Excel worksheets that allow convenient use of the many equations given in this text to solve typical optomechanical interface design and analysis problems. Some of these equations are relatively complex, so the worksheets have been developed to facilitate equation use and to reduce the chance of improper parameter application. The 102 files included in each worksheet correspond to designs and/or numerical examples worked out in the text. Input values pertaining specifically to those examples are listed. The two worksheets on the disk are different versions of the same program. In Version 1, data inputs are in U.S. Customary units while in Version 2 inputs are in metric units. In both cases, all data are presented in both sets of units. A table of files (with hyperlinks) is provided in each worksheet to assist in finding the proper file for a specific computation. The examples in the text are cross referenced to the applicable worksheet files. Custom solutions to problems similar to the examples in the text can be obtained by revising the input data in the file as appropriate for the case to be evaluated. The program will then automatically solve the problem using those inputs and the appropriate equations from the text. This tool should be especially useful when parametric analysis of variations of key parameters is needed to obtain an optimum design.

I sincerely wish for the users of this book and of the CD-ROM a deepening understanding of the technologies discussed and success in the application of the concepts, designs, and analysis techniques presented here.

1. Yoder, P.R., Jr., *Mounting Lenses in Optical Instruments*, TT21, SPIE Press, Bellingham, 1995.
2. Yoder, P.R., Jr., *Design and Mounting of Prisms and Small Mirrors in Optical Instruments*, TT32, SPIE Press, Bellingham, 1998.
3. Yoder, P.R., Jr., *Opto-Mechanical Systems Design*, 2nd ed., Marcel Dekker, New York, 1993.

Paul R. Yoder, Jr.
Norwalk, Connecticut

TERMS AND SYMBOLS

This list of the terms and symbols used in this book is intended to help the reader sort through the shorthand language of the various technical topics and the equations used to express the relationships so useful in the design process and the analysis of designs. The author has attempted to be consistent in the use of symbols for variables throughout the text, but there are occasions where the same symbol has more than one meaning. To some extent, customary usage in the field of optomechanics has dictated the use of a specific term or terms, The symbol α is a good example since it is used to represent the coefficient of thermal expansion for a material when the common abbreviation CTE is not appropriate, as in equations. Subscripts are frequently used to identify the specific application of a symbol to a specific material (as in the use of α_M to designate the CTE for a metal as distinguished from α_G for a glass). We list here fundamental parameters and their units, frequently used prefixes, Greek symbol applications, acronyms, abbreviations, and other terms found in the text.

Units of Measure

Parameter	SI or metric	U.S. and Canadian
Angle	rad, radian	°, degree
Area	m^2, square meter	$in.^2$, square inch
Conductivity, thermal	W/mK, watt/meter-kelvin	Btu/hr-ft-°F, British thermal unit per hour-foot-degree Fahrenheit
Density	g/m^3, gram per cubic meter	$lb/in.^3$, pound per cubic inch
Diffusivity, thermal	m^2/s, meter squared per second	$in.^2/s$, inch squared per second
Energy	J, joule	ft-lb, foot-pound
Force	N, newton	lb, pound
Frequency	Hz, hertz	Hz, hertz
Heat	Btu, British thermal unit	ft/lb, foot-pound
Length	m, meter	in., inch
Mass	kg, kilogram	lb, pound
Moment of force (torque)	N/m, newton-meter	lb-ft, pound-foot
Pressure	Pa, pascal	$lb/in.^2$, pound per square inch
Specific heat	J/kg-K, joule/kilogram-Kelvin	Btu/lb-°F, British thermal unit per pound-degree Fahrenheit
Strain	$\mu m/m$, micrometer/meter	$\mu in.$ per in., microinch per inch
Stress	Pa, pascal	$lb/in.^2$, pound per square inch
Temperature	K, kelvin; °C, degree Celsius	°F, degree Fahrenheit
Time	s or sec, second	s or sec, hr, second, hour

Velocity	m/s or m/sec, meter/second	mph, mile per hour
Viscosity	P, poise; cP, centipoise	lb-s/ft^2, pound-sec per square foot
Volume (solid)	m^3, cubic meter	in.^{3}, cubic inch

Prefixes

mega	M	million
kilo	k	thousand
centi	c	hundredth
milli	m	thousandth
micro	μ	millionth
nano	n	billionth

Greek Symbol Applications

α	CTE; angle
β	angle; term used in equation for shear stress in a bonded optic
β_G	rate of change in refractive index with change in temperature (dn/dT)
γ	shape factor for a resilient pad in a prism mounting
γ_G	thermo-optical coefficient for a glass
δ	decentration of an elastomeric-supported optic; ray angular deviation
δ_G	glass coefficient of thermal defocus
Δ	spring deflection; finite difference (change)
Δ_E	eyepiece focus motion per diopter
θ	angle
λ	wavelength; thermal conductivity in Schott catalog
μ	Poisson's ratio in Schott catalog
μ_M, μ_G	coefficient of sliding friction of metal, glass
ξ	ratio of shortest to longest dimensions of a rectangular mirror
π	3.14159
ρ	density
σ	standard deviation
Σ	summation
σ_i	tensile yield strength of components in a bonded joint
υ	Poisson's ratio
ϕ	angle
φ	cone half-angle

Acronyms and Abbreviations

A/R	antireflection
ANSI	American National Standards Institute
AWJ	abrasive water jet
AXAF	Advanced X-ray Astrophysical Facility

CA	clear aperture
CCD	charge-coupled device
CG	center of gravity
CNC	computer numerically controlled
CR	resistance to humidity in Schott catalog
CRES	corrosion-resistant (stainless) steel
CTE	coefficient of thermal expansion
CVD	chemical-vapor-deposited
DOF	degrees of freedom
EDM	electric discharge machining (process for contouring metal)
ECM	electro-chemical machining (process for contouring metal)
EFL	effective focal length (as of a lens or mirror)
ESO	European Southern Observatory
FEA	finite-element analysis
FLIR	forward-looking infrared sensor
FUSE	Far Ultraviolet Spectroscopic Explorer
GOES	Geostationary Operational Environmental Satellite
HeNe	helium-neon laser
HIP	hot isostatic pressing
HRMA	high-resolution mirror assembly
ID	inside diameter
IPD	interpupillary distance
IR	infrared
IRAS	Infrared Astronomical Satellite
ISIM	Integrated Science Instrument Module
KAO	Kuiper Airborne Observatory
LAGEOS	Laser Geodynamic Satellite
LLTV	low light-level television
LOS	line of sight
LRR	lower rim ray at maximum semifield angle
MLI	multilayer insulation
MMT	Multiple Mirror Telescope
MTF	modulation transfer function
NASA	National Aeronautics and Space Administration
NGST	Next-Generation Space Telescope
OBA	optical bench assembly
OD	outside diameter
OFHC	oxygen-free high-conductivity
OPD	optical path difference
OTF	optical transfer function
p-v	peak to valley
RH	relative humidity
rms	root mean square
RTV	room-temperature vulcanizing
SOFIA	Stratospheric Observatory of Infrared Astronomy
SPDT	single-point diamond turning
TIR	total internal reflection; total indicator runout
tpi	threads per inch
ULE	Corning's ultra-low expansion material

URR	upper rim ray at maximum semifield angle
UV	ultraviolet
VLT	Very Large Telescope

Other Terms

a, b, c, etc.	dimensions
A	aperture, area
-A-, -B-, etc.	reference surface designation
A_C	area of elastically deformed region at an interface
a_G	acceleration factor (interpreted as "times ambient gravity")
A_T	annular area of a thread
AVG	as subscript, indicates average value
C	center of curvature
C	as subscript, indicates circular shape for a bonded area
C_K	mirror mount type factor used to determine gravitational effect
C_p	specific heat
C_R, C_T	spring constants in radial, tangential directions
C_T	center of curvature of a toroidal surface
C_X, C_Y	spring constants in X, Y directions
CYL	as subscript, indicates cylindrical shape
d	diameter of a screw head
D	thermal diffusivity; diopter
D_B	diameter of a bolt circle
D_G	OD of a circular optic
D_M	ID of a metal component
dn/dT	rate of change in refractive index with change in temperature
D_P	diameter of a resilient pad
D_R	OD of a compressed snap ring
D_T	pitch diameter of a thread
E/ρ	specific stiffness
E	Young's modulus
f	focal length
F	force
f_E	focal length of an eyepiece
f_S	safety factor
g	acceleration due to gravity
H	thread crest-to-root height
I, I'	angle of incidence, refraction
J	strength of an adhesive bond
k	thermal conductivity
K	stress optic coefficient
K_1, K_A, etc.	constant term in an equation
L	length of a spring that is free to bend; width or diameter of a bond
$L_{j, k}$	axial length of a lens spacer
ln (x)	natural logarithm of x
m	reciprocal of Poisson's ratio
n	refractive index

N	number of springs
n_d	refractive index for $\lambda = 546.074$ nm
N_E, N_1, N_2	number of threads per unit length of differential thread
p	thread crest-to-crest pitch; linear preload
P	preload force; optical power
P_i	preload force per spring
q	heat flux per unit of area
Q	torque; bonding area
Q_{MAX}	maximum bonding area within face dimension
Q_{MIN}	minimum bonding area for strength of joint
r	snap ring cross-sectional radius
R	surface radius
R_λ	reflectance of a surface at wavelength λ
r_C	radius of elastically deformed region at an interface
roll	component tilt about transverse axis
r_S	radius to center of a spacer
R_S	reflectance of a coated surface
R_T	cross-section radius of toroidal surface
RT	as subscript, indicates racetrack shape for bond area
S_{AVG}	average contact stress in an interface
S_B	stress in a bent component such as a spring
S_C	contact stress at an optic-to-mount interface
SC	as subscript, indicates sharp corner interface
S_e	shear modulus of an elastomer
S_f	fracture strength of a window material
S_j, S_k	sagittal depth of surface j, k
S_M	tangential tensile (hoop) stress in a mount's wall
S_{MY}	microyield strength
S_{PAD}	average stress in a pad-to-optic interface
SPH	as subscript, indicates spherical interface
S_R	radial stress at an optic-to-mount interface
S_S	shear stress developed in a bonded joint from a temperature change
S_T	tensile stress
S_W	yield strength for window material
S_Y	yield strength
t	thickness (as of spring or flange)
T_λ	transmittance of a surface at wavelength λ
T_A	assembly temperature
TAN	as subscript, indicates a tangential interface
tanh	hyperbolic tangent function
t_C	cell wall thickness
T_C	temperature at which assembly preload reduces to zero
t_e	thicknes of an annular elastomer layer
t_E	edge thickness of a lens
TOR	as subscript, indicates a toroidal interface
U, U′	angles of marginal ray with respect to the axis in object, image space
V	volume; lens vertex
v_d	Abbe number for $\lambda = 546.074$ nm
W	weight

w_S	wall thickness of a spacer
X, Y, Z	coordinate axes
y_C	contact height on an optical surface
y_S	ID/2 for a lens mounting

Mounting Optics
in Optical Instruments

CHAPTER 1
Introduction

This chapter addresses general issues that typically must be considered by designers or engineers during the evolution of an optical instrument design. Subsequent chapters delve more deeply into specific design issues involving mounting the common types of optics.

The effective engineering design of optical instruments requires advance knowledge of the adverse environments under which the product is expected to operate successfully as well as those it must survive. In this chapter, we summarize ways in which temperature, pressure, vibration, shock, moisture, corrosion, contamination, fungus, abrasion, erosion, and high-energy radiation can affect an instrument's performance and/or useful life. We also offer some very general suggestions for designing an apparatus to withstand these adverse conditions. More specific design guidelines are included in later sections as parts of descriptions of successful instrument designs. Because careful selection of materials is vital for maximizing environmental resistance and ensuring the proper operation of the product, we review the attributes of some of the most frequently used optical and mechanical materials.

1.1 Applications of Optical Components

Lenses serve many functions in optical instruments. In general, they are used to form real or virtual images of large or small objects at various distances, or they redirect rays to form pupils of the optical system. In addition, some lenses serve as correctors that differentially refract rays over their apertures in order to modify (read "correct") aberrations introduced by other image-forming components.

The most common forms of lenses are objectives, relay or erecting lenses, eyepieces, field lenses, magnifiers, and corrector plates. Most lenses have polished spherical or aspherical surfaces that refract rays in accordance with Snell's law. Some lens surfaces are configured to diffract rays. Here we will limit our attention to refracting lenses since we are primarily concerned with mounting principles rather than image-forming considerations. Diameters are limited by difficulties in making high-quality optical glass in large sizes and in fabricating precision surfaces larger than about 20 in. (0.5 m).*

Windows, filters, shells, and domes serve one or more of the following functions:

• They separate and seal the interior of the instrument from the outside environment,
• They adapt the spectral characteristics of the transmitted (or reflected) beam,
• They correct aberrations (as in the case of Maksutov corrector shells).

Shells are meniscus-shaped windows, while domes are deep shells, with apertures subtending meridional angles as large as 180° from their centers of curvature. Hyperhemispheres are domes that extend beyond a hemisphere.

---

* See Appendix A for a list of conversion factors.

1

Mirrors may have flat (plano) or curved surfaces. The latter are termed "image-forming mirrors" since they have optical power because of their curved reflecting surfaces. They can function similarly to lenses in the above-mentioned roles. Since refraction is not involved, chromatic aberration is absent when images are formed by mirrors.

Reflecting optics can be made with aperture sizes far larger than lenses primarily because the absence of a need to transmit light allows substantial support to be provided over the full extent of the back side of the optic rather than solely around the rim as in most lenses. Furthermore, the stiffness of the mirror substrate can be enhanced by choosing its thickness for mechanical reasons rather than optical ones. The availability of substrate materials with suitable mechanical characteristics, such as high stiffness (i.e., Young's modulus) and/or a low coefficient of thermal expansion (CTE), also contributes to the advantage of mirrors over lenses in large sizes.

The principal applications for most prisms, beamsplitters or beamcombiners, and flat mirrors, i.e., components that do not contribute optical power and hence cannot form images, are as follows:

- Deviating or bending the system axis,
- Displacing the system axis laterally,
- Folding an optical system into a given shape or package size,
- Providing proper image orientation,
- Adjusting optical path length,
- Dividing or combining beams by intensity or aperture sharing (at a pupil),
- Dividing or combining images at an image plane,
- Scanning a beam,
- Dispersing light spectrally (gratings or prisms), and
- Modifying the aberration balance of the optical system.

The number of reflections provided in a system that includes mirrors and/or prisms is important, especially in visual and photographic or video applications. An odd number of reflections produces a "left-handed" (reversed or reverted) image that is not directly readable, while an even number gives a normal, "right-handed" image. The latter is readable even if it is inverted (see Fig. 1.1). Vector techniques, summarized well by Walles and Hopkins,[1] are powerful tools for determining how a particular combination of reflecting surfaces will affect the location and orientation of an image.

(a)   (b)

Fig. 1.1 (a) Left- and (b) right-handed images.

In this book we describe in considerable detail various design configurations for lenses, windows, filters, shells, domes, prisms, and mirrors that accomplish their intended functions, as well as typical ways in which these components can be mounted and analyzed for stress buildup and/or surface distortion caused by mounting forces.

1.2 Key Environmental Considerations

It is essential in a serious discussion of any instrument design to identify the environmental conditions under which the end item is expected to perform in accordance with given specifications, as well as the extreme conditions that it must survive without permanent damage. The most important conditions to be considered are temperature, pressure, vibration, and shock. These external influences exert static and/or dynamic forces on hardware members that may cause deflections or dimensional changes. These changes may result in misalignment, buildup of adverse internal stresses, birefringence, or even breakage of components. In some applications, "crash safety" (the instrument or portions of it must not pose a hazard to personnel in an otherwise survivable violent-shock event) is also specified. Other important considerations include humidity, corrosion, contamination, fungus growth, abrasion, erosion, and high-energy radiation, which can affect performance or lead to progressive deterioration of the instrument. It is important for intended users and system engineers to define the expected exposures of the instrument to adverse environments under operating, storage, and transportation conditions as early in the design process as possible so appropriate provisions can be made to minimize their effects in a timely manner.

Different environments exist for operation, storage, and shipment conditions. The significance of these environments differs according to the intended use of the system, since an instrument to be used in the controlled environment of a laboratory would be expected to experience a different set of conditions than one designed for military or space applications. For nonspaceborne military applications, general information on the expected extreme and typical values of natural climatic conditions for hot, basic, cold, severe cold, and sea surface and coastal regions of the earth, as well as the worldwide air environment to a 80-km (262,000-ft) altitude may be derived from U.S. MIL-STD-210, "Climatic Information to Determine Design and Test Requirements for Military Systems and Equipment."[2] ISO 10109, "Environmental Requirements,"[3] issued by the International Standards Organization, provides similar guidance (see Parks[4] and Yoder[5]). Much of the data contained in these standards are also applicable to nonmilitary equipment.

The environmental conditions encountered in space also vary in severity, depending on spacecraft location relative to the sun, Earth, and other celestial bodies. The low-Earth-orbit environment is rather well known, having been explored through instrumented probes and manned missions (see, for example, Musikant and Malloy[6]). Higher orbits such as those encountered by synchronous satellites also are fairly well defined. Ventures to the moon and the nearby planets have revealed harsh environments that challenge payload designers to select materials and configure hardware to protect sensors long enough to accomplish the mission. Detailed considerations of the problems of designing optical instruments to cope with such extreme environments are beyond the scope of this book.

1.2.1 Temperature

Key temperature effects to be considered include high and low extremes, thermal shock, and gradients. Military equipment is usually designed to withstand extreme temperatures of - 62°C (- 80°F) to 71°C (160°F) during storage or shipment. It usually must operate adequately at temperatures of - 54°C (- 65°F) to 52°C (125°F). Commercial equipment generally is designed for smaller ranges of temperatures. Special-purpose equipment such as a spaceborne infrared sensor payload may experience temperatures approaching absolute zero, while sensors intended to function in the interior of a furnace may have to operate at temperatures of several hundred degrees Celsius.

Rapid changes in temperature occur when an electro-optical sensor on a spacecraft leaves or reenters the Earth's shadow or when a camera is taken directly from a warm room to a frigid arctic location. These "thermal shocks" can significantly affect performance or even cause damage to the optics. Thermal diffusivity is a characteristic of all materials that affects how quickly parts of an optical instrument respond to temperature changes. Most optical materials have low thermal conductivities, so heat is not transferred rapidly through them. Slower changes of temperature affect performance mainly by introducing temperature gradients, changing the dimensions of parts, or causing instrument parts to move relative to each other. Materials that have inhomogeneous thermal expansion coefficients, such as those sometimes used in mirror substrates, change dimensions under temperature changes differently at various locations within a component and hence modify critical dimensions or the surface figure. Common effects of misalignments are loss of system resolution or quality as a result of focus errors or asymmetry of images, loss of calibration in measuring devices, and pointing errors. Gradients can degrade the uniformity of the refractive index in transmitting materials such as glass and cause similar effects. Focus compensation techniques, such as those summarized in Sect. 12.1 of this book, help reduce some of these adverse thermal effects. However, they generally cannot correct problems that are due to gradients.

1.2.2 Pressure

Pressure manifests itself in optical instrument design chiefly because the refractive index of air changes with altitude; gases, moisture, or other contaminants "pump" through small leaks in instrument housings whenever outside pressure changes; and optical components exposed to pressure differentials may distort elastically or, in the extreme case, be damaged. Optical components experiencing aerodynamic or hydrodynamic overpressures in moving vehicles can also deflect excessively if they are not properly designed and mounted for these conditions. An example is a thin window on a forward-looking infrared (FLIR) sensor exposed to ram air pressure in an aircraft (see Sect. 5.3 of this book). Everyday changes in ambient barometric pressure can degrade the performance of high-resolution optical devices such as the optical lithography projectors used to make microcircuits because the refractive index of the air adjacent to optical surfaces changes sufficiently to cause errors in focus or in magnification. The optics of some sealed instruments, such as submarine periscopes or missile-tracking telescopes, may also suffer from air pressure variations when the temperature changes or the vehicle dives to great depths.

Other pressure-related effects include outgassing in a vacuum of certain materials (plastics, elastomers, lubricants, brazed joints, surface platings, etc.) and permeation of water vapor through seals and seemingly impervious walls, such as castings. Very careful selection of materials and precise control of manufacturing processes help significantly in these instances.

1.2.3 Moisture and other contamination

In order to maximize an optical instrument's resistance to humidity, corrosion, and contamination, it is important to use compatible materials in the design (i.e., materials that do not naturally form a galvanic couple when in contact with each other); to assemble the instrument in a clean, dry environment; and to seal all paths where leakage could otherwise occur between the instrument's interior and the outside world. Techniques for sealing optical instruments are discussed briefly in Sects. 2.3 and 4.9 of this book. Once sealed, the interior cavities of the instrument may be purged with a dry gas (such as nitrogen or helium) through valves or removable seal screws to remove traces of moisture that could condense on optical surfaces or other sensitive component surfaces. In some cases, the pressure of the residual gas within the instrument will intentionally be somewhat above ambient external pressure. Raising internal pressure does not reduce the entry of moisture, but helps prevent contamination by particulates. Diffusion of water into the instrument is determined by the partial pressure of water and the permeability of the walls and seals. Partial pressure is governed by the difference in relative humidity (RH) inside and outside the device and by temperature. Drying the inside increases the time required for the gas inside to reach RH equilibrium with the outside environment.[7]

In some instruments, the optics are sealed to the housing, but a leakage path is intentionally provided so that pressure differentials do not build up. In such cases, the leakage path is through a desiccator and a particulate filter that deter moisture, dust, and other undesirable matter from entering.

The performance of optical instruments using ultraviolet (UV) light, such as lithography systems working at a 157-nm wavelength, is degraded by the presence of seemingly insignificant quantities of certain contaminants in the optical path. These may be in the form of deposits of hydrocarbons and/or silicones on optical surfaces or water vapor in the surrounding gas. Interaction of the UV radiation with molecules of the contaminant plays a strong role in these effects. The presence of small amounts of diatomic oxygen in the gas reduces the effects of some potential surface contaminants by converting them into less harmful chemicals. Excessive amounts of this oxygen can reduce transmission of the system. The quantities of all potential contaminating materials in and around the instrument need to be controlled to predetermined allowable levels to ensure the success of these instruments.[8]

1.2.4 Vibration and shock

Vibration and shock environments both involve application of mechanical forces to the instrument. These forces cause the entire instrument or portions of it to be displaced from their normal equilibrium positions. The displaced member tends to return to equilibrium under the action of restoring forces that may include internal elastic forces, as in the case of a mass attached to a spring, or gravitational forces, as in the case of a pendulous mass. If the driving force is periodic, the member oscillates about the equilibrium position under a condition of sustained vibration. If that force is sudden and temporary, the member is said to be experiencing a shock impulse.

Any physical structure has characteristic natural frequencies at which its members oscillate mechanically in specific vibrational modes. Application to that structure of a driving force at or near one of these particular frequencies (or a harmonic of it) can cause a condition of resonance in which the amplitude of the member's oscillation increases until it is limited by internal or external damping, or damage occurs. Usually the amplitude, frequency, and direction of the forces externally applied to an instrument cannot be controlled by the designer, so the only corrective action possible is to make the instrument's components stiff enough so that their lowest natural frequency is higher than that of the driving forces. Steinberg reported that it is good engineering practice for an instrument to be designed so the fundamental frequency of a component increases by a factor of 2 at each interface (structure to mount, mount to optic, etc.) to limit resonant coupling.[9] Some designs include a means for damping vibrations.

It is important to recognize that microscopic changes in dimension and/or contour can occur in an optical component as a result of the applied load, either by gravity or by acceleration. These changes may be temporary under low (operational) loading or permanent under higher (survival) loading that exceeds the breaking point for brittle (glass-type) materials or the elastic limit* of mechanical materials. Englehaupt indicated that stress may need to be kept at least one order of magnitude lower in optical components than in conventionally engineered mechanical hardware.[10]

Design techniques that can be used to increase the resistance of an optical instrument to vibration and shock include ensuring adequate support for fragile optical members (such as lenses, windows, shells, prisms, and mirrors); providing adequate strength for all structural members to minimize the risk of distortion beyond their elastic (or perhaps their microyield**) limit; and reducing the mass to be supported.

Key to achievement of a successful design under specified vibration and shock conditions is knowledge of how the instrument will react to the imposed forces. Analytical (i.e., software) tools of ever-increasing capability using finite-element analysis (FEA) methods are available for modeling the design and predicting its behavior under variable imposed time- and spatial-loading.[11-14] Some of these tools interface with optical design software so that degradation of optical performance under specific adverse conditions can be evaluated directly. The effects of temperature changes, thermal gradients, and pressure changes also can be evaluated with these same analytical tools.

---

* Defined as that level of stress that causes a strain per unit length of 2 parts per thousand.
** Defined as that stress that causes 1 part per million (ppm) of plastic, i.e., nonelastic, strain.

1.2.5 Radiation

Limited protection can be provided for optics exposed to high-energy radiation in the form of gamma and x-rays, neutrons, protons, and electrons by shielding them with materials that absorb these radiation types; by using optical materials, such as fused silica, that are relatively insensitive to such radiation; or by using radiation-protected optical glasses. The latter suffer from a slight reduction in blue-end visible and UV light transmission before exposure to radiation, but maintain their transmission characteristics over a broad spectral range after such exposure much better than unprotected glasses.

Several types of glass incorporating cerium oxide to increase their resistance to radiation are available from suppliers as Schott Glass Technologies, Inc. These materials differ only slightly in their optical and mechanical properties compared with the equivalent standard glasses (see Marker [15]).

1.2.6 Fungus

The potential for damage to optics and coatings by fungus is greatest when the instrument is exposed simultaneously to high humidity and high temperature, conditions that primarily exist in tropical climates. The use of organic materials, such as cork and leather, in optical instruments is specifically forbidden by military specifications. This is generally good practice also for nonmilitary applications unless the environment will be very well controlled. Inorganic materials also may support the growth of fungus because of residual contaminants on supposedly clean surfaces. Even glass may support fungus growth under certain conditions.[4] In the long term, this growth may stain the glass and adversely affect transmission and image quality.

1.2.7 Abrasion and erosion

Abrasion and erosion problems occur most frequently in devices with optical surfaces that are exposed to wind-driven sand or other abrasive particles or to raindrops or ice and snow particles moving at high relative velocity. Usually the former damage occurs on land vehicles or helicopters, while the latter occurs on aircraft traveling at high speed [>200 m/s, (447 mph)]. Softer optical materials, such as infrared-transmitting crystals, are most affected by these conditions.[4,16] A limited degree of protection can be afforded by thin coatings of harder materials. In the space environment, exposure to micrometeorites and debris may cause damage to optics, such as unprotected telescope mirrors. Retractable or disposable covers are used in some cases to provide temporary protection.

1.3 Extreme Service Environments

In addition to MIL-STD-210[2] mentioned earlier, representative environmental conditions are listed in Table 1.1.[17] Examples are given for each category to illustrate the general type of instrumentation expected to undergo the extreme exposures. Additional data pertinent to vibration levels that optical instruments may experience in common applications are given in Table 1.2.[17] The latter data are vibrational power spectral

Table 1.1 - Typical values for selected adverse environmental conditions

Environment	Normal	Severe	Extreme	Example of Instrumentation Undergoing Extreme Condition
Low temperature (T_{MIN})	293 K (20°C)	222 K (-51°C)	2.4 K (-271°C)	Cryogenic satellite payload
High temperature (T_{MAX})	300 K (27°C)	344 K (71°C)	423 K (150°C)	White cell for combustion study
Low atmospheric pressure	88 kPa (0.9 atm)	57 kPa (0.5 atm)	0 kPa (0 atm)	Satellite telescope
High atmospheric pressure	108 kPa (1.1 atm)	1 MPa (9.8 atm)	138 MPa (1361 atm)	Window on submersible vehicle
Relative humidity (RH)	25-75%	100%	Under water	Submerged camera
Acceleration factor (a_G)	2	12	11,000	Gun-launched projectile
Vibration	200×10^{-6} m/s rms $f \geq 8$ Hz	0.04 g^2/Hz $20 \leq f \geq 100$ Hz	0.13 g^2/Hz $30 \leq f \geq 1500$ Hz	Satellite launch

Adapted from Vukobratovich.[17]

Table 1.2 - Typical vibrational power spectral densities characteristic of military and aerospace environments

Environment	Frequency (Hz)	Power spectral density (PSD)	Environment	Frequency (Hz)	Power spectral density (PSD)
Navy warships	1 – 50	0.001 g^2/Hz	Ariane launch vehicle	5 – 150 150 – 700 700 – 2000	+6 dB/octave 0.04 g^2/Hz -3 dB/octave
Minimum integrity test (MIL-STD-810E)	20 – 1000 1000 – 2000	0.04 g^2/Hz -6 dB/octave	Space shuttle (orbiter keel location)	15 – 100 100 – 400 400 — 2000	+6 dB/octave 0.10 g^2/Hz -6 dB/octave
Typical aircraft	15 – 100 100 – 300 300 – 1000 ≥1000	0.03 g^2/Hz +4 dB/octave 0.17 g^2/Hz -3 dB/octave			
Thor-Delta launch vehicle	20 – 200	0.07 g^2/Hz			
Titan launch vehicle	13 – 30 30 – 1500 1500 – 2000	+6 dB/octave 0.13 g^2/Hz -6 dB/octave			

Adapted from Vukobratovich.[17]

densities and frequency ranges of typical military and aerospace environments. Neither of these sets of data is exhaustive or absolute. More severe conditions may apply.

1.4 Environmental Testing

Environmental testing of hardware is intended to ensure that it has been designed and manufactured to withstand all pertinent environmental conditions to which it might reasonably be subjected, alone or in combination, throughout the equipment's planned life cycle. Whenever possible, the test item should be in the final configuration and interfaced with the related support structure, if any. In some cases, testing of portions of the equipment or representative prototype versions may be permitted.

Guidelines for planning and conducting environmental tests to determine the ability of military equipment to withstand the anticipated climatic exposures may be found in U.S. MIL-STD-810, "Environmental Test Methods and Engineering Guidelines." [18] These guidelines also may apply, within limits, to nonmilitary equipment. Another excellent source of guidance regarding testing of optical instruments is contained in International Standard ISO 9022, "Environmental Test Methods." [19] This detailed specification defines the required types and severity of tests in a variety of methods. Summaries of this document have been given by Yoder [4] and by Parks. [5]

1.5 Key Material Properties

Key terms and mechanical properties of materials in the context of optical instrument design and the symbols and units used to represent them in this book are as follows:

Force (F) is an influence applied to a body that tends to cause that body to accelerate or to deform. The force is expressed in newtons (N) or pounds (lb).

Stress (S) is force imposed per unit area. It may be internal or external to a body and is expressed in pascals (Pa) [equivalent to newtons per square meter (N/m^2)] or pounds per square inch $(lb/in.^2)$.

Strain ($\delta L/L$) is an induced dimensional change per unit length. It is dimensionless, but is commonly expressed in micrometers per meter ($\mu m/m$) or microinches per inch ($\mu in./in.$).

Young's modulus (E) is the rate of change of unit tensile or compressive stress with respect to linear strain within the proportional limit. It is expressed in pascals (N/m^2) or pounds per square inch $(lb/in.^2)$.

Yield strength (S_Y) is the stress at which a material exhibits a specified deviation from elastic behavior (proportional stress vs. strain). It usually equals a 2×10^{-3} or 0.2% offset.

Microyield strength (or precision elastic limit) (S_{MY}) is the stress that causes one part per million (ppm) of permanent strain in a short time.

Thermal expansion coefficient (CTE or α) is change in length per unit length per degree of temperature change. It is commonly expressed in millimeters per millimeter per degree Celsius [mm/(mm°C)] or inches per inch per degree Fahrenheit (in./in.-°F). It may also be expressed as ppm per degree.

Thermal conductivity (k) is the quantity of heat transmitted per unit of time through a unit area per unit of temperature gradient. It is commonly expressed in watts per meter Kelvin [W/(mK)] or British thermal units per hour-foot-degree Fahrenheit (Btu/hr-ft-°F).

Specific heat (C_p) is the ratio of the quantity of heat required to raise the temperature of a body by 1 degree to that required to raise the temperature of an equal mass of water by 1 degree. It commonly is expressed in joules per kilogram Kelvin (J/kg-K) or British thermal units per pound-degree Fahrenheit (Btu/lb-°F).

Density (ρ) is mass per unit volume and is expressed in grams per cubic centimeter (g/cm^3) or pounds per cubic inch ($lb/in.^3$)

Thermal diffusivity (D) quantifies the rate of heat dissipation within a body. It is a derived property expressed as thermal conductivity divided by the product of density and specific heat [$k/(\rho C_p)$].

Poisson's ratio (υ) is the dimensionless ratio of a lateral unit strain to a longitudinal unit strain in a body under uniform longitudinal tension or compression. Its maximum value is 0.5.

Stress optic coefficient (K) relates internal stress to the optical path difference for polarized components of light in refractive materials. It is expressed as squate millimeters per newton (mm^2/N).

The materials of greatest importance to us here are optical glasses, plastics, crystals, and mirror substrate materials; metals and composites used for cells, retainers, spacers, lenses, mirror and prism mounts, and structures; adhesives; and sealants. These materials are discussed at some length by Paquin.[20] Appendix B contains tables of the key optomechanical properties of selected materials. A few general comments follow.

1.5.1 Optical glasses

Several hundred varieties of optical-quality glass are available from manufacturers worldwide. The "glass map" shown in Fig. 1.2 includes most of the glasses produced by Schott Glass Technologies, Inc. in the United States and/or Germany. Other manufacturers produce essentially the same glasses. These are typically plotted by refractive index n_d (ordinate) and Abbe number v_d (abcissa) for yellow (helium) light as shown in the figure. They fall into 22 groups based upon chemical constituents. Figure 1.3 shows a page from the Schott catalog[21] for a representative glass type (BK7) and illustrates the types of technical information available about each glass for optomechanical design purposes. Most mechanical properties of interest are listed under "Other Properties." The $\alpha_{-30/+70}$ item is the material's CTE for the temperature range of concern in instrument design; λ (here k) is thermal conductivity, ρ is density, E is Young's modulus, and μ (here υ) is Poisson's ratio. Resistance to humidity is indicated on a scale of 1 (high) to 4 (low) by the parameter CR. The rates of change with temperature in the refractive index (dn/dT) are of interest in temperature-compensated systems.

Table B1 in Appendix B lists selected mechanical properties of 68 optical glasses made by Schott Glass Technologies and designated by Walker as the types he considered most useful to lens designers. These glasses "span the most common range of index and dispersion and have the most desirable characteristics in terms of price, bubble content, staining characteristics and resistance to adverse environmental conditions" (Ref. 22, p. H-356). The glasses are listed in order of increasing six-digit "glass code" (n_d - 1 followed by 10 times v_d). The maximum and minimum values for each parameter are indicated by a superscript "a." It is interesting to note that these extreme values typically

12

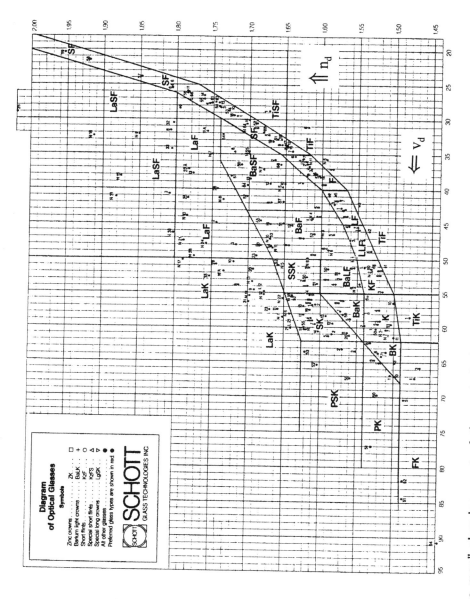

Fig. 1.2 "Glass map" showing most of the optical glasses available from one major manufacturer. (Courtesy of Schott Glass Technologies, Inc., Duryea, PA.)

BK7	517642		$n_d = 1.51680$ $\quad v_d = 64.17$	$n_F - n_C = 0.008054$
			$n_e = 1.51872$ $\quad v_e = 63.96$	$n_F - n_{C'} = 0.008110$

Refractive Indices

	λ [nm]	
$n_{2325.4}$	2325.4	1.48921
$n_{1970.1}$	1970.1	1.49495
$n_{1529.6}$	1529.6	1.50091
$n_{1060.0}$	1060.0	1.50669
n_t	1014.0	1.50731
n_s	852.1	1.50980
n_r	706.5	1.51289
n_C	656.3	1.51432
$n_{C'}$	643.8	1.51472
$n_{632.8}$	632.8	1.51509
n_D	589.3	1.51673
n_d	587.6	1.51680
n_e	546.1	1.51872
n_F	486.1	1.52238
$n_{F'}$	480.0	1.52283
n_g	435.8	1.52668
n_h	404.7	1.53024
n_i	365.0	1.53627
$n_{334.1}$	334.1	1.54272
$n_{312.6}$	312.6	1.54862
$n_{296.7}$	296.7	
$n_{280.4}$	280.4	
$n_{248.3}$	248.3	

Constants of Dispersion Formula

B_1	1.03961212
B_2	$2.31792344 \cdot 10^{-1}$
B_3	1.01046945
C_1	$6.00069867 \cdot 10^{-3}$
C_2	$2.00179144 \cdot 10^{-2}$
C_3	$1.03560653 \cdot 10^2$

Constants of Formula for dn/dT

D_0	$1.86 \cdot 10^{-6}$
D_1	$1.31 \cdot 10^{-8}$
D_2	$-1.37 \cdot 10^{-11}$
E_0	$4.34 \cdot 10^{-7}$
E_1	$6.27 \cdot 10^{-10}$
λ_{TK} [μm]	0.170

Temperature Coefficients of Refractive Index

[°C]	$\Delta n_{rel}/\Delta T$ [10^{-6}/K]			$\Delta n_{abs}/\Delta T$ [10^{-6}/K]		
	1060.0	e	g	1060.0	e	g
$-40/-20$	2.4	2.9	3.3	0.3	0.8	1.2
$+20/+40$	2.4	3.0	3.5	1.1	1.6	2.1
$+60/+80$	2.5	3.1	3.7	1.5	2.1	2.7

Internal Transmittance τ_i

λ [nm]	τ_i (5 mm)	τ_i (25 mm)
2500.0		
2325.4	0.89	0.57
1970.1	0.968	0.85
1529.6	0.997	0.985
1060.0	0.999	0.998
700	0.999	0.998
660	0.999	0.997
620	0.999	0.997
580	0.999	0.996
546.1	0.999	0.996
500	0.999	0.996
460	0.999	0.994
435.8	0.999	0.994
420	0.998	0.993
404.7	0.998	0.993
400	0.998	0.991
390	0.998	0.989
380	0.996	0.980
370	0.995	0.974
365.0	0.994	0.969
350	0.986	0.93
334.1	0.950	0.77
320	0.81	0.35
310	0.59	0.07
300	0.26	
290		
280		
270		
260		
250		

Color Code

λ_{80}/λ_5		33/30

Remarks

Relative Partial Dispersion

$P_{s,t}$	0.3098
$P_{C,s}$	0.5612
$P_{d,C}$	0.3076
$P_{e,d}$	0.2386
$P_{g,F}$	0.5349
$P_{i,h}$	0.7483
$P'_{s,t}$	0.3076
$P'_{C',s}$	0.6062
$P'_{d,C'}$	0.2566
$P'_{e,d}$	0.2370
$P'_{g,F'}$	0.4754
$P'_{i,h}$	0.7432

Deviation of Relative Partial Dispersions ΔP from the "Normal Line"

$\Delta P_{C,t}$	0.0216
$\Delta P_{C,s}$	0.0087
$\Delta P_{F,e}$	-0.0009
$\Delta P_{g,F}$	-0.0009
$\Delta P_{i,g}$	0.0036

Other Properties

$\alpha_{-30/+70\,°C}$ [10^{-6}/K]	7.1
$\alpha_{20/300\,°C}$ [10^{-6}/K]	8.3
T_g [°C]	557
$T_{1013.0}$ [°C]	557
$T_{107.6}$ [°C]	719
c_p [J/(g·K)]	0.858
λ [W/(m·K)]	1.114
ρ [g/cm³]	2.51
E [10^3 N/mm²]	82
μ	0.206
K [10^{-6} mm²/N]	2.77
$HK_{0.1/20}$	610
B	0
CR	2
FR	0
SR	1
AR	2.0
PR	2.3

SCHOTT Optical Glass

Nr. 10 000 9/92

Fig. 1.3 A page from an optical glass catalog showing optical and mechanical properties of a typical glass (BK7). (Courtesy of Schott Glass Technologies, Inc., Duryea, PA.)

differ only by a factor of about 2. So, as a rule of thumb, drastic mechanical differences do not occur when glass type is changed.

Table B2 compares 11 lightweight Schott glasses (these are not included in Fig. 1.2 or Table B1) with the nearest optically equivalent standard-weight types.[23] These glasses might well be chosen over the corresponding standard glasses for use in prisms and second-surface mirrors if weight is a prime concern. The mechanical properties of the lightweight varieties (other than density) are not greatly different from those of the standard varieties. The properties of radiation-resistant glass types are available from Schott.[24] These glasses are not included in Fig. 1.2 or Table B1.

1.5.2 Optical plastics

A few types of commercially available plastics are suitable for use as optical components in some applications. Key types are identified and selected mechanical properties are listed in Table B3.

In general, optical plastics are softer than glasses, so they tend to scratch easily and are hard to polish to a precise surface figure. Their CTEs and dn/dTs are larger than those of glasses and of most crystals. Plastics tend to absorb water from the atmosphere. This changes their refractive indices. Their specific stiffnesses (E/ρ) are lower than those for glasses. The biggest advantages of using plastic optical components are their low densities and ease of manufacture in large quantities by low unit-cost molding techniques. It is relatively simple to mold integral mechanical mounting features into plastic components such as lenses, windows, prisms, or mirrors during manufacture. This facilitates mounting these components and eliminates the need for some mechanical parts, thereby reducing overall costs.

1.5.3 Optical crystals

A variety of natural and synthetic crystalline materials are available for use in optics when transmission in the infrared or ultraviolet spectral regions is required. A few also transmit in the visible region, but usually not as well as glasses. Crystals are also used to provide special optical characteristics such as increased dispersion for some specific wavelengths. They fall into four groups: alkali and alkaline earth halides, infrared-transmitting glasses and other oxides, semiconductors, and chalcogenides. Mechanical properties are given in Tables B4 through B7 for the crystals commonly used as optics.

1.5.4 Mirror materials

Mirrors consist of a reflecting surface (usually a thin-film coating) attached to or integral with a supporting structure or substrate. Their sizes can range from a few millimeters to many meters. The substrates can be made of glasses, low-expansion ceramics, metals, composites, or (rarely) plastics. Tables B8a and B8b list some mechanical properties of the most common mirror materials. Table B9 quantifies structural figures of merit for most of the same materials.[20] The figures of merit allow direct comparisons between candidate materials for a given application. For example, a commonly used figure of merit in mirror design is specific stiffness, E/ρ, which helps us determine which material would have the least mass or self-weight deflection for a mirror of a given geometry and size. The various figures of merit listed in Table B9 relate to the comparisons in the headings. The choice of which figure of merit to apply in a particular case depends upon the design requirements and constraints. Tables B10a through B10d list the characteristics of aluminum alloys, aluminum matrix composites, several grades of beryllium, and major silicon carbide matrix types used in mirrors.

The method used in manufacturing a given mirror depends largely upon the type of material involved. Table B11 correlates common machining, surface finishing, and coating methods for various common materials.[10] It is important that the manufacturing processes, including plating or coating, do not introduce excessive internal or surface stress into the mirror substrate or coating.

1.5.5 Materials for mechanical components

The materials typically used for the mechanical components of optical instruments, such as instrument housings, lens barrels, cells, spacers, retainers, and prism and mirror mounts, are metals (typically aluminum alloys, beryllium, brass, Invar, stainless steel, and titanium). Composites (metal matrices, silicon carbide, and filled plastics) may be used in some structural applications. Some of these materials are also used as mirror substrates. The mechanical properties of selected versions of the metals and one metal matrix may be found in Table B12. The general qualifications of the metals in the context of optical component mounting applications are as follows:

Aluminum alloys: Alloy 1100 has low strength, is easily formed by spinning or deep-drawing, and can be machined and welded or brazed. Alloy 2024 has high strength and good machinability, but is hard to weld. Alloy 6061 is a general-purpose structural aluminum alloy with moderate strength, good dimensional stability, and good machinability. It is easily welded and brazed. Alloy 7075 has high strength and machines well, but is not suited for welding. Alloy 356 is used for moderate- to high-strength structural castings. It machines and welds easily. Most aluminum alloys are heat treated to differing degrees of hardness, depending on the application. Their surfaces oxidize quickly, but can be protected by chemical films or anodic coatings. The latter may produce significant dimensional buildup. A black anodized finish reduces light reflections, so this type of finish is frequently used on aluminum parts for optical instruments. The CTE match of aluminum alloys to glasses, ceramics, and most crystals is not close. Table B10a compares the characteristics of several aluminum alloys used for mirror substrates.

Beryllium is light in weight, has high stiffness, conducts heat well, resists corrosion and radiation effects, and is fairly stable dimensionally. It is relatively expensive to purchase and to process, so it is used primarily in optical instruments intended for sophisticated applications such as structures and mirror or grating substrates for use at cryogenic temperatures. It also is the material of choice in some space applications where radiation resistance or weight savings are vital and monetary costs are of lesser importance. Table B10c compares the characteristics of several common beryllium grades. Paquin has countered claims about the extreme hazards of working with beryllium by pointing out that simple exhaust systems with suitable filters for particulate material and conventional means for the collection and disposal of loose abrasive grinding and polishing slurry are very effective as safety precautions.[25]

Brass is used where high corrosion resistance, good thermal conductivity, and/or ease of machining are required, but weight is not critical. It is popular for screw-machined parts and marine applications. Brass can be blackened chemically.

Invar, an iron-nickel alloy, is used most freqeuently in high-performance instruments for space and/or cryogenic applications to take advantage of its low CTE. It is quite heavy, and machining sometimes affects its thermal stability. Annealing is advised. A version called Super-Invar has an even lower CTE over a limited temperature range. It is not recommended for use at temperatures below - 50°C (- 58°F). To prevent oxidation, Invar frequently is chrome plated.

Stainless steels [sometimes called corrosion-resistant steels (here abbreviated CRES)] are used in optical mounts primarily for their strength and their fairly close CTE match to some glasses. They are relatively dense, so a weight penalty must be paid to achieve these advantages. A chromium oxide layer that forms on exposed surfaces makes these steels resistant to corrosion. In general, these steels are harder to machine than aluminum alloys. Type 416 is the most easily machined and can be blackened chemically or with black chrome plating. Type 17-4PH has good dimensional stability. Stainless steels can be welded to like materials or brazed to many different metals.

Titanium is the material of choice in many high-performance systems where a close CTE match to crown glass is essential. Flexures are sometimes made of titanium because of its high yield strength (S_Y). It is about 60% heavier than aluminum. Titanium is somewhat expensive to machine. It can be cast. Brazing is easy, but welding is more difficult; electron beam or laser welding techniques work best. Parts can also be made by powder metallurgy methods. Corrosion resistance is high.

Some plastics, particularly glass- or carbon fiber-reinforced epoxies and polycarbonates, are used in structural parts such as housings, spacers, prism and mirror mounts, and lens barrels for cameras, binoculars, office machines, and other commercial optical instruments. They are relatively lightweight, and most can be machined conventionally or by single-point diamond turning (SPDT). Some can be cast. Generally, plastics feature low cost. Unfortunately, they are not as stable dimensionally as metals and tend to absorb water from the atmosphere and to outgas in a vacuum. The CTEs of filled varieties can be customized to some extent.

1.5.6 Adhesives and sealants

Optical cements used to hold the refracting surfaces of lenses or prisms together as, for example, in forming cemented doublets, triplets, or beamsplitters, must be transparent in the spectral region of interest, have good adhesion characteristics, have acceptable shrinkage, and (preferably) be able to withstand exposure to moisture and other adverse environmental conditions. The most popular optical cements are thermosetting and photosetting (ultraviolet light curing) types. Some mechanical properties of interest are given in Table B13 for a generic type of optical cement.

Structural adhesives most frequently used to hold optics to mounts and to bond mechanical parts together are one- and two-part epoxies, polyurethanes, and acrylics. Most cure best at elevated temperatures and suffer some (up to 6%) shrinkage during curing. Their CTEs are about 10 times those of structural materials and glasses, while stiffnesses are about two orders of magnitude lower than those for structural materials and glasses. Some adhesives emit volatile ingredients during curing or if exposed to a vacuum or elevated temperatures. The emitted material may then condense as a contaminating film on nearby cooler surfaces, such as lenses or mirrors. A few adhesives have low shrinkage and low volatilities. The typical properties of representative types are summarized in Table B14.

The sealants used today are usually room-temperature-vulcanizing (RTV) elastomers that cure into flexible, form-fitting masses with reasonably good adherence properties. They are typically poured or injected into gaps between lenses and mounts or between mounting components to seal leaks and/or to help hold the optics in place under vibration, shock, and temperature changes. Some outgas or emit effluents (typically acetic acid or alcohol) during curing or in vacuum more than others. Use of primers prior to application of the sealants is recommended by the manufacturers for many of these products. Typical physical characteristics and mechanical properties of a few representative sealants are given in Tables B15a and B15b. At least one of these (DC 93-500) is accepted by the National Aeronautical and Space Administration (NASA) as a low volatility sealant for space applications. Unfortunately, it is relatively expensive. The curing times, colors, and certain physical properties of sealants can be modified significantly through the use of additives and/or catalysts.

1.6 Dimensional Instability

Paquin has defined dimensional instability as "the change that occurs in response to internal or external influences" (Ref. 26, p. 160) In order to create a dimensionally stable instrument, one must control these changes (i.e., strains) in optomechanical components to levels that do not compromise performance requirements. In situations requiring a stability on the order of normal machining tolerances, strain must be controlled to about 1 part in 10^3. This is relatively easy to accomplish. In high-precision applications, tolerances of $1:10^6$ apply and strain must be controlled to the same degree. Even higher precision is possible, but tolerances may be as small as $1:10^9$, and finding materials and manufacturing processes to achieve such tolerances requires the utmost care at all stages of design and production. A considerable amount of luck would also be helpful.

The dimensional changes of concern here are due to externally applied forces that cause plastic deformation; internal (residual) stresses that relieve themselves (usually unpredictably) with time, with temperature change, or under vibration and/or shock; microstructural changes such as phase transformations or recrystalization within the materials; and inhomogeneity and anisotropy of the materials. Paquin[25,26] and Jacobs[27] deal with these potential causes of problems at much greater length than we can here. It is important to recognize the possibility that microscopic changes will occur within the parts of an optical instrument so provisions can be made to avoid or at least minimize these changes whenever possible.

References

1. Walles, S. and Hopkins, R.E., "The orientation of the image formed by a series of plane mirrors," *Appl. Opt.* Vol. 3, 1447, 1964.

2. U.S. MIL-STD-210, "Climatic Information to Determine Design and Test Requirements for Military Systems and Equipment," Superintendent of Documents, U.S. Government Printing Office, Washington.

3. ISO Standard 10109, "Environmental Requirements," International Organization for Standardization, Geneva.

4. Yoder, P.R., Jr., "Opto-Mechanical Systems Design, 2nd ed., Marcel Dekker, New York, 1993.

5. Parks, R.E., "ISO environmental testing and reliability standards for optics," *SPIE Proceedings* Vol. 1993, 32, 1993.

6. Musicant, S. and Malloy, W.J., "Environments stressful to optical materials in low earth orbit," *SPIE Proceedings* Vol. 1330, 119, 1990.

7. Vukobratovich, D., private communication, 2001.

8. McCay, J., Fahey, T., and Lipson, M., "Challenges remain for 157-nm lithography," *Optoelectronics World, Supplement to Laser Focus World,* Vol. 23, S3, 2001.

9. Steinberg, D.S., *Vibration Analysis for Electronic Equipment,* Wiley, New York, 1973.

10. Englehaupt, D., "Fabrication Methods," Chapt. 10 in *Handbook of Optomechanical Engineering*, CRC Press, Boca Raton, 1997.

11. Genberg, V., "Structural Analysis of Optics", Chapt. 8 in *Handbook of Optomechanical Engineering*, CRC Press, Boca Raton, 1997.

12. Hatheway, A.E., "Review of finite element analysis techniques: capabilities and limitations," *SPIE Critical Review* Vol. CR43, 367, 1992.

13. Hatheway, A.E., "Unified thermal/elastic optical analysis of a lithographic lens," *SPIE Proceedings* Vol. 3130, 100, 1997.

14. Genberg, V. and Michels, G., "Design optimization of actively controlled optics", *SPIE Proceedings* Vol. 4198, 158, 2000.

15. Marker, A.J. III, Hayden, J.S., and Speit, B., "Radiation resistant optical glasses," *SPIE Proceedings* Vol. 1485, 55, 1991.

16. Harris, D.C., *Materials for Infrared Windows and Domes*, SPIE Press, Bellingham, 1999.

17. Vukobratovich, D., "Optomechanical Design Principles," Chapt. 2 in *Handbook of Optomechanical Engineering*, CRC Press, Boca Raton, 1997.

18. U.S. MIL-STD-810, "Environmental Test Methods and Engineering Guidelines," Superintendent of Documents, U.S. Government Printing Office, Washington.

19. ISO Standard ISO 9022, "Environmental Test Methods," International Organization for Standardization, Geneva.

20. Paquin, R.A., "Materials for Optical Systems," Chapt. 3 in *Handbook of Optomechanical Engineering*, CRC Press, Boca Raton, 1997.

21. Schott Optical Glass Catalog, Schott Glass Technologies, Inc., Duryea.

22. Walker, B.H., "Select optical glasses," in *The Photonics Design and Applications Handbook*, Lauren Publishing, Pittsfield, H-356, 1993.

23. Schott Product Information 2106/91, Lightweight Optical Glasses, Schott Glass Technologies, Inc., Duryea, 1991.

24. Schott Product Information 10017e, Radiation Resistant Glasses, Schott Glass Technologies, Inc., Duryea, 1990.

25. Paquin, R.A., "Metal Mirrors," Chapt. 4 in *Handbook of Optomechanical Engineering*, CRC Press, Boca Raton, 1997.

26. Paquin, R.A., "Dimensional instability of materials: how critical is it in the design of optical instruments?" *SPIE Critical Review* Vol. CR43, 160, 1992.

27. Jacobs, S.F., "Variable invariables: dimensional instability with time and temperature," *SPIE Critical Review* Vol. CR43, 181, 1992.

CHAPTER 2
The Optic-to-Mount Interface

The prime purpose of the optic-to-mount interface is to hold the component (lens, window, filter, shell, prism, or mirror) in its proper position and orientation within the optical instrument throughout use. This implies the presence of mechanical constraints, i.e., external forces, that limit component motion when the temperature changes or when external mechanical disturbances occur. The application of these constraints is the first topic considered in this chapter. The advantages of kinematic-type mounting techniques are explained and typical impacts of dimensional tolerances on lens alignment are summarized. We then explore how the applied forces may cause stresses to build up or birefringence to develop within the component. The generalizations on mounting stresses given here are discussed in more detail and quantified in Chapter 11. This chapter closes with brief considerations of the cost and manufacturability of optical components and their mounts.

2.1 Mechanical Constraints

2.1.1 General considerations

Under all operating conditions, it is important that each optical component be constrained so it remains within decentration, tilt, and axial spacing budgets and that induced stresses, surface deformations, and birefringence are tolerable. Both lateral and axial constraints are needed for each component. Preferably, the mechanical interfaces should be kinematic so all six degrees of freedom (DOF; three translations and three rotations) are independently constrained without redundancy. A true kinematic interface applies six forces at infinitesimal areas (points) so that no moments can be transferred to the optic. In such cases, stress (force per unit area) can be large. A semikinematic interface is one with the same six constraints, but each of these acts over a small area to distribute the force and reduce the stress.

Semikinematic support of optics generally is practical only if that optic is relatively rigid. This is the case for most prisms and some mirrors where the smallest dimension is at least one fifth of the largest dimension. Rotational symmetry of most optical system apertures leads to corresponding symmetry in most lens and window mounts and in many mirror mounts. This usually simplifies the design of the associated mechanical housings. Some thick lenses and small stiff mirrors can be mounted semikinematically. Rotation of a symmetrical lens or mirror about the optical axis is critical only in high-performance applications, so this particular degree of freedom generally does not need to be specifically constrained. Most prisms are amenable to semi-kinematic mounting.

A rigid body with more than six constraints is called "overconstrained" and is nonkinematic. The location of an overconstrained body may be uncertain and it may be deformed by the forces. Mountings for circular optics such as lenses are most often designed so that the contact areas are as large as practical and the forces are uniformly distributed outside the edges of the apertures. The mechanical interfaces are machined so the forces exerted are as nearly symmetrical as possible. This approach distributes the forces so they are not overly concentrated. Multiple-contact supports frequently are used as axial and transverse, i.e., radial, supports for large mirrors. Various types of these supports will be discussed in Chapter 9.

2.1.2 Lens interfaces

Radial positioning of lenses is traditionally obtained from contact between the lens rim and the cylindrical inside diameter (ID) of the mount. Such an interface is called "rim contact." Constraint can also come from the radial components of axial force (preload) exerted against curved lens surfaces; radial preload produced by such means as radially directed clamps, or setscrews; radial forces imposed by induced mechanical interferences (such as shrink fitting with or without use of shims); or differential contraction of lens and mounting materials as a result of temperature changes.

With rim contact, a poorly edged lens may be tilted or decentered. Figure 2.1 illustrates conditions in which the lens rim is tilted or decentered with respect to its optical axis (the line connecting the surface centers of curvature). Axial forces applied to a lens mounted in this manner will introduce nonsymmetrical internal stresses.

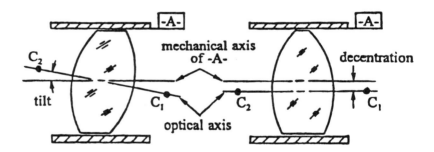

Fig. 2.1 Registering a poorly edged lens by its cylindrical rim may result in tilt or decentration of the optical axis. (a) Tilted rim, (b) decentered rim.

Axial constraint is provided by clamping the lens near its rim between a mounting feature such as a shoulder or spacer and some retaining means. Figure 2.2(a) shows an example involving a biconvex lens element. The surface (R_1) registers against the edge of the cylindrical surface (-A-) so its center of curvature (C_1) is automatically located on the mechanical axis of -A-. If there is radial clearance between the lens rim and the mount's inner diameter (ID) and if, during the assembly process, the lens is caused to slide laterally while maintaining contact with the edge of -A-, C_2 also can be made to lie on the mechanical axis. An axial preload applied to an annular region near the edge of the polished surface (as indicated by the arrows in the figure) will center the lens if the slopes of the spherical surfaces at the contact height are sufficient to provide a difference in opposing radial force components [see Fig. 2.2(b)] that is sufficient to overcome friction and slide the lens laterally. When the optical axis is centered, all radial components balance each other and tend to hold the lens in the aligned condition.

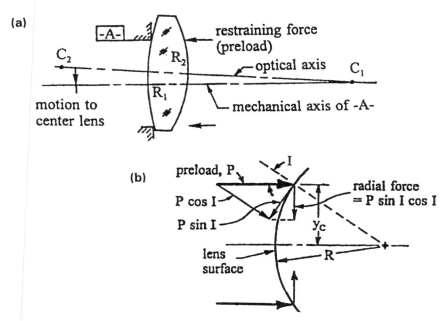

Fig. 2.2 (a) Interfacing the mount to the lens at the lens' polished surfaces is called "surface contact." (b) Geometry showing opposing radial force components that tend to center the lens.

Hopkins [1] indicated that a net difference in slopes of the front and back lens surfaces at the contact height of at least 17° is needed to achieve centering by means of reasonable axial preload. The following equation, based on Shannon,[2] applies to the same situation.

$$(y_C/2R)_1 - (y_C/2R)_2 \geq 0.07 \tag{2.1}$$

where the parameters are as shown in Fig. 2.2. The usual sign convention for radii applies.

Example 2.1: Self-centering effect that is due to axial preload.

Two biconvex lenses, each with a diameter of 50.00 mm (1.968 in.), have surface radii R_i of (a) 500.00 mm (19.685 in.) and -367.00 mm (-14.449 in.) and (b) +254.00 mm. (+10.00 in.) Should these lenses self-center with a preload applied at a height y_C of 24.00 mm (0.945 in.)?

Applying Eq. (2.1):
(a) [24.00/(2)(500.00)] - [24.00/(2)(-367.00)] = 0.057
This is < 0.07, so the lens may not self-center.

(b) [24.00/(2)(254.00)] - [24.00/(2)(-254.00)] = 0.094
This is > 0.07, so the lens should self-center.

If the lens is constrained by large axial forces and also touches the ID of the mount, warpage of the lens and asymmetrical stress concentrations will occur. This will not happen if considerable radial clearance is provided and mechanical contact occurs only on the polished lens surfaces, as indicated in Fig. 2.3. Errors in the orientation of the rim are then not significant since the rim does not touch the mount's ID.

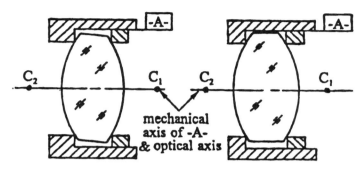

Fig. 2.3 If the glass-to-mount registration occurs at the polished surfaces, lens edging errors are not critical. (a) Tilted rim, (b) decentered rim.

If the interface surfaces in the mount are not well located, the lens can be decentered or tilted with respect to the overall optical system axis. Figure 2.4 illustrates four typical cases in which: (a) the bore -A- and shoulder -C- are tilted with respect to the cell outside diameter (OD), which is assumed to be properly aligned to the system axis; (b) the bore -A- is decentered with respect to the cell OD; and (c) the spacer is wedged so surface -C- is tilted with respect to bore -A-. In the latter case, the axial preload will be unsymmetrical and tend to decenter and/or tilt (sometimes called "roll") the lens within any existing radial clearance to the cell ID. Warpage and concentrated stress buildup also may occur if the axial force is large.

If the lens surfaces are not sufficiently curved for the preload to center the lens, some external means can be employed for this purpose. Shims can be inserted locally to adjust the radial separation between the lens and the mount, or radial forces can be exerted by such means as setscrews. Figure 2.5 illustrates the latter mechanism. The moveable cell containing the lens rests against a flat surface in the fixed cell. It can be pushed laterally and is constrained axially by setscrews acting against a conical cell rim. The use of four screws is prefered over three to minimize "crosstalk" between adjustments.

Since there must always be some finite clearance between the mount ID and the lens OD for assembly, tolerances on these parts are typically specified as "minus 0, plus something" for the mount ID and "minus something, plus 0" for the lens. The nominal radial clearance also is defined. For example, the following combination might be specified: mount ID = 50.8000 - 0 + 0.0250 mm (2.0000 - 0 + 0.0010 in.), lens OD = 50.7200 - 0.0500 + 0 mm (1.9969 - 0.0020 + 0 in. The nominal radial clearance will then be 0.040 mm (0.0015 in.) and the lens decentration will be between 0.040 mm (0.0016 in.) and 0.0775 mm (0.0030 in.) at assembly temperature. If the temperature changes, this preload also changes. This preload also changes as a result of differential

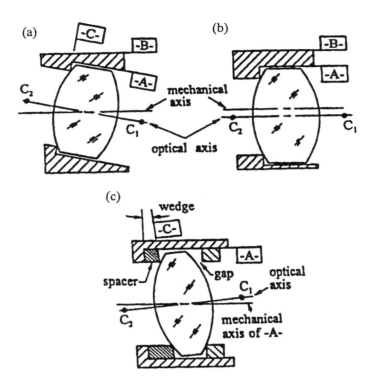

Fig. 2.4 Perfect lenses pressed against imperfect interfaces will be misaligned. (a) Bore and shoulder tilted, (b) bore decentered, (c) spacer wedged, (d) retainer wedged.

expansion between the lens material and the mounting material. The equations for estimating the rate of change in the preload with temperature for single and multiple lens assemblies are given in Chapter 12.

2.1.3 Prism interfaces

Figure 2.6, adapted from Smith,[3] indicates how the required six constraints might be applied to a rectangular parallelepiped-type body such as a simple cube prism. In Fig. 2.6(a), six identical balls are attached to three mutually perpendicular flat surfaces. The dashed construction lines indicate how the balls are located symmetrically. If the prism is held in contact with all six balls, it will be uniquely constrained. The bottom of the prism rests on the three contacts parallel to the X-Z plane so it cannot translate in the Y direction or tilt about the X- or Z-axes. Two contacts parallel to the Y-Z plane prevent translation along the X-axis and rotation about the Y-axis. The single contact at the X-Y plane controls translation along the Z-axis. A single force applied to the near corner of the prism and aimed toward the origin would hold the prism in place. Ideally, this force should pass through the center of gravity (CG) of the prism.

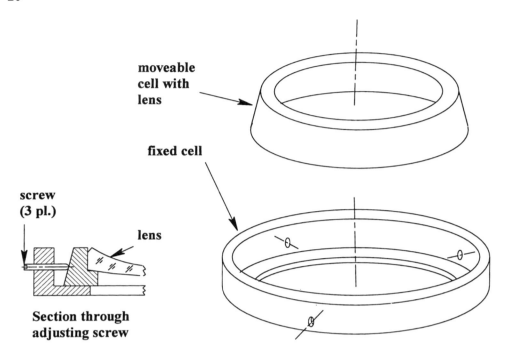

Fig. 2.5 Radial setscrews used to center a lens. Screws bearing against a conical cell surface allow lateral adjustment and constrain the moveable cell axially.

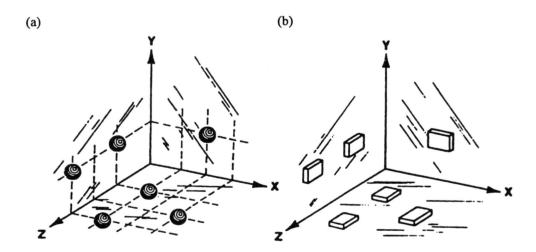

Fig. 2.6 (a) Kinematic and (b) semikinematic position-defining registration surfaces intended for interfacing with a cube-shaped prism (not shown). (Adapted from Smith.[3])

Three forces, each applied normal to one of the exposed prism surfaces and directed toward a contact point or toward a point midway between adjacent contact points also would hold the prism. Unfortunately, this particular multiple-force configuration is not very practical for an optical application since all prism faces would be at least partially obscured. By increasing the separations of some of the balls, it may be possible to clear the apertures without destroying symmetry or the kinematic condition. However, this would not help the stress concentration problem inherent with the point contacts.

Figure 2.6(b) shows conceptually how the point contacts on balls could be replaced by small areas on raised flat pads to distribute the mechanical preload forces on the prism surfaces. The design now is semikinematic. The pads may have any practical shape such as square (as shown) or perhaps circular. If the pads are machined or lapped coplanar and mutually perpendicular, introduction of stress at the contacts with a perfect cube prism is minimized. Distortion of the prism also is minimized. In practice, it is very difficult (read "expensive") to make the pads touching any prism surface as coplanar as the polished optical surface, which typically has shape imperfections that are no larger than a small fraction of the wavelength of light. If the pad surfaces are not accurately aligned to each other and the prism is forced into intimate contact with them, the prism could be distorted by introduced moments, or one or more interfaces could degenerate into line or point contacts, thereby causing stress to increase. Figure 2.7 illustrates these conditions for three possible pad-to-prism surface mismatches. Assuming that the mount is more rigid than the prism, the dashed lines in each view show typical distortions of the adjacent optical surface that are caused by imposed moments. Combinations of the errors shown here can be expected to occur. This may accentuate the prism distortions.

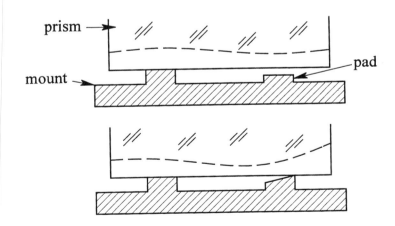

Fig. 2.7 Effects of coplanarity errors on a prism forced into contact with two registration pads of a small area.

To keep the optical performance of the prism within allowable bounds, the tolerances on coplanarity errors for the pads must be essentially the same as the allowable surface figure errors for that prism. Typically, careful lapping of the mechanical surfaces on a flat surface can achieve coplanarity within about 20×10^{-6} in. (0.5 µm). Single-point diamond turning can reduce these errors to less than 4×10^{-6} in. (0.1 μm).

The means used to clamp the prism against its reference pads in a semi-kinematic mount include a variety of spring types, such as cantilevered clips and "straddling" springs. These constraints are discussed in detail in Sects. 7.1 and 7.2.

Frequently it is necessary for optical subassemblies, including their mounts, to be removed from the optical instrument and replaced in the identical location and orientation. Semikinematic interfaces allow this to be accomplished with high accuracy. Figure 2.8(a) shows (schematically) one such interface as described by Strong.[4] It consists

(a)   (b)

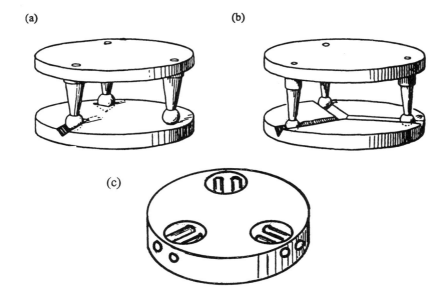

(c)

Fig. 2.8 (a) and (b). Concepts for zero degree of freedom separable interfaces. (From Strong.[4]) (c) Concept for providing "vees" with multiple parallel rods. (From Kittel.[5])

of lower and upper plates; the optic is attached to the upper plate (thereby forming the removable subassembly) and the lower plate is permanently attached to the instrument's structure. Attached to the bottom of the upper plate are three balls, symmetrically located on a given "bolt circle" diameter. The lower plate has two "sockets" (a "vee" and a trihedral-shaped hole) and a flat surface. This is sometimes referred to as a "Kelvin clamp." The balls fit repeatably into the sockets, establishing six positional constraints whenever the plates are clamped together. The three balls and the three sockets can be manufactured or purchased with posts that can be pressed into holes drilled in the plates. A conical socket can be substituted for the trihedral with slight loss of accuracy (because contact occurs on a line rather than three points). Figure 2.8(b) shows a similar interface mechanism in which the three balls mate with three radially directed "vees." Kittel has shown how "vees" can be formed by pressing dowel pins into three pairs of holes drilled into the lower plate. The pins form three parallel grooves, [see Fig. 2.8(c)]. This construction is less expensive than machining the "vees" directly into the plate.[5]

A nonkinematic technique frequently used for mounting prisms involves glass-to-metal bonds with thin layers of adhesives. These designs generally result in reduced interface complexity and compact packaging while providing mechanical strength that is adequate for withstanding the severe shock, vibration, and temperature changes characteristic of military and aerospace applications. This mounting technique is described in Sect. 7.3. Glass-to-metal bonding is also used in some less rigorous applications because of its inherent simplicity and reliability.

A stress-free technique for mounting prisms inserts a series of flexures between the prism and the mount. These flexures can be of a variety of configurations; their prime purpose is to isolate the optic from temperature effects on dissimilar materials and to prevent the introduction of moments. This mounting technique is discussed in Sect. 7.4.

2.1.4 Mirror interfaces

Semikinematic clamped and adhesive-bonded mechanical mounts typically are used to support small (i.e., stiff) mirrors, while the mounts for larger mirrors always are nonkinematic because the latter optics tend to be thin relative to their maximum dimension and are relatively flexible. Multiple axial and radial supports must be provided for larger mirrors to minimize the self-weight deflection of optical surfaces between supports. These mountings are discussed in Chapters 9 and 10.

2.1.5 Interfaces with other optical components

Windows, shells, and domes are mounted nonkinematically by such techniques as potting them into their mounts with an elastomeric material. This establishes the (usually) desired moisture, dust, and pressure seal and reduces stresses. Filters also are mounted nonkinematically using techniques similar to those used for mounting lenses. Examples of all of these optical component mountings are described in Chapter 5.

2.2 Consequences of Mounting Forces

Preloads applied to the surfaces of optical components compress (or strain) the optic and produce corresponding elastic stresses within the material. In Chapter 11, we show how to estimate the magnitudes of these stresses and to determine if they appear to be tolerable. As mentioned earlier, forces concentrated on small surface areas cause localized stresses of high magnitude. These are particularly undesirable since they can lead to excessive distortion of malleable materials such as plastics or some crystals, or breakage of brittle materials such as glass or other crystals. Reaction forces are also exerted on the mount. These can distort the mount temporarily or permanently or, in extreme cases, cause the mount to fail.

Applied forces may introduce birefringence (inhomogeneity of the refractive index) into normally isotropic optical materials. Birefringence affects the propagation speeds of the perpendicular and parallel components of polarized light passing through the material, so these components become out of phase. The magnitude of birefringence occurring per unit length in a particular sample of material under a given level of stress depends on the stress optic coefficient of the material. This parameter can be found in manufacturer's catalogs for optical glasses and elsewhere in the literature for some crystals. Birefringence is most important in optical systems using polarized light, such as polarimeters, most interferometers, many laser systems, and high-performance cameras.

Even low levels of applied force can cause optical surfaces to deform, especially if the forces are not applied symmetrically. Minute surface deformations (measured in fractions of a wavelength of light) affect system performance. The significance of a given deformation depends strongly on the location of the surface in the optical system and the performance requirements of the system containing the optical surface in question. Larger departures from perfection can be tolerated on surfaces near an image than near a system pupil. Because of these system- and application-dependent factors, no general methods of estimating surface deformations, or guidelines in regard to how much surface deformation can be tolerated, are given here.

2.3 Sealing Considerations

Optical instruments intended for military or aerospace applications and many intended for more environmentally benign commercial or consumer applications need to be sealed against entry of moisture or other contaminants from the surrounding environment. This means that minute gaps between windows and/or lenses and mechanical parts of the instrument must be sealed shut. The sealing materials include flat or convoluted gaskets, O-rings, and formed-in-place elastomeric seals. Moving components such as those used in focusing mechanisms such as camera lenses or eyepieces are sometimes sealed to fixed members with flexible bellows-type dynamic seals.[6] The castings used for housings should be impregnated to fill pores and minute holes that otherwise can leak.

Figure 2.9 illustrates two standard techniques for sealing a lens into a cell. In Fig. 2.9(a), a compressed O-ring fills the radial gap between the lens rim and the cell wall. Fig. 2.9(b) shows a design with a formed-in-place gasket in which a sealant is injected with a hypodermic syringe through several access holes in the cell wall to fill an annular groove machined into the cell's ID adjacent to the lens rim. During the injection process, the lens axis should be horizontal and the injection started at the bottom. As the gap is filled, air escapes through holes at the top, and filling continues until sealant starts to emerge from all the holes. Extra radial holes may be added to the design to assist in monitoring the filling process in larger versions of this type of mounting. In some other designs, cell-mounted optics are sealed in place with an elastomeric sealant applied through a thin hypodermic needle into a gap around the rim of the component before a mechanical retaining means is attached.

In all these designs, the sealant effectively fills the space between the optic and the mount with a slightly flexible material that adheres well to the adjacent surfaces. In general, the same techniques can be applied to lenses, windows, filters, shells, and domes as discussed and illustrated by several examples in Chapters 3 through 5.

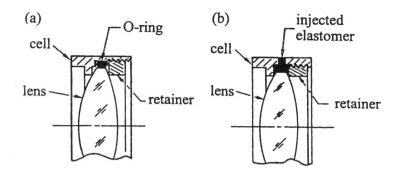

Fig. 2.9 Two techniques for sealing a lens into its mount: (a) an O-ring around the lens rim. (b) an injected (formed-in-place) elastomeric seal.

Flushing and pressurizing housings and assemblies with a dry gas (such as nitrogen or helium) are common techniques for minimizing internal damage caused by humidity, dust, and other contaminants that can pass through microscopic holes in the walls and joints as temperature and air pressure vary. Some instruments are vented through desiccators and dust filters to keep their interiors clean without completely sealing them to atmospheric changes. This approach is especially valuable in thin-walled devices or those with thin exposed optics that cannot withstand pressure differentials.

2.4 Cost and Manufacturability

The cost and manufacturability of the optical and mechanical components of an optical instrument are determined largely by the physical dimensions of the optic (because extremely large or extremely small parts are hard to make and test), the dimensional tolerances assigned during the design process, and the complexity of assembly and alignment. They are also driven, usually to a lesser extent, by choices of material. Very soft or very hard optical materials are hard to grind and polish. A few glasses and many crystals fall into the former category, while fused silica, sapphire, and diamond fall into the latter. Similarly, most aluminum alloys and brass are easy to machine, while titanium and Invar are more difficult. Some materials are easily machined to very high accuracy by single-point diamond turning so this is a popular technique for making high-performance optical and mechanical components even though it may be more expensive than using conventional machines and tool bits.

Smith[3,7] and others[8-11] have discussed their philosophies for assigning tolerances. Willey and Parks[12] have detailed techniques and algorithms useful in evaluating assigned tolerances in terms of their impact on the cost of lens elements and interfacing mechanical parts. These latter techniques allow designers to predict whether a given design can be built to specified tolerances and to estimate the manufacturing costs of the optical components used.

One question that arises frequently during the early stages of instrument development is the number of adjustments to be built into the design. Having too many adjustments leads to instability and the strong possibility of crosstalk between supposedly independent adjustments, as well as a situation where nothing in the optical train acts as a fixed reference. On the other hand, the absence of adjustments frequently demands excessively tight tolerances. The compromise philosophy is one in which the basic performance of the instrument is achieved by selective close tolerancing and use of a minimum number of adjustments. These adjustments allow the reduction of residual misalignments during assembly. The ideal tolerance budget should relax tolerances on parameters that are very difficult to control or for which errors are not especially harmful. The parameters that do not fall into these categories would then be toleranced more tightly. This concept leads in many cases to the most cost-effective design.

It should be obvious to the reader that if it is known that some tolerances are excessively tight in terms of available fabrication technology, then it is sensible to redesign the instrument based on the tolerance data. The alternative is to discover the need for redesign after failing in the attempt to make parts that meet these requirements. Review of the design by individuals skilled in the applicable manufacturing procedures well before that design is released for manufacture also tends to prevent unfortunate surprises during fabrication, inspection, assembly, or testing.

References

1. Hopkins, R. E., "Lens Mounting and Centering," Chapt. 2 in *Applied Optics and Optical Engineering*, Vol. VIII, Academic Press, New York, 1980.
2. Shannon, R.R., "How to design a lens for manufacturing," *OSA How-To Program, Boston*, Optical Society of America, Washington, 1990.
3. Smith, W.J., "Optics in Practice," Chapt. 15 in *Modern Optical Engineering*, 3rd. ed., McGraw-Hill, New York, 2000.
4. Strong, J., *Procedures in Applied Optics*, Marcel Dekker, New York, 1988.
5. Kittel, D., "Precision mechanics," *SPIE Short Course Notes*, SPIE Press, Bellingham, 1989.
6. Yoder, P. R., Jr., *Opto-Mechanical Systems Design*, 2nd. ed., Marcel Dekker, New York, 1993.
7. Smith, W. J., "Fundamentals of establishing an optical tolerance budget," *SPIE Proceedings*, Vol. 531, 196, 1985.
8. Plummer, J. L., "Tolerancing for economies in mass production of optics," *SPIE Proceedings* Vol. 181, 90, 1979.
9. Parks, R., "Optical specifications and tolerances for large optics", *SPIE Proceedings,* Vol. 406, 1983.
10. Adams, G., "Selection of tolerances," *SPIE Proceedings*, Vol. 892, 173, 1988.
11. Willey, R. R. and Durham, M. E., "Maximizing production yield and performance in optical instruments through effective design and tolerancing," *SPIE Proceedings*, Vol. CR43, 76, 1992.
12. Willey, R.R., and Parks, R., "Optical Fundamentals", Chapt. 1 in *Handbook of Optomechanical Engineering*," CRC Press, Boca Raton, 1997.

CHAPTER 3
Mounting Individual Lenses

In this chapter, we consider several techniques for mounting individual lenses in optical instruments. These techniques are most applicable to optics with apertures in the range of approximately 6 to 406 mm (0.25 to 16 in.). Although most of the discussions deal with glass lenses interfaced with metal mountings, the designs are generally applicable to lenses made of optical crystals and plastics. Numerous examples are included to illustrate the use of given design equations.

We include inexpensive, lower-precision techniques as well as more costly and more precise designs intended for higher-performance applications. Two examples of designs involving simple spring clips are shown. The burnished cell design, the circular-section snap ring, and the pressed-in-place rectangular-section ring are then described, as is a design with a circular ring resting in a ramped-cell ID. Designs with threaded retaining rings, with bolted-on or clamped-on flanges, and ones with cantilevered springs are considered next. Then we describe the common types of glass-to-metal interfaces: "sharp-corner," tangential, toroidal, spherical, and flat and step bevels. The chapter concludes with descriptions of the elastomeric mounting, several designs usable with lenses having nonsymmetrical apertures, and brief considerations of ways to mount plastic lenses.

3.1 Spring Mountings for Lenses and Filters

Optical components that do not need precise positioning and that must not be excessively constrained throughout large temperature changes, such as condensing lenses and heat-absorbing filters used in close proximity to heat sources in slide projectors, are frequently mounted by spring clips. These low-cost designs allow free flow of air across the optical surfaces to help minimize temperature rise while maintaining adequate alignment at all temperatures. They also provide some shock and vibration resistance.[1-3]

Figure 3.1 illustrates one example. It shows a lens made of heat-resistant glass (such as Pyrex) held in detents on three flat springs spaced at 120° intervals about the lens rim and cantilevered from a metal mounting ring. The symmetry of the cantilevered springs tends to keep the lens centered. A variant of this design has two such lenses held convex-to-convex in springs appropriately shaped with multiple detents to maintain the needed axial separation and to support both lenses.

Figure 3.2 shows the mounting for a heat-absorbing filter and a biconvex condensing lens as used in the Kodak Ektagraphic slide projector Model EF-2. The rims of the optics fit partway into appropriately shaped cutouts in the sheet-metal baseplate and are held down by a spring-loaded, notched dual clip that fits over the component's rims at the top. Separation of the elements is maintained by the separation of the cutouts in the baseplate and of the notches in the clip. Notches in the sheet-metal bracket shown at left in the figure hold the optics against rotation about a vertical axis. The shape of the baseplate cutout for the lens can be designed so a lens with different first and second curvatures cannot be inserted backward without calling attention to that fact. The

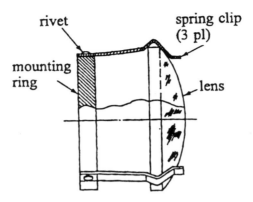

Fig. 3.1 A technique for mounting a lens on three leaf springs located at 120° intervals around the rim. (From Yoder.[1])

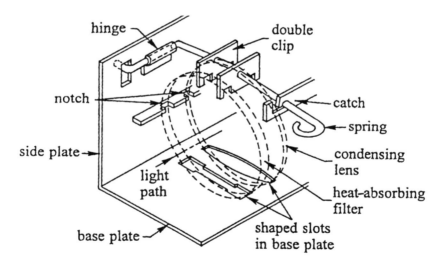

Fig. 3.2 Conceptual schematic of a spring-loaded mounting for a heat-absorbing filter and a biconvex condensing lens in a Kodak Ektagraphic projector. The optics are shown by dashed outlines.

spring holding the clip over the optics is designed for ease of engagement and disengagement to facilitate servicing. Many other variations on the spring-mounting technique exist; all are intended to minimize design and hardware production cost while meeting technical goals, such as promoting cooling, preservation of low-level alignment, and ease of replacement.

3.2 Burnished cell mountings

The burnished cell technique is most frequently used for mounting small lenses such as those for microscope or camera objectives or for tiny lenses used in endoscopes where space constraints restrict the use of separate retainers and a need for disassembly is not anticipated. This type of mounting is made of malleable material such as brass or certain aluminum alloys. It is designed with a protruding lip that is to be mechanically deformed around the rim of a lens at assembly. This secures the lens against an internal cell shoulder or spacer.[1,3,4] Figure 3.3 shows a typical example. Figure 3.3(a) shows the cell and the lens prior to assembly. The optional chucking thread facilitates installation of the cell on a lathe spindle. In some designs, the cell lip is tapered to facilitate intimate contact with the lens bevel.

The cell lip is deformed by pressing one, but preferably three or more, hardened rod-shaped tools or rollers simultaneously and symmetrically against the lip at an oblique angle while the cell is slowly rotated. The lens should be held axially against the cell shoulder by external means (not shown in the figure) during the burnishing procedure to help keep it centered. If the radial fit between the lens and cell wall is close and the lens rim is accurately ground, this technique results in a well-aligned subassembly. Preload is uncertain in this mounting configuration. Once completed [see Fig. 3.3(b)], the subassembly is essentially permanent, since it would be very difficult to unbend the metal. In a slightly different assembly method, the cell lip is deformed around the lens rim by a swaging process in which a concave conical tool is pressed axially against that lip, bending it uniformly around its periphery toward the lens. Rotation of the subassembly about an axis is not required.

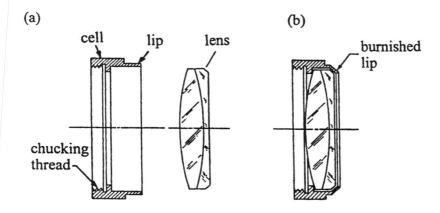

Fig. 3.3 A lens burnished into a cell made of malleable metal. (a) Cell and lens configurations, (b) the completed subassembly.

In some designs, a thin narrow "gasket" of resilient material such as a thin rubber O-ring is inserted between the lens and the shoulder or, preferably, between the lens and the burnished lip (to maintain glass-to-metal registration for alignment). This softens the interface and provides some measure of sealing. In the latter case, it is important for the lip to be long enough to trap the seal all the way around the lens rim.

Other designs may incorporate a coil spring between the lens and the shoulder to offer a more predictable axial preload and flexibility during temperature changes. Figure 3.4 shows an example. The spring ends should be ground flat to promote uniform contact all around the edge of the lens aperture. Jacobs[4] has suggested using a thin brass tube that is slotted transversely as the spring. In designs of this type, we gain some of the advantages of spring mounting as well as simplicity of the burnished-rim mounting technique. If the spring force (axial preload) is not sufficient to hold the lens against the lip under extreme shock and vibration, rebound may damage the polished surfaces.

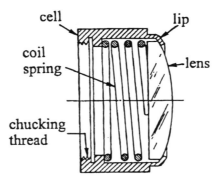

Fig. 3.4 A spring-loaded version of the burnished-in lens mounting. (Adapted from Jacobs.[4])

3.3 Snap and "Interference Fit" Rings

A discontinuous (i.e., cut) ring that drops into a groove machined into the ID of a cell is commonly termed a "snap ring" since it acts as a spring.[1,2] This ring usually is made of spring steel wire and so has a circular cross-section as shown in Fig. 3.5. Rings with rectangular or trapezoidal cross-sections are less frequently used. The cut in the ring allows it to be compressed slightly while sliding into the groove; this cut usually is made wide enough for a tool to be inserted for ring removal. The groove cross section can be rectangular (the most popular), vee-shaped, or curved.

It is difficult to ensure contact between the lens surface and the ring using this technique since the thickness, diameter, and surface radius of the lens as well as ring dimensions, groove location and dimensions, and temperature changes all affect the degree of mechanical interference, if any, existing between the lens surface and the ring. For this reason, this technique is used only where the location and orientation of the lens are not critical. It is virtually impossible to provide a specific axial preload to the lens.

To assist the reader who might need to design this type of lens-to-mount interface, Fig. 3.6 illustrates (to an exaggerated scale) the pertinent geometry for a convex

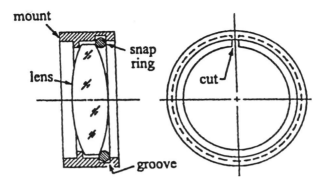

Fig. 3.5 Technique for constraining a lens with a cut circular cross-section snap ring located in a groove in the mount ID. (Adapted from Yoder.[1])

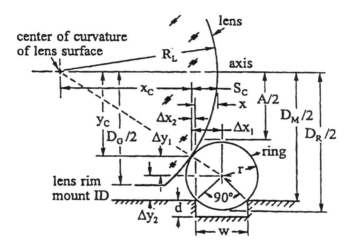

Fig. 3.6 Design geometry for the circular snap ring lens constraint.

lens surface of radius R_L, diameter D_G, and clear aperture A with a circular ring of cross-sectional diameter $2r$ and (compressed) OD of D_R when mounted in a cell with an ID equal to D_M. The following equations define the contact height y_C and the axial location x of the inner edge of the groove relative to the vertex of the lens. The dimensions (width w and depth d) of the nominal rectangular groove that allow the ring to just touch the lens while seating against both edges of the groove are also defined. This design is based on the reasonable but somewhat arbitrary specification that the angular subtense of the groove width as seen from the center of the ring cross section equals 90°.

$$y_C = (D_G + A)/4 \tag{3.1}$$

$$x_C = (R_L^2 - y_C^2)^{1/2} \tag{3.2}$$

$$S_C = R_L - x_C \tag{3.3}$$

$$\Delta y_1 = y_C r / R_L \tag{3.4}$$

$$\Delta x_1 = x_C r / R_L \tag{3.5}$$

$$\Delta y_2 = (D_M / 2) - y_C - \Delta y_1 = w/2 \tag{3.6}$$

$$\Delta x_2 = \Delta x_1 - \Delta y_2 \tag{3.7}$$

$$x = S_C - \Delta x_2 \tag{3.8}$$

$$d_{MINIMUM} = r - \Delta y_2 \tag{3.9}$$

$$d_{RECOMMENDED} = 1.25 \, d_{MINIMUM} \tag{3.9a}$$

$$w = 2 \Delta y_2 \tag{3.10}$$

$$D_R = 2(y_C + \Delta y_1 + r) \tag{3.11}$$

Note that $(D_R - 4r)$ should be at least equal to the required lens aperture A. If not, a new (smaller) value for ring cross-sectional diameter 2r should be chosen and the computations repeated until this is so.

Example 3.1: Convex surface interface with a snap ring.
(For design and analysis, use File 1.1 of the CD-ROM)
Design a lens snap ring mounting with the following dimensions: D_G = 25.4 mm (1.0 in.), A = 22.0 mm (0.8661 in.), R_L = 50.8 mm (2.0 in.), D_M = 25.6 mm(1.0079 in.), and r = 1.0 mm (0.0394 in.).

From Eqs. (3.1) through (3.11):
   y_C = (25.4 + 22.0)/4 = 11.8500 mm (0.4665 in.)
   x_C = $(50.8^2 - 11.85^2)^{1/2}$ = 49.3986 mm (1.9448 in.)
   S_C = 50.8 - 49.3986 = 1.4014 mm (0.0552 in.)

Δy_1 = (11.85)(1.0)/50.8 = 0.2333 mm (0.0092 in.)
Δx_1 = (49.3986)(1.0)/50.8 = 0.9724 mm (0.0383 in.)
Δy_2 = (25.6/2) - 11.85 - 0.2333 = 0.7167 mm (0.0282 in.)
Δx_2 = 0.9724 - 0.7167 = 0.2557 mm (0.0101 in.)
x = 1.4014 - 0.2557 = 1.1457 mm (0.0451 in.)
$d_{MINIMUM}$ = 1.0 - 0.7167 = 0.2833 mm (0.0111 in.)
$d_{RECOMMENDED}$ = (1.25)(0.2833) = 0.3541 mm (0.0139 in.)
w = (2)(0.7167) = 1.4334 mm (0.0564 in.)
D_R = (2)(11.85 + 0.2333 + 1.0) = 26.1666 mm (1.0302 in.)

Check: $(D_R - 4r)$ = 26.1666 - (4)(1.0) = 22.1666 mm (0.8727 in.) This is greater than A, therefore acceptable.

Figure 3.7 shows what happens if a nominally dimensioned lens is properly seated in the cell, the groove has nominal dimensions and the ring cross-sectional diameter 2r is nominal (the ring just touches the lens), oversized (the ring contacts the groove only on its outer edge and tends to rise out of that groove), and undersized (the ring seats in the groove, but clearance exists between the lens and the ring). Only in the case of an oversized ring is the lens subject to any axial preload. Analytical means for predicting this preload are not available at present. This problem can occur if the groove is mislocated axially, has the wrong width, or has the wrong depth.

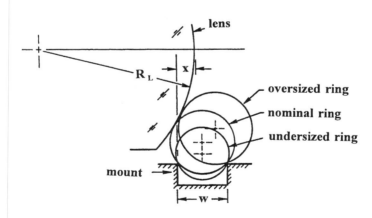

Fig. 3.7 Effect of variation in ring cross-sectional diameter in the mounting configuration of Fig. 3.6.

While the surface-contacting-type of interface could be used with a concave lens surface, it is more common to place a flat bevel on the surface and locate the snap ring so it just touches that bevel at its midpoint. Figure 3.8 and the following equations then apply. The bevel width is b. The suitability of the cross-sectional diameter 2r should be checked by calculating $(D_R - 4r)$; this should equal or exceed A.

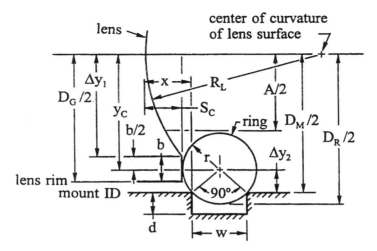

Fig. 3.8 Configuration for snap-ring constraint of a lens with a concave surface having a flat bevel.

$$y_C = (D_G/2) - (b/2) \tag{3.12}$$

$$\Delta y_1 = (D_G/2) - b \tag{3.13}$$

$$\Delta y_2 = (d_M/2) - y_C \tag{3.14}$$

$$S_C = R_L - (R_L^2 - \Delta y_1^2)^{1/2} \tag{3.15}$$

$$d_{MINIMUM} = r - \Delta y_2 \tag{3.9}$$

$$d_{RECOMMENDED} = 1.25\, d_{MINIMUM} \tag{3.9a}$$

$$w = 2\Delta y_2 \tag{3.10}$$

$$x = S_C + r - (w/2) \tag{3.16}$$

$$D_R = 2(y_C + r) \tag{3.17}$$

Figure 3.9 shows what happens if a lens with a beveled concave surface is properly seated in the cell, the groove has nominal dimensions, and the ring cross-sectional diameter 2r is nominal (the ring just touches the lens); oversized (the ring contacts the groove only on its outer edge and tends to rise out of that groove); and undersized (the ring seats in groove, but clearance exists between the lens and the ring). As for a convex surface, only in the case of an oversize ring is the lens subject to any axial preload, and analytical means for predicting this preload are not available.

Example 3.2: Concave surface interface with a snap ring.
(For design and analysis, use File 1.2 of the CD-ROM)

Design a snap ring mount for a lens with a concave surface and flat bevel per Fig. 3.8. Let D_G = 25.4 mm (1.0 in.), A = 22.0 mm (0.8661 in.), R_L = 50.8 mm (2.0 in.), D_M = 25.6 mm (1.008 in.), r = 1.0 mm (0.039 in.), and b = 1.0 mm (0.039 in.).

From Eqs. (3.9) through (3.10) and (3.12) through (3.17):

y_C = (25.4 / 2) - (1.0 / 2) = 12.2 mm (0.480 in.)
Δy_1 = (25.4 / 2) - 1.0 = 11.7 mm (0.461 in.)
Δy_2 = (25.6 / 2) - 12.2 = 0.6 mm (0.024 in.)
S_C = 50.8 - $(50.8^2 - 11.7^2)^{1/2}$ = 1.3657 mm (0.054 in.)
$d_{MINIMUM}$ = 1.0 - 0.6 = 0.4 mm (0.016 in.)
$d_{RECOMMENDED}$ = (1.25)(0.4) = 0.5 mm (0.020 in.)
w = (2)(0.6) = 1.2 mm (0.047 in.)
x = 1.3657 + 1.0 - (1.2/2) = 1.7657 mm (0.069 in.)
D_R = (2)(12.2 + 1.0) = 26.4 mm (1.039 in.)

Check: $(D_R - 4r)$ = 26.4 - (4)(1.0) = 22.4 mm (0.882 in.).
This is > A and therefore acceptable.

If the cell is designed without a groove in its cylindrical ID, a cut snap ring with a rectangular cross-section can be inserted against the lens. The spring must compress slightly as it is pressed in place. Some degree of constraint will then be offered by friction between the ring and the ID. Disassembly is possible if means (such as radially oriented holes) are provided in the ring to allow attachment of a tool. However, the design may be excessively sensitive to shock and vibration.

A configuration for a ring-constraint design with a different form of groove is shown in Fig. 3.10. Here a circular cross-section ring rests against a tapered or ramped inside surface of the cell wall. The ring is pressed in place and the cell is plastic, so it is somewhat resilient. Spring action holds the ring between the lens surface and the ramp. This design is less sensitive to dimensional errors and temperature changes than those with conventional grooves. Preload is hard to predict.

A lens can also be constrained by a continuous ring as shown in Fig. 3.11. The OD of the ring is made very slightly oversized with respect to the ID of the cell for an interference fit. After the lens is installed, the ring is pressed into the cell. It is difficult to determine exactly when the ring touches the lens surface, so it would be impossible to

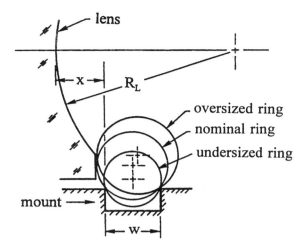

Fig. 3.9 Effect of variation in ring cross-sectional diameter in the mounting configuration of Fig. 3.8.

achieve a particular preload on the lens and hard even to ensure that contact is made.

A preferred assembly technique would be to heat the cell (and perhaps cool the ring) so the ring slips easily into place against the lens surface. It is theoretically possible to achieve a specific preload by calculating the dimensional changes that are due to the temperature change and ensuring that the ring contacts the lens at the start of the temperature equalization process. In this design, the cell and ring materials should have similar CTEs to prevent loosening or excessive internal stress buildup at extreme low temperature as a result of differential contraction. Publication B4.1-1967 of the American National Standards Institute (ANSI) defines the appropriate dimensions for force/shrink fits using thin sections (Class FN-1).[6] Assembly by an interference fit technique is quite permanent, since it is virtually impossible to remove the ring without damaging either the ring or the lens.

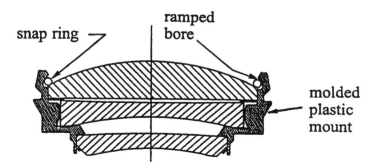

Fig. 3.10 A snap-ring-loaded lens-mounting configuration featuring a ramped seat for the ring. (Adapted from Plummer.[5])

MOUNTING INDIVIDUAL LENSES

MOUNTING INDIVIDUAL LENSES

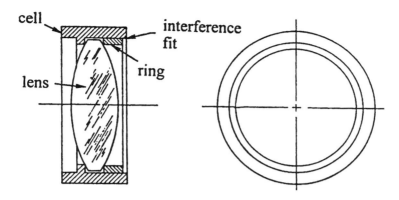

Fig. 3.11 A lens constraint design with a continuous ring pressed in place with an interference fit. (Adapted from Yoder.[1])

3.4   Retaining Ring Constraints

The most frequently used technique for mounting lenses is to clamp the lens near its rim between a shoulder or spacer and a retaining ring. The ring may be threaded or configured as an annular flange. When mounting larger lenses, it is sometimes advantageous to use multiple cantilevered spring clips to serve as an "interupted" constraining flange.

Manufacturing variations in the axial dimensions of lenses and cells can be compensated for with any of these constraints. The continuous ring configurations are compatible with environmental sealing with a cured-in-place elastomer or an O-ring. These designs are easily incorporated into multiple-component lens systems that are separated by spacers as discussed in Chapter 4.

The total axial force (preload), P, in pounds, that should be exerted on the lens by any means of constraint to hold it in place may be calculated as $P = W\Sigma a_G$ where W is the weight of the lens and Σa_G is the vector sum of the maximum anticipated externally-applied accelerations, such as those due to constant acceleration, random vibration (3σ), amplified resonant vibration (sinusoidal), acoustic loading, and shock. These accelerations can be expressed as multiples, a_G, of ambient gravity. Since all types of external accelerations do not generally occur simultaneously, the magnitude of the summation term does not need to be taken literally. For simplicity, we here consider a_G to be a single-valued, worst-case number. Equation (3.18) then applies.

$$P = W a_G \tag{3.18}$$

Note that if the lens weight is expressed in kilograms, Eq. (3.18) must include a multiplicative factor of 4.448 to convert units. The preload is then in newtons (N). Friction and moments imposed at the interfaces are ignored.

3.4.1 Threaded retaining ring

Figure 3.12 illustrates a typical threaded retaining ring mounting design for a biconvex lens. Contact between the lens and the mount occurs on both polished surfaces as recommended earlier for precise centering of the lens and to minimize the need for precise edging or close tolerances on the diameter of the lens.[1] To minimize bending of the lens, contact should occur at approximately the same height from the axis on both

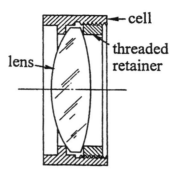

Fig. 3.12 Typical configuration of a lens secured in its mount with a threaded retaining ring. (From Yoder.[7])

sides of the lens[8] (see Sect. 11.2.2). The fit of the ring threads into the cell threads should be loose (Class-1 or -2 per ANSI Publication B1.1-1982) so the ring can tilt slightly, if necessary, to accommodate residual wedge angle in the lens when the lens is properly centered optically. This helps to ensure that the preload is distributed uniformly around the lens periphery. A rule-of-thumb criterion for suitability of the fit of the threaded version is to assemble the ring in the mount without an optic in place, hold it to the ear, and shake it. One should be able to hear the ring rattle in the mount.

Sets of holes or transverse slots are sometimes machined into the exposed face of the retainer to accept pins or rectangular lugs on the end of a cylindrical wrench that is used to tighten the retainer. Alternatively, a flat plate-type tool that spans the retainer can be used as the wrench. The cylindrical wrench is easier to use and is more conducive to measurement of torque applied to the ring.

An equation for the approximate magnitude of the axial preload (P) produced by tightening a threaded retainer with pitch diameter D_T (see Fig. 3.13) to a torque Q against a lens surface can be derived as shown in Appendix C. The first term results from the classical equation for a body sliding slowly on an inclined plane (i.e., the thread), while the second represents the friction effects at the circular interface between the lens surface and the end of the rotating retainer. This equation is

$$P = Q/[D_T(0.577\mu_M + 0.500\mu_G)] \tag{3.19}$$

where μ_M is the coefficient of sliding friction of the metal-to-metal interface in the

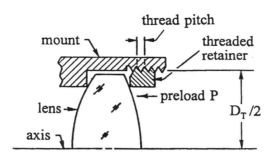

Fig. 3.13 Geometry for relating torque applied to a retainer to the resulting axial preload.

thread and μ_G is the coefficient of sliding friction of the glass-to-metal interface. Some designs place a thin "slip ring" between the lens and the retainer to prevent rotation of the lens as the retainer is tightened. Then, μ_M is used in both terms.

Equation (3.19) is an approximation because of small factors neglected in the derivation and larger uncertainties in the values of μ_M and μ_G. The latter values depend strongly on the smoothness of the metal surfaces (which depends, in part, upon the machined finish as well as how many times the thread has been tightened) and whether the surfaces are dry or moistened by water or a lubricant. Laboratory physics-type measurements of the angle at which a dry anodized aluminum block just begins to slide down an inclined dry anodized aluminum surface have indicated that μ_M is about 0.19, while similar experiments with polished glass and dry anodized aluminum indicated μ_G to be about 0.15. Substituting these values into Eq. (3.19), we obtain $P = 5.42Q/D_T$. This corresponds to within about 8% to the commonly accepted approximation of the P to Q relationship, which is [9,10]

$$P = 5Q/D_T \qquad (3.19a)$$

Note that like metals (aluminum on aluminum, etc.) should never be in contact in a threaded joint without lubrication (such as a dry film) or some form of coating or plating since they will gall and possibly seize.

Example 3.3: Preload obtained from a torqued retainer.
(For design and analysis, use File 2.1 of the CD-ROM)
Assume that a 2.1-in. (53.3-mm) OD lens is to be clamped with a total preload of 12.5 lb (55.60 N) delivered by a retainer screwed into a cell on a thread of pitch diameter 2.2 in. (55.88 mm). Using Eq. (3.19a), approximately what torque should be applied?

Rearranging Eq. (3.19a), $Q = PD_T/5 = (12.5)(2.2)/5 = 5.5$ lb-in. (0.62 N-m).

An aspect of threaded retainer design that has, to the best knowledge of this author, escaped consideration in the literature on optical instrumentation design is the question of preferred dimensions for the threads and the stress developed in those threads by an applied axial preload. Intutitvely, one might expect that a coarse thread would withstand axial force better than a fine one. Dimensional or "packaging" constraints might, on the other hand, require the use of fine threads in order to minimize wall thickness and overall diameter of the mount. We recognize that extra care must be exercised in assembling a fine-threaded retainer to prevent "crossing" the threads and rendering the parts unusable.

Figure 3.14 shows the commonly used terminology for screw threads, while Fig. 3.15 shows the basic profile of a thread.[11] The dimension designations apply to a metric bolt (i.e., the retainer's threads) and its matching nut (i.e., the internal thread in the mount). The profile of a thread with inch dimensions is essentially the same as that shown in Fig. 3.15. These fall into the unified thread system, with two major series called "UNC" and "UNF" for coarse and fine pitches, respectively.

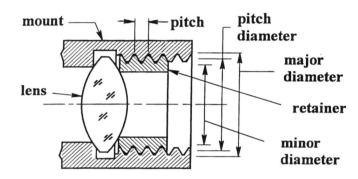

Fig. 3.14 Schematic showing terminology for retainer screw threads.

We are interested here in determining the average stress in the threads as the total axial preload divided by the annular area over which that force is distributed. We then compare that stress with the yield stress of the materials used since stripping of the threads is the chief concern. From the geometry of Fig. 3.15, the crest-to-root thread height, H, is related to the thread pitch, p, by the following equation:

$$H = (0.5)(\sqrt{3})(p) = 0.866p \qquad (3.20)$$

We also see from the figure that the annular area actually in contact has a radial dimension of (5/8)H. Hence, the annular area per thread is

$$A_T = (\pi)(D_2)(5H/8) = (1.700)(D_T)(p) \qquad (3.21)$$

where D_T is the pitch diameter of the thread.

Internal threads

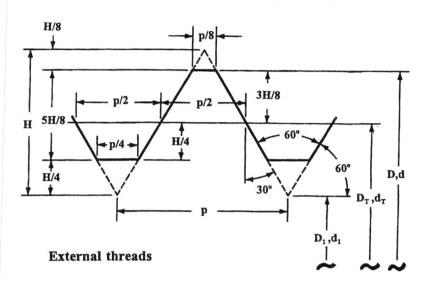

External threads

Fig. 3.15 Basic thread profile where D, (d) = major diameter, D_1 (d_1) = minor diameter, D_T (d_T) = pitch diameter, p = pitch. Capital and lower-case letters represent external and internal threads, respectively. (Adapted from Shigley and Mischke.[11])

It is well known that the first few (typically three) threads on a bolt carry most of the tensile load developed when the bolt is tightened. Assuming this is also the case for a threaded lens retainer, the total annular area in contact is $3A_T$ (at least before exposure to high accelerations at low temperature when some distortion of thread shape might occur). Hence, the stress in the threads, S_T, is approximately

$$S_T = P/(3A_T) = 0.196P/(D_T p) \tag{3.22}$$

It should be noted that for those designs in which the mount has a higher CTE than the lens, the thread stress should be estimated at the lowest survival temperature since then the preload is the greatest and this represents a worst-case situation. In Sect. 12.2.3, we show how to estimate the preload change in typical lens mounting configurations as the temperature drops to its minimum expected value.

Example 3.4: Stress in retainer threads that is due to axial preload. (For design and analysis, use File 2.2 of the CD-ROM)
(a) Estimate the stress in the threads of the retainer from Example 3.3 and the applicable safety factor if the thread size is 32 threads per inch (tpi) (1.26 threads/mm) at minimum temperature and worst case acceleration when the preload increases to 935 lb (4161 N). Assume that the metal parts are 6061 aluminum with a minimum yield strength of 8000 lb/in.^{2} (55.2 MPa)? (b) What is the finest thread that produces a safety factor of 2 for this low temperature condition?

(a) From Eq. (3.22), $S_T = (0.196)(935)/[(2.2)(1/32)] = 2666$ lb/in.^{2} (18.4 MPa)
  Safety factor = f_S = 8000/2666 = 3.0

This stress level is sufficiently below the yield strength of the metal used, so we would not be concerned about thread failure.

(b) $S_T = 8000/f_S = 8000/2.0 = (0.196)(935)/(2.2)(1/p)$
Hence, p = (2.2)(4000)/(0.196)(935) = 48.0 tpi (1.89 threads/mm)

This thread would be suitable for use in the retainer design.

3.4.2 Clamping (flange) ring

A typical design for a lens mounting involving a clamped (flange-type) retaining ring is shown in Fig. 3.16. Flange-type retainers are most frequently used with large-aperture lenses where manufacture and assembly of a threaded ring would be difficult. Their functions are essentially the same as that of the threaded ring described earlier.

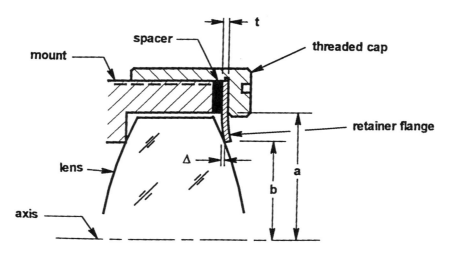

Fig. 3.16 Schematic configuration of a flange-type retainer axially constraining a lens in a mount.

The magnitude of the preload produced by a given axial deflection of the flange shown in the figure can be approximated by considering the flange to be a perforated circular plate with its outer edge fixed and an axially directed load applied uniformly along the inner edge to deflect that edge. The applicable equation relating inner edge deflection, Δ, to total preload as given by Roark[12] can be rewritten as follows:

$$\Delta = (K_A - K_B)(P/t^3) \tag{3.23}$$

where:

$$K_A = \frac{3(m^2 - 1)[a^4 - b^4 - 4a^2b^2\ln(a/b)]}{4\pi m^2 E_M a^2} \tag{3.24}$$

$$K_B = \frac{3(m^2 - 1)(m + 1)[2\ln(a/b) + (b^2/a^2) - 1][b^4 + 2a^2b^2\ln(a/b) - a^2b^2]}{(4\pi m^2 E_M)[b^2(m + 1) + a^2(m - 1)]} \tag{3.25}$$

and

P = total preload
t = thickness of flange cantilevered section
a = outer radius of cantilevered section
b = inner radius of cantilevered section
m = reciprocal of Poisson's ratio (υ_M) of the flange material
E_M = Young's modulus of the flange material.

The spacer under the flange can be ground at assembly to the particular axial thickness that produces the predetermined flange deflection when firm metal-to-metal contact is achieved by tightening the clamping screws. Variations in as-manufactured lens thicknesses are accommodated by customizing the spacer. The flange material and thickness are the prime design variables. The dimensions a and b, and hence the annular width (a - b), can also be varied, but these are usually set primarily by the lens aperture, mount wall thickness, and overall dimensional requirements.

An important factor to be considered in designing a flange retainer for a lens is the stress S_B built up in the bent portion of the flange. This must not exceed the yield stress S_B of the material. The following equations adapted from Roark[12] apply:

$$S_B = K_C P/t^2 = S_Y/f_S \tag{3.26}$$

or, solving for t,

$$t = \sqrt{(f_S K_C P/S_Y)} \tag{3.26a}$$

where:

$$K_C = \left(\frac{3}{2\pi}\right)\left[1 - \frac{2mb^2 - 2b^2(m+1)\ln(a/b)}{a^2(m-1) + b^2(m+1)}\right] \quad (3.27)$$

Example 3.5: Deflection of a clamping flange. (For design and analysis, use File 3 of the CD-ROM)

Consider a 15.75-in. (400.05-mm)-diameter corrector plate for a telescope that is to be held in place with a total preload P of 120 lb (534 N) distributed uniformly around and near the edge of the plate by a titanium (Ti6Al4V) flange that limits the aperture of the plate to 15.500 in. (393.700 mm). A radial clearance Δr of 0.010 in. (0.254 mm) is to be provided between the plate and the mount ID. Dimensions are

a = (15.750/2) + 0.010 = 7.885 in. (200.279 mm) $\upsilon_M = 0.340$
b = 15.500/2 = 7.750 in. (196.850 mm) m = 1/0.340 = 2.941
$E_M = 16.5\times10^6$ lb/in.^{2} (11.4×10^{10} Pa) S_Y = 120,000 lb/in.^{2} (827 MPa)

Calculate (a) the required flange thickness, t, for a safety factor f_S of 2 and (b) the flange inner edge deflection Δ.

(a) From Eqs. (3.27) and (3.26a):

$$K_C = (3/2\pi)\left[1 - \frac{(2)(2.941)(7.750^2) - (2)(7.750^2)(2.941+1)(\ln(7.885/7.750))}{(7.885^2)(2.941-1) + (7.750^2)(2.941+1)}\right]$$

$$= 0.0164$$

$$t = \sqrt{[(2)(0.0164)(120)/120{,}000]} = 0.0057 \text{ in. } (0.1455 \text{ mm})$$

(b) From Eq. (3.24, (3.25) and (3.23):

$$K_A = \frac{(3)((2.941^2 - 1)(7.885^4 - 7.750^4 - (4)(7.885^2)(7.750^2)(\ln(7.885/7.750)))}{(4\pi)(2.941^2)(7.885^2)(16.5\times10^6)}$$

$$= 1.0556\times10^{-11} \text{ in.}^4/\text{lb}$$

$$K_B = \frac{(3)(2.941^2 - 1)(2.941+1)(2\ln(7.885/7.750)) + (7.750^2/7.885^2) - 1)\;(7.750^4 + (2)(7.885^2)(7.750^2)(\ln(7.885/7.759)) - (7.885^2)(7.750^2))}{(4\pi)(2.941^2)(16.5\times10^6)((7.750^2)(2.941+1) + (7.885^2)(2.941-1))}$$

$$= 1.8321\times10^{-13} \text{ in.}^4/\text{lb}$$

$$\Delta = (1.0554\times10^{-11} - 1.8321\times10^{-13})(120/0.0057^3) = 0.0067 \text{ in. } (0.1707 \text{ mm})$$

To check using Eq. (3.26):

$$S_B = (0.0164)(120)/0.0057^2 = 60,572 \text{ lb/in.}^2 \ (417.6 \text{ MPa}) \quad \text{(within 1\% of target)}$$

It is important for the end of the mount to which the flange is referenced to be flat and that the clamped portion of the flange be stiff enough for the deflection Δ measured between the attachment points (screws) to be essentially the same as that at the screws. A simple means for accomplishing this is to add a back up ring between the screw heads and the flange as shown in Fig. 3.16. This ring can be made of aluminum if it is thick enough to ensure uniform clamping of the flange. A stiffer material such as titanium could be thinner. If the flange is machined from a thicker blank, the clamping ring can be incorporated in it as an integral feature. This may be less expensive than adding a separate part.

A great advantage of the flange-type constraint over the threaded retainer is that it can be calibrated, so we can know quite precisely what preload will be delivered when the flange is deflected by a particular amount. This measurement of the spring constant of the flange can be done offline using a load cell or other means to measure the force produced by various deflections. This refines the performance prediction made during design using the above equations. Since the test is nondestructive, we can safely assume that during actual use the hardware will behave as measured.

Another technique for holding the flange of Fig. 3.16 against the end of the mounting wall is shown in Fig. 3.17. Here a threaded cap is used instead of multiple screws. The prime benefit is that the cap tends to hold the flange uniformly all around its periphery, while the screws hold it intermittantly. The shoulder machined into the cap must be flat. As in the case of threaded retainers, the fit of these threads should be Class-1 or -2 per ANSI Publication B1.1-1982 so the cap can square itself to the flange as necessary. Slots or holes for a pin wrench should be provided to facilitate tightening the cap.

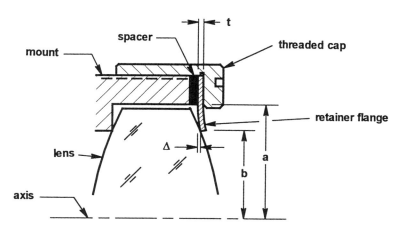

Fig. 3.17 Using a threaded cap rather than a set of screws to secure a flange.

3.4.3 Distributing preload uniformly

Very stiff flanges or threaded retainers would tend to contact the lens at the three highest points at low preload and at more points at higher preload because either the lens or the retainer (or both) then bend. Stress concentrations at the contacts and/or optical surface deformations caused by lack of conformity of the interfacing surfaces result. Various means that can be used to equalize preload around the lens with flange-type constraints and with threaded retainers are shown in Fig. 3.18. Each mechanical part touching the lens provides some measure of axial resiliency. One surface of the lens registers against the shoulder in all cases. We will consider the effects of different shapes of the mechanical interface with the lens in Sect. 3.6 and in Chapter 11.

In Fig. 3.18(a), several flexures are built into a separate pressure ring.[8] In Fig. 3.18(b), an O-ring is compressed against the lens surface. Vukobratovich[10] has indicated that O-rings should have a hardness of about 70 durometer and that the interfaces should be dimensioned so the ring is nominally compressed after assembly to about 50% to 70% of the full level of compression recommended by the manufacturer. More or less compression can then take place as the temperature changes without losing sealing capability or causing undue stress. O-rings harden with time. Their spring rates have been described by Martini as exponential.[13]

In the design shown in Fig. 3.18(c), the dimension "x" is machined at assembly to cause a predetermined amount of displacement of the flexure corner when the retainer is firmly seated. This design is intended to be used with a concave surface. The configuration shown in Fig. 31.8(d) serves the same function for a convex surface. Again,

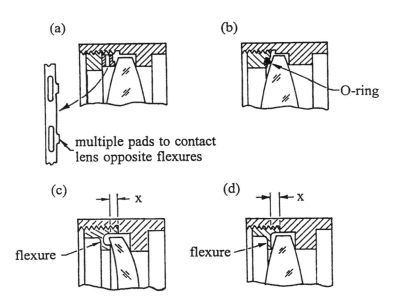

Fig. 3.18 Four design techniques for distributing axial preload uniformly around the edge of a lens surface. (a) Multiple flexures, (b) O-ring contact, (c) flexure retainer on a concave surface, (d) flexure retainer on a convex surface.

dimension "x" is machined at assembly for a specific flexure displacement. Spacers inserted between the retainer and cell in the designs of Figs. 3.18(c) and 3.18(d) would allow simpler adjustment of dimension "x" on a surface grinder.

3.5 Constraining the Lens with Multiple Spring Clips

A simple way to clamp a lens into its mount is illustrated by Fig. 3.19. Here the lens rests against three thin Mylar shims (shown with exaggerated thickness) attached to

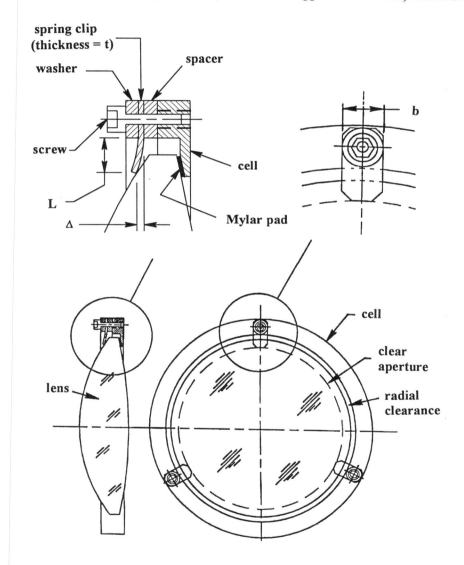

Fig. 3.19 Concept for a lens mounting using three radially oriented cantilevered springs to provide preload against pads on a cell shoulder.

a shoulder in the cell. The shims are located at 120° intervals and serve as semikinematic registration surfaces. Preload is applied by three metal clips that act as cantilevered springs. The outer ends of the clips are attached to the cell with screws. Spacers between the clips and the cell are machined to impart specific deflections to the clips, thereby providing preload for the lens. The clips are located so the preload is directed through the lens directly toward the pads. This minimizes bending moments that otherwise could be applied to the optic. The use of the Mylar pads reduces the need to machine the shoulder as a geometrically accurate and smooth surface. The cell shoulder might well be configured to provide an appropriately shaped interface for the lens such as a conical surface tangent to a convex lens surface, a toroidal interface for a concave lens surface, or a flat interface for a lens with a flat surface or one with a flat bevel. These types of interfaces are discussed in detail in the next section.

In some lens mounting designs, additional clips are used; they are usually spaced equally around the lens periphery. By doing so, the portion of the preload derived from each clip is reduced. This may reduce the bending stress developed within each clip.

The following equation (adapted from Roark[12]) can be used to calculate the deflection Δ required of each of N clips from its relaxed (undeflected) condition to provide a specific total preload:

$$\Delta = (1 - v_M^2)(4PL^3)/(E_M b t^3 N) \tag{3.28}$$

where:

v_M is Poisson's ratio for the clip material
P is the total preload
L is the free (cantilevered) length of the clip
E_M is Young's modulus for the clip material
b is the width of the clip
t is the thickness of the clip
N is the number of clips employed.

Example 3.6: Cantilevered spring lens mounting.
(For design and analysis, use File 4 of the CD-ROM)

Assume a lens is to be constrained axially with a preload of 60 lb (267 N) by three Ti6Al4V titanium spring clips with dimensions L = 0.3125 in. (7.937 mm), b = 0.375 in. (9.525 mm), and t = 0.0408 in. (1.036 mm). How much should each clip be deflected?

From Table B12, $v_M = 0.34$ and $E_M = 16.5 \times 10^6$ lb/in.^{2} (1.14×10^5 MPa)

From Eq. (3.8): $\Delta = (1 - 0.34^2)(4)(60)(0.3125^3)/[(16.5 \times 10^6)(0.3750)(0.0408^3)(3)]$
                    $= 0.0051$ in. (0.1295 mm)

Assuming that this deflection can be measured to $\pm$ 0.0005 in. ($\pm$ 0.013 mm) or $\pm$ 10%, the desired preload should be achieved within $\pm$ 6 lb (27 N).

Equation (3.2) quantifies the bending stress S_B in the clip material that is due to the deflection imposed when the optic is held in place with the preload, P:

$$S_B = 6PL/(bt^2N) \qquad\qquad (3.29)$$

This stress should not exceed about one-half the yield strength of the material used (i.e., a safety factor, f_S, of about 2 applies). According to Roark,[12] the bending stress from Eq. (3.29) could be reduced by a factor of about 3 if the fixed end of the clip were clamped in place rather than perforated for attachment to the mount with screws.

Example 3.7: Stress in a cantilevered spring.
(For design and analysis, use File 4 of the CD-ROM)
Calculate the stress in each of the springs used in Example 3.6 using Eq. (3.29).

$$S_B = (6)(60)(0.3125)/[(0.3750)(0.0408^2)(3)] = 60,073 \text{ lb/in.}^2 \text{ (414 MPa).}$$

From Table B12, the minimum yield strength of titanium is approximately 120×10^3 lb/in.^{2} (82.7×10^7 Pa). The desired safety factor f_S of about 2 therefore exists.

To see how a variation in dimensions might affect a specific lens mounting design, let us choose titanium for the spring clips and require that $f_S = 2$. Keeping b constant, one can easily determine from the above equations that a longer spring should be thicker to obtain a specific preload. Similarly, with length constant, a wider spring should be thinner to obtain a specific preload. The rate of change of deflection with spring length is greater than that for varying spring width. For reliability of measuring deflection and achieving a desired preload within about 10%, Δ should be at least 0.005 in. (0.127 mm).

Referring once again to Fig. 3.19, we see that the spring clip length, L, affects the overall diameter of the mount. If contact occurs just outside the lens clear aperture, A, the OD will be approximately $A + 2L + 2t_C$, where t_C is the cell wall thickness.

In some optical systems, such as laser diode beam collimators, optical correlators, anamorphic projectors, and some scanning systems, the natural aperture shapes of some lenses, windows, prisms, and mirrors are rectangular, racetrack, trapezoidal, etc., because their fields of view are different in the vertical and horizontal meridians. Cylindrical, toroidal, and nonrotationally symmetrical aspheric optical surfaces are frequently used in such optical systems to create other desired beam shapes or to introduce different magnifications in orthogonal directions. These lenses have nonrotationally symmetrical surface shapes and may have noncircular apertures, so they cannot be mounted conventionally in circular cells or held in place by threaded retainers since the surface sagittas at a given distance from the axis are not equal. Mounts for these optics are usually customized for the particular needs of the component under consideration.

A simple example of such a mounting design is shown in Fig. 3.20. The lens is a plano-concave cylindrical lens with a 2:1 aperture aspect ratio. The lens is clamped with four spring clips into a rectangular recess machined into a flat plate. The plate is circular, so it can be attached conventionally to the structure of the instrument. Note that a slot is provided to align the lens to the system axis as represented by a pin or key (not shown). The clips provide localized preload to hold the lens in the recess under the anticipated acceleration forces. Four Mylar pads are attached to the mount shoulder interface with the flat side of the lens directly opposite the clips. These pads must be accurately coplanar in order not to bend the lens by overconstraint from the clips, so the shoulder must be accurately machined flat. With small optics, three pads probably would provide

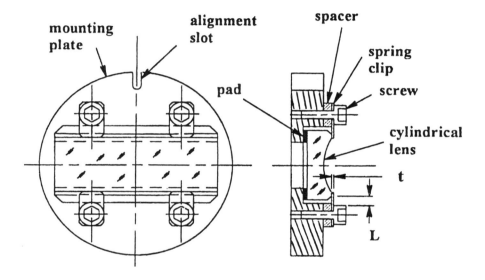

Fig. 3.20 Schematic diagram of a mounting technique for a cylindrical lens.

adequate support and function semikinematically. The design of the clips follows that described for circular lenses.

Lenses with cylindrical surfaces can be registered against off-center parallel rods as shown schematically in Fig. 3.21. The rods are pressed into parallel holes bored through the mount at the appropriate distance from the mount axis. This technique can be applied to convex or concave surfaces. Some means of preloading for maintaining axial contact between the lens and the rods, such as spring clips or a retaining flange, would be needed. This type mounting facilitates rotational alignment of the cylinder axis.

3.6 Geometry of the Lens-to-Mount Interface

3.6.1 The "sharp-corner" interface

The "sharp-corner" interface is created by the intersection of a cylindrical bore

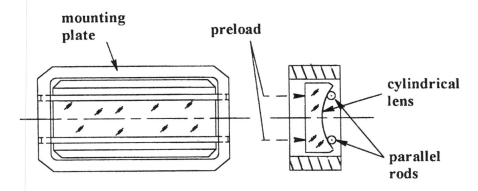

Fig. 3.21 A parallel-rod type of registration interface for cylindrical lenses.

in a lens mount and a plane machined perpendicular to the axis of that bore. It is the interface easiest to produce and is used in the vast majority of optical instruments. Hopkins[14] indicated that the machinist is more likely to achieve a smooth edge on a sharp corner, and the chance of damage to that edge during handling, storage, or assembly is minimized, if the angle between the intersecting machined surfaces is greater than 90°.

In reality, the sharp corner is not actually a knife edge. Delgado and Hallinan[15] quantified it as one in which the intersection of the machined surfaces on the metal part has been burnished in accordance with good shop practice to a radius on the order of 0.002 in. (0.05 mm). This small radius surface contacts the glass at a height y_C. Figure 3.22 illustrates the interface on a convex spherical lens surface.

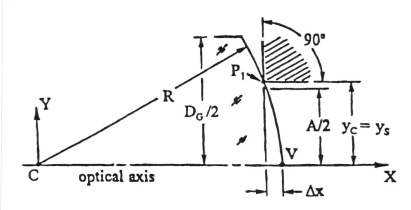

Fig. 3.22 Schematic of a 90° sharp-corner interface on a convex spherical surface.

Design geometries for sharp-corner interfaces for 90° and 135° angles and for convex and concave surfaces of radius R, clear aperture A, and diameter D_G are shown schematically in Figs. 3.22 through 3.25.[16] The axial location of the contact point P_1 with respect to the surface vertex V (here defined as Δx) is of interest since it provides a

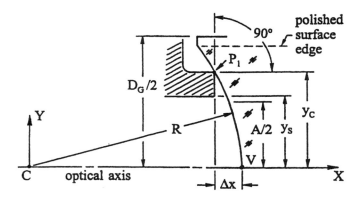

Fig. 3.23 Schematic of a 90° sharp-corner interface on a concave spherical surface.

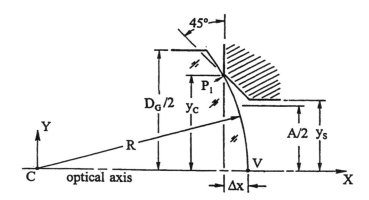

Fig. 3.24 Schematic of a 135° sharp-corner interface on a convex spherical surface.

basic reference for locating and dimensioning the mechanical parts. In the four cases shown here, Δx is simply the sagittal depth of the spherical surface at the contact height y_C, or:

$$\Delta = (R - (R^2 - y_C^2)^{1/2} \tag{3.30}$$

We define y_S as the inside radius of the mount at the interface. It may equal $A/2$, but this is not always true. Frequently, y_S is defined as $A/2$ plus 0.5% of A (i.e., 0.505A). Then, if there is no compelling reason to do otherwise, we would place P_1 at $(A + D_G)/4$, as specified by Eq. (3.1). In Fig. 3.22, $y_C = y_S$. In other cases, $y_C > y_S$, so a larger mount OD would be required for a given aperture and mounting wall thickness.

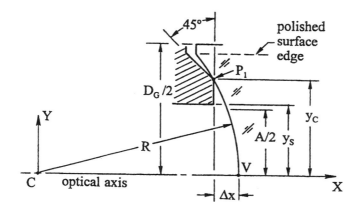

Fig. 3.25 Schematic of a 135° sharp-corner interface on a concave spherical surface.

Example 3.8: Location of mount corner P_1 with respect to a convex lens vertex with a sharp-corner interface.
(For design and analysis, use File 5.1 of the CD-ROM)

Let a lens surface radius be 20.0 in. (508.0 mm) and y_C = 2.0 in. (50.8 mm). What is Δx?

By Eq. (3.30): $\Delta x = 20.000 - (20.000^2 - 2.000^2)^{1/2} = 0.100$ in. (2.540 mm)

Note that this calculation applies equally well to a convex or concave lens surface and to 90° or obtuse-angle sharp-corner designs.

3.6.2 The tangential (conical) interface

If the spherical lens surface contacts a conical surface in the mount, the design is called a "tangential interface" (see Fig. 3.26). The tangential interface is not feasible with a concave lens surface, but it is generally regarded as the nearly ideal interface for convex surfaces. Easily made by modern machining technology, the conical interface tends to produce smaller contact stress in the lens for a given preload than the sharp-corner interface. This attribute of the conical interface is discussed in Sect. 11.2.

The cone half-angle, φ, is determined by the following equation:

$$\varphi = 90 - \arcsin(y_C/R) \tag{3.31}$$

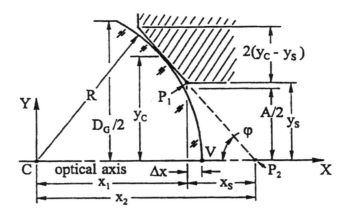

Fig. 3.26 Schematic of a tangential interface on a convex spherical surface.

We again define y_C as the midpoint between the clear aperture and the rim of the lens per Eq. (3.1). The tolerance for φ in a given design depends primarily on the desired radial width of the conical annulus, or land, on the metal part and the allowable error in axial location of the lens vertex. Typically, this tolerance is about ± 1°.

Equations (3.32) through (3.35) can be used to establish Δx, the axial distance from P_1 to V, as shown in Fig. 3.26.[16] Example 3.9 illustrates the use of these equations.

$$x_s = y_s / \tan \varphi \qquad\qquad (3.32)$$

$$x_2 = R / \sin \varphi \qquad\qquad (3.33)$$

$$x_1 = x_2 - x_s \qquad\qquad (3.34)$$

$$\Delta x = R - x_1 \qquad\qquad (3.35)$$

3.6.3 The toroidal interface

A toroidal interface can be used with either convex or concave surfaces and is particularly useful on concave lens surfaces where the tangent interface cannot be used. The reasons for this (which have to do with minimizing contact stress) will be explained further in Sect. 11.2. Figure 3.27(a) shows a toroidal (donut-shaped) mechanical surface contacting a convex spherical lens surface of radius R at height y_C .

Example 3.9: Location of mount corner with respect to a convex lens vertex with a tangential interface.
(For design and analysis, use File 5.2 of the CD-ROM)
Assume R = 20.0 in. (508.0 mm), A = 2.0 in. (50.8 mm), and D_G = 2.1 in. (53.34 mm). Locate the point P_1 with respect to the vertex.

By Eq. (3.1) and the geometry of Fig. 3.26:

y_C = (2.100 + 2.000)/4 = 1.025 in. (26.035 mm)
y_S = 1.025 - [(2.100 - 2.000) / 4] = 1.000 in. (25.4 mm).

By Eqs. (3.32) through (3.35):
φ = 90° - arc sin (1.025/20.000) = 87.062°
x_S = 20.000/tan 87.062° = 1.026 in. (26.060 mm)
x_2 = 20.000/sin 87.062° = 20.026 in. (508.668 mm)
x_1 = 20.026 - 1.026 = 19.000 in. (482.600 mm)
Δx = 20.000 - 19.000 = 1.000 in. (25.4 mm).

The center of the toroidal surface with cross-sectional radius R_T is at C_T as shown in Fig. 3.27(b). From the geometry of these figures, we can derive equations for locating P_1 with respect to V for the convex surface.[16] The X-coordinate of P1 is found by solving the analytical equation for the circle representing the toroidal section with its center displaced by h and k in the X and Y directions, respectively, from the origin at C when $y_1 = y_S$. Considering all radii as positive, then:

$$\theta = \arcsin(y_C/R) \qquad (3.36)$$

$$h = (R + R_T)\cos\theta \qquad (3.37)$$

$$k = (R + R_T)\sin\theta \qquad (3.38)$$

$$x_1 = h - [R_T^2 - (y_S - k)^2]^{1/2} \qquad (3.39)$$

$$\Delta x = R - x_1 \qquad (3.35)$$

Figure 3.28 shows a toroidal interface at a concave spherical lens surface. Note that R_T is smaller than R. Equations (3.36), (3.40) through (3.42) and (3.35) can be used to find Δx.[16] Example 3.10 shows the computations for a typical design.

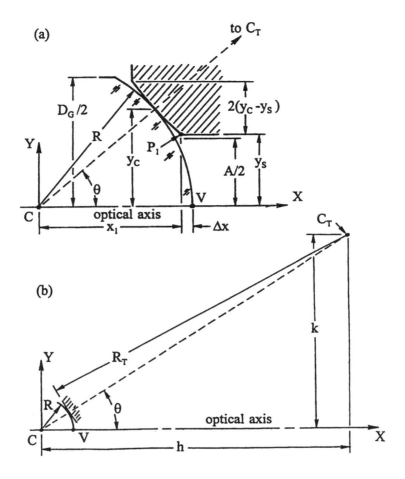

Fig. 3.27 Schematics of a toroidal interface on a convex spherical surface. (a) Detailed view, (b) expanded view.

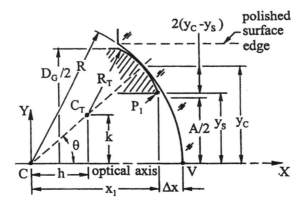

Fig. 3.28 Schematic of a toroidal interface on a concave spherical surface.

Example 3.10: Location of mount corner with respect to a convex lens surface vertex with a toroidal interface.
(For design and analysis, use File 5.3 of the CD-ROM)
Let $R = 10.0$ in. (254.0 mm), $y_C = 1.025$ in. (26.035 mm), $y_S = 1.0$ in. (25.4 mm), and $R_T = 10R = 100.0$ in. (2540.0 mm). Locate the point P_1.

By Eqs. (3.36) through (3.39) and Eq. (3.35):
θ = arc sin $(1.025/10.000) = 5.883°$
$h = (10.000 + 100.000)(\cos 5.884°) = 109.420$ in. (2779.280 mm)
$k = (10.000 + 100.000)(\sin 5.884°) = 11.277$ in. (286.436 mm)
$x_1 = 109.420 - [100.000^2 - (1.000 - 11.277)^2]^{1/2} = 9.949$ in. (252.705 mm)
$\Delta x = 10.000 - 9.949 = 0.051$ in. (1.295 mm).

$$\theta = \arcsin(y_C/R) \tag{3.36}$$

$$h = (R + R_T)\cos\theta \tag{3.40}$$

$$k - (R + R_T)\sin\theta \tag{3.41}$$

$$x_1 = h - [R_T^2 - (y_S - k)^2]^{1/2} \tag{3.42}$$

$$\Delta x = R - x_1 \tag{3.35}$$

The radial extent of the toroidal land against which the lens can touch in each case can be seen from Figs. 3.27 and 3.28 to be $2(y_C - y_S)$. In the last two numerical examples, this annular width is $2(1.025 - 1.000) = 0.050$ in. (1.270 mm). Knowledge of this dimension is useful when defining tolerances for the mechanical parts to prevent degeneration of the interface into line (sharp-corner) contact at the inner or outer edges of this land. Sharp-corner contact rather than toroidal contact would, in those cases, increase the stress for a given level of axial preload.

Either of these toroidal surfaces can be cut on a numerically controlled lathe or diamond turning machine with little difficulty. The exact cross-sectional radius produced is not particularly critical. Tolerances of - 0, +100 % are not uncommon. The reason for this will be evident from our considerations of contact stress for this type of interface in Sect. 11.2.

3.6.4   The spherical interface

Figures 3.29 and 3.30 show, respectively, spherical mounting surfaces

Example 3.11: Location of mount corner with respect to a concave lens surface vertex with a toroidal interface.
(For design and analysis, use File 5.4 of the CD-ROM)
Let R = 10.0 in. (254.0 mm), y_C = 1.025 in. (26.035 mm), y_S = 1.0 in. (25.4 mm) and R_T = 0.5R = 5.0 in. (127.0 mm). Locate the point P_1.

By Eqs. (3.36), (3.40 through (3.42), and (3.35):

θ = arc sin (1.025/10.000) = 5.883°
h = (10.000 - 5.000)(cos 5.883°) = 4.974 in. (126.331 mm)
k = (10.000 - 5.000)(sin 5.883°) = 0.512 in. (13.017 mm)
x_1 = 4.974 + [(5.000^2 - (1.000 - 0.512)^2]$^{1/2}$ = 9.950 in. (252.731 mm)
Δx = 10.000 - 9.950 = 0.050 in. (1.270 mm)

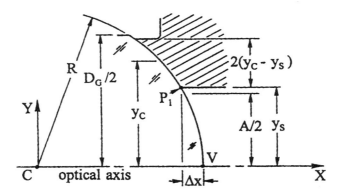

Fig. 3.29 Schematic of a spherical interface on a convex spherical surface.

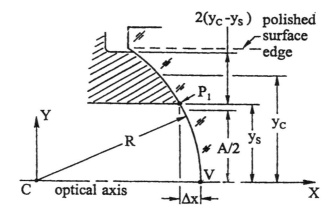

Fig. 3.30 Schematic of a spherical interface on a concave spherical surface.

contacting convex and concave spherical lens surfaces. Once again, the contact height y_C is at the midpoint of the land contacting the lens. If we substitute y_S for y_C, Eq. (3.30) can be used to find Δx in either case.

The mechanical interface surfaces must be accurately ground and lapped to match the radii of the lenses within a few wavelengths of light. Each mechanical part that is to touch a lens surface must be designed with access for lapping. The final stages of manufacture of these surfaces must be done in the optical shop using the same tools used to make the corresponding glass surface. Since the manufacture and testing of these surfaces are expensive, the spherical interface mounting technique is hardly ever used. This author can recall only one example from his personal experience. It involved spherical seats against which the spherical back surface of a meniscus-shaped mirror was pressed. That example is described in Sect. 13.16 and is illustrated in Figs. 13.27 and 13.29.

The spherical interface does have the distinct advantage that axial mechanical forces are distributed over large areas so they cause relatively low contact stresses under normal preloads, and very high acceleration loads can be survived. They also facilitate heat transfer.

3.6.5 Interfaces on bevels

It is standard optical shop practice to lightly bevel all sharp edges of lenses. The main reason for this is to minimize the danger of chipping, so this is called a "protective bevel." Larger bevels or chamfers are used to remove unneeded material when weight is critical or packaging constraints are tight, and/or to provide mounting surfaces. Usually all these secondary surfaces are ground with progressively finer abrasives. If the lenses are likely to have to endure severe stress, the bevels and the lens rims may also be given a crude polish by buffing with polishing compound on a cloth or felt-covered tool. These procedures tend to strengthen the lens material by reducing subsurface damage from the grinding operations.

Figure 3.31 shows three lenses with bevels. The planoconvex element of Fig.3.31(a) has minimum protective bevels that typically might be specified as "0.5 mm maximum face width @ 45°" or "0.4 ± 0.2-mm face symmetric to surfaces." Each surface of the biconcave lens of Fig.3.31(b) has a wider bevel oriented perpendicular to the lens' optical axis. This lens cannot be centered by applying axial preload; some external means such as that suggested by Fig. 2.5 must be applied. Tight tolerances on this perpendicularity must be specified if both centers of curvature of the lens surfaces are to be brought to the mount's mechanical axis simultaneously by translation of the lens. Tolerances for this 90° angle of ±30 arcsec or less are common for precision lenses.

Figure 3.31(c) shows a meniscus lens with a wide 45° bevel on the concave side and a step ground into the rim on the other (convex) side to form a flat bevel recessed into the lens. A conventional retainer or a spacer can be brought to bear against this bevel. Either a sharp corner or, preferably, a toroidal surface-contact interface can be used on the concave side. It should be noted that protective bevels are needed at the edges of these larger bevels. It is not good practice to apply an axial preload directly against an angled

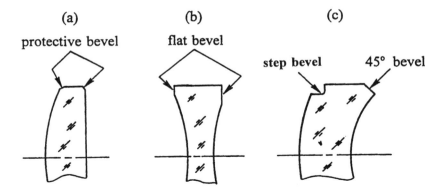

Fig. 3.31 Typical bevels applied to lens edges during manufacture. (a) Protective bevels, (b) flat bevels perpendicular to the axis, (c) 45° and stepped bevels.

bevel since that surface may not be precisely located.

A generous bevel or radius should be built into the inner leading edge of the retainer so that it does not interfere with a rounded inside corner that usually is created in a step bevel during manufacture. Figure 3.32 illustrates this design feature as well as the use of a judiciously placed undercut in the mechanical mount that facilitates cutting the internal thread in the mounting wall.

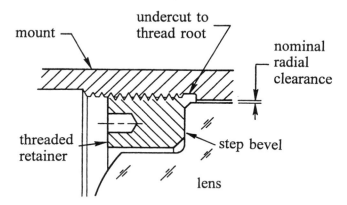

Fig. 3.32 Special provisions in some mechanical parts that interface with lenses.

3.7 Elastomeric Mountings

A relatively simple technique for mounting lenses, windows, filters, and mirrors is illustrated schematically in Fig. 3.33. This figure shows a typical design for a lens constrained by an annular ring of a resilient elastomeric material (typically epoxy, urethane, or RTV) within a cell.[1] Hopkins[14] reported that Dow Corning RTV732 is an appropriate material for this purpose, while Bayar[8] indicated that Dow Corning RTV3112 has frequently been used in aerial cameras. General Electric RTV8112 is representative of materials meeting U.S. military specification MIL-S-23586E. EC2216B/A epoxy made by 3M has been used for this purpose (see the design of Fig. 4.13) and is representative of that class of elastomer. Characteristics of the elastomers are given in Tables B15a and B15b. The epoxy is described in Table B14.

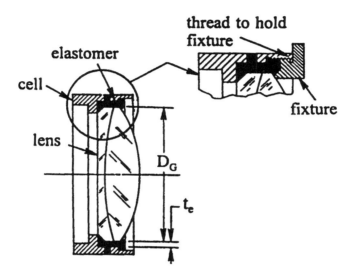

Fig. 3.33 Technique for mounting a lens with an annular ring of cured-in-place elastomer. The detail view shows one means for holding the lens and constraining the elastomer during curing.

One side of the elastomeric ring is intentionally left unconstrained so the material can deform under compression or tension caused by temperature changes. Registry of one optical surface against a machined mounting surface aligns the lens within the mount. Centration can be established prior to curing and maintained throughout the curing cycle with shims or external fixturing. The detail view of Fig. 3.33 shows one means for holding the lens in place and constraining the elastomer during curing. The fixture, which is made of Teflon or a similar plastic or metal coated with a mold release, can be removed after curing. The elastomer is typically injected with a hypodermic syringe through radially oriented access holes in the mount until the space around the lens is filled. Shims can be used to center the lens. They are removed after curing. If the annular elastomer layer has a particular thickness, t_e, the assembly will, to a first-order approximation, be athermal in the radial direction. This minimizes stress buildup within the optomechanical components that is caused by differential radial expansion or contraction of the lens, cell, and elastomer under temperature changes. This thickness is[8]

$$t_e = (D_G/2)(\alpha_M - \alpha_G)/(\alpha_e - \alpha_M) \qquad (3.43)$$

where α_G, α_M, and α_e are the CTEs of the lens, mount, and elastomer respectively and the other terms are as shown in Figure 3.33.

The axial length of the elastomer layer approximately equals the edge thickness of the lens. Because Eq. (3.43) neglects the effects of this length, Poisson's ratio, Young's modulus, and shear modulus, it should be considered an approximation. The application of Eq. (3.43) does not make the assembly athermal in the axial direction. When the temperature changes, the same nominal length of mounting wall, elastomer, and lens change at different rates that are proportional to the applicable CTEs. Some amount of shear is then introduced into the elastomer layer.

If the elastomer layer is completely encapsulated (as it would be if it is injected to completely fill a closed annular space between a lens rim, mount ID, shoulder, and a retainer), the elastomer will try to expand at elevated temperatures to a volume greater than the space available. The lens may then become radially stressed since most elastomers have a high Poisson's ratio of about 0.490 to 0.499. This problem can be minimized by keeping the amount of elastomer used in any such design as small as possible while still producing the desired seal.

Miller[17] described a finite-element analysis of three generic elastomerically mounted lens designs involving germanium lenses of the same [2.051-in. (52.095-mm)] diameter and with meniscus, biconvex, and biconcave shapes (see Fig. 3.34). The lenses were all mounted in aluminum cells with a silicone rubber. Example 3.12 determines the elastomer layer thickness with the help of Eq. (3.43).

Example 3.12: Athermal elastomer thickness for a lens per Eq. (3.43). (For design and analysis, use File 6 of the CD-ROM)

One of the 2.051-in. (52.095-mm) diameter germanium lenses of Miller's study[17] is to be mounted by an annular elastomeric ring in an aluminum cell. Apply Eq. (3.43) to determine the approximate value for the athermal thickness t_e. Assume the material properties to be:

$\alpha_G = 3.33 \times 10^{-6}$ /°F (6.0×10^{-6} /°C) $\alpha_M = 12.78 \times 10^{-6}$ /°F (23.0×10^{-6} /°C)
$\alpha_e = 138 \times 10^{-6}$ /°F (248.0×10^{-6} /°C)

From Eq. (3.43): $t_e = (2.051/2)(12.78 - 3.33)(10^{-6})/[(138 - 12.78)(10^{-6})]$
                        $= 0.078$ in. (1.981 mm).

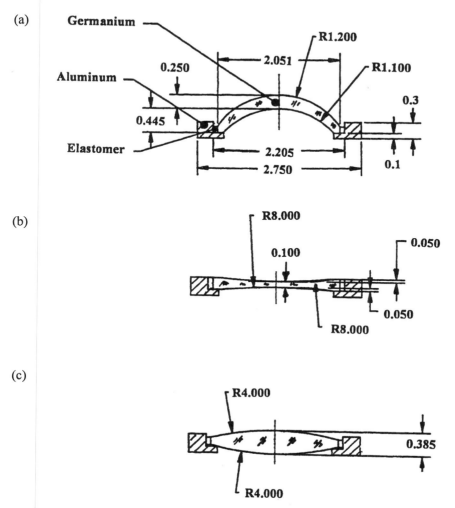

Fig. 3.34 Schematics of lens configurations studied by Miller.[17] (a) Meniscus, (b) biconcave, and (c) biconvex shapes.

In his study, Miller varied t_e from the nominal "athermal" value of 0.077 in. (1.956 mm) just calculated to 0.065 times that value [0.005 in. (0.127 mm)] and determined by FEA the stresses within the lenses and within the cells, as well as the resonant frequencies and first vibrational modes of the assemblies. Figure 3.35 shows the stress distributions at elevated temperature (50° C) for each lens type at two values of t_e. The maximum stress levels (darkest ends of gray scales) are indicated for each case. The contours of the lenses and the elastomer layers have been emphasized here to make those shapes more visible. Fidelity of reproduction is poor in the figures, but definite changes in stress patterns are visible. The highest stresses are found, as might be expected, with the thinner layers. Note that the elastomer bulges outward at high temperature for the "athermal" thickness, but is obviously in tension, as shown by its concave boundaries, at the 0.010-in. (0.254-mm) thickness. It can be seen that the elastomer does not completely fill the available space between the lens and the cell wall at this elevated temperature.

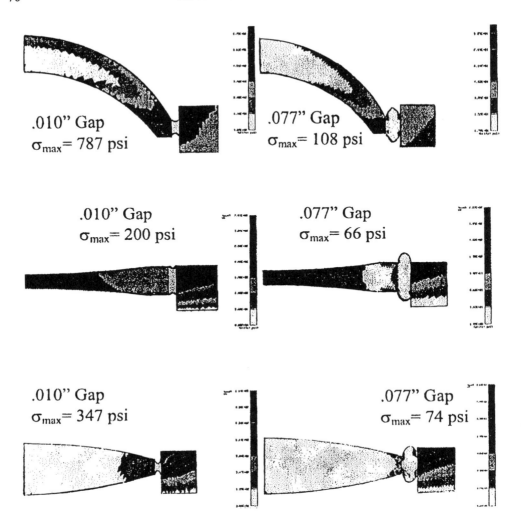

.010" Gap
σ_{max}= 787 psi

.077" Gap
σ_{max}= 108 psi

.010" Gap
σ_{max}= 200 psi

.077" Gap
σ_{max}= 66 psi

.010" Gap
σ_{max}= 347 psi

.077" Gap
σ_{max}= 74 psi

Fig. 3.35 Stress magnitudes and distributions for the lenses of Fig. 3.34 at 50°C for elastomer layers with 0.077-in. (1.956-mm) (approximately "athermal") and 0.010-in. (0.254-mm) radial thicknesses. (Adapted from Miller.[17])

Figure 3.36 shows the variations of maximum stresses with t_e for all three lens types. The most interesting general conclusions to be drawn from this figure are that reducing the thickness by as much as a factor of 2 has little effect on stress; Eq. (3.43) does not give the lowest stress; and the stress is dependent upon lens shape. Although it is not specifically discussed by Miller, increasing t_e from the "athermal" value would tend to decrease thermally induced stress and increase the flexibility of the joint. From a stress viewpoint, the tolerance for the thickness of the elastomer layer can obviously be quite large.

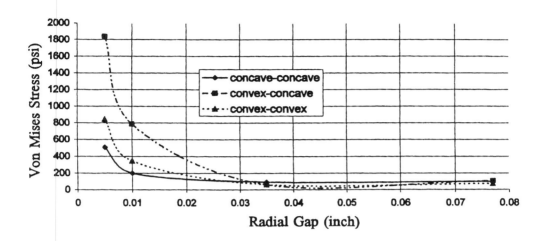

Fig. 3.36 Variations of the maximum stress with thickness of the elastomer layer in the lenses of Fig. 3.34 at 50°C. (From Miller.[17])

Figure 3.37 shows the variation in the lowest resonant frequency of the lens/cell assemblies as functions of lens shape and elastomer thickness. Again, we see small changes for rather large decreases in layer thickness and dependence on lens shape. The expected increase in frequency for thinner (i.e., stiffer) layers is apparent. The biconvex and biconcave lenses have essentially the same resonant characteristics, while the meniscus-shaped lens shows a greater variation.

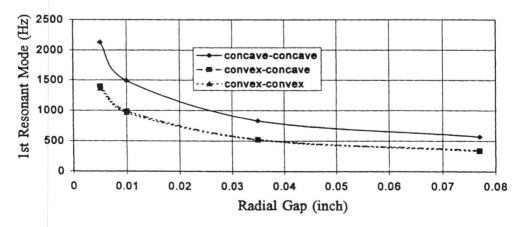

Fig. 3.37 Variations of the resonant frequency with thickness of the elastomer layer in the lens assemblies of Fig. 3.34 at 50°C. (From Miller.[17])

Vukobratovich[18] quoted a more accurate equation for t_e, derived by Muench,[19] that takes the Poisson's ratio of the elastomer into consideration. This is Eq. (3.44), which is applied in Example 3.13.

$$t_e = \frac{(D_G/2)(1 - \nu_G)(\alpha_M - \alpha_G)}{(\alpha_e - \alpha_M + (\nu_e)(\alpha_G - \alpha_e)}$$ (3.44)

Example 3.13: Athermal elastomer thickness for a lens per Eq. (3.44). (For design and analysis, use File 7 of the CD-ROM)
Recompute Example 3.12 using Eq. (3.44). All listed design and material parameters remain the same. Assume $\nu_e = 0.49$.

From Eq. (3.44):
$$t_e = \frac{(2.051/2)(1 - 0.49)(12.78 - 3.33)(10^{-6})}{(138 - 12.78 + (0.49)(3.33 - 138))(10^{-6})} = 0.083 \text{ in. } (2.119 \text{ mm})$$

This thickness is about 10% larger than that obtained with Eq. (3.43) and significantly different from Miller's value of about 0.045 in. (1.143 mm) for minimum stress in the same lens as determined by FEA and shown graphically in Fig. 3.37.

Hatheway[20] indicated that thin elastomer layers used for bonding or encapulating optics are considerably stiffer than thick ones. He derived the relationship indicated graphically in Fig. 3.38 in which a material's "apparent modulus" increases dramatically from Young's modulus for thick sections to its bulk modulus for thin sections. This is compatible with the resonant frequency increase for thin elastomer joints as shown in Fig. 3.37.

Valente and Richard[21] have reported an analytical technique for estimating the decentration, δ, of a lens mounted in a ring of elastomer when subjected to radial gravitational loading. Their equation was extended very slightly here to include more general radial acceleration forces by adding an acceleration factor a_G as follows:

$$\delta = \frac{2 a_G W t_e}{\pi D_G t_E \{[E_e/(1 - \nu_e^2)] + S_e\}}$$ (3.45)

where:

W = lens weight	t_e = elastomer layer thickness
D_G = lens diameter	t_E = lens edge thickness
ν_e = elastomer Poisson's ratio	E_e = elastomer Young's modulus

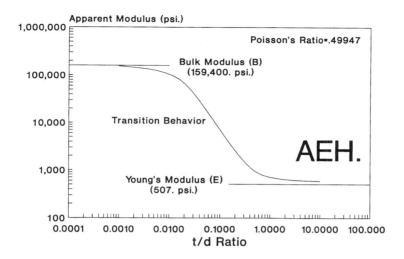

Fig. 3.38 The apparent stiffening of an elastomer layer in thin layers. (From Hatheway.[20])

S_e = elastomer shear modulus as determined from Eq. (3.46)

$$S_e = E_e / [(2)(1 + \nu_e)] \tag{3.46}$$

The decentrations of modest-sized optics corresponding to normal gravity loading are generally quite small, but may grow significantly under shock and vibration loading (see Example 3.14). A resilient material is naturally elastic and so will tend to restore the lens to its unstressed location and orientation when the acceleration force dissipates. A lens assembly mounted in this manner is described in Sect. 13.12.

Example 3.14: Decentration of a lens in a radially athermal elastomeric mounting. (For design and analysis, use File 8 of the CD-ROM)

Consider a BK7 lens with diameter $D_G = 10.0$ in. (254.0 mm), thickness $t_E = 1.0$ in. (25.4 mm), and weight $W = 7.147$ lb (3.242 kg) mounted in a DC3112 elastomeric ring inside a titanium cell. Assume the following properties for the materials:

$\alpha_G = 3.94 \times 10^{-6} /°F$ $(7.1 \times 10^{-6} /°C)$ $\qquad$ $\alpha_M = 4.90 \times 10^{-6} /°F$ $(8.8 \times 10^{-6} /°C)$
$\alpha_e = 167 \times 10^{-6} /°F$ $(300.6 \times 10^{-6} /°C)$
$E_e = 500$ lb/in.^{2} (3.447 MPa) $\qquad$ $\upsilon_e = 0.499$

From Eq. (3.46), $S_e = 500/[(2)(1 + 0.499)] = 167$ lb/in.^{2} (1.150 MPa)

(a) What should be the elastomer thickness t_e using Eq. (3.44)?

From Eq. (3.44):

$$t_e = (10.0/2)(\frac{(1 - 0.499)(4.90 - 3.94)(10^{-6})}{[167 - 4.90 + (0.499)(3.94 - 167)](10^{-6})}) = 0.030 \text{ in. } (0.762 \text{ mm})$$

(b) How much should the lens decenter under radial accelerations of 1 and 250 times gravity?

From Eq. (3.45), for $a_G = 1$ and 250:

$$\delta_1 = \frac{(2)(1.0)(7.147)(0.030)}{(\pi)(10.0)(1.0)[(500/(1 - 0.499^2)) + 167]} = 1.6 \times 10^{-5} \text{ in. } (4.1 \times 10^{-4} \text{ mm})$$

$$\delta_{250} = (250)(1.6 \times 10^{-5}) = 0.004 \text{ in. } (0.102 \text{ mm})$$

The self-weight deflection seems negligible, but the high acceleration deflection probably would be significant if full performance is expected under that acceleration.

Elastomeric constraint is a good technique for mounting nonsymmetrical optics such as lenses and windows with rectangular apertures since threaded retainers and continuous-ring clamps do not adapt well to noncircularly symmetrical applications. Elastomeric constraint also may be appropriate for optical components lacking rotational symmetry of their optical surfaces. See, for example, the planoconcave lens shown in Fig. 3.39. One edge of the lens involving a portion of the aperture that is not needed to transmit useful rays to the image has been cut away. Removal of this unneeded material reduces weight and provides clearance needed for other system components. The plano surface should be in contact with a registration shoulder of the mounting plate and centered mechanically. Elastomer is then inserted into the annular gap between the lens rim and the mount ID and cured.

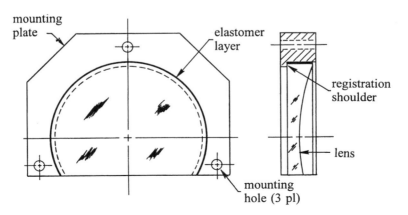

Fig. 3.39 A typical technique for mounting a lens with noncircular aperture by potting it into a mount with an elastomeric layer.

Equations (3.43) or (3.44) can be used to estimate the elastomer layer thicknesses required in this design to make the configuration athermal in the height or width direction. The appropriate overall linear dimension of the lens (height or width) is substituted for D_G. As pointed out earlier, this thickness need not be tightly tolerard.

The surfaces of a lens mounted in this manner can be curved or aspherical (including wild "potato-chip" types) if specific points on those surfaces can be identified as registration points for alignment purposes and convex mechanical pads (such as segments of spherical surfaces) are provided to contact those points. Without such registration features, the lens must be aligned optically and held by shims or other means until the elastomer has cured.

3.8 Advantages of a Spherical Lens Rim

Figure 3.40 illustrates a design feature that minimizes potential problems in installing lenses in cell inside diameters when radial clearances are small.[22] Here the lens rim is ground spherically with the radius approximately equal to one-half the lens diameter. The rim is then a short centralized section of the surface of a ball that fits easily into the cell at any angular orientation. With this technique, a lens can be inserted into an opening that is only a few micrometers larger than the lens diameter without jamming in place from unavoidable tipping before it is properly seated. Close radial fits such as these might be appropriate for applications in which the lens will experience high acceleration loading. The lens shown in Fig. 3.40 has a precision flat bevel on its concave side to interface with the cell shoulder. A tangential interface is provided on the retainer contacting the polished convex surface.

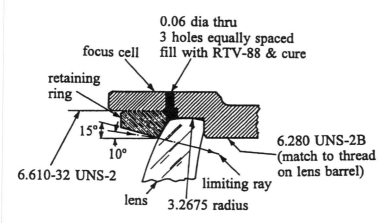

Fig. 3.40 A spherical-rim lens in a cell. Dimensions are inches. (Adapted from Yoder.[22])

Although this spherical rim requires some special optical fabrication steps, it increases tooling and labor costs only slightly since the surface contour does not need to be precise and tolerances on all but the lens OD are loose. The spherical rim has been found to be worthwhile in preventing damage such as chipping of lens edges at the assembly stage when the lenses have maximum value and replacement could be expensive and affect production schedule. This is especially true if the lens is part of a matched set, i.e., lenses made to a design optimized for specific glass-melt parameters, for as-manufactured thicknesses of other components in the system, or if the cell ID has been customized for the particular lens being installed. See Sect. 4.3 for a discussion of the latter procedure.

Another feature of the design shown in Fig. 3.40 is provision for injecting elastomer (RTV88) through several (here three) holes equally spaced around the lens rim to seal the lens to the cell and to add extra insurance that the lens will not shift under extreme shock or vibration. The sealant also helps prevent the retainer from turning.

If the radius of the curved rim is larger than one-half the lens diameter, that feature is sometimes called a "crowned" rim. It still facilitates inserting the lens with a small radial clearance, but the range of tilt accepted without binding is reduced. Spacers and lens cells for high-precision lens assemblies frequently are made with crowned rims.

The design shown in Fig. 3.10 also has a spherical rim interface.[5] The cell ID adjacent to the rim of the center element has a convex toroidal shape instead of the usual cylindrical shape. The lens rim is cylindrical, but it can be inserted into the cell while it is tipped significantly. It straightens out on contact with the shoulder and is held by the preload exerted by the snap ring. If the cell is machined of metal or molded of plastic, provision of curved surfaces such as the toroidal ID requires only minor additional machining operations or that the outer surface of the inside mold for the plastic case have the appropriate machined contour. With molded mountings it also is not difficult to provide tangential, toroidal, or even spherical mechanical surfaces to interface with lens surfaces. Features such as these can also be machined into metal mountings at some increased cost.

3.9 Flexure Mountings

In order to achieve optimum image quality, very high performance lenses must be assembled to extremely tight axial (despace), tilt, and decentration tolerances relative to other lenses in an optical assembly or to some other component within the assembly, such as one or more mechanical reference(s). Alignment must then be fully retained under operational levels of shock, vibration, pressure, and temperature variations. Furthermore, misalignments occurring during exposure to survival levels of these environments must be reversible. Mounting techniques that involve mechanical clamping of a lens component or elastomeric encapsulation do not always prevent the relative motion of a lens with respect to the mount to the degree that is required under all these adverse conditions. It may then be advantageous to attach the lens to symmetrically disposed flexures so that differential expansion of materials caused by temperature changes does not affect tilt or centration. Although they may be similar in appearance, a flexure is not the same as a spring. A flexure is an elastic element that provides controlled relative motion of components, while a spring provides controlled force through elastic deformation. In the present context, the lens is supported on flexures in the manner depicted schematically in Fig. 3.41.

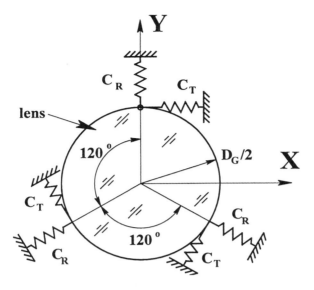

Fig. 3.41 Schematic for a "three-point" flexure support for a lens. (Adapted from Vukobratovich.[23])

The compliances of the three radially oriented flexures keep the lens centered in spite of differential expansion that is due to temperature changes and allow the lens to decenter during extreme (survival-level) shock and vibration exposure yet return to the correct location and orientation after those dynamic disturbances have subsided. They also minimize stress within the optic during such exposures. The symbols C_R and C_T in Fig. 3.41 represent the spring constants (stiffnesses) of the radial and tangential flexures. Typically, the flexures are stiff tangentially and soft radially. They also are stiff axially (perpendicular to the plane of the figure). Vukobratovich[23] gives the following relationship for the X and Y spring constants:

$$C_X = C_Y = (3/2)(C_R + C_T) \tag{3.47}$$

We next describe several configurations of flexure mounts designed to maintain radial alignment of the individual lens.

Figure 3.42 schematically illustrates a design by Ahmad and Huse[24] in which the rim of the lens is bonded with an adhesive such as epoxy to the ends of three thin blades that are parts of flexure modules. Those blades are compliant radially, but stiff in all other directions. When the dimensions of the mount (here shown as a simple cell) and lens change with temperature, any mismatch in CTEs causes the flexures to bend. Since this action is symmetrical with respect to the axis, the lens stays centered.

The detail in Fig. 3.42(a) shows flexure modules manufactured separately and attached to the mount with screws so the bonded subassembly comprising the lens and the three flexures can be removed and replaced without damage. Since they are separate, the

78

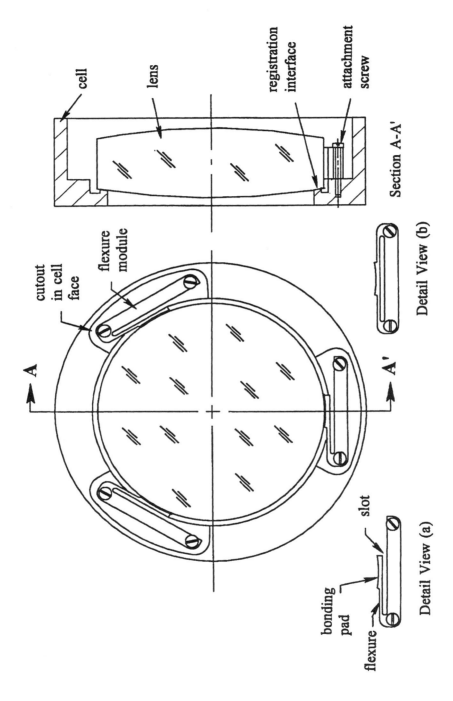

cell

lens

registration
interface

attachment
screw

Section A-A'

cutout
in cell
face

flexure
module

A

A'

bonding
pad

flexure

slot

Detail View (a)

Detail View (b)

Fig. 3.42 A mounting concept in which the rim of a lens is bonded to three removable flexure modules. (Adapted from Ahmad and Huse.[24])

three flexures can be removed and replaced without damage. Since they are separate, the flexure modules can be made from a material appropriate for the application, such as titanium or beryllium copper, while the mount can be made of a different material, such as stainless steel. The metal surface adjacent to the lens rim can be shaped as a concave cylinder to approximate the curvature of that rim, or localized flats can be ground onto the rim to match the flexure shape. In either case, the thickness of the adhesive layer will then be uniform over the joint. This is desirable for maximum strength of the bond.

Not shown in Fig. 3.42, but mentioned in the original authors' description, are dabs of epoxy applied around the edges of the flexure modules after they are are screwed in place to secure the modules to the cell in the plane of the figure. In other versions of this concept, mechanical pins are used to lock the modules in place.

The detail (b) in Fig. 3.42 shows a different configuration for the flexure module in which the flexible portion is attached at both ends and the lens is bonded to a pad in the middle of the blade. The function of this design is basically the same as the single-ended design discussed earlier.

Another configuration for a flexure mounting, described by Bacich,[25] is shown in Fig. 3.43. Here the flexure blades are formed integrally with the cell, so they cannot be removed. The cell material must be chosen in part so the integral flexures function reliably throughout the many temperature cycles inherent in the desired long useful life of the instrument. As in the design shown in Fig. 3.42, these flexures must be accurately machined with a specific and uniform thickness. Precisely curved slots are easily created by the electric discharge machining (EDM) process. In this process a wire of an appropriate diameter is passed through a hole and then raised to an electric potential significantly higher than the cell so an arc is formed that eats away at the metal while the wire is moved in the desired path; this motion usually is under computer control.

Two versions of the basic mount design are depicted in Fig. 3.43. In Fig. 3.43(a) and 3.43(b), the rim of the lens is bonded to the flexures in the same general manner as in the design of Fig. 3.42. Figures 3.43(c) and 3.43(d) show the bottom surface of the lens bonded to shelves built into the flexure blades.

Yet another flexure mounting is shown in Fig. 3.44. This design also uses integral flexure blades. They are formed in a box-shaped cell by locally machining the corners from the top and bottom rims of the box in the region where the flexure is to be located. The blades are then attached at both ends in the general configuration of the design shown in the detail (b) of Fig. 3.42. As in the flexure mountings of Ahmad and Huse and Bacich described earlier, their function is to allow dimensional changes between lens and cell when the temperature changes without disturbing the centration of the lens.

The description by Steel et al.[26] of this mounting configuration includes a discussion of the manner in which the angular subtense ϕ of the bonded region was determined. Using finite-element analysis, 30° and 45° angles were compared. The larger angle was selected because it resulted in a smaller degree of distortion of the lens surfaces at the extreme operational temperature, had a higher natural frequency, and produced less stress in the cell and adhesive (RTV) joint. These attributes of the design were all within the tolerances allowed for the application.

80

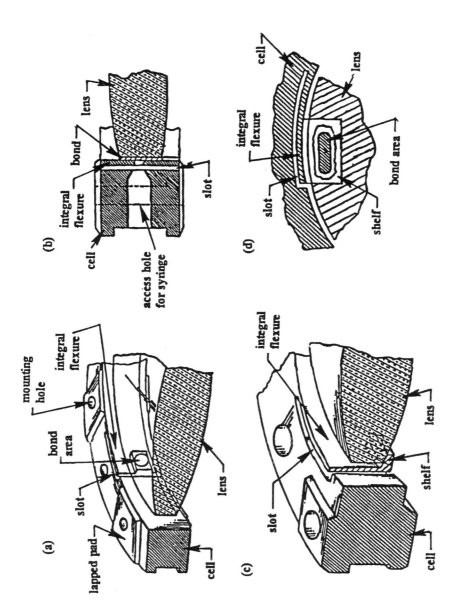

Fig. 3.43 Flexure mountings with the lens bonded to integral flexures. In (a) and (b) the bonds are on the lens rim while, in (c) and (d), the bonds are on local areas in the lens' face. (Adapted from Bacich.[25])

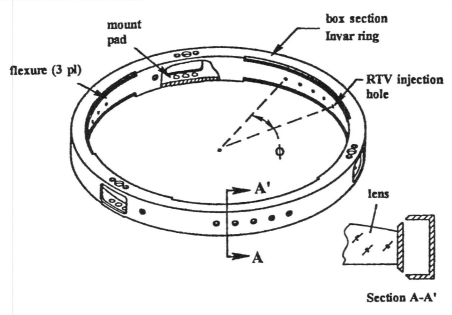

Fig. 3.44 A flexure-type lens mounting in which the lens is bonded to three flexure blades machined into a box-section cell. (Adapted from Steel et al.[26])

3.10 Aligning the Lens in Its Mount

In all the flexure mounts just discussed, it is assumed that the lens has been properly centered before it is bonded to the flexure blades. The same may be assumed to apply to many of the previously described mounting configurations that do not have flexures. The way this is accomplished is very important. Since high-precision mounting techniques are used only when performance expectations are very demanding, considerable care must be exercised in the centering process, and the instrumentation required is generally complex. One cannot rely on radial components of an axial force to center the surface-contacted lens perfectly because friction is hard to overcome when the differences between the opposing radial forces become small. Smith indicated the lower limit on residual centration error to be 0.0005 in. (12.5 μm).[2] In some of the most accurate centering techniques, the lens is held in a fixture of some sort and adjusted to the proper orientation and location relative to some external reference such as a mechanical surface, to a prealigned light beam, or to an interferometer cavity. Once the associated metrology instrumentation verifies that the lens is adequately aligned, it is clamped mechanically, potted into the mount with elastomer, or bonded to flexures to preserve that alignment. The fixture can then be removed.

We will consider here four basic techniques for precision centering of individual lenses. In these, the lens is (1) mounted directly onto an interface provided in an instrument and adjusted so as to be centered and squared on to the optic axis of some other lens(es) or some other critically controlled feature(s); (2) the lens is mounted in its own cell and then the cell is mounted and aligned in the instrument; (3) the lens is aligned and squared on to mechanical surfaces of its own cell, which has precisely controlled premachined interfaces to the instrument references; or (4) the lens is mounted in its own cell and then the appropriate mechanical surfaces of the cell are precisely machined to interface directly with reference surfaces in the instrument and thus to correctly position the optic axis of the lens.

To illustrate the first alignment technique, Fig. 3.45(a) schematically shows a lens barrel into which the meniscus lens (also shown) is to be mounted with the concave spherical surface touching a toroidal interface inside the barrel. The barrel is positioned on a precision spindle (such as one with an air bearing), with its axis of rotation vertical so the premachined toroidal surface runs true as the spindle is slowly rotated. A high-quality mechanical or electronic indicator can be used as the testing means for this adjustment. Alternatively, the barrel OD can be positioned relative to the spindle axis and then a finish cut made on the toroidal surface to true it to the rotation axis. The single-point diamond turning method produces the most accurate surfaces.

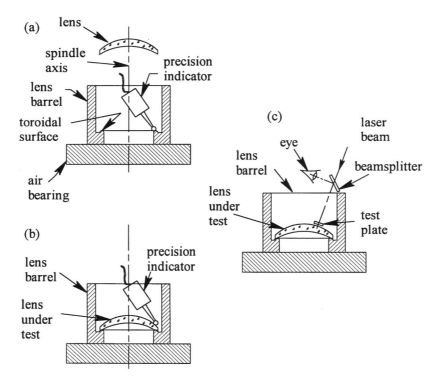

Fig. 3.45 Schematics of a technique for centering a lens to an interface within a lens barrel or cell as in alignment technique 1 in the text.

The lens is inserted as indicated in Fig. 3.45(b). Note that the lower surface is now automatically aligned to the spindle axis. The lens is moved laterally until the indicator shows that the top spherical surface runs true as the spindle rotates. The lens is then secured to the mount in one of several ways. These include mechanical clamping as previously described or bonding with adhesive. If the latter technique is to be employed, success has been achieved by securing the lens with a few localized dabs of UV-curing epoxy and following curing of that adhesive, a more permanent bond is achieved with room temperature-curing epoxy. This two-step bonding technique allows the lens and barrel to be removed from the spindle before the second application of epoxy has cured, thus freeing the spindle for another use.

The mechanism used to move the lens laterally during alignment may be as shown in Fig. 2.5 or as shown conceptually in Fig. 3.46. In both cases, radially directed push screws provide the desired motion. Ball-tipped setscrews are frequently used to ensure a smooth interface with the moveable component. Four screws arranged orthogonally minimize crosstalk between movements. Greater precision can be achieved if ball-tipped micrometers are substituted for the screws. Springs may be used in lieu of two of the screws or micrometers to provide restoring forces in opposition to the two remaining orthogonal adjustments. Commercial spring-loaded ball-plunger setscrews are often used as the restoring devices. After radial alignment is completed, the lens is secured in position and the screws can be removed.

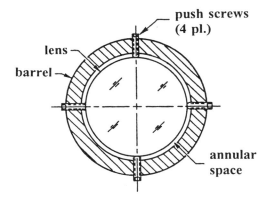

Fig. 3.46 Radially oriented setscrews used to center a lens to a spindle axis.

A more accurate means for sensing optical surface runout on a precision spindle is shown in Fig. 3.45(c). Here a planoconcave "test plate" with nearly the same radius of curvature as the surface to be tested is mounted near the latter's surface.[27] The two surfaces must be nearly parallel. The uncoated (or partially reflecting) concave surface then forms a Fizeau interferometer, with the convex top surface of the lens being aligned. Fringes created by interference of a HeNe laser light beam passing through the test plate are viewed through a beamsplitter plate (or cube) as shown. As the spindle is rotated, the fringes will move as long as the surface of the rotating lens wobbles. When the lens is properly centered, the fringes will appear stationary. If another test plate of appropriate curvature is used, fringes formed between that surface and the lower surface of the lens being aligned can be observed through the top surface of that lens to verify the centration of the lower surface. Variations of this test method have been described by Hopkins[14] and by Yoder.[1]

In another means for judging proper lens alignment, a target is imaged through the lens and the motion of that image is observed under magnification as the spindle is rotated. Yet another technique passes an appropriately converged or diverged interferometer beam through the lens under test. That lens does not rotate. The quality of the transmitted wave front is evaluated to detect alignment errors. A null lens may be needed in this test setup in order to compensate for the inherent aberrations of the test lens. Note that a hollow shaft type of air-bearing table is needed if the beam is to pass through that component.

Figure 3.47 shows a setup that might be employed in aligning a lens and then bonding it to three flexure blades in a lens barrel. The barrel design shown here is of the type shown in Fig. 3.42, but may be as shown in Figs. 3.43 or 3.44 or some other configuration involving tangentially oriented flexures. The alignment fixture with a linear stage attached is secured to the table. The orientation of this fixture must be such that the stage motion is parallel to the spindle's axis. The lens barrel is aligned mechanically so its centerline is aligned to the spindle's axis and is then secured to the spindle table. The lens is placed on the vacuum chuck, the chuck is activated, and the chuck/lens subassembly is attached to the fixture with two springs. Two orthogonal adjustment mechanisms are needed. Only one is shown in the figure. Initially, the lens will not be aligned to the flexures or to the tangent interface in the barrel. Using a centration monitor such as the Fizeau interferometer shown in the figure, the lens is moved with the adjustment screws until it runs true as the spindle is rotated back and forth through its free range of motion, which is limited by the presence of the alignment mechanisms. When this adjustment is completed, the lens is lowered onto the barrel interface with the stage. The centration is then checked and refined as necessary.

At this point, the lens rim should be located symmetrically with respect to the flexure blades and a short distance away from the bonding pads. If the spacing is not

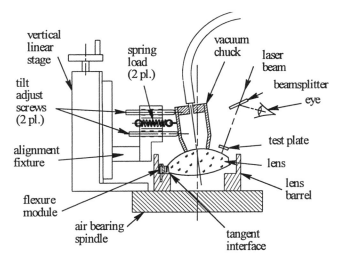

Fig. 3.47 Schematic of an alignment setup for bonding a lens to flexures in a barrel as in alignment technique 1 in the text.

flexure blades and a short distance away from the bonding pads. If the spacing is not quite right to provide the proper adhesive layer thickness, the flexure modules can be released and moved so this spacing becomes acceptable. The adhesive is injected into these spaces through holes in the flexure blades (not shown) and allowed to cure. After the alignment is checked once more, the vacuum can be released and the fixture removed. The barrel and the attached lens can then be removed from the table.

Note that if the flexure blades are not provided as separable (and therefore adjustable) modules, the alignment of the barrel to the spindle axis becomes more difficult. Proper clearances between the bonding pads and the lens rim can be provided only by holding manufacturing tolerances closely on the mount's ID and the lens' OD.

To illustrate the second centering technique given here, the lens is first mounted conventionally in an individual cell and then that subassembly is inserted into the lens barrel, which is in turn attached to an air-bearing spindle as shown in Fig. 3.48. Three pins arranged at 120° intervals around the barrel and oriented parallel to the barrel axis protrude through three holes provided in the cell. One pin and one hole are shown. The ID of each hole is slightly larger than the OD of the corresponding pin. The lens/cell subassembly is adjusted laterally and tilted within the clearances between the pins and their holes until both lens surfaces run true to the spindle's axis [see Fig.3.48(b)]. The axial location of the lens also can be adjusted at this time using the linear slide.

Centration testing is best done optically in this case since the lower surface of the lens is not accessible for contact with an indicator. When alignment is satisfactory, the spaces around the pins are filled with epoxy and the epoxy is cured. The pinning process described here is sometimes called "liquid pinning" or "plastic dowelling." It achieves the same result as mechanical pinning in which holes are drilled and reamed and pins pressed in place, but it does not involve the hazards of those operations.

It is not essential that the lens/cell subassembly be held on a vacuum chuck as shown in Fig. 3.48. A mechanical tool attached directly to the cell and configured to interface with the adjusting screws and springs would serve the same purpose. Another possible modification of this concept uses three threaded rods (studs) instead of smooth pins and threads on the inside surfaces of the three holes into which these rods protrude. The cured epoxy would then lock into the opposing threads and provide greater strength in resisting axial movement of the adjusted subassembly.

In the third lens alignment technique described here, a cell is premachined to close tolerances on its OD, circularity of that OD, and perpendicularity of both the top and bottom cell faces to the mechanical axis of the OD. A suitable interface for the lens also is machined into the cell in the same machine setup as used to finish the OD. Single-point diamond turning is best for these machining operations because of its inherent precision. The setup of Fig. 3.49 can be used to align the lens to the cell.

Figure 3.49(a) shows the premachined cell with its OD centered to the rotation axis of the spindle using a precision indicator and secured to the spindle table. The convex surface of the meniscus lens is to be interfaced with the mechanical surface of the cell. The latter surface is shown as toroidal, but it could be conical in this example. The lens is to be secured with a threaded retainer [shown in (b)] or other suitable means. The lens

(a)

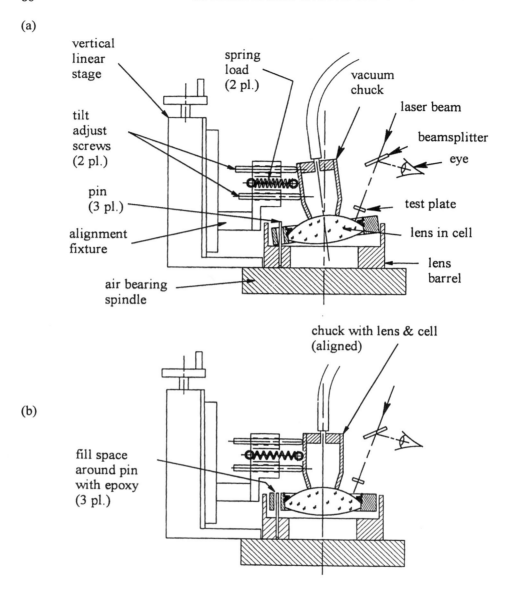

Fig. 3.48 Schematic of an alignment setup for centering a lens/cell subassembly to a lens barrel as in alignment technique 2 in the text.

lens is moved on the interface with adjustment screws (not shown) until the top surface runs true as the table is rotated. The retainer is then carefully clamped down and the alignment checked again. Note that an optical test for centration such as the type shown in Figs. 3.47 and 3.48 could be used to advantage here.

       Once the lens is properly clamped, the lens/cell subassembly can be removed from the spindle table and inserted into the lens barrel. This barrel has a carefully

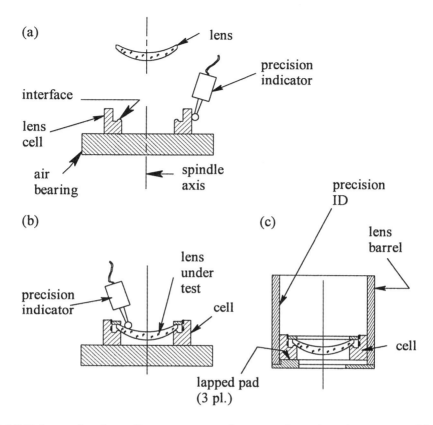

(a)

lens

precision
indicator

interface

lens
cell

air
bearing

spindle
axis

(b)

precision
indicator

lens
under
test

cell

(c)

precision
ID

lens
barrel

cell

lapped pad
(3 pl.)

Fig. 3.49 Schematic of an alignment setup for centering a lens in a premachined cell and then installing it in a barrel with a precision ID as in alignment technique 3 in the text.

machined, truly cylindrical ID that is very slightly larger than the OD of the lens cell. This ensures that the lens will be aligned to the axis of that barrel. As might be concluded from the configuration shown for the barrel, this technique lends itself to stacking several such lens/cell subassemblies in the same barrel. This configuration is discussed in more detail in the next chapter.

The fourth alignment technique is illustrated by Fig. 3.50. Here the lens cell [Fig. 3.50(a)] is premachined so its top and bottom faces are parallel, flat, and separated by a specific thickness "y." A surface with shape appropriate to interface with the lens also is machined into the cell so as to be parallel to the cell faces and at dimension "x" from surface -A-. The cell is placed on a precision plane-parallel spacer attached to an air-bearing table. The lens is inserted against the interface provided in the cell, [see Fig.3.50(b)]. The lens is adjusted laterally until it is aligned to the rotation axis and secured in place. The rim of the cell is then machined in situ to have the proper OD and to make that OD cylindrical and perpendicular to surface -A-. The lens/cell subassembly can then be removed and inserted into a barrel that has a cylindrical bore with ID only slightly larger than the cell OD.

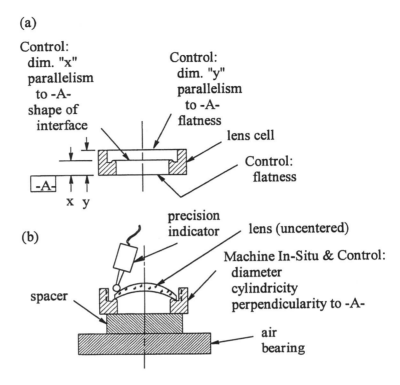

Fig. 3.50 Schematic of an alignment setup for centering a lens in a partially premachined cell, installing and aligning the lens, and completing the cell machining as in alignment technique 4 in the text.

3.11 Mounting Plastic Components

Injection and compression molding at high temperature and high pressure are the most common techniques for manufacturing lenses from plastics. Polymethylmethacrylate, polystyrene, polycarbonate, styrene acrylonitrile, polyetherimide, polycyclohexylmeth-acrylate, or one of the newer materials such as cyclic olefin copolymer are the most commonly used materials. Windows and filters also can be fabricated from plastic. Plastic prisms and mirrors are used only in low-performance applications. Diamond turning techniques are frequently used for short production runs and prototype quantities of plastic optics. The resulting products may be configured in the same manner as conventionally manufactured glass optics with cylindrical rims, bevels, and convex or concave surfaces, or they can have all these plus Fresnel or diffractive surfaces, aspheres, or integral mounting features such as flanges, tabs, holes, locating pegs, brackets, or spacers. Plastic lenses can also be configured to nest together, eliminating separate spacers and facilitating centration. These features greatly simplify assembly and reduce the number and complexity of mechanical interfacing parts (see the example in Sect. 4.6).

Plastic optics can be assembled by clamping, adhesive or solvent bonding, heat staking, or welding with ultrahigh-frequency sound. All these assembly means are applied well outside the optical apertures. Plastics are not very well suited for making cemented doublets, since optical cements may soften the plastic and destroy the surfaces. The materials used to make the lenses have large CTEs, so temperature changes may cause excessive internal or surface stress as a result of differential expansion or contraction. Plastic materials tend to absorb moisture from the atmosphere; dimensions and refractive index then change with time.

Figure 3.51 shows section views through several molded plastic lenses that according to Altman and Lytle[28] demonstrate favorable and unfavorable characteristics. The lens in Fig. 3.51(a) is a conventional glass meniscus lens while Fig. 3.51(b) shows the equivalent plastic lens. The latter has slightly shorter radii because of the lower refractive index of the plastic relative to that of the glass and is thicker to facilitate the flow of the raw material into the mold before heating and compression. The thin lens of Fig. 3.51(d) has a poor design for plastic molding since the material will not flow easily into the central region. That shown in Fig. 3.51(c) would be better in this regard. Figures 3.51(e) and 3.51(f) show a lens molded with a protruding rim that forms a recess into which a companion lens can fit to make a nested air-spaced doublet. Centration and spacing are ensured by close dimensioning of the molds to compensate for any shrinkage during curing. Figures 3.51(g) and 3.51(h) show a cemented doublet (lens materials and cement not specified) and a well-proportioned meniscus lens.

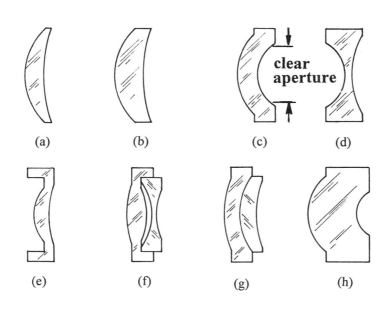

(a)   (b)   (c)   (d)

(e)   (f)   (g)   (h)

Fig. 3.51 Sectional views of typical plastic lenses. (a) Glass lens for reference, (b) equivalent plastic lens, (c) strongly curved lens with integral flat beveled rim, (d) lens with inadequate axial thickness, (e) positive lens with recess for companion lens to make doublet as shown in (f), (g) cemented doublet, (h) thick lens with high curvatures. (From Altman and Lytle.[28])

Nonspherical surfaces can be molded on plastic optics nearly as easily as spherical ones. The trick is in making the molds to the negative contour of the desired surface. Plummer[29] has described the high-order nonrotational polynomial aspherics built into the refracting corrector plate, concave mirror, and eye lens of the viewfinder for the unique single-lens reflex Polaroid SX-70 camera. Each element was made by injection molding. The molds were made by hand correcting steel surfaces shaped initially by single-point diamond turning. A customized measuring machine capable of at least 0.1-μm precision while sliding a 0.8-mm diameter sapphire ball lightly over the surface to be measured provided error maps that defined where correction was required and and how large the correction should be. This same technique can be applied to make molds for nearly any aspheric surface to be used in other applications.

Plastic lenses with or without rotational symmetry and other types of optical components are produced by numerous manufacturers. Figure 3.52 shows selections of components made by one vendor. Mounting features are clearly visible in some items.

References

1. Yoder, P.R., Jr., *Opto-Mechanical Systems Design*, 2nd ed., Marcel Dekker, New York, 1993.
2. Smith, W.J., "Optics in Practice," Chapt. 15 in *Modern Optical Engineering*, 3rd ed., McGraw-Hill, New York, 2000.
3. Horne, D.F., *Optical Production Technology*, Adam Hilger Ltd., Bristol, England, 1972.
4. Jacobs, D.H., *Fundamentals of Optical Engineering*, McGraw-Hill, New York, 1943.
5. Plummer, W.T., "Precision: How to achieve a little more of it, even after assembly," *Proceedings of the First World Automation Congress (WAC '94), Maui*, 193, 1994.
6. Baldo, A.F., "Machine Elements," Chapt. 8.2 in *Marks' Standard Handbook for Mechanical Engineers*, E.A. Avallone and T. Baumeister III, eds., McGraw-Hill, New York, 8, 1987.
7. Yoder, P.R., Jr., "Lens mounting techniques", *SPIE Proceedings* Vol. 389, 2, 1983.
8. Bayar, M., "Lens barrel optomechanical design principles," *Opt. Eng.* Vol. 20, 181, 1981.
9. Kowalski, B.J., "A user's guide to designing and mounting lenses and mirrors," *Digest of Papers, OSA Workshop on Optical Fabrication and Testing, North Falmouth*, 98, 1980.
10. Vukobratovich, D., "Optomechanical Systems Design," Chapt. 3 in *The Infrared & Electro-Optical Systems Handbook,* Vol. 4, ERIM, Ann Arbor, and SPIE, Bellingham, 1993.
11. See Chapt. 8, "The Design of Screws, Fasteners, and Connections", in Shigley, J.E. and Mischke, C.R., *Mechanical Engineering Design,* 5th ed., McGraw-Hill, New York 1989.
12. Roark, R.J., *Formulas for Stress and Strain*, 3rd ed., McGraw-Hill, New York, 1954. See also Young, W.C., *Roark's Formulas for Stress & Strain,* 6th ed., McGraw-Hill, New York, 1989.
13. Martini, L.J., *Practical Seal Design*, Marcel Dekker, New York, 1984.
14. Hopkins, R.E., "Lens Mounting and Centering", Chapt. 2 in *Applied Optics and Optical Engineering,* Vol. VIII, Academic Press, New York, 1980.
15. Delgado, R.F., and Hallinan, M., "Mounting of optical elements," *Opt. Eng.,* Vol. 14, S-11, 1975. (Reprinted in *SPIE Milestone Series,* Vol. 770, 173, 1988.)

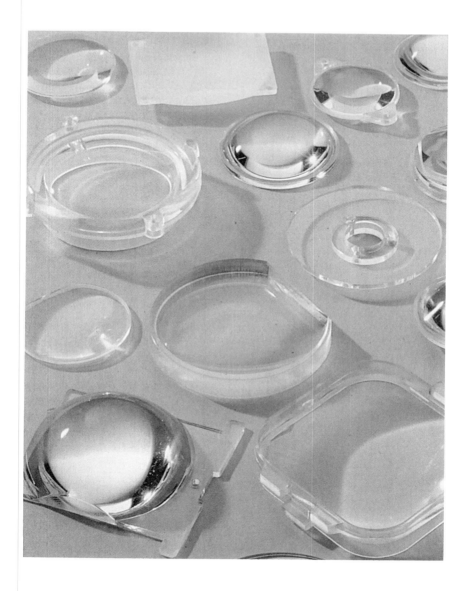

Fig. 3.52 Some typical plastic lenses manufactured by injection or compression molding techniques. Note the variety of shapes and mounting features. (Courtesy of Corning Precision Lens, Inc., Cincinnati, OH)

16. Yoder, P.R., Jr., "Location of mechanical features in lens mounts," *SPIE Proceedings* Vol. 2263, 386, 1994.

17. Miller, K.A., "Nonathermal potting of optics," *SPIE Proceedings* Vol. 3786, 506, 1999.

18. Vukobratovich, D., "Bonded mounts for small cryogenic optics", *SPIE Proceedings* Vol. 4131, 228, 2000.

19. Muench, T., Internal report, Lockheed Martin, Co., Palo Alto.

20. Hatheway, A.E., "Analysis of adhesive bonds in optics," *SPIE Proceedings* Vol. 1998, 2, 1993.

21. Valente, T.M., and Richard, R.M., "Interference fit equations for lens cell design using elastomeric lens mountings," *Opt. Eng.* Vol. 33, 1223, 1994.

22. Yoder, P.R., Jr., "Optomechanical designs of two special-purpose objective lens assemblies," *SPIE Proceedings* Vol. 656, 225, 1986.

23. Vukobratovich, D., "Flexure mounts for high-resolution optical elements", *SPIE Proceedings* Vol. 959, 18, 1988.

24. Ahmad, A. and Huse, R.L., "Mounting for high resolution projection lenses", U.S. Patent No. 4,929,054, issued May 29, 1990.

25. Bacich, J.J., "Precision lens mounting", U.S. Patent No. 4,733,945, issued March 29, 1988.

26. Steele, J.M., Vallimont, J.F., Rice, B.S., and Gonska, G.J., "A compliant optical mount design", *SPIE Proceedings* Vol. 1690, 387, 1992.

27. Carnel, K.H., Kidger, M.J., Overill, A.J., Reader, R.W., Reavell, F.C., Welford, W.T., and Wynne, C.G., "Some experiments on precision lens centering and mounting," *Optica Acta,* Vol.21, 1974, 615 (Reprinted in *SPIE Proceedings* Vol.770, 207, 1988).

28. Altman, R.M., and Lytle, J.D., "Optical-design techniques for polymer optics," *SPIE Proceedings* Vol. 237, 380, 1980.

29. Plummer, W.T., "Unusual optics of the Polaroid SX-70 Land Camera," *Appl. Opt.* Vol. 21, 196, 1982.

CHAPTER 4
Multiple-Component Lens Assemblies

The assembly of two or more optical components such as lenses, windows, or filters into a common mechanical surround generally involves multiple applications of the basic mounting techniques discussed in Chapter 3. We discuss here several technical requirements unique to multiple-component optical assemblies, but not previously considered. Topics include the design and fabrication of spacers that are commonly used to separate adjacent components in a mount; assembly techniques (drop-in, "lathe," "poker-chip," and modular) that provide varying degrees of control over intercomponent centering; methods and instrumentation for precision alignment; techniques for sealing and purging completed assemblies; and mechanisms for moving one or more lenses relative to other lenses for focus adjustment, focal length variation, magnification change, etc. Numerous examples of hardware design illustrate the various types of construction.

4.1 Spacer Design and Manufacture

The separation of multiple lenses in assemblies generally requires the presence of one or more spacers to establish the proper axial separations of adjacent optical surfaces and to provide a means for registering the lenses for alignment purposes. Alternatively, these functions may be accomplished by one or more shoulders machined integrally into the mount. For simplicity, we refer here to either as a spacer. Figure 4.1 shows an example. The parameters indicated are those needed to find the length $L_{j,k}$ of the spacer between the contact points P_j and P_k at heights y_j and y_k on the spherical surfaces of absolute radii $|R_j|$ and $|R_k|$ to produce the separation $t_{j,k}$ between the adjacent vertices. The sagittal depths of the surfaces are S_i and S_j respectively. These are calculated by the following equations and assigned positive signs if contact occurs to the right of the vertex and negative signs if contact occurs to the left of the vertex.

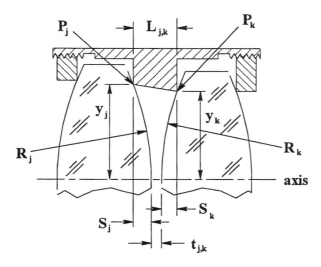

Fig. 4.1 Geometry for dimensioning a spacer or shoulder between two lenses.

$$S_j = |R_j| - (R_j^2 - y_j^2)^{1/2} \tag{4.1}$$

$$S_k = |R_k| - (R_k^2 - y_k^2)^{1/2} \tag{4.2}$$

$$L_{j,k} = t_{j,k} - S_j + S_k \tag{4.3}$$

In the figure, S_j is negative while S_k, $t_{j,k}$, and $L_{j,k}$ are positive.[1]

Example 4.1: Calculation of spacer length.
(For design and analysis, use File 9 of the CD-ROM)
Assume that two bi-convex lenses with radii $R_2 = 30.0$ in. (762.0 mm) and $R_3 = 7.5$ in. (190.5 mm) are to be separated axially by 0.0750 in. (1.905 mm). If the contact heights are $y_2 = 1.5$ in. (38.1 mm) and $y_3 = 1.667$ in. (42.342 mm), what length of spacer is needed?

From Eqs. (4.1) and (4.2):
$\qquad S_i = -[30.0 - (30.0^2 - 1.5^2)^{1/2}] = -0.0375$ in. (- 0.953 mm)
$\qquad S_j = 7.5 - (7.5^2 - 1.667^2)^{1/2} = 0.1876$ in. (4.765 mm)
From Eq. (4.3)
$\qquad L_{3,4} = 0.0750 + 0.0375 + 0.1876 = 0.3001$ in. (7.622 mm).

As mentioned in Sect. 2.1.1, a distinct advantage of surface contact interfaces is that the lenses can have decentered or tilted rims without affecting the alignment of their optical axes. This is illustrated in Fig. 4.2, where three lenses with obvious rim errors have been aligned to a common axis using two spacers that contact the spherical surfaces. Note that the spacers also need not be perfect, nor must they be centered to the axis. Centration of the lenses using the spacers and some form of metrology apparatus that senses alignment errors will minimize the axial distance between the outer surfaces. Hopkins[2] described a technique for assembling and aligning the lenses and spacers in such an assembly as well as one form of error-measuring apparatus to be used to ensure that this is the case. Once aligned, the components are secured to maintain that alignment. We summarize the method and a variation on the apparatus here.

Figure 4.3 shows the lens assembly of Fig. 4.2 schematically in a mechanical housing with two additional (top and bottom) spacers and the alignment sensing apparatus. The latter is a laser autocollimator based on one described by Brockway and Nord.[3] The lenses and spacers can each be moved transversely in two orthogonal directions by mechanisms not shown. The beam from the autocollimator is aligned normal to the upper surface of the slightly wedged glass reference plate forming the base of the housing. The first spacer is centered approximately to the beam and anchored to the plate with clamps or wax. The first lens is then placed on that spacer. Ring patterns will be seen through the eyepiece; two result from interference between the reference surface and each spherical

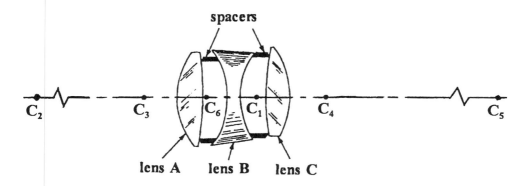

Fig. 4.2 A surface-contacted triplet lens that is perfectly centered while neither the lens rims nor spacers are perfect or centered. (Adapted from Hopkins.[2])

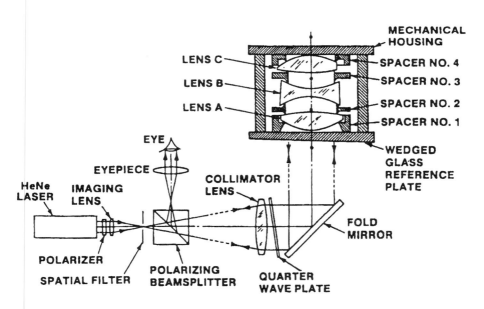

Fig. 4.3 Setup for monitoring and adjusting centration of multiple lenses as they are assembled. (Adapted from Hopkins[2] and Brockway and Nord.[3])

surface of the lens, while a third comes from interference between the lens surfaces. The lens is moved until the patterns are centered to each other using a translation mechanism such as that shown in Fig. 2.5. The lens is then clamped or bonded to the spacer with adhesive. The next spacer is added and clamped or bonded to the first lens. The second lens is added and manipulated until the interference rings formed from its surfaces are centered. That lens is then secured in place. The process is repeated for the third spacer and the third lens. The fourth spacer is added and the entire assembly is clamped together axially to retain the alignment.

There are cases where some interference rings will appear too large or too small for accurate centration. In those cases, refocusing of the autocollimator and/or addition of an auxiliary lens to the beam may adjust the apparent sizes of the rings sufficiently to facilitate alignment of the surfaces producing the interference.

A potential difficulty with this technique is that the ODs of the lenses and those of the spacers will not, in general, be concentric, so it may be difficult to secure these components in a lens barrel. We consider ways to avoid this problem in Sect. 4.3.

Since the annular widths of most spacers are small compared with their diameters (see Fig. 4.4 for a typical case), their manufacture can be difficult. If turned on a lathe, they may end up out of round and have nonparallel faces. To minimize these problems, a stress-free manufacturing procedure such as that described by Westort[4] should be employed. His technique ensures the correct IDs and ODs, roundness, parallelism of faces, and squareness of faces for any reasonably proportioned spacer.

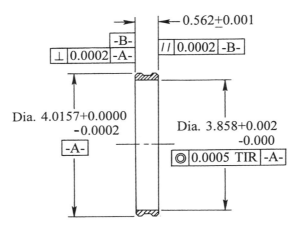

Fig. 4.4 A typical lens spacer. Dimensions are in inches. (From Westort.[4])

Figure 4.5 illustrates the main steps of this procedure. The material used is a 400 series stainless steel that matches that in the lens cell, which was in turn chosen to provide a reasonable thermal match to the lenses to be mounted. The spacer is first rough machined from a blank [dashed outline in Fig. 4.5(a)] to near finished dimensions and heat treated to relieve stresses. The spacer is then potted with a low-temperature melting alloy into a fixture [Fig. 4.5(b)] and bored to the final ID. After unpotting, multiple spacers are then installed onto a precision arbor and ground to the final OD [Fig. 4.5(c)]. This ensures the concentricity as well as the dimensional correctness of these surfaces. Each spacer is then inserted into a fixture with a precision bore that matches and squares on to the spacer OD [Fig. 4.5(d)]. The top surface is ground flat and its edges burnished. The spacer is then turned over and the top surface is ground flat and to the final spacer thickness. Once the edges of that face are burnished, the spacer is completed.

This procedure results in a spacer with 90° sharp-corner interfaces to the lenses. One or both faces could be ground conically with minor modifications of this procedure

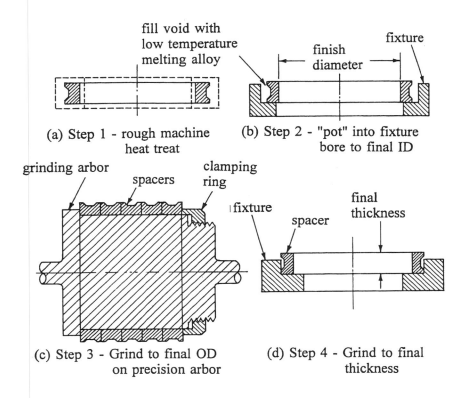

Fig. 4.5 Sequence of major steps (described in text) in one method for making precision spacers. (From Westort.[4])

if the facing operations were done on a precision spindle with the grinding wheel set at the appropriate angle. Toroidal interfaces could also be made on a spindle; the grinding wheel then needs to move in the correct curve. This is quite feasible on a modern computer numerically controlled (CNC) lathe or when using SPDT machining.

Figure 4.6 shows a cell in which the spacer of Fig. 4.4 is intended to fit. The complete assembly is shown in Fig. 4.7. The latter spacer is the first on the left. The maximum clearance between the spacer OD and the cell ID is 0.0008 in. (20.3 μm). Care must be employed during assembly to keep the spacer from binding as it is inserted. The rim of the spacer could be ground spherically or crowned in the manner described for lenses in Sect. 3.8 to prevent this potential problem. Each spacer would then have to be ground individually on a spindle instead of in groups as shown in Fig. 4.5(c).

The other spacers in the assembly of Fig. 4.7 are worth mentioning. The thickness of the second spacer is shown exaggerated for clarity. Typically, such spacers are die-cut rings of metal, such as stainless steel of a specific thickness as required by the lens design, but probably are in the region of 0.002 in. (50 μm). These spacers are

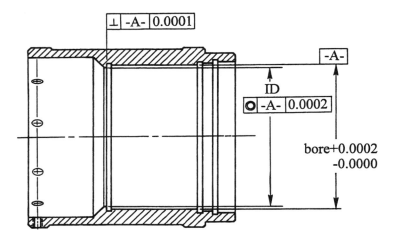

Fig. 4.6 Cell in which the spacer shown in Fig. 4.4 is used. Dimensions are inches. (Adapted from Westort.[4])

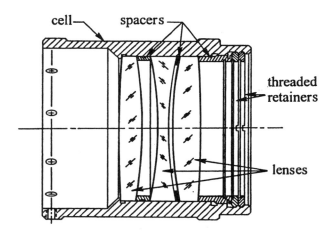

Fig. 4.7 High-performance relay lens assembly for submarine periscope use. (Adapted from Westort.[4])

flexible enough that they conform to a "best fit" to the adjacent glass surfaces (which usually are quite close in radius) when preloaded by a retainer. The spacers must be thick enough to ensure that the surfaces do not contact at the axis if the sagittal depth of the convex face exceeds that of the concave face.

The third spacer of Fig. 4.7 serves two purposes. It acts as a slip ring so rotation of the retaining ring does not drag the lens with it and disturb the rotational alignment around the axis of the last lens. In precision assemblies, lenses frequently are manually rotated ("clocked" or "phased") during installation so that their residual optical wedges tend to cancel each other and produce the best possible image. This spacer also is long enough to bring the retainer to a conveniently accessible location. Note that two retaining rings are used. The second locks the first to help prevent loosening under vibration (which can be quite severe when the periscope is moving through water). In addition, the threads of both rings should be treated with locking compound.

Figure 4.8(a) shows a die-cut plastic spacer shaped with three tabs that can be inserted between two lenses that need a small axial air space. Addis described such spacers, made of polyester film, as a viable and inexpensive means for separating air spaced doublets.[5] The outer ring supports the tabs and lies outside the lens ODs. The tabs protrude between the lens surfaces to the clear apertures of the elements. An advantage pointed out by Addis is that air or nitrogen can easily flow into the space between the lens surfaces when the assembly is purged to remove moisture. A continuous shim would not allow this to happen unless grooves were cut into the spacer or the lens rims.

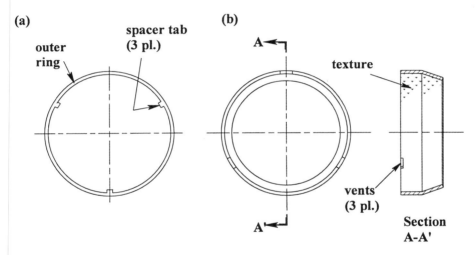

Fig. 4.8 (a) A thin plastic spacer with tabs to separate the surfaces. (b) A molded plastic spacer with ventilation grooves. (Adapted from Addis.[5])

Figure 4.8(b) shows a typical molded plastic spacer with grooves of this type.[5] Contact with the lens occurs most of the way around the assembly to distribute preload. Molded spacers are advantageous from the cost viewpoint in quantity production; they can be made accurately enough for applications in which extreme accuracy is not required. If the spacers are made of black plastic and textured internally as indicated schematically in the figure, stray light can be attenuated.

Before we leave the subject of lens spacers, we should consider the appropriateness of edge-contacting lens surfaces without any spacer. Figure 4.9 shows a typical configuration. Here the adjacent surfaces are strongly curved and the convex side of the left lens element touches the bevel of the concave surface. Usually when this is encountered, the size of the axial air space is a strong driver of some aberration, so it must be controlled accurately. Either of two techniques can be used to establish the

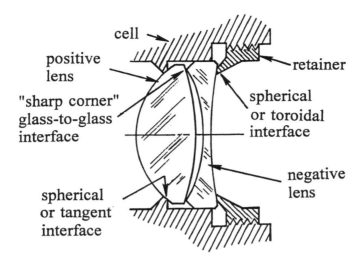

Fig. 4.9 Schematic mounting for an edge-contacted doublet in which the positive element is centered between a shoulder and a bevel on the negative element. (Adapted from Price.[6])

contribution of each element to this air space: the sagittal depth of each surface from the plane of the contact can be measured directly using, for example, a ring spherometer with an appropriately sized ring, or the diameter of the contact (i.e., that of the bevel on the concave surface) can be measured and the sagittal depths of each surface corresponding to that diameter calculated from Eqs. (4.1) and (4.2) using the known radii of curvature of each surface. In either case, the difference between these dimensions is the air space.

The real issue here is not design, but manufacture of the edge-contacted lens assembly. Price stated the usual reaction of optical shop personnel to such designs rather humorously as follows: "You want to put that sharp bevel on a flint glass, right? Where do you think flint glass got its name? You're right, it chips easily, and especially at the edge of a bevel. Further, if you have to move one lens on the other to align the two, you can scratch the coating on the second lens. What do you get? High scrap losses." (Ref. 6, p. 469). These disadvantages must be balanced against the advantages: no spacer is needed and one element may self-center.

The logical approach then is to evaluate each design on its own merits, considering the relative radii of the adjacent surfaces, the ability to set the contact at a reasonable diameter, the brittleness and hardness of the glasses, the ratio of radius to diameter at the contact diameter, the sensitivity of the design to air space variations and element tilts, the ability of the design to achieve self-centering, and the sizes of the lenses and their their resulting weights.[6] To this list, this author suggests adding consideration of the potential for damage to the lenses from extreme stress buildup at the sharp-corner glass-to-glass interface, especially at low temperatures.

4.2 Drop-in Assembly

Designs in which all lenses and the interfacing surfaces of the mount are fabricated to specified dimensions within specified tolerances and assembled without further machining and without adjustment are called "drop-in" assemblies. Low cost, ease of assembly, and simple maintenance are prime criteria for these designs. Typically, relative apertures are f/4.5 or slower, and performance requirements are not high.

An example is shown in Fig. 4.10. This is a fixed-focus eyepiece for a military telescope.[7] Both lenses (identical doublets oriented crown to crown) and a spacer fit into the ID of the cell with 0.003 in. (0.075 mm) radial clearance. A threaded retainer holds these components in place. Sharp-corner interfaces are used throughout. The accuracy of centration depends primarily upon the accuracy of the lens edging and the ability of the axial preload to "squeeze out" differences in edge thickness (i.e., wedge) before the rims of the lenses touch the cell ID. The axial air space between the lenses depends upon the spacer dimensions, which typically are held to design values within 0.010 in. (0.25 mm).

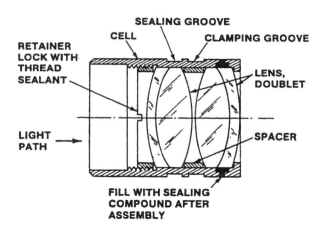

Fig. 4.10 Example of a drop-in assembly. (From Yoder.[7])

Lens assemblies for many military and commercial applications with modest performance requirements traditionally follow the drop-in design concept. Most involve high-volume production and many are intended for assembly by "pick-and-place" robots. Cost is of prime importance. Careful tolerancing, guided by knowledge of standard optical and mechanical shop practices is essential, since parts are usually selected from stock at random, and few, if any, adjustments at the time of assembly are feasible. It is expected that a small percentage of the end items will not meet all performance requirements. Those that fail are discarded, since that is generally more cost-effective than troubleshooting and fixing the problem affecting any individual "out-of-tolerance" component.

4.3 Lathe Assembly

A "lathe-assembled" lens is one in which each seat in the mount is custom machined on a lathe or diamond turning machine to fit closely to the measured OD of a specific lens.[7] Furthermore, the axial position of each seat is usually determined during this operation. For this to be successful, all components should have a high degree of roundness. The tolerances on lens ODs can be relatively loose (say ±0.01 in. [±0.25 mm]). The corresponding seat IDs are initially machined undersize so that significant material can be removed during the final machining process. Radial clearances between a lens and its seat of 0.0002 in. (5.1 µm) are common; clearances as small as 50×10^{-6} in. (1.3 µm) are feasible. With such small clearances, these lens mountings are referred to as "hard mounts." Spherical or crowned rims may be appropriate if the edge thicknesses are large. This design feature, described in Sect. 3.8, is intended to facilitate the assembly of lenses into closely fitting mount IDs without jamming from lens tilts.

Figure 4.11 illustrates the measurement and fitting sequence. Figure 4.11(a) shows an air-spaced doublet in a cell. Measurements to be made on the as-manufactured lenses are indicated by the circled numbers 1 through 5 in Fig. 4.11(b). Actual values can be written in the boxes below the numbers on a copy of this figure to create a record for a given assembly. Lens surface radii must be obtained from test plate or interferometric measurement during manufacture. They also must be made part of the recorded data. The mechanical surfaces designated by the letters A through E are machined to suit this specific set of lens measurements and to position the lenses axially within specified tolerances. Machining of surface D, which provides a tangential interface for lens 1, is an iterative process, with trial insertions of the lens and measurement of its vertex location relative to flange surface B to ensure achievement of the 57.150-mm axial dimension within the specified ±10-µm tolerance. The spacer thickness is also machined iteratively, with trial assembly and measurement of overall axial thickness to ensure meeting the design tolerance for this dimension.

Figure 4.12 shows a 24-in. (61-cm) focal length, f/3.5 aerial camera objective lens designed for lathe assembly.[8] The titanium barrel was made in two parts so a shutter and iris could be inserted between lenses 5 and 6. The machining of the lens seats to fit the measured lens ODs and to provide proper air spaces began with the smaller diameter components and progressed toward the larger ones. Each lens was held with its own retaining ring, so no spacers were required. The lenses were fitted into the front and back barrel components in single lathe setups to maximize centration. These optomechanical subassemblies were mechanically piloted together (the pilot diameters were machined in the same setups as the lens seats) so their mechanical and optical axes coincided. An O-ring was used to seal the barrel-to-barrel interface with metal-to-metal contact between the flanges. Tangent surfaces were used in the convex surface interfaces. Flat bevels were ground on the concave surfaces with accurate perpendicularity to the lens' optical axes to ensure proper centration. Because of space constraints between lenses 2 and 3, and 3 and 4, step bevels were ground into the lens rims to provide spaces for the retainers. Injected elastomer rings (not shown) sealed lenses 1, 5, 6, and 7 to the barrel. All internal air spaces were interconnected with ducts (not shown) to facilitate purging with dry nitrogen to minimize condensation of internal moisture at low temperatures.

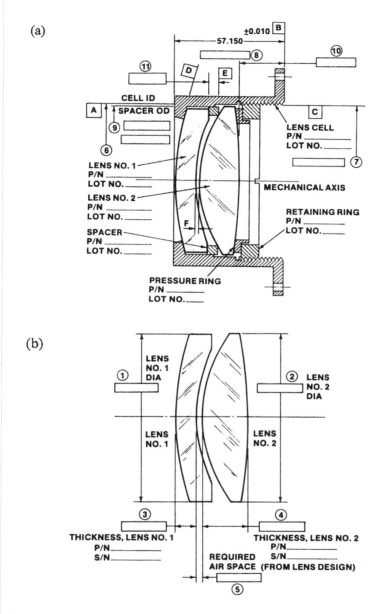

Fig. 4.11 An air-spaced doublet assembly made by the lathe-assembly process. (a) Complete assembly, (b) measurements made on lenses. (From Yoder.[7])

This technique is also often used in the assembly of lenses for high-performance optical systems such as might be used in military or space systems.[9] Examples of such designs may be found in Sects. 13.2 and 13.6. The application for the above-discussed air-spaced doublet is described in Sect. 13.16. The technique may also be used to advantage (perhaps without the elaborate data retention) if the assembly is to be subjected to severe vibration and/or shock conditions.

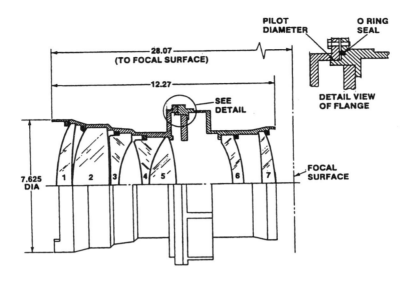

Fig. 4.12 Sectional view of a lathe-assembled aerial camera lens assembly. Dimensions are given in inches. (From Bayar.[8])

4.4 Poker-Chip Assembly

Optomechanical subassemblies with the lenses mounted and aligned precisely within individual subcells that were inserted in sequence into precisely machined IDs of lens barrels (in the manner of a stack of poker chips) have been described by several authors.[1,2,11-15] Assembly and alignment techniques 3 and 4 of Sect. 3.10 are used. One such design is shown in Fig. 4.13.[13] The lenses of this low-distortion, telecentric projection lens were aligned within their respective stainless steel cells to tolerances as small as 0.0005 in. (12.7 μm) of decentration, a 0.0001-in. (2.5-μm) edge thickness total indicator runout due to wedge, and a 0.0001-in. (2.5-μm) surface edge runout due to tilt. They then were potted in place with 0.015-in. (0.381-mm) thick annular rings of 3M 2216B/A epoxy adhesive injected through radial holes in the subcells to secure the lenses in place. The subcell thicknesses were machined so that the air spaces between lenses were within design tolerances without adjustment. After curing, the subcells were inserted into the stainless steel barrel and secured with retainers.

Vukobratovich[14] discussed the last-described technique for mounting lenses within subcells and illustrated it with examples in which each lens was burnished or epoxied into its own subcell. In one case, the cylindrical outer surface of each cell was machined on a spindle to be concentric with and parallel to the optical axis of the lens after the lens was installed. The cell ODs were machined to the proper OD for insertion along with similarly machined subcells into a common barrel. In another case, the cells were machined to the proper ODs; then the lenses were installed, centered to those ODs, and epoxied in place. In yet another Vukobratovich design (see Sect. 13.14), subcells with prealigned and elastomerically supported lens components were press fitted into a barrel

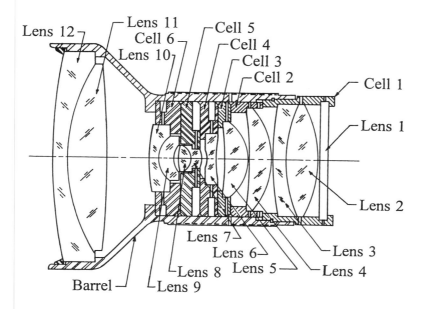

Fig. 4.13 A high-performance projection lens assembled by the poker-chip technique. (From Fischer.[13])

with slight radial mechanical interference fits.[15]

The assembly of lenses in the poker-chip configuration facilitates performance optimization by fine transverse adjustment of one or more lenses during the final stage of assembly. Figure. 4.14 shows an example of such an assembly in which the third element can be transversely adjusted with three screws to allow modification of its aberration contributions to compensate for residual aberrations of the optical system.[14] When this technique is employed, the moveable lens must have sufficient sensitivity to the specific aberration to be compensated for so that reasonable movement produces the desired effect. On the other hand, it must not be too sensitive to this and other aberrations, for this would make the adjustment too critical. The choice of which element to move is usually made by the lens designer during the tolerance analysis. In some lens assemblies, multiple components are chosen as "compensators," with each affecting one specific aberration more than others.

A vital aspect of the aberration compensation technique is the availablity of a suitable real-time means for measuring aberrations during the adjustment process. Figure 4.15 shows a test setup involving a lens barrel containing many lenses, three of which act as aberration compensators. These lenses are located at the axial locations indicated by the "access holes." Push rods driven by two micrometers penetrate such holes at each location to move each lens laterally by sliding its moveable poker-chip subassembly

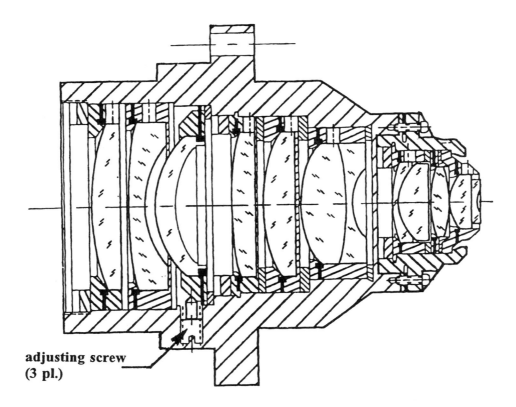

**adjusting screw
(3 pl.)**

Fig. 4.14 Sectional view of a lens assembly with one lens element acting as an aberration compensator for performance optimization during assembly. (From Vukobratovich.[14])

relative to all the others. A restoring force is exerted by a spring (not shown) acting through a third hole symmetrically located with respect to the motions of the micrometers in their plane of action. This allows the micrometers to operate essentially in a simple "push-pull" mode.

In the setup of Fig. 4.15, the lens barrel is clamped to a "vee" block fixture which is in turn installed in an interferometer (not shown). The interferometer allows the effects of the movement of each lens on overall performance to be assessed. Optimization is accomplished by successive approximations. When the system's performance is maximized, the moveable lenses are locked in place by some internal mechanisms (not shown) to preserve the alignment. The access holes are then sealed to keep moisture and dirt out.

To optimize the performance of some lens assemblies, small movements of one or more poker chips in the axial direction are necessary in addition to lateral adjustments. The use of threaded cells turning in mating threads in the barrel (similar to some eyepiece focus adjustments) for axial positioning of the lens is not practical here because the

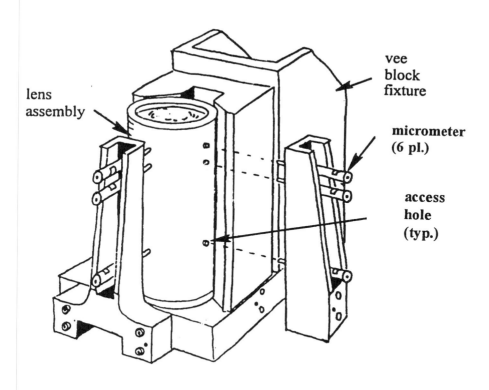

Fig. 4.15 Schematic of a test fixture with a lens assembly in which three lenses are transversely adjustable for performance optimization.

threads are too coarse, even they are if designed to act differentially (see Sect. 4.10.1). Furthermore, the cells must not be turned about their axes during axial adjustment because residual wedge defects in the optical and/or mechanical components can then affect centration of the optics and increase aberrations.

Bacich[16] described some mechanisms for making fine axial adjustments that are easily accessed from the outside of the lens barrel. Figure 4.16 shows two such mechanisms. In Fig. 4.16(a), three balls distributed at 120° intervals slide in vertical holes in the lens cell (poker chip) and rest on cone-point setscrews penetrating the wall of the cell. Another lens cell (not shown) rests on top of the three balls. By accessing the screws through holes in the barrel wall and turning them by equal amounts, one can increase or decrease the air space between adjacent lenses by small amounts. In Fig. 4.16(b), the same effect is obtained by setscrews driving into three wedged slots in the cell wall. Half-balls attached to the tops of the cantilevered wedges touch the next cell (not shown). In either case, when the cells are locked together axially, the adjustments are secured. One technique for locking cells together is described in the next section. The use of these adjustment means to differentially tilt a lens is recommended only if the assembly design does not require the cell rims to be aligned to each other.

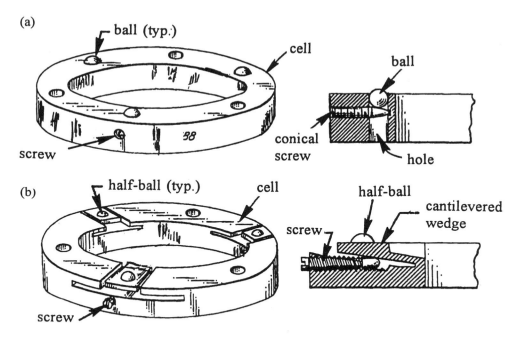

Fig. 4.16 Typical mechanisms that can be used to adjust air spaces between adjacent "poker-chip" lens subassemblies. (Adapted from Bacich.[16])

4.5 Precision Alignment of Multiple-Lens Assemblies

In Section 3.10 we discussed several techniques for mounting and aligning an individual lens to optical and/or mechanical references in a cell or lens barrel. Those techniques can be extended directly to alignment of multiple lenses. The lenses can be individually aligned in sequence to the same reference(s) or aligned to different references, depending upon the specific design configuration. We consider here some examples of applications of these techniques to high-precision lens assemblies.

Figure 4.17 is a simplified sectional view of a lens system requiring nearly perfect centration of several lenses and described by Carnell et al.[12] The assembly was intended to serve as a wide-field (110°) telecentric objective lens for bubble-chamber photography. A large amount of barrel distortion with a specific variation in magnitude with field angle was designed into the lens and was to appear very precisely (i.e., within a few micrometers of the design values) in the completed lens over the entire image. The design also had significant coma to increase the entrance pupil diameter with field angle. The lens was aligned using alignment technique 3 from Sect. 3.10 as follows.

Each lens was mounted individually in a brass cell whose OD and faces had been machined true by diamond turning on a precision air bearing (see Fig. 4.18). A 0.25-mm (0.010-in.)-radius "knife-edge" seat (actually a toroidal interface as defined in Sect. 3.6.3) was machined inside each cell to contact one convex or concave spherical lens surface.

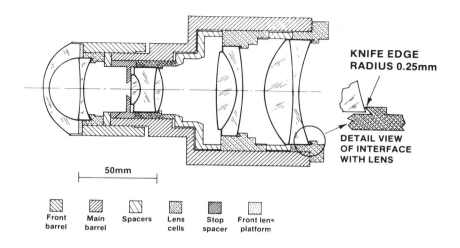

KNIFE EDGE
RADIUS 0.25mm

DETAIL VIEW
OF INTERFACE
WITH LENS

50mm

Front barrel | Main barrel | Spacers | Lens cells | Stop spacer | Front lens platform

Fig. 4.17 Optomechanical configuration of a lens assembly requiring extremely precise centration of several lens components. (Adapted from Carnell et al.[12])

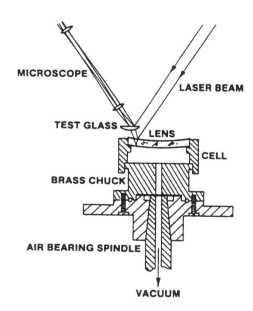

MICROSCOPE

LASER BEAM

TEST GLASS

LENS

CELL

BRASS CHUCK

AIR BEARING SPINDLE

VACUUM

Fig. 4.18 Instrumentation used to monitor centration of each optical surface in the assembly of Fig. 4.17. (Adapted from Carnell et al.[12])

All machining, lens assembly, and alignment were completed before removing the cell from the spindle. The lens was held in place during alignment by a light vacuum of about

0.8 atm absolute. Centering was monitored by observing interference fringes between the lens surfaces and a spherical test glass held close to the exposed surface of the lens. Centration was judged to be correct when the fringe pattern appeared to remain stationary as the spindle was slowly rotated. This indicated that the rotating surface ran true to the cell axis within a fraction of a wavelength of the laser beam used ($\lambda = 0.633$ µm). The lens was cemented to the cell with a room-temperature curing epoxy (3M 2216B/A). The epoxy formed an annular layer of thickness of about 0.1 mm (0.004 in.) between the rim of the lens and the ID of the cell. The individual cemented subassemblies were assembled in a barrel with carefully bored cylindrical IDs. Spacers determined the air spaces. Air pressure relief holes (not shown in the figure) were provided at strategic locations to permit the cells to be inserted with almost an interference fit.

The doublets and the triplet of the design were cemented together with a variation of this technique. One element was attached to a trued vacuum chuck on the air-bearing spindle with the concave surface up and centered as described earlier. The appropriate amount of optical cement was added and then the second element was lowered into place. The cement layer was squeezed until testing with the test plate interferometer indicated that the inner surfaces were parallel. The upper element was then positioned so the top surface ran true. Any wedge introduced in the cement layer was then removed by differential application of axial pressure and the top element's centering was refined as necessary. The referenced paper by Carnell et al.[12] mentioned that a sufficient index of refraction difference occurred in the glass-to-cement interface at the test wavelength to give about 1% Fresnel reflectance at each surface, allowing the fringes to be seen by the unaided eye. This process was used repeatedly for the triplet.

Carnell et al.[12] reported that upon evaluation the system aberrations were essentially as expected. When the assembly was rotated in a vee-block, the axial image moved by no more than 1 µm (4×10^{-5} in.), indicating that excellent rotational symmetry about the mechanical axis had been achieved. It was concluded that the alignment of the optics was at least an order of magnitude better than the alignment that could be achieved by previously available, more conventional techniques.

Figure 4.19 shows another high-precision lens assembly. It is assembled and aligned in accordance with alignment technique 4 of Sect. 3.10. On the right side, one can clearly see the lenses. All are singlets made of fused silica. As shown on the left side of the figure, they are each attached to flexures machined integrally with their cells in the fashion of Fig. 3.43. The cells and the lens barrel are made of stainless steel so there is a significant CTE mismatch between the lenses and the mechanical parts. Hence the flexures are used to keep the lenses centered over a significant temperature range.

The lens elements are attached to the flexures with epoxy as shown in Fig. 3.43. The cells are then diamond turned in situ as illustrated in Fig. 3.50(b). The ODs of all but two cells are a few micrometers smaller than the ID of the barrel into which they are to be inserted. The two special cases are those for the third and fifth lenses from the top, which are transversely adjustable with radially directed screws to optimize performance at the final stage of alignment. The cell ODs are sufficiently undersized to allow the adjustments to be made. The adjustment mechanism is similar to that shown in Fig. 2.5. A thick annular spacer is provided between the third and fourth lenses to determine the corresponding air space. Thin annular spacers (shims) of appropriate thicknesses (shown

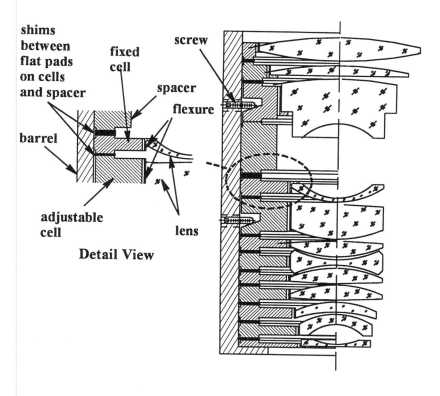

Fig. 4.19 Schematic partial section view of a lens assembly with two laterally adjustable cells. The lenses are assembled and aligned in their cells and the cells machined precisely to fit the barrel ID.

exaggerated in the figure) are located between the cells to allow those air spaces to be set within tolerances. These typically would be made of the same material as the cells and barrel for thermal expansion compatability.

Figure 4.20 illustrates an interferometric setup that might be used to monitor alignment of the lens assembly during adjustment of the two sliding lenses of Fig. 4.19. Fringes formed in double-pass through the lens assembly between a reference flat surface and the retrodirective mirror are observed using a video camera located above the beamsplitter cube. The quality of the image is recorded after each iterative adjustment of the moveable lenses.

After the lens assembly's perfomance has been maximized, it is clamped together using the means shown in Fig. 4.21. Here three rods pass through clearance holes in each cell and shim and thread into holes in the barrel's lower endplate. Nuts are attached to the upper threaded ends of the rods. By tightening the nuts, the rods are put in tension and clamp the cells together axially without disturbing centration because all interfacing pads on the cells are flat and perpendicular to the axis of the system.

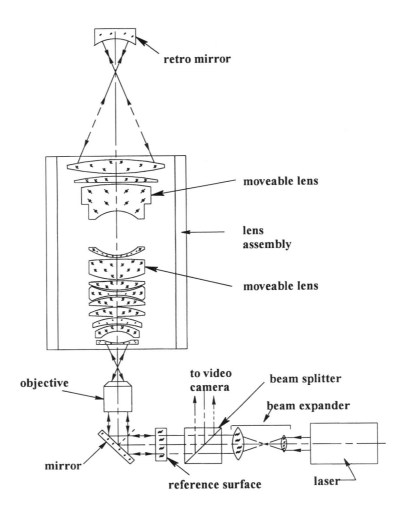

Fig. 4.20 A test setup that might be used to evaluate the performance of the assembly shown in Fig. 4.19 during adjustment of the laterally moveable lenses.

Yet another concept for alignment and clamping together of poker chip lens subassemblies is shown in Fig. 4.22. Here three cells with their lenses installed (but not included in the figure) are shown in exploded view. These cells are part of a stack of poker-chip subassemblies that make up a complex lens assembly for imaging a mask onto silicon wafers to create computer chips with submicrometer feature resolution. Each cell has flat pads on its top and bottom faces. These pads are coplanar and parallel. Shims are used between the cell pads, as shown in Figs. 4.19 and 4.21. Alternatively, the pads may contact each other to provide the proper air spaces between lens vertices when the cells are assembled into a stack. In the latter case, the heights of the pads would be carefully controlled. The lenses are flexure mounted and aligned in the cells so their optic axes are at the geometric centers of the cell ODs and perpendicular to the pad's faces.

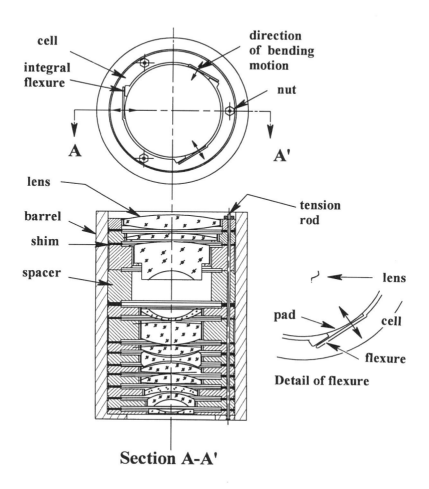

Fig. 4.21 Schematic of a means for axially clamping the lens cells in the assembly of Fig. 4.19 after alignment is completed using tension rods at 120° intervals. Some details of the flexures also are shown.

The lower cell in Fig. 4.22 has three rods pressed into or threaded into holes in the cell so as to be perpendicular to the plane defined by the pads on the cell's top surface. These rods protrude through clearance holes in the middle and top cells when they are brought together. During assembly, the lower cell acts as the reference and the middle cell is aligned by sliding it laterally until the optic axis of that second cell is colinear with that of the lower cell. This adjustment would be made on an air-bearing spindle using interferometric sensing of errors. When the adjustment is completed, the spaces between the rods and the holes in the upper cell are filled with epoxy and cured. The third cell is then placed on top and aligned in the same manner as the second. It too is epoxied in place. The same process could be followed to build a stack of all the lens cells in the assembly.

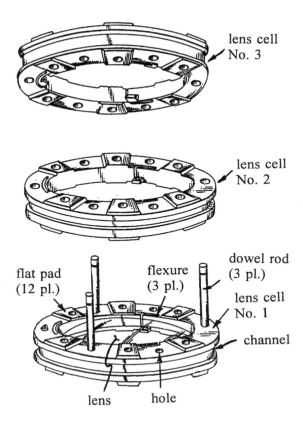

Fig. 4.22 "Exploded" view of three lens cells that illustrate a technique for affixing one cell to another by liquid pinning rods in clearance holes after alignment. (Adapted from Bacich.[16])

Figure 4.23 shows a schematic sectional view through a stack of 12 cells, each containing a lens or acting as a major spacer. Once precisely aligned to each other, they form a complete optical assembly. Two cells (5 and 10) are to be adjusted axially and radially to optimize the performance of the whole optical system. A test setup of the type shown in Fig. 4.20 might be used. A fixture of the type shown in Fig. 4.15 could provide a means for making the lateral adjustments. Custom-ground shims located between precision pads on the faces of the cells would be one means for adjusting the air spaces. These shims and pads are not shown in Fig. 4.23, but would be used as indicated in Figs. 4.19 and 4.21. Mechanisms of the types shown in Figs. 4.16 could be used in some other assemblies to provide the axial adjustment.

As may be noted from Fig. 4.23, all cells except those to be adjusted are shown epoxied to the dowel rods that are firmly attached to cells 1, 2, 6, 7, and 11. At this stage during assembly, the nonadjustable components have previously been aligned to a common axis and the adjacent air spaces corrected before the epoxy was inserted around the rods and cured. As shown, the assembly is ready for final positioning of the moveable cells and epoxying them to the rods. Once this is accomplished, the entire stack would be

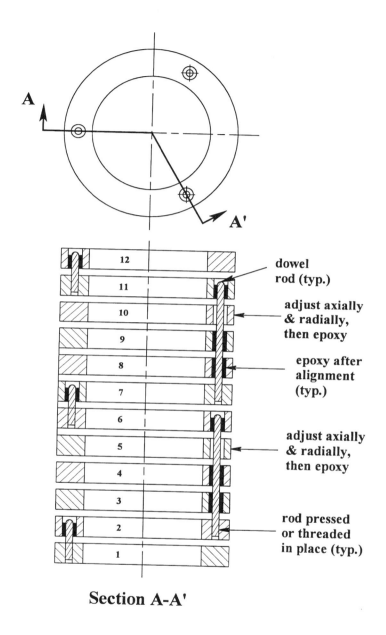

Fig. 4.23 Schematic of lens cells stacked, aligned, and epoxied to dowel rods in preparation for final alignment of two adjustable cells. After alignment, those cells are epoxied in place. (Adapted from Bacich.[16])

clamped together axially with tension rods as in Fig. 4.21 or by some equivalent technique. A housing would then be added to enclose the assembly. This would be done so as not to affect the optical system alignment.

4.6 Assemblies with Plastic Housings and Lenses

In Sect. 3.10, we mentioned the design and manufacture of plastic lenses for optical instrument applications. Typical of these applications are camera viewfinders and objectives, magnifiers, television projection systems, compact disc players, night vision goggles, and head-mounted displays. In hardware requiring the lowest cost and low to moderate performance, mechanical parts also can be made of plastic. For such cases, Lytle advocated the parallel design of the housings into which plastic lenses are to be mounted and the lenses themselves.[17] Low-cost housings can be molded of plastic using techniques similar to those employed in making optics. Their configurations may be traditional, innovative, or even impossible to manufacture using common machine tool methods. Figure 4.24 shows a collet-type housing in which four molded lenses with integral tabs are inserted so the tabs fit into slots in the housing. End caps are slipped over the ends of the housing, thereby compressing the housing around the lens rims. The caps are then secured by ultrasonic bonding. Disassembly of such a unit is not generally considered practical or desirable in view of its relatively low cost compared with conventional glass and metal construction.

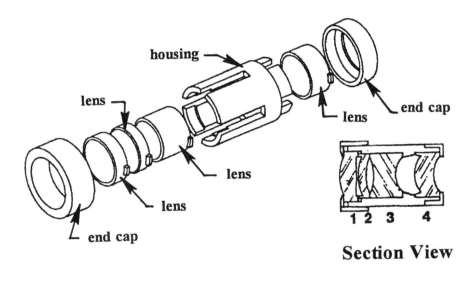

Section View

Fig. 4.24 Lens assembly featuring all-plastic construction. The four lenses are constrained by a colletlike compression of the slotted housing by end caps that are secured by ultrasonic bonding after assembly. (Adapted from Lytle.[17])

The upper diagram of Fig. 4.25 illustrates a mounting arrangement in which lenses are located in separate cylindrical housings. These housings are joined during assembly. The joint is shown next to the negative lens. The aperture stop is integral with the second housing. A spacer separates the left two lenses and both positive lenses are secured with retainers. The retainers might be bonded in place with adhesive or heat sealed to the housing. In the design represented by the lower diagram, the joint is between

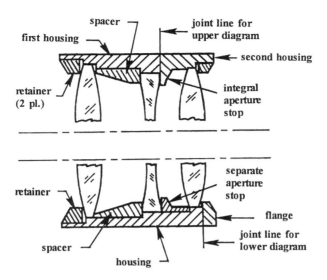

Fig. 4.25 Schematics of two all-plastic, three-lens assemblies with identical optics. The upper design (with two axially joined housings) would have a lower cost, but the lower one (with one housing and a flange) would have better lens centration. (Courtesy of Corning Precision Lens, Inc., Cincinnati, OH)

a cylindrical housing and an attached flange. This flange is outside the right positive lens. Here all lenses are mounted in the same housing, thereby achieving better centration since all lens seats are molded into the same part. The aperture stop must be a separate part, so the cost of the bottom design would probably be somewhat higher than that of the top design. The tradeoff is then between cost and centration (i.e., performance).

Several all-plastic lens assemblies are illustrated in Fig. 4.26. Focus is achieved in some by turning an inner cell (containing the lenses) inside an outer housing, with axial motion driven by a pin riding in a helical cam slot in that housing. Other assemblies have two axially adjustable cells with lenses. Each of these cells has a pin that rides in its own cam slot. The two motions allow adjustment of magnification as well as focus. One such assembly is described in more detail in Sect. 13.8.

4.7 Modular Assembly

The assembly, alignment, and maintenance of optical instruments are simplified if groups of related optomechanical components are constructed as prealigned and interchangeable modules. In some cases, the individual modules are considered to be nonmaintainable, and the instrument is repaired by replacing defective modules, usually without requiring system realignment. Vukobratovich reviewed alignment accuracy and structural stiffness resulting from modular design and fabrication methods.[18]

The manufacture of modular designs is somewhat more complex than the

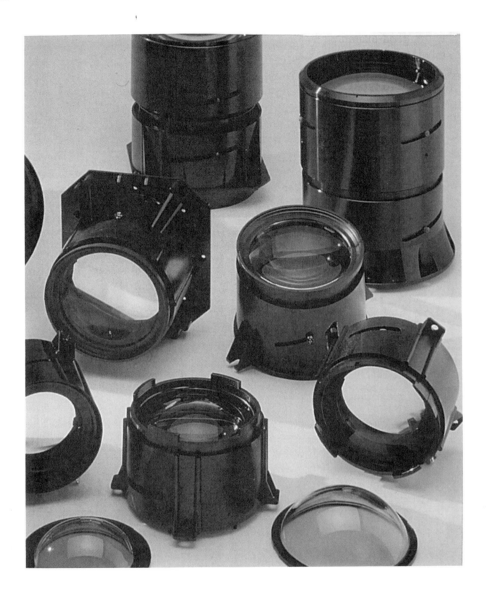

Fig. 4.26 Photographs of all-plastic lens assemblies. (Courtesy of Corning Precision Lens, Inc., Cincinnati, OH.)

equivalent nonmodular versions because of the added requirement for interchangeability without compromising performance. To meet the last requirement in some cases, adjustments may be made within the module during assembly. In other cases, mounting surfaces are machined to specific orientations and/or locations with respect to optical axes and focal planes. The achievement of performance goals is greatly facilitated by the design and fabrication of optomechanical fixtures specifically intended for manufacture and alignment of the modules.[18]

A good example of modular design as used in a military 7×50 binocular [19] is illustrated in Fig. 4.27. This instrument has prealigned and parfocalized (i.e., preset back focal distance) objective and eyepiece assemblies, as well as left and right housings with prealigned Porro-type erecting prisms. The housings are identical until the final machining stage. The objective assembly is described in Sect. 13.4. It has many advantages over adjustable designs, such as that described in Sect. 13.3.

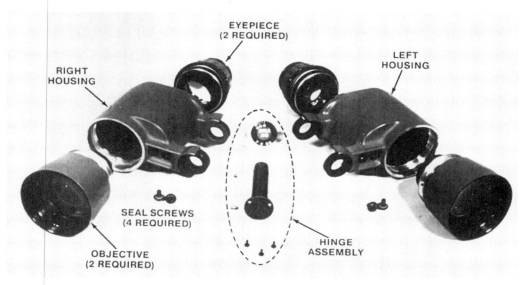

Fig. 4.27 A military binocular with modular construction. (From Yoder.[1])

Many photographic and video camera lenses, microscope objectives, and telescope eyepieces are essentially optomechanical modules. See, for example, the microscope objective assembly described in Sect. 13.9. In photographic applications, a variety of modular lens assemblies can be interchanged on a single camera body or moved from one camera to another of similar type. These lens modules are parfocalized so their calibrated infinity focal planes automatically coincide with the camera's film plane.

Modern injection-molding techniques allow complex optomechanical assemblies to be fabricated from plastic materials in modular form. Figure 4.28 shows such a module designed for use in an automatic coin-changer mechanism. It is made of polymethyl-methacrylate (acrylic) and has two lens elements (one aspheric) molded integrally with a mechanical housing having prealigned mounting provisions and interfaces for attaching two detectors. When manufactured in large quantities, this type of module is inexpensive. Since it requires no adjustments, it is easy to install and virtually maintenance free.

Single-point diamond turning techniques facilitate the creation of self-aligning optomechanical modules that involve precisely located and contoured optical component mounting interfaces and integral mounting features. Although they are most frequently

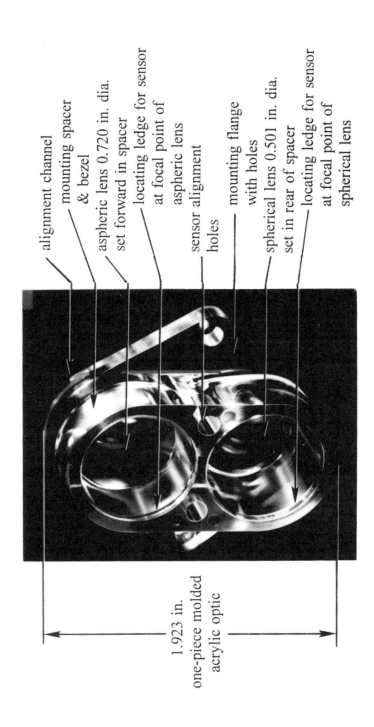

alignment channel
mounting spacer
& bezel
aspheric lens 0.720 in. dia.
set forward in spacer
locating ledge for sensor
at focal point of
aspheric lens
sensor alignment
holes

mounting flange
with holes
spherical lens 0.501 in. dia.
set in rear of spacer
locating ledge for sensor
at focal point of
spherical lens

1.923 in.
one-piece molded
acrylic optic

Fig. 4.28 One-piece molded acrylic optical assembly with two integral prefocused lenses, interfaces for detectors, and a mounting flange. (Courtesy of Corning Precision Lens, Inc., Cincinnati, OH.)

used with reflecting optics, these methods and machines are also applicable to fabricating precision mounts for lenses and to helping to achieve the part interchangeability needed in modular instruments. For infrared applications, optical surfaces can be created directly in crystalline lens substrates and in metal mirrors in the same SPDT machine setup used to create precision mechanical mounting and alignment features on the module.

4.8 Catadioptric Systems

A catadioptric optical system is one that has both refracting (lens) and reflecting (mirror) components. Most are adaptations of classic all-reflecting (catoptric) designs such as the Cassegrain or Gregorian types. Usually the refractive (dioptric) components are added to improve performance or to increase the usable field of view. The catadioptric system usually works at a faster relative aperture, is physically shorter, and has a larger field than the equivalent catoptric version. Although a reflecting system with field lenses added near the focal plane is technically catadioptric, this term is more frequently associated with systems having full-aperture refracting components such as in Schmidt or Maksutov objectives or derivatives of the Schmidt–Cassegrain system.

Full-aperture lenses of catadioptric systems are usually called "correctors" or "corrector plates," since they usually have near- zero total optical power and serve primarily to correct aberrations that cannot be corrected by the associated mirrors. Mounting and sealing of these correctors follow the same general guidelines as for their smaller counterparts discussed earlier. Larger components have greater weights and frequently have reduced structural strength, so they suffer more from gravitational, acceleration, and thermal effects than smaller components. As mentioned in Sect. 3.4.2, large-diameter threaded retaining rings are difficult to make and install, so flange-type retainers are more frequently employed. Some designs use multiple cantilevered clips as described in Sect. 3.5 to secure and preload large correctors. Sealing by elastomeric formed-in-place gaskets usually is best for the larger correctors. Smaller ones can be sealed with O-rings.

To illustrate a typical catadioptric system, Fig. 4.29 shows schematically one of the 20-in. (50.8-cm) focal length, f/1 "Satrack" cameras developed in the mid-1950s to photograph orbiting satellites. The optical design, created by James G. Baker, is an enhancement of the Schmidt objective. The single corrector plate of the classic Schmidt is replaced here by a full-aperture air-spaced triplet (black profiles). Note that this figure is a composite of two sectional views.

The best available description of this system is found in MIL-HDBK-141 entitled *Optical Design*.[20] A portion of that description follows:

> It will be noted that the aperture of the system is very close to the center of curvature of the primary mirror, but the single corrector plate, which normally is located there, is split up into a color corrected triplet for the purpose of eliminating the small amount of residual axial color in the single Schmidt plate. The four inner surfaces of this system are aspheric.

122

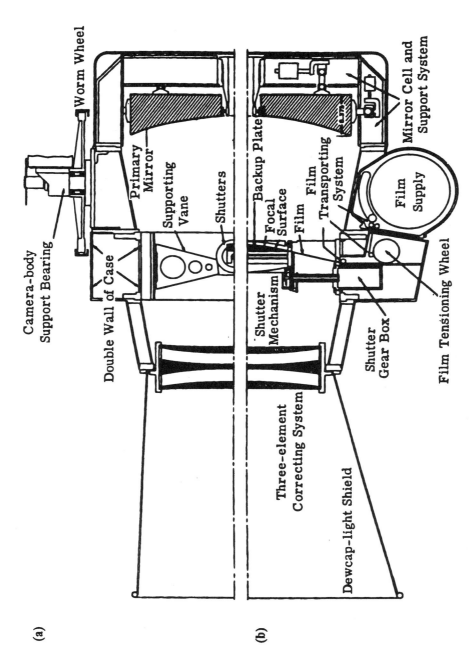

Fig. 4.29 Half-section views of the "Satrack" camera assembly. (a) Plan view, (b) elevation view. (From MIL-HDBK-141.[20])

It is presumed that, because of the high relative aperture of this system (f/1), the curvature of the Schmidt plate required would be more exreme than usual, leading to more axial color than the designer could tolerate. The splitting up of the single plate into three, with the central glass different from the outside, and the distribution of the Schmidt curvature among four surfaces would tend to alleviate this situation.

It will be noted from [Fig. 4.29] that the film is transported over a spherically curved gate, which matches the curved focal plane of the image. The curvature in the plane at right angles must necessarily be zero, because of the mechanical impossibility of bending the moving film into a compound curve. Consequently, the field coverage in this direction is limited to only 5 degrees, while in the direction of film travel it reachs the amazing value of 31 degrees. It was found that at the edges of this extreme field the focal surface departs slightly from a spherical shape, so the film runners are not quite circular. The combination of careful design and excellent execution resulted in a system wherein 80 percent of the point energy anywhere in the field is within a circle 0.001 inch in diameter. This instrument was conceived for the purpose of tracking the U.S. Vanguard satellite, and the first instrument arrived just in time to be used for the original Sputniks. (Ref. 20, p. 19-14)

Although not much optomechanical detail can be derived from Fig. 4.29, one can see that the primary mirror is supported radially and axially on counterbalanced lever mechanisms. Supports of this type are described in Sect. 10.3. The diameter of the mirror is about 31 in. (79 cm) to prevent vignetting at the edges of the field.

Several of these cameras were built and used with great success at various locations around the world. Periodic maintenance kept them operational for many years. The most serious repair needed was repolishing of the exposed plano surface of the outer corrector plate, which became stained over time by deposits from visiting birds. The aluminum/silicon monoxide coatings on the primary mirror also needed to be replaced occasionally, and the aspheric film runners (i.e., film platen) needed to be repolished because of wear from the film passage.

Other catadioptric instruments are discussed in Sects. 13.15 through 13.17.

4.9 Sealing and Purging Considerations

As discussed briefly in Sect. 2.3, sealing is an important aspect of optical instrument design. The primary purpose is, of course, to keep moisture, dust, and other contaminants from entering and depositing on optical surfaces, electronics, or delicate mechanisms. The need for protection from adverse environments depends on the intended use. Military and aerospace optical equipment is subjected to very severe environmental exposures, whereas the optics used in scientific or clinical laboratories and in commercial and consumer applications (such as in interferometers, spectrographs, microscopes, cameras, surveyor's transits, binoculars, laser copiers and printers, and compact disc players) usually experience much more benign environments. Low-cost instruments may have few, if any, provisions for sealing.

Static protection from the environment at normal temperatures and pressures is provided by sealing exposed windows and lenses with cured-in-place elastomeric gaskets or O-rings. Seals for hard-vacuum applications can be created with preformed gaskets made of resilient metals such as lead, gold, indium, or gold-plated Inconel.[21,22] Some examples involving window seals are shown in Sect. 5.2. Nonporous materials are preferred for housings and lens barrels. Castings usually need impregnation with plastic resins to seal pores. O-rings made of Viton are the best for long-term reliability.

Exposed sliding and rotating parts are frequently sealed to fixed members of the instrument with dynamic seals such as O-rings, glands with formed lips, rolling diaphragms, or flexible bellows made of rubber or metal. In the eyepiece shown in Fig. 4.30, a dual-purpose rubber bellows seals the focusing lens cell to a fixed housing at the left (not shown) as well as to the innermost lens at the left of the cell, while the outermost lens at the right of the cell is sealed statically with elastomer. The moving inner subassembly (cell and lenses) slides rather than turns when the focusing ring is turned. Rotation is prevented by a fixed pin riding in a slot in the moving part. A portion of the bellows fits into a groove in the mounting flange to seal the entire eyepiece to the instrument.[23]

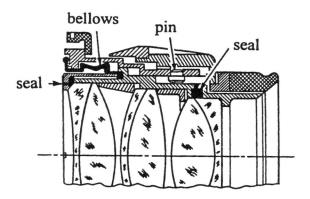

Fig. 4.30 Schematic diagram of an eyepiece with static and dynamic seals. (Adapted from Quammen et al.[23])

Many sealed instruments are flushed with dry gas, such as purified nitrogen or helium, during assembly. A pressure differential above ambient of perhaps 5 lb/in.^{2} (3.4×10^4 N/m^2) is sometimes generated within the instrument to help prevent intrusion of contaminants. Access through the instrument walls may, in this case, be provided by a spring-loaded valve that is basically similar in function to those used on automobile tires. Access for flushing nonpressurized instruments can be provided by threaded through-holes into which seal screws (typically round or pan head machine screws with O-rings under the head) are inserted after flushing. Applications of seal screws, O-rings, and injected elastomers as seals in a binocular are shown in Fig. 4.31.

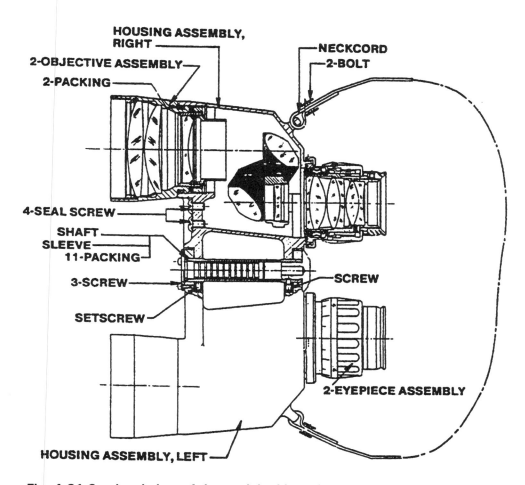

HOUSING ASSEMBLY, RIGHT
2-OBJECTIVE ASSEMBLY
2-PACKING
NECKCORD
2-BOLT
4-SEAL SCREW
SHAFT
SLEEVE
11-PACKING
3-SCREW
SCREW
SETSCREW
2-EYEPIECE ASSEMBLY
HOUSING ASSEMBLY, LEFT

Fig. 4.31 Sectional view of the modular binocular shown in Fig. 4.27. Sealing provisions include static (O-ring and elastomeric) seals and a bellows-type eyepiece dynamic seal as shown in Fig. 4.30. (Courtesy of the U.S. Army.)

The internal cavities of sealed instruments, such as the housings of an aerial camera lens, should be connected by leakage paths to the main cavity (small bored or cast-in holes inside housing walls, grooves through the edges of lenses, spacers with tabs or vents, etc.) in order for the flushing process to work properly. An example is discussed in Sect. 13.12 and shown in Fig. 13.18.

Removal of air, moisture, and/or products of outgassing from these ancillary cavities is facilitated if the instrument is evacuated and backfilled two or three times with the dry gas. Baking the instrument at a slightly elevated temperature for several hours also tends to vaporize moisture and expedite stabilization of outgassing of volatile materials. To prevent potentially harmful pressure changes that are due to temperature changes, sealed instruments that do not have sturdy walls can be allowed to "breathe" through desiccators.[1] An example of the latter construction is discussed in Sect. 13.18.

4.10 Internal Mechanisms

4.10.1 Focus mechanisms

In many optical instruments, internal adjustments are required during normal operation. Examples are focusing a camera or binocular on objects at different distances, changing the focal length of a zoom lens, or adjusting a telescope eyepiece to suit the focus requirements of the observer's eye. Most of these adjustments involve axial motions of certain lenses or groups of lenses within the instrument. A few applications, such as the range compensator of a camera range finder or rectification of converging images of parallel lines in architectural photography, may involve decentration or tilting of lenses.

In some cameras focus is changed by moving the entire objective lens relative to the film, while in others it is changed by moving one or more lens components within the objective relative to the rest of the components. The required motions may be small or large, depending on the lens focal length and object distance, but these motions must always be made precisely and with minimum decentration or tilt of the moving components.

Figure 4.32 illustrates a typical mechanism used in a camera lens module to couple rotation of an external knurled focus ring through a differential thread to move all the lens elements axially as a group. The differential thread consists of a coarse pitch

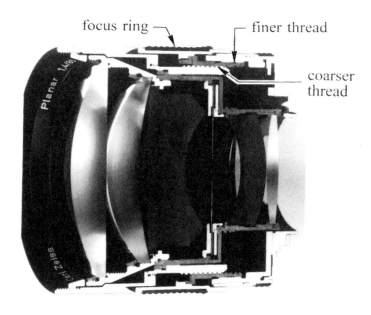

Fig. 4.32 Example of a camera lens assembly with a differential thread focus mechanism. (Courtesy of Carl Zeiss, Inc., Germany.)

thread and a finer one on outer and inner surfaces of a cylindrical part of the focus ring. When that ring is turned, the threads act together to move the lens subassembly axially as if it were driven by a thread of a pitch significantly finer than that actually used in the mechanism.

A differential combination of threads with N_1 and N_2 threads per inch (tpi) results in an equivalent thread of N_E tpi in accordance with the equation

$$N_E = N_1 N_2 / (N_2 - N_1) \tag{4.4}$$

Cutting internal and external threads of, say, 28 and 32 tpi on the actuating member and mating parts of a focus mechanism such as that shown in Fig. 4.32 would not be particularly difficult. Equation (4.4) indicates that the threads would subtract when turned and this would result in a differential motion equivalent to a single thread of 224 tpi. Experience has demonstrated that the manufacture of a 224-tpi thread would be difficult and that problems could occur at assembly since it is hard to engage very fine threads without crossing the threads and possibly destroying the mating parts. These problems associated with the manufacture, assembly, and short lifetime of very fine threads are avoided by use of the differential thread mechanism.

Since they are customarily used to observe objects at long distances, the objectives of most military telescopes, binoculars, and periscopes traditionally are not designed to be refocused for nearby objects. The angular calibration of reticle patterns used for weapon fire control then remains constant since the image distance to that pattern equals the objective focal length. If the magnification of such an instrument is greater than three power, its eyepiece(s) should be individually focusable to suit the user's eye accommodation. Refocusing the eyepiece(s) will have no effect on reticle calibration since the image of the target and the pattern are axially coincident at the eyepiece's object plane.

A focus adjustment (commonly called the "diopter adjustment") of at least ±4 diopters (D) is common for military instruments, while a range of +2 to - 3 D is common on consumer equipment. A scale calibrated in 1/2 or 1/4 D increments usually is placed on the eyepiece focus ring for ease of setting. Assuming that the entire eyepiece is moved axially to make this adjustment, the axial displacement Δ_E for a 1 D change in collimation of the beam entering the eye is approximated by

$$\Delta_E = f_E^2 / 1000 \quad \text{or} \quad f_E^2 / 39.37 \tag{4.5}$$

where f_E is the eyepiece focal length in millimeters or inches, respectively.

Example 4.2: Multiple lead thread for eyepiece focus.
(For design and analysis, use File 10 of the CD-ROM)

The focus of an eyepiece with f_E = 1.110 in. (28.194 mm) is to be changed by ± 4 D. (a) What axial motion is required? (b) If this motion is to be produced by rotating the focusing ring 240° to prevent ambiguity in reading the focus scale, what should be the pitch of the thread?

(a) By Eq. (4.5), $\Delta_E = 1.110^2 / 39.37 = 0.031$ in. (0.795 mm) for a 1 D change
so $\pm 4\Delta_E = \pm 0.250$ in. (6.350 mm) for a ± 4 D change.

(b) For the entire motion to take place in a ±240° ring rotation, a thread pitch of (360/240)(0.250) = 0.375 in./thread or 2.667 threads per inch would be needed. The corresponding metric thread would be 9.54 mm/thread or 0.105 thread per millimeter.

The thread defined in this example is very coarse. Additive differential threads (combination of a right-handed thread and a left-handed thread turning simultaneously) or multiple-lead threads (such as a set of four to six individual coarse threads in parallel) can be used to advantage here. Cams with cam followers also can be used in such cases.

Figure 4.33 shows the mating threaded parts for a 6-lead, 16-tpi eyepiece focusing mechanism. The lenses move 6/16 = 0.375 in. per turn or 0.250 in. (6.350 mm) in 240° rotation. This multiple-lead thread thus has precisely the characteristics required for the eyepiece focus mechanism described in Example 4.2. The pitch diameter of each thread is approximately 1.18 in. (29.97 mm), while the axial length of the thread engagement is about 0.28 in. (7.11 mm). With six threads engaged, much averaging of minor manufacturing errors takes place so that the motion feels smooth to the user.

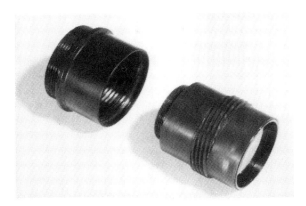

Fig. 4.33 Mating threaded parts for a multiple-lead eyepiece focusing mechanism with six parallel grooves spaced at 0.0625-in. (1.587-mm) intervals. Axial motion is 0.375 in. (9.525 mm) per turn.

Nonmilitary telescopes and binoculars utilize different means for focusing on objects at different distances. Since there is usually no reticle pattern to keep in focus, either the eyepiece(s) or the objective(s) can be moved for this purpose. The classic design for focusable binoculars, as exemplified by Fig. 4.34, moves both eyepieces

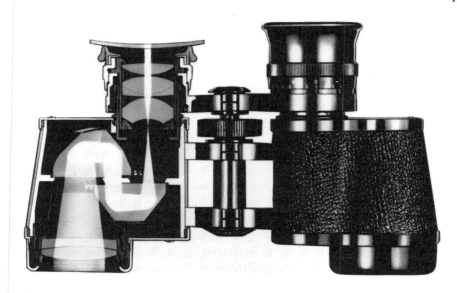

Fig. 4.34 A commercial binocular of traditional design with focusable eyepieces. (Courtesy of Carl Zeiss, Inc., Germany.)

simultaneously along their axes as the knurled ring located on the central hinge is rotated. One eyepiece has individual focus capability to allow accommodation errors between right and left eyes to be balanced. The eyepieces in this design slide in and out of holes in the cover plates on the prism housings. It is very difficult to seal the gaps between the eyepieces and these plates adequately. Most commercial instrument designs make no attempt to do so.

Figure 4.35 shows an individually focusable eyepiece for a low-cost commercial binocular in which the entire internal lens cell rotates on a coarse thread to move axially

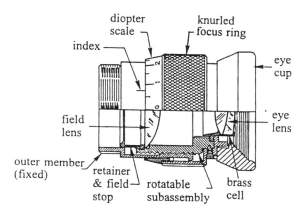

Fig. 4.35 A simple focusing eyepiece in which the lens cell rotates on a coarse thread. (Adapted from Horne.[24])

for diopter adjustment.[24] In the eyepiece shown in Fig. 4.30, the entire internal lens cell slides axially without turning. The latter configuration has the performance advantage of maintaining better lens centration when refocused and can be sealed (with a bellows) better than one with a rotating cell, but it is more complex and therefore more expensive.

A more elegant contemporary approach for focusing a binocular is illustrated in Fig. 4.36. Here rotation of a focus ring on the central hinge moves the internal lens elements of both objectives axially to adjust the focus. Rotation of another knurled ring adjacent to the focus ring biases the position of the focusable lens of one objective to provide the required diopter adjustment. Improved sealing is provided with this design, since all external lenses can be sealed to the instrument housings. Rotary seals are provided on the adjustment shafts.

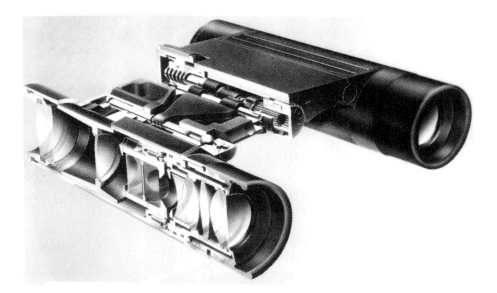

Fig. 4.36 A commercial 8 × 20 pocket binocular with internal focusing mechanisms. (Courtesy of Swarovski Optik K.G., Austria.)

4.10.2 Zoom mechanisms

Most camera zoom lenses have two lens groups that move axially in accordance with specified mathematical relationships to vary the focal length and maintain image focus. Adjustment for different object distances is usually accomplished by moving a third lens group, although some more sophisticated designs do this by modifying the zoom motions. Lens motions are usually controlled by mechanical cams driven manually by the operator or by a small motor. Some operate under control of an internal microprocessor.[25] Smoothness of motion is critical, and lost motion (backlash) in the mechanism must be minimized.

A representative zoom lens assembly is shown in Fig. 4.37. This lens, described by Ashton,[26] had a 5:1 zoom range and a 20- to 100-mm (0.787- to 3.937-in.) focal length. It operated at f/2.8 and was designed for use in a cine (motion picture) application involving 35-mm film. The lens was about 330 mm (11.8 in.) long and 150 mm (5.9 in.) in diameter. The field of view of this lens was 58° horizontally and about 40° vertically at its wide-angle (shortest focal length) setting. The object distance (focus), zoom, and iris mechanisms were designed for motorized or manual gear drive, but the driving means are not shown in the figure.

The first lens group (an air-spaced doublet) was fixed in place, while the second group (the focus cell F) was moved axially to focus on objects from infinity to as close as 35 cm (13.8 in.). Two lens groups (Z1 and Z3) were mounted in the same structure (outer zoom carriage) so they moved together axially. A third lens group (Z2) moved axially in another structure (inner zoom carriage) in synchrony with the other zoom groups. Each carriage had two pairs of rollers located 120° apart that rode on smoothly SPDT-machined IDs of the lens housing. A third roller, at 120° to both the others, rode on a flat spring attached to the inside of the lens housing. Pressure exerted by the spring-loaded rollers kept the carriages in contact with the diamond-machined surfaces. The movements of the zoom lens groups were controlled by a multiple-slot cylindrical cam cut into a separate drive ring that fitted over the outside of the housing and ran on ball bearings (not shown). Cam followers attached to the zoom carriages passed through axially oriented slots in the housing to engage the cam slots. Each cam follower used dual rollers spring loaded apart to engage both sides of the cam slot, thereby eliminating backlash that could make the image jump whenever the direction of zoom was reversed.

The lenses were mounted in steel cells chosen to approximate the CTEs of the glasses. This permitted the use of minimal radial clearances between lenses and cells and improved thermal stability compared with designs using aluminum cells. During assembly, the cells were first aligned to the carriage and roller ODs by means of jigs. They then were bonded in place with a flexible adhesive (not specified by the author). Retaining rings were added after the adhesive had cured to ensure that the lenses were securely clamped in place axially.

Another example of a zoom lens mechanism may be found in Sect. 13.20.

References

1. Yoder, P.R., Jr., *Opto-Mechanical Systems Design*, 2nd ed., Marcel Dekker, New York, 1993.
2. Hopkins, R.E., "Some thoughts on lens mounting," *Opt. Eng.* Vol. 15, 428, 1976.
3. Brockway, E.M., and Nord, D.D., "Lens axial alignment method and apparatus," U.S. Patent No. 3,507,597, issued April 21, 1970.
4. Westort, K.S., "Design and fabrication of high-performance relay lenses," *SPIE Proceedings* Vol. 518, 21, 1984.
5. Addis, E.C., "Value engineering additives in optical sighting devices", *SPIE Proceedings* Vol. 389, 36, 1983.

132

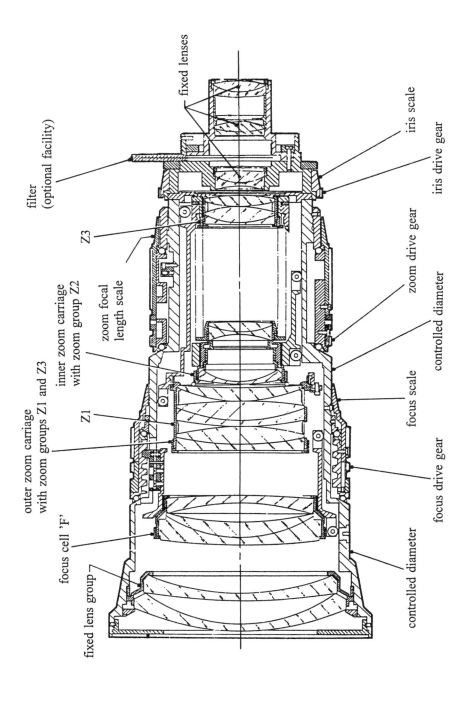

Fig. 4.37 Sectional view of a 20- to 100-mm (0.787- to 3.937-in.) focal length, f/2.8 zoom lens assembly. (From Ashton.[26])

6. Price, W.H., "Resolving optical design/manufacturing hang-ups," *SPIE Proceedings* Vol. 237, 466, 1980.

7. Yoder, P. R., Jr., "Lens mounting techniques," *SPIE Proceedings* Vol. 389, 2, 1983.

8. Bayar, M., "Lens barrel optomechanical design principles," *Opt. Eng.* Vol. 20, 181, 1981.

9. Yoder, P.R., Jr., "Optomechanical designs of two special-purpose objective lens assemblies," *SPIE Proceedings* Vol. 656, 225, 1986.

10. Richey, C.A., "Aerospace mounts for down-to-earth optics," in *Machine Des.* Vol. 46, 121, 1974. (Reprinted in *SPIE Proceedings* Vol. 770, 133, 1988.)

11. Hopkins, R.E., "Lens Mounting and Centering," Chapt. 2 in *Applied Optics and Optical Engineering,* Vol VIII, Academic Press, New York, 1980.

12. Carnell, K.H., Kidger, M.J., Overill, M.J., Reader, A.J., Reavell, F.C., Welford, W.T., and Wynne, C.G., "Some experiments on precision lens centering and mounting," *Optica Acta* Vol. 21, 615, 1974. (Reprinted in *SPIE Proceedings* Vol.770, 207, 1988.

13. Fischer, R.E., "Case study of elastomeric lens mounts," *SPIE Proceedings* Vol. 1533, 27, 1991.

14. Vukobratovich, D., "Optomechanical Systems Design," Chapt. 3 in *The Infrared & Electro-Optical Systems Handbook,* Vol. 4, ERIM, Ann Arbor and SPIE, Bellingham, 1993.

15. Vukobratovich, D., "Design and construction of an astrometric astrograph," *SPIE Proceedings* Vol. 1752, 1992, 245.

16. Bacich, J.J., "Precision lens mounting," U.S. Patent No. 4,733,945, issued March 29, 1988.

17. Lytle, J.D., "Polymeric Optics," Chapt. 34 in *OSA Handbook of Optics* Vol. II, Optical Society of America, Washington, 34.1, 1995.

18. Vukobratovich, D., "Modular optical alignment,", *SPIE Proceedings* Vol. 376, 427, 1999.

19. Trsar, W.J., Benjamin, R.J., and Casper, J.F., "Production engineering and implementation of a modular military binocular," *Opt. Eng.* Vol. 20, 201, 1981.

20. Section 19.5.1 in MIL-HDBK-141, *Military Standardization Handbook, Optical Design*, Defense Supply Agency, Washington, DC, 1962.

21. Manuccia, T.J., Peele, J.R., and Geosling, C.E., "High temperature ultrahigh vacuum infrared window seal," *Rev. Sci. Instr.* Vol. 52, 1981, 1857.

22. Kampe, T.U., Johnson, C.W., Healy, D.B., and Oschmann, J.M., "Optomechanical design considerations in the development of the DDLT laser diode collimator," *SPIE Proceedings* Vol. 1044, 46, 1989.

23. Quammen, M.L., Cassidy, P.J., Jordan, F.J., and Yoder, P.R., Jr., "Telescope eyepiece assembly with static and dynamic bellows-type seal," U.S. Patent No. 3,246,563, issued April 19, 1966.

24. Horne, D.F., *Optical Production Technology*, Adam Hilger, Bristol, England, 1972.

25. Fischer, R.E., and Kampe, T.U., "Actively controlled 5:1 afocal zoom attachment for common module FLIR," *SPIE Proceedings* Vol. 1690, 137, 1992.

26. Ashton, A., "Zoom lens systems," *SPIE Proceedings* Vol. 163, 92, 1979.

CHAPTER 5
Mounting Optical Windows, Filters, Shells, and Domes

The optical components considered in this chapter do not form images. They are intended either to act as a transparent barrier between the outside environment and the interior of the instrument or, in the case of a filter, to modify the spectral characteristics of the transmitted (or reflected) beam. Typically they have the form of plane parallel plates or meniscus-shaped elements (shells and domes). Materials include optical glass, fused silica, optical crystal, or plastic. With the exception of filters, these optics have as their prime purposes excluding dirt, moisture, and other contaminants and/or supporting a pressure differential between interior and exterior atmospheres. Critical aspects of mountings for these components include mechanically or thermally induced surface distortions, contact stresses, and sealing. Since most filters are plane parallel plates, their mountings are usually the same as those for flat windows. Location within the optical system of a window or a filter is important because the tolerances on defects such as surface deformation, wavefront tilt, and homogeneity of the index of refraction are more stringent near pupils than near images. Tolerances on component cleanliness, material inclusions, and surface blemishes (scratches and digs) are tighter near images than near pupils. In this chapter, we discuss typical mountings for various configurations of the optics of interest. The significance of component size relative to mounting technique is indicated where appropriate.

5.1 Simple Window Mountings

Figures 5.1 and 5.2 show typical mounting designs for round aperture windows used to seal the interiors of optical systems from the outside world.[1,2] In Fig. 5.1, the window is a 20-mm (0.79-in.) diameter by 4-mm (0.16-in.) thick disk of BK7 glass. It is intended to be used in the f/10 beam of a military telescope reticle projection subsystem near an image plane. The surfaces need only be flat to ±10 waves peak-to-valley (p-v) of visible light and parallel to 30 arcmin. The window is sealed in a stainless steel (303 CRES) cell with a polysulfide base sealing compound (EC801 made by 3M) according to U.S. military specification MIL-S-11031. This secures the window and forms an effective seal. Note that the glass references axially against a flat annular shoulder inside the cell and that the adhesive fills the space created by undercutting that shoulder. Uniformity of the encapsulating adhesive layer's radial thickness can easily be achieved by inserting shims between the glass and metal before the adhesive is injected. Ideally, any pressure differential should have the higher pressure on the left to avoid the possibility of applying excessive shear stress to the sealant joint.

An alternative configuration for this subassembly that has only slightly less reliability (because of the increased chance of pinholes in the seal) does not have the sealant injection holes. The sealant would then be carefully applied to the window rim and/or the cell inside diameter before inserting the window into the cell. With either design, any excess sealant should be cleaned from the window surfaces before it cures. The suitability of the seal can be inferred from observation of sealant bead continuity around the window rim or, preferably, checked by pressure proof testing.

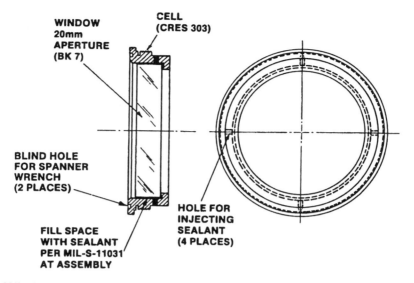

Fig. 5.1 Window subassembly with an elastomerically sealed-in-place glass optic. (From Yoder.[1])

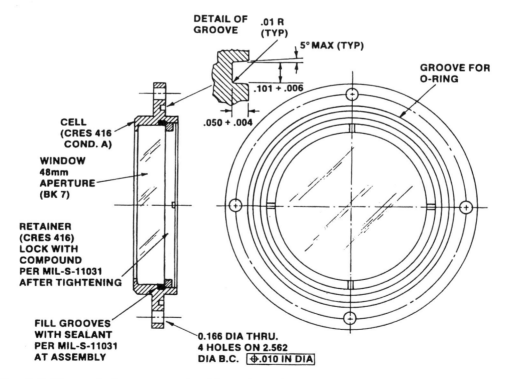

Fig. 5.2 Glass window constrained by a threaded retaining ring and sealed with elastomer. Dimensions are in inches. (From Yoder.[2])

The external thread on the cell mates with a threaded hole in the instrument housing. A flat gasket or O-ring would typically be used between the cell's flange and the housing to seal the interface.

The subassembly shown in Fig. 5.2 has a BK7 window of 50.8 mm (2.0 in.) diameter and 8.8 mm (0.346 in.) thickness sealed with military specification sealant in a stainless steel (416 CRES) cell and secured with a threaded retainer that also is made of stainless steel. This window is intended to be used as an environmental seal in front of the objective of a 10-power telescope.[2] The light beam transmitted through this window is collimated and nearly fills the clear aperture at all times, so the critical optical specifications are the transmitted wave-front error (±5 waves spherical power and 0.05 wave p-v irregularity for green light) and wedge angle (30 arcsec maximum).

In this design, the maximum and minimum radial clearances between glass and metal at ambient temperature are 0.265 mm (0.010 in.) and 0.110 mm (0.004 in.), respectively. As can be shown using equations to be found in Sect. 12.4, this clearance is sufficient to prevent excessive radial force from being exerted on the glass at the anticipated extreme low temperature of - 80°F (- 62°C).

The cell is provided with an annular groove for an O-ring that is used to seal the cell to the instrument housing at the next level of assembly. The dimensions of the groove are shown in the detail view. Note that the mounting holes are outside this seal. Screws used to attach the subassembly would thread into blind holes in the instrument housing. All the seals are designed to hold at least 5 lb/in.^{2} (3.45×10^4 N/m^2) positive pressure of dry nitrogen inside the telescope for an extended period. Since the retainer is on the inside, this pressure differential presses the window against the shoulder. Once again, pressure testing is advised to confirm the seal's integrity.

A compact vacuum-tight window assembly developed for cryogenic applications in a double-walled dewar was described by Haycock et al.[3] It is illustrated in Fig. 5.3. The window was germanium and had a racetrack-shaped aperture of about 5.25 by 1.30 in. (133.3 by 33.0 mm). Since a hermetic seal was required, a gasket of indium was compressed by a spring-loaded piston onto the heavily beveled rim of the window as shown in Fig. 5.4. Deflection of the spring plate provided sufficient total preload [(on the order of 530 lb (2350 N)] to hold the window in place at all temperatures between 77 K and 373 K and to create a peak compressive stress in the indium of about 1200 lb/in.^{2} (8.27 MPa).

The spring plate was slit radially at its inner boundary to distribute the force evenly around the edge of the window. Titanium was used for the spring because of its low CTE, high Young's modulus, and high strength. This plate resembles the circular flange discussed as a lens constraint in Sect. 3.4.2. The window frame was Nilo 42 (Ni_{42} Fe_{58}) which approximated the CTE of the germanium. The piston was aluminum for ease of fabrication to its unusual shape.

One important design parameter was the width at the narrower end (bottom) of the triangular gap into which the indium was pressed. A small dimension was needed to maintain the required pressure within the seal, but if too small, it would be difficult to

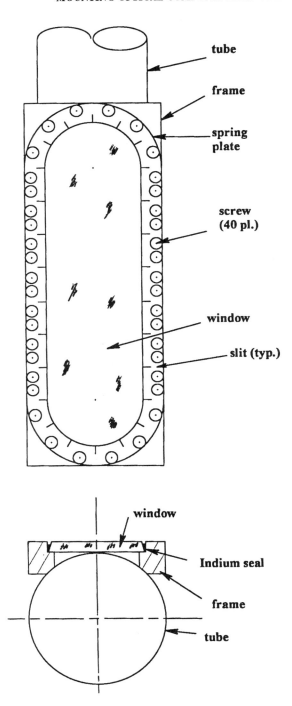

Fig. 5.3 Plan and end views of a cryogenic window assembly with pressure-loaded indium seal. (Adapted from Haycock et al.[3])

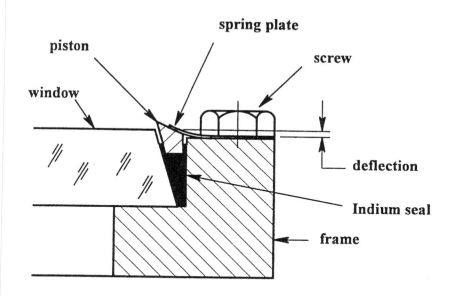

Fig. 5.4 Detail view of the pressure-loaded indium seal for the window assembly of Fig. 5.3. (Adapted from Haycock et al.[3])

assemble the seal with complete packing of the indium into the volume. It was found that a dimension of 0.010 in. (0.254 mm) was satisfactory for this application. Another critical dimension was the gap on either side of the piston under spring load. A value of 0.001 in. (25 μm) was appropriate to sufficiently minimize extrusion of the indium at higher temperatures so the seal would remain intact over time periods of the order of 1 week. Testing of the assembly at cryogenic temperature indicated that it was leakproof to the accuracy of the test apparatus (10^{-10} std atm cc/s) during and after repeated cycling (> 200 cycles) throughout the temperature range of 293 K to 77 K.

After reading the paper by Haycock et al.,[3] this author conjectured that a modification of their design in which an elastomeric "gasket" formed in place at the bottom of a triangular gap between a beveled window and its mount, or an O-ring in that same location, might be spring loaded with a piston in a manner similar to that described here. This would provide radially directed compression of the elastomer onto the rim of the window and seal it adequately for some noncryogenic applications such as those experienced in an aerospace-type apparatus. Because the rim of the window is heavily beveled, this would have the advantage of not requiring a separate means for providing preload normal to the window surface to press the window against its mounting interface.

5.2 Mounting "Special" Windows

In this "special" category we include windows for military electro-optical sensors [such as forward-looking infrared (FLIR) systems, low-light-level television (LLLTV) systems, laser range finder/target designator systems], for aerial and space-based reconnaissance and mapping cameras, and for optical systems in deep submergence vehicles. We do not consider windows used in high-energy laser systems because space limitations do not permit an adequate explanation of their complex design and their unique mounting problems. Readers interested in this type of window are referred to the voluminous literature on laser-induced effects on optical materials, including papers by Holmes and Avizonis,[4] Loomis,[5] Klein,[6-10] Klein and DeSalvo,[11] Palmer,[12] Weidler,[13] and the published reports from the annual symposium on laser-induced damage in optical materials (commonly known as the Boulder Damage Conference).

Most airborne electro-optical sensors and cameras are located within environmentally controlled equipment bays in the aircraft fuselage or in a wing-mounted pod. Typically, an optical window is provided to seal the bay or pod and to provide aerodynamic continuity of the enclosure. Its quality must be high and long lasting in spite of exposure to adverse environments. Single- and double-glazed configurations are used as dictated by thermal considerations. Both types are discussed here.

Figure 5.5 shows a window subassembly for a typical LLLTV camera utilizing light in the spectral region of 0.45 to 0.90 μm. Two plane parallel plates of crown glass are laminated together to form a single 19-mm (0.75-in.) thick glazing with an elliptical aperture measuring approximately 25 by 38 cm (9.8 by 15.0 in.). It is mounted in a

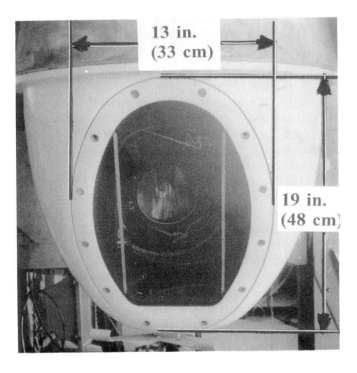

Fig. 5.5 An elliptically shaped laminated glass window used in a low-light-level television system mounted in an aircraft pod. (Adapted from Yoder.[1])

cast aluminum frame. The frame interfaces with the curved surface of the camera pod and is held in place by twelve screws as shown in the figure. The internal construction of this subassembly is shown schematically in the exploded view in Fig. 5.6. The wires connect to an electrically conductive coating applied to one glass plate before lamination. This coating provides heat for anti-icing and defogging purposes during a military mission. It also attenuates electromagnetic radiation. The exposed window is susceptible to erosion from impacts of particulate matter, rain, and/or ice, so it is designed so the optic can be replaced if it is damaged. The assembled window is sealed to allow no more than 0.1 lb/in.^{2} (6.9×10^2 Pa) air leakage each minute when the pod is pressurized at about 7.5

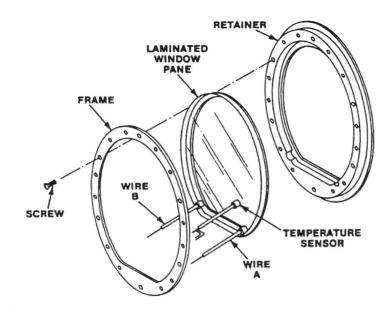

Fig. 5.6 Exploded view of the window subassembly shown in Fig. 5.5. (From Yoder.[1])

lb/in.^{2} (5.2×10^4 Pa) above ambient. The design is also capable of withstanding, without damage, a proof pressure differential of 11 lb/in.^{2} (7.6×10^4 Pa) in either direction. Both exposed surfaces of the window are broadband antireflection coated.

The multiaperture window assembly shown in Fig. 5.7 is designed for use in a military application involving a FLIR sensor operating in the spectral region 8 to 12 μm and a laser range finder/target designator system operating at 1.06 μm. The larger window is used by the FLIR system and is made of a single plate of chemical vapor-deposited (CVD) zinc sulfide (ZnS) approximately 1.6 cm (0.63 in.) thick. Its aperture is 30 by 43 cm (11.8 by 16.9 in.). The smaller windows are similar and have elliptical apertures of 9 by 17 cm (3.5 by 6.7 in.). They are used by the laser transmitter and receiver systems and are made of BK7 glass 1.6 cm (0.63 in.) thick. All surfaces are appropriately antireflection coated for maximum transmission at the specified wavelengths at a 47°±5° angle of incidence. Robinson et al.[14] indicated that the coatings also resist erosion caused by rain at a rate of 1 in. (2.5 cm) per hour with an impact velocity approaching 500 mi/hr (224 m/sec) for at least 20 min. The specifications for transmitted wave-front quality are 0. 1 wave p-v at 10.6 µm over any 2.5 cm (1 in.) diameter instantaneous aperture for the FLIR window and 0.2 wave p-v power, plus 0. 1 wave irregularity at 0.63 µm over the full apertures for the laser windows.

The CVD ZnS used in this design is not an easy material with which to work. Fortunately, it transmits in the visible adequately enough for the optician to identify the volume within an oversized raw material blank where the element should be located in order to avoid the worst inclusions and bubbles.

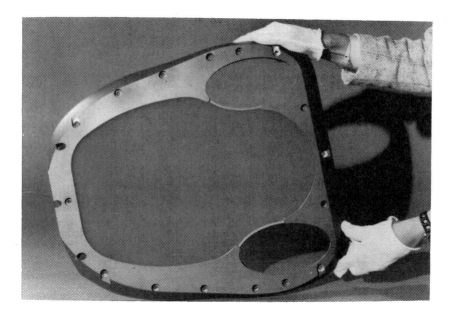

Fig. 5.7 A multi-aperture window subassembly. The larger element is IR-transmitting zinc sulfide while the smaller ones are BK7 optical glass. (From Yoder[2])

The mechanical strength of the ZnS and BK7 glazings is maximized by controlled removal of material using progressively finer abrasives during grinding as described by Stoll et al.[15] to ensure that all subsurface damage caused by previous operations has been removed. This process is called "controlled grinding." The wedge is brought within specified limits (66 arcsec maximum for the ZnS element and 30 arcsec maximum for the BK7 elements) during this grinding process. The edges of all windows are control ground and cloth polished, primarily to maximize strength. This multistep grinding followed by polishing minimizes the risk of breakage from forces imposed by the mounting, shock and vibration, or temperature changes. All three glazings are bonded with adhesive into a lightweight frame made of 6061-T651 aluminum plate anodized after machining to the complex contours shown in Fig. 5.7. The bonded assembly is attached to the aircraft pod by screws through several recessed holes around the edge of the frame. The mating surfaces of the frame and pod must match closely in contour in order not to deform the optics or disturb the seals.

Figure 5.8 illustrates a segmented window subassembly typical of those used with panoramic aerial cameras designed to photograph from horizon to horizon transverse to the flight path of an aircraft. The size of the window required for use with such a camera is determined primarily by the location and size of the lens's entrance pupil and the camera's field of view. In this case, these dimensions are 4.5 in. (11.4 cm) and ±7.125°, respectively.

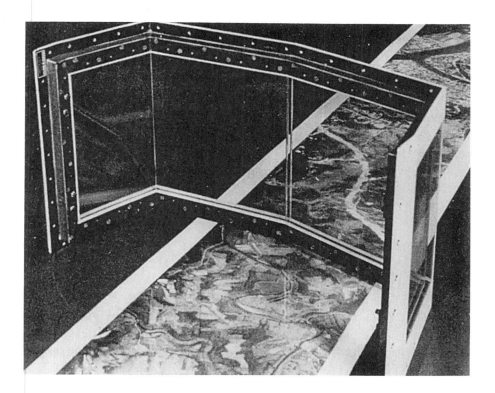

Fig. 5.8 Segmented window subassembly used with a military panoramic aerial camera to photograph horizon to horizon. A simulated strip photo of the type taken through such a window is also shown. (From Yoder.[1])

The window in Fig. 5.8 is of dual-pane construction with fused silica glazings outside and BK7 glass glazings inside. Since the aircraft flies at high velocity, the most critical design problem here is thermal. Boundary-layer effects heat the outer window glazing and since that material is a good blackbody with an emissivity of about 0.9, it would normally radiate heat into the camera and its surrounding equipment. To combat this deleterious effect, the inside surfaces of the outer glazings are coated with a low-emissivity (gold) coating. All other window surfaces are conventionally antireflection coated to maximize transmission in the film sensitivity spectral region.

The square elements in the center of the window subassembly have dimensions of approximately 12.6 by 13.0 in. (32 by 33 cm) and are 0.4 in. (1.0 cm) thick. The side glazings are somewhat smaller in one dimension. The glazings are separated by a few millimeters. Conditioned air from the aircraft is circulated through the space between the glazings before and during flight.

The adjacent edges of the individual elements in each of the inner and outer glazings of this segmented window are beveled and polished. These edges are cemented with flexible adhesive. As indicated in Fig. 5.9, the glass elements are sealed into recesses machined into the aluminum frame with an elastomeric-type adhesive and secured by a metal retainer. The contours of the subassembly and its mounting hole pattern are made to match those of the aircraft interface by reference to special tooling and fixtures.

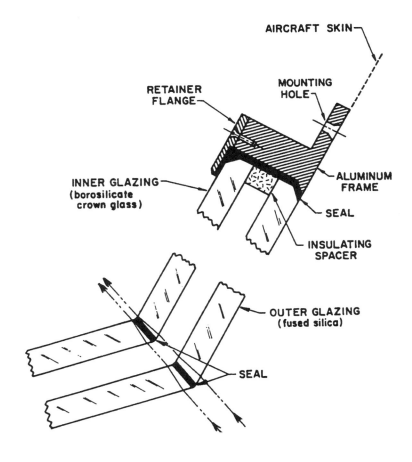

Fig. 5.9 Partial schematic of a double-glazed, multisegment aerial camera window of the type shown in Fig. 5.8. Note how refraction minimizes the obscuration at the joints. (From Yoder.[1])

5.3 Windows Subject to Pressure Differential

When a plane parallel circular window is subjected to a pressure differential ΔP applied uniformly over an unsupported aperture A, the minimum value for its thickness t_w to provide a safety factor of f_S over the material's yield strength S_F should be as given by Eq. (5.1): [16]

$$t_w = [0.5 A_w][(K_w f_s \Delta P_w)/S_F]^{1/2} \qquad (5.1)$$

where:

$\quad$ K_w = a support condition constant = 1.25 (if unclamped)
$\quad$ $\qquad\qquad\qquad\qquad\qquad\qquad$ = 0.75 (if clamped)

Figure 5.10 illustrates the two types of constraint at the window's edge. The unclamped condition applies approximately if the window is supported by an annular ring of elastomer as described in Sect. 3.7. Maximum stress occurs at the center of this window. The clamped condition applies if a retainer or circular flange is used. Maximum stress then occurs at the edge of the clamped area. The customary value for f_S is 4. Typical minimum values for S_F at room temperature for some commonly used infrared window materials as given by Harris[16] are listed in Table B16.

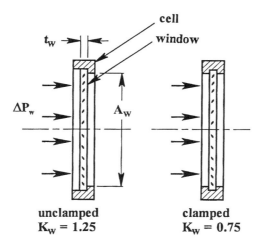

unclamped
$K_W = 1.25$

clamped
$K_W = 0.75$

Fig. 5.10 Schematic diagrams of (a) an unclamped circular window and (b) a clamped circular window. (Adapted from Harris.[16])

Example 5.1: Thickness required of a circular window to safely withstand a given pressure differential.
(For design and analysis, use Files 11.1 & 11.2 of the CD-ROM)
A sapphire window with an unsupported aperture of 14 cm (5.51 in.) is subjected

to a pressure differential of 10 atm (147 lb/in.^{2} or 1.01 MPa). Assuming a safety factor f_S of 4, (a) what should its thickness be if it is potted into its mount with a ring of RTV elastomer (i.e., unclamped)? (b) what should its thickness be if it is clamped?

(a) From Table B16, the minimum S_F for sapphire is approximately 300 MPa (43,511 lb/in.^{2}).

By Eq. (5.1), $t_w = [(0.5)(14)][(1.25)(4)(1.01))/300]^{1/2} = 0.909$ cm (0.358 in.)

(b) By examination of Eq. (5.1), $t_{w\ CLAMPED}/t_{w\ UNCLAMPED} = (0.75/1.25)^{1/2} = 0.775$

Therefore, clamping the window allows the thickness to be reduced to:

$(0.775)(0.909) = 0.704$ cm (0.277 in.)

Dunn and Stachiw[17] investigated the thickness-to-unsupported diameter ratio t_w/A_w for the relatively thick plane parallel plate and conical-rim windows typically used in deep submergence vehicles that experience large pressure differentials. The material they considered was Rohm and Haas grade B Plexiglas (polymethylmethacrylate). The parameters varied included diameter, thickness, pressure differential, mounting flange configuration, and in the case of the conical windows, the included cone angle (from 30° to 150°). During testing, the pressure was increased at a rate of 600 to 700 lb/in.^{2} (4.13×10^6 to 4.83×10^6 Pa) per minute to failure. The cold-flow displacement (extrusion) of the window material into the lower-pressure space was also measured. The strength of conical windows was found to increase nonlinearly with the included cone angle, the greatest improvements coming at the lower end of the angular range. Flat windows and 90° conical windows of the same t_w/A_w ratio were found to fail at approximately the same critical loading. Typically, a 1.0-in. (2.5-cm) diameter 90° window of $t_w/A_w = 0.5$ failed at about 16,000 lb/in.^{2} (1.10×10^6 Pa). It was concluded from this study that the failure pressure differential scales as the t_w/A_w ratio.

Two typical high pressure window design configurations are shown in Fig. 5.11. The 90° conical window of Fig. 5.11(a) is supported along its entire rim, and its inner surface is flush with the smaller end of the conical mounting surface. The retainer compresses the neoprene gasket enough to constrain the window at low pressure differentials. The flat window in Fig. 5.11(b) is sealed with an O-ring midway along its rim and it is kept from falling out at zero pressure differential by a retaining ring. The rims of both windows were coated with vacuum grease prior to assembly. Dunn and Stachiw did not specify complete details for these operational designs, but one can infer that the tolerances reported for the experimental versions would also apply. Accordingly, the conical angles were held to ±30 arcmin, minor diameters of conical windows were held to ±0.001 in. (25 µm), window rims and mating metal surfaces were finished to a rms finish of 32. A radial clearance of 0.005 to 0.010 in. (0.13 to 0.25 mm) was typically provided around flat windows.

These parametric study results typically indicate that for $A_w = 4.0$ in. (10.2 cm),

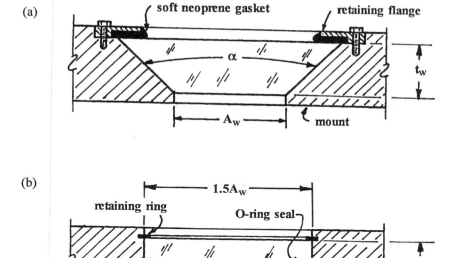

Fig. 5.11 Typical high-pressure plane parallel polymethylmethacrylate window configurations for deep submergence vehicles. (a) 90° conical rim and (b) cylindrical rim. (Adapted from Dunn and Stachiw.[17])

the windows should be 2.0 in. (5.1 cm) thick. Failure would be anticipated at about 4000 lb/in.^{2} (2.70×10^7 Pa). The window's material would be expected to extrude through the aperture of the mount by about 0.5 in. (1.3 cm) at the time of failure. The authors wisely recommended proof-testing all windows intended for man-rated applications.

5.4 Filter Mountings

Glass and better-quality plastic absorption filters are employed extensively in photography, photometers, chemical analysis equipment, and slide projectors. Glass interference filters used singly or in combination with absorption (blocking) filters are convenient means for isolating specific narrow transmission bands in systems such as those using lasers. These filters generally require temperature control. Gelatine filters are noted for their low cost and wide variety. Inhomogeneities of optical quality, thickness variations, and surface figure errors, as well as low mechanical strength and poor durability, limit their use to rather low-performance applications. They are generally used in protected environments. If the gelatine is sandwiched between transparent plates of a more durable material such as glass, physical strength and durability can be greatly improved.

Many applications for optical filters require only that the component be supported approximately centered in and roughly aligned normal to the transmitted light beam. In fixed laboratory instruments, the filter can be simply dropped into a slot and held by gravity. Cell mountings such as the burnished, snap-ring, elastomeric, and retaining ring designs described in Chapter 3 for lens elements are frequently employed to hold filters in other instruments. Heat-absorbing filters for projectors and other high-temperature applications are typically restrained by spring clips that allow thermal expansion. Interference filters require precise angular orientation to the beam so strict attention must be paid to that aspect of their mounting design.

Some thin filters are cemented to a refracting substrate (i.e., a window) that provides mechanical rigidity or environmental protection to the subassembly. A typical example is shown in Fig. 5.12. In this case, a 1.2-mm (0.05-in.)-thick sheet of red filter glass is cemented with conventional optical cement to a crown glass window of 7.5 mm (0.30 in.) axial thickness. The 88-mm (3.46-in.)-diameter subassembly serves two purposes: It transmits properly in the spectral region characteristic of the filter and it is sufficiently stiff to function as a window to seal an optical instrument against a 0.5-atm

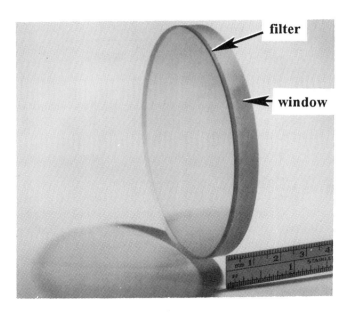

Fig. 5.12 A laminated filter and pressure window. (Adapted from Yoder.[1])

pressure differential. The composite construction was chosen to avoid the excessive light loss that would occur if the entire 8.70-mm (0.342-in.) thickness were made of filter glass. The maximum pressure-induced sag of the filter was specified to be one wave of red light. This amount of bending would not be sufficient to damage the cemented interface.

If we consider the laminated component to be a homogeneous disk, we can verify the window design with the help of Eq. (5.2), which was adapted from Roark as given

$$\Delta y = K_w D_G^4 / (16 t_w^3) \qquad\qquad (5.2)$$

where:

$$K_w = 0.1875(1 - v^2)\Delta P_w / E_G \qquad\qquad (5.3)$$

and:

Δy = sag of deformed surface at its center
D_G = diameter of window that is exposed to the pressure differential
t_w = window thickness
υ = Poisson's ratio of the glass
ΔP_w = unit applied load = $(a_p)(14.7 \text{ lb/in.}^2)$ or $(a_p)(0.1014 \text{ MPa})$
a_p = pressure differential factor (times 1 atm)
E_G = Young's modulus of the glass

Example 5.2: Deflection of a clamped circular window under a specified pressure differential.
(For design and analysis, use File 12 of the CD-ROM)
The filter/window of Fig. 5.12 is clamped around its edge, leaving a diameter of 3.250 in. (82.550 mm) exposed to a pressure differential of 0.5 atm. Assume that the window is homogeneous BK7 glass and 0.342 in. (8.700 mm) thick. What is its central deflection? Compare this deflection to a tolerance of 1.0 wave at $\lambda = 0.633$ μm (2.492×10^{-5} in.).

From Table B1: $E_G = 1.17 \times 10^7$ lb/in.^{2} (8.067×10^4 MPa) $\upsilon_G = 0.208$

From Eq. (5.3): $K_w = 0.1875(1 - 0.208^2)(14.700/2)/1.17 \times 10^7 = 1.127 \times 10^{-7}$

$a_p = 0.5$
$\Delta P_w = (0.5)(14.7) = 7.350$ lb/in.^{2} (0.051 MPa)

From Eq. (5.2): $\Delta y = (1.127 \times 10^{-7})(3.250/2)^4 / [(16)(0.342^3)]$
$= 1.964 \times 10^{-5}$ in. (4.989×10^{-4} mm)

Dividing by the wavelength, we find that $\Delta y = 0.788$ wave

The filter/window would be expected to meet the stated deflection requirement.

Another laminated filter is shown in Fig. 5.13. This is a composite filter consisting of a mosaic of narrow bandpass interference filter elements cemented between two 290-mm (11.4-in.) diameter crown glass plates. The thicknesses of the plates and of the filters were nominally 6 mm (0.24 in.) and all had the same thickness within 0.1 mm

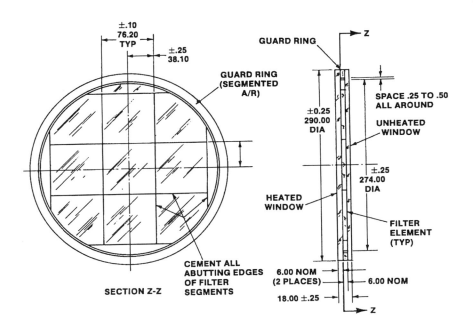

Fig. 5.13 Composite filter design consisting of a laminated and heated mosaic of interference filter elements. (From Yoder.[1])

(0.004 in.). Rather than controlling the wedge angles of the filter elements to an extremely tight tolerance, they were made to a "reasonable" wedge tolerance and oriented variously at assembly to minimize average deviation. This was permissible since the filter was intended for a nonimage-forming application. The outside diameter of the filter mosaic was made somewhat smaller than the outside diameters of the windows so that an annular "guard ring" made up of crown glass segments could be cemented between the windows to protect the edges of the interference filter coatings from the environment. The outside diameter of the assembly was edged after cementing.

Since a narrow-bandpass filter is temperature sensitive, wire heater conductors were built into the double-laminated window in the form of a grid, and a temperature sensor (mounted on one window surface outside the clear aperture) was used to drive a temperature control electrical circuit in the instrument. The temperature setting was slightly above the anticipated ambient for the application.

The cemented filter assembly described here was mounted in an aluminum cell and clamped around its edge by a retaining flange secured to the cell with several screws. Two O-rings and a flat gasket sealed the assembly. Figure 5.14 shows a sectional view through the mount. The assembly was not intended to be exposed to a significant pressure differential. The cell was insulated thermally with G10 phenolic from the body of the optical instrument of which it was a part, and heat was supplied to the cell by the strip heater indicated in the figure. The filter was designed for a nominal temperature of 45°C (113°F) and to have a spectral passband with a nominal full-width-to-half-maximum of

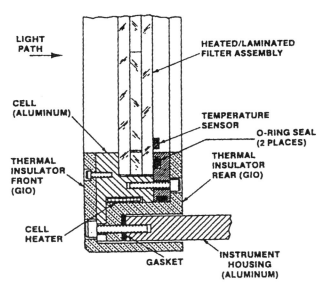

Fig. 5.14 Schematic sectional view of the mount for the filter subassembly shown in Fig. 5.13. (From Yoder.[1])

30 Å centered at a specific near-infrared laser wavelength. Out-of-passband radiation was blocked with a separate absorption filter of conventional design elsewhere in the system.

5.5 Mounting Shells and Domes

Meniscus-shaped windows are usually called "shells" or "domes." They are commonly used on electro-optical sensors requiring access to large fields of view by scanning a line of sight over a large conical space and in wide-field astronomical telescope objectives such as the Bouwers, Maksutov, or Gabor types (see Kingslake[19]). They also are frequently used as protective windows for underwater vehicles. Hyperhemispheres are domes that extend beyond 180° angular extent. An example is shown in Fig. 5.15. The outside diameter of this optic is 127 mm (5.0 in.), the dome thickness is 5 mm (0.2 in.), and the angular aperture is approximately 210°. This dome is made of crown glass; many other domes are made of infrared-transmitting materials such as fused silica, zinc sulfide, zinc selenide, silicon, magnesium fluoride, sapphire, spinel, and CVD diamond. With the exception of fused silica and diamond, which are relatively durable, these materials are susceptible to erosion and other damage caused by exposure to moisture and contaminants in the atmosphere, especially at high velocity.

Domes are typically mounted on instrument housings by potting them with elastomers or clamping them through soft gaskets with ring-shaped flanges. Figure 5.16 illustrates three of these techniques. Hard mounting of these optics against metal mechanical interfaces and constraint by metal retainers is generally not attempted.

Harris[14] discussed methods for designing a dome that would be resistant to the magnitude of pressure load that would be experienced if the dome were at the leading edge of a missile or airborne sensor in high-velocity flight. He also explained why domes

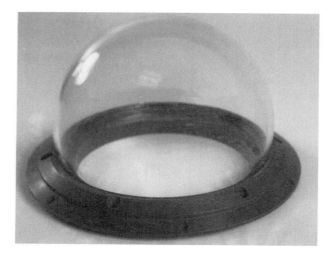

Fig. 5.15 A crown glass hyperhemispheric dome potted with elastomer into a metal flange. Dimensions are given in the text.

reach high temperatures during such flights.

References

1. Yoder, P.R., Jr., *Opto-Mechanical Systems Design*, 2nd ed., Marcel Dekker, New York, 1993.

2. Yoder, P.R., Jr., "Non-image forming optical components," *SPIE Proceedings* Vol. 531, 1985, 206.

3. Haycock, R.H., Tritchew, S., and Jennison, P., "A compact Indium seal for cryogenic optical windows." *SPIE Proceedings* Vol.1340, 165, 1990

4. Holmes, D.A. and Avizonis, P.V. (1976). "Approximate Optical System Model", *Appl. Opt.* Vol. 15, 1075, 1976.

5. Loomis, J.S., "Optical quality of laser windows", *Proceedings 4th Conference on Infrared Laser Window Materials*, Air Force Material Labs., Wright Patterson AFB, 1976.

6. Klein, C.A., "Methodology for designing high-energy laser windows," in *Proceedings International Conference on Lasers '78*, STS Press, McLean, 1978.

7. Klein, C.A. "Thermally induced optical distortion in high energy laser systems", *Opt. Eng.* Vol. 18, 591, 1979.

8. Klein, C.A. "Mirrors and windows in power optics," *SPIE Proceedings* Vol. 216, 204, 1980.

9. Klein, C. A. "Optical distortion coefficients of laser windows - one more time," *SPIE Proceedings* Vol. 1047, 58, 1989.

10. Klein, C.A., "Pulsed laser-induced damage to diamond," *Diamond Films and Technology* Vol. 5, 141, 1995.

11. Klein, C.A., and DeSalvo, R., "Thresholds for dielectric breakdown in laser-irradiated diamond," *Appl. Phys. Lett.,* Vol. 63, 1895, 1993.

153

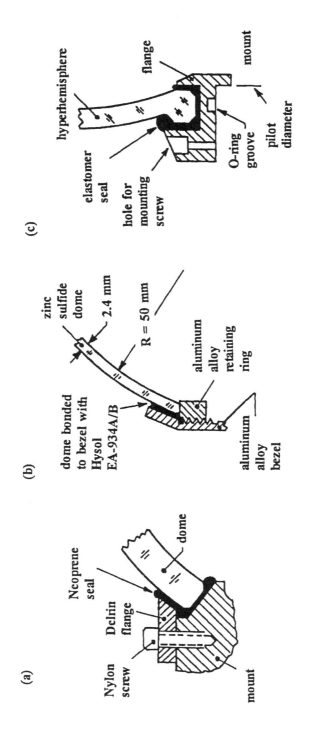

Fig. 5.16 Three configurations for dome mountings. (a) Dome clamped through a soft gasket with a flange. (Adapted from Vukobratovich.[20]) (b) Dome constrained by an internal retainer. (Adapted from Speare and Belloli.[21]) (c) Hyperhemisphere potted with elastomer, (Adapted from Yoder.[1])

12. Palmer, J.R., "Thermal shock: catastrophic damage to transmissive optical components in high power CW and repetitive pulsed laser environments," *SPIE Proceedings* Vol. 1047, 87, 1989.

13. Weidler, D.E., "Large exit windows for high power beam directors," *SPIE Proceedings Vol. 1047*, 153, 1989.

14. Robinson, B., Eastman, D.R., Bacevic, J., Jr., and O'Neill, B.J., "Infrared window manufacturing technology," *SPIE Proceedings* Vol. 430, 302, 1983.

15. Stoll, R., Forman, P.F., and Edleman, J. "The effect of different grinding procedures on the strength of scratched and unscratched fused silica," *Proceedings of Symposium on the Strength of Glass and Ways to Improve It*, Union Scientifique Continentale du Verre, Charleroi, Belgium, 1, 1961.

16. Harris, D.C., *Materials for Infrared Windows and Domes, Properties and Performance*, SPIE Press, Bellingham, 1999.

17. Dunn, G., and Stachiw, J., "Acrylic windows for underwater structures," *SPIE Proceedings* Vol. 7, D-XX-1, 1966.

18. Young, W.C., *Roark's Formulas for Stress & Strain*, 6th ed., McGraw-Hill, New York, 429, 1989.

19. Kingslake, R., *Lens Design Fundamentals*, Academic Press, New York, 311, 1978.

20. Vukobratovich, D., "Introduction to Opto-Mechanical Design," *SPIE Short Course Notes*, SPIE Press, Bellingham, 1986.

21. Speare, J., and Belioli, A. "Structural mechanics of a mortar launched IR dome," *SPIE Proceedings* Vol. 450, 182, 1983.

CHAPTER 6
Prism Design

Many types of prisms have been designed for use in various optical instrument applications. Most have unique shapes as demanded by the geometry of the ray paths, reflection and refraction requirements, compatability with manufacture, weight reduction considerations, and provisions for mounting. Before we consider how to mount these prisms, we should understand how they are designed. Our first topics in this chapter are refractive effects, total internal reflection, and the construction and use of tunnel diagrams. We then see how to determine aperture requirements and reference analytical means for calculating third-order aberration contributions from prisms. The chapter closes with design information for 27 types of individual prisms and prism combinations frequently encountered in optical instrument design.

6.1 Geometric Considerations

6.1.1 Refraction and reflection

The laws of refraction and reflection of light govern the passage of rays through prisms and mirrors. In Fig. 6.1, we see a comparison of ray paths from an object passing

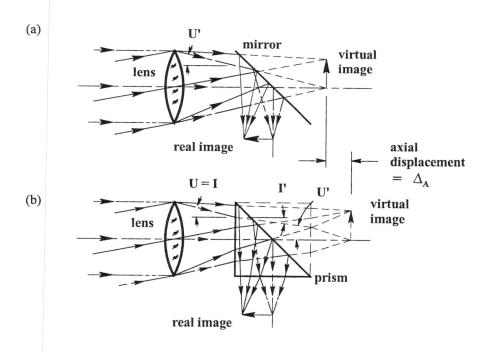

Fig. 6.1 Illustrations of 90° deviations by reflection of rays (a) at a 45° mirror and (b) in a right-angle prism. In (b), angles U, U', I, and I' pertain to the first surface of the prism.

155

through a lens and a reflector en route to the image. In Fig. 6.1(a), the reflector is a flat mirror while in Fig. 6.1(b) it is a right-angle prism in which reflection occurs at an internal surface. The most significant differences are the ray deviations that occur at the prism's refracting surfaces and the axial displacement of the image caused by the replacement of air by glass in part of the path. Refraction, of course, follows Snell's law, which may be written as:

$$n_j \sin I_j = n'_j \sin I'_j \tag{6.1}$$

where n_j and n'_j are the refractive indices in object and image spaces of surface "j", and I_j and I'_j are the ray angles of incidence and refraction, respectively, at that surface. Reflection follows the familiar relationship:

$$I'_j = I_j \tag{6.2}$$

where I_j and I'_j are the values of the ray angles of incidence and reflection at surface "j." The angles in these equations are measured with respect to the surface normal at the point of incidence of the ray on the surface or the axis. The algebraic signs of the angles are not shown in either of these equations.

The entrance and exit faces of most prisms are oriented perpendicular to the optical axis of the optical system since this promotes symmetry and reduces aberrations for noncollimated beams passing through the prism. Notable exceptions are the Dove prism, the double-Dove prism, wedge prisms, and prisms used to disperse light in monochromators and spectrographs.

A prism with faces normal to the optical axis refracts rays exactly as would a plane parallel plate oriented normal to the axis. The geometrical path length, t_A, through the prism measured along the axis is the same as the thickness of the plate. Any reflections occurring inside the prism do not affect this behavior. The axial displacement, Δ_A (see Fig. 6.1), of an image formed by rays passing through the prism is given by:

$$\Delta_A = t_A(1 - \frac{\tan U'}{\tan U}) = \frac{t_A}{n}(n - \frac{\cos U}{\cos U'}) \tag{6.3}$$

For small angles, this equation reduces to the paraxial version:

$$\Delta_A = (n - 1)t_A/n \tag{6.4}$$

Example 6.1: Image axial displacement due to insertion of a prism.
(For design and analysis, use File 13, of the CD-ROM)
Assume that an aplanatic lens images a distant object with a f/4 beam. How much does the image move axially (a) exactly and (b) paraxially when a right-angle prism

made of FN11 glass with thickness t_A = 38.1 mm (1.50 in.) is inserted in the beam?

(a) The marginal ray angle for this f/4 beam is sin U' = 0.5/(f-no.) = 0.5/4
= 0.1250   Hence, U' = 7.1808°

From Table B2, the refractive index for FN11 glass is 1.621.

Since the entrance face of the prism is normal to the axis, I = U' so, by Eq. (6.1),
sin I' = sin 7.1808°/1.621 = 0.07711   and I' = 4.4226°

By Eq. (6.4), the image moves by
Δ_A = (38.1/1.621)[1.621 - (cos 7.1808°/cos 4.4226°)]
= 14.711 mm (0.579 in.)

(b) By Eq. (6.5), the paraxial approximation of this displacement is
Δ_A = (1.621 - 1)(38.1)/1.621 = 14.596 mm (0.575 in.)

Reflection within a prism folds the light path. In Fig. 6.1(b), the object (an arrow, not shown) is imaged by the lens through the prism as the indicated virtual image. After reflection, the real image is located as shown. If the page were to be folded along the line representing the reflecting surface, the real image and the solid-line rays would coincide exactly with the virtual image and the dashed-line rays. A diagram showing both the original prism (ABC) and the folded counterpart (ABC') is called a "tunnel diagram" (see Fig. 6.2). The rays a-a' and b-b' represent actual reflected paths, while rays a-a" and b-b" appear to pass directly through the folded prism with proper refraction, but without the reflection. Multiple reflections are handled by successive folds of the page. This type of diagram, which can be drawn for any prism, is particularly helpful when designing an optical instrument using prisms since it simplifes the estimation of required apertures and hence the size of those prisms.

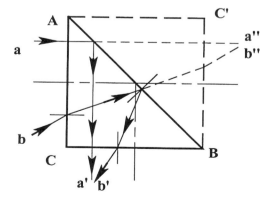

Fig. 6.2 Illustration of a tunnel diagram for a right-angle prism.

To illustrate the use of a tunnel diagram, let us consider the telescope optical system of Fig. 6.3. This could be a spotting telescope or one side of a binocular. The pair

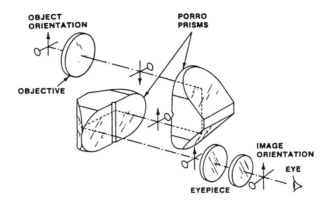

Fig. 6.3 Optical system of a typical telescope with a Porro prism erecting system. (From Yoder.[1])

of Porro prisms serve to erect the image as indicated by the "arrow crossed with a drumstick" symbols at various locations in the figure. Figure 6.4(a) shows the front portion of the same system with the Porro prisms represented by tunnel diagrams. Folds in the light path are indicated by the diagonal lines. We designate all the prism apertures as "A"; the axial path length of each prism is then 2A. In Fig. 6.4(b) the prism path lengths are shown as 2A/n; these are the thicknesses of air optically equivalent to the physical paths through the prisms. The air-equivalent thickness is sometimes called the "reduced thickness." In a reduced thickness diagram, the marginal rays converging to the axial image point can be drawn as straight lines (i.e., without refraction). The ray heights at each prism surface (including the reflecting surfaces) are paraxial approximations of the true values that would be obtained by trigonometric ray tracing. Paraxially, angles in radians replace the sines of the angles. In most applications, this degree of approximation is adequate. For example, an angle of 7° is 0.12217 radians and its sine is 0.12187. The differences between these values are not significant for prism design purposes.

Smith used tunnel diagrams to illustrate the determination of the minimum Porro prism apertures required for use in a typical prism erecting telescope.[2] With a diagram similar to Fig. 6.4(b), he noted that the proportion of face width A_i to reduced thickness was A_i: $(2A_i/n_i)$ or $n_i/2$. He then redrew the diagram in the form shown in Fig. 6.5 to facilitate calculating the minimum value for A_1 and A_2. The dashed lines drawn from the top front prism corners to the opposite vertices both have slopes, m, equalling one-half the ratio just derived or $n_i/4$. These lines are loci of the corners of a family of prisms with the proper proportions. The intersections of these two dashed lines with the outermost full-field ray (frequently called the "upper rim ray" or URR) locate the corners of the two Porro prisms. Note that the air spaces between optical components must be known for this procedure to succeed.

(a)

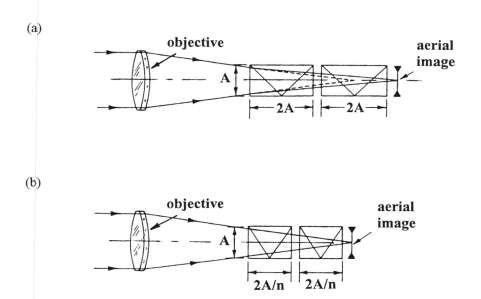

(b)

Fig. 6.4 Lens and Porro prisms from Fig. 6.3 with prisms shown (a) by conventional tunnel diagrams and (b) by tunnel diagrams with reduced (air equivalent) thicknesses. (Adapted from Smith.[2])

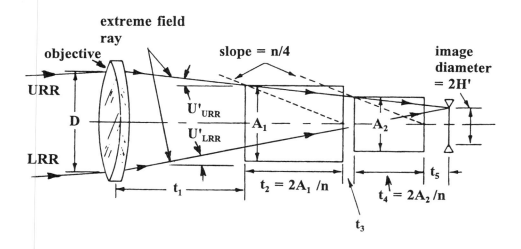

Fig. 6.5 Determination of minimum prism apertures from geometric proportions and the outermost unvignetted upper full-field (rim) ray (URR). The corresponding lower field (rim) ray (LRR) is used to determine the ability of the prisms to function by total internal reflection (TIR). (Adapted from Smith.[2])

It is easy to see from Fig. 6.5 that the slope of the URR is

$$\tan U'_{URR} = \frac{[(D/2) - H']}{EFL_{OBJ}} \tag{6.5}$$

and that the semiaperture of the second prism is $A_2/2 = H' + (t_4 + t_5)(\tan U')$. This semiaperture also is given by the expression $A_2/2 = (m)(t_4) = (n_i)(t_4)/4$. Equating these expressions for A_2 , we find that the thickness of the second prism is

$$t_4 = \frac{(t_5)(\tan U'_{URR}) + H'}{(n_i/4) - \tan U'_{URR}} \tag{6.6}$$

and

$$A_2 = (n_i)(t_4)/2 \tag{6.7}$$

By similar logic, we can write expressions for the axial thickness and aperture of the first Porro prism:

$$t_2 = \frac{(t_3 + t_4 + t_5)(\tan U'_{URR}) + H'}{(n_i/4) - \tan U'_{URR}} \tag{6.8}$$

and

$$A_1 = (n_i)(t_2)/2 \tag{6.9}$$

The apertures derived by these calculations should be confirmed by more precise techniques, such as ray tracing, especially if a specific amount of vignetting is needed for off-axis aberration control. To allow for protective bevels and dimensional tolerances, we might need to increase the apertures of both prisms by small amounts, such as a few percent of their apertures.

Example 6.2: Calculation of prism size.
(For design and analysis, use File 14 of the CD-ROM)
Find the minimum apertures of both prisms in a system as in Fig. 6.5 if EFL_{OBJ} = 177.800 mm (7.000 in.), objective aperture = 50 mm (1.968 in.), image diameter = 15.875 mm (0.625 in.), t_3 = 3.175 mm (0.125 in.), t_5 = 12.7 mm (0.500 in.), and prism index = 1.500.

By Eq. (6.5), $\tan U'_{URR}$ = [(50.000/2) - (15.875/2)]/177.800 = 0.09596

$U'_{URR} = 5.481°$

By Eq. (6.6), $t_4 = [(12.700)(0.09596) + (15.875/2)]/[(1.5/4) - 0.09596]$
                     $= 32.801$ mm (1.291 in.)

By Eq. (6.7),
                 $A_2 = (1.5)(32.813)/2 = 24.601$ mm (0.968 in.)

By Eq. (6.8), $t_2 = [(3.175 + 32.801 + 12.700)(0.09596)$
                       $+ (15.875/2)]/[(1.5/4) - 0.09596] = 45.185$ mm (1.779 in.)

By Eq. (6.9), $A_1 = (1.5)(45.185)/2 = 33.889$ mm (1.334 in.)

The general geometric technique just described can be adapted to determine the required apertures of other types of prisms used in converging or diverging beams.

6.1.2 Total internal reflection

A special case of refraction can occur when a ray is incident upon an interface where n is greater than n' as, for example, at the hypotenuse surface (surface 2) inside a right-angle prism. In the last section we assumed that all rays would reflect, as indeed they would if the surface had a reflective coating such as silver or aluminum. If that surface is uncoated, however, Snell's law [Eq. (6.1)] says that for small angles of incidence and low values of prism index, a ray can refract through that surface into the surrounding air, (see ray a-a' in Fig. 6.6). This ray is vignetted and does not contribute to the image formed below the prism. If we increase the ray angle I_2, the angle I'_2 also increases. For some value of I_2, I'_2 can reach 90°. Then sin I'_2 is unity. Since this sine cannot exceed unity, we find that for still larger values of I_2, the ray reflects internally

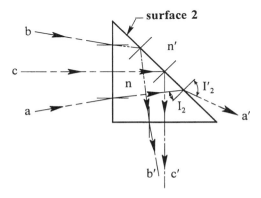

Fig. 6.6 Ray paths through an unsilvered right-angle prism of low refractive index. Ray a-a' is at an angle of incidence I_2 smaller than I_c so it "leaks" through the surface, while I_2 for each of rays b-b' and c-c' exceeds I_c so they "totally reflect" internally.

just as if the surface were silvered. The particular value of I_2 corresponding to $I'_2 = 90°$ is called the "critical angle," I_C. This angle is calculated from the equation:

$$\sin I_C = n'_2 / n_2 \tag{6.10}$$

Usually, the medium beyond surface 2 is air, so n'_2 is unity and $\sin I_C = 1/n_2$.

We can take advantage of total internal reflection (TIR) in prisms by choosing the refractive index high enough that all rays that we want to reflect exceed I_C at the surface in question. Then the reflections take place without photometric loss, and reflective coatings are not needed on that surface. It is important to note that TIR occurs only at clean surfaces, so special care must be taken not to let the surface become contaminated with condensed water, fingerprints, or other foreign matter that can change the refractive index outside that surface.

Example 6.3: Unvignetted field of view for TIR in a prism erecting telescope. (For design and analysis, use File 15 of the CD-ROM)
Assume that the prisms of Example 6.2 are not silvered and are made of F2 glass with a refractive index of 1.620. What field of view can the prisms transmit without vignetting caused by a loss of TIR?

From Eq. (6.10), $\sin I_C = 1/1.620 = 0.61728$, so $I_C = 38.1181°$
From the geometry of Fig. 6.6, I' at the prism entrance face is $(45° - I_C) = 6.8819°$

From Eq. (6.1), the ray angle in front of each prism is
$\sin I = (1.620)(\sin 6.8819°) = 0.19411$, so $I = 11.1930°$

This ray angle equals the slope of the lower rim ray (LRR) passing from the bottom of the lens aperture to the top of the image. Hence,
$U'_{LRR} = 11.1930°$ and $\tan U'_{LRR} = 0.19788$

Modifying Eq. (6.5) to apply to the LRR (by changing the minus sign to a plus sign in the numerator), we get:
$\tan U'_{LRR} = [(D/2) + H']/EFL_{OBJ} = [(50.000/2) + H']/177.800 = 0.19788$

Solving for the image height, we get $H' = 10.18277$ mm

Since $H' = (EFL_{OBJ})(\tan U'_{PR})$, we find that the unvignetted telescope field of view is $\pm$ arc-tan $(H'/EFL_{OBJ}) = \pm 3.2778°$

6.2 Aberration Contributions of Prisms

As mentioned earlier, prisms usually are designed so their entrance and exit faces are perpendicular to the optical axis of the transmitted beam. If that beam is collimated, no aberrations are introduced. Aberrations do result if the beam is not collimated. In a converging or diverging beam, a prism introduces longitudinal aberrations (spherical, chromatic, and astigmatic) as well as transverse aberrations (coma, distortion, and lateral chromatic). Smith provided exact and third-order equations for calculating the aberration contributions of a plane parallel plate or the equivalent prism.[2] Ray-tracing programs give the aberration contributions of prisms in a given design on a surface-by-surface basis.

6.3 Typical Prism Configurations

Chapter 13 of MIL-HDBK-141 *Optical Design*[3] gives generic dimensions, axial path lengths, and tunnel diagrams for many types of common prisms. Most of these designs were described earlier in ORDM 2-1, *Design of Fire Control Optics*, a two-volume treatise on telescope design written by Frankford Arsenal's long-time chief lens designer, Otto K. Kaspereit, and published by the U.S. Army in 1953. Since copies of the latter book are hard to find and both, like later excerpts,[2,4,5] do not always include all the information we need to design mounts for the prisms, we include here design data for 27 types of prisms, some of which were not included in any of these references. Included are orthographic projections, generic dimensions, axial path length, and in many cases, isometric views, tunnel diagrams, approximate prism volume, and bonding area information (see Sect. 7.4). The following parameter definitions apply:

A	= aperture for collimated beam passage
B, C, D, etc.,	= other linear dimensions
a, b, c, etc.,	= typical bevels
δ, θ, φ, etc.,	= angular dimensions
t_A	= axial path length
V	= prism volume (neglecting small bevels)
ρ	= glass density
a_G	= acceleration factor measured as "times gravity"
Q_{MIN}	= minimum bond area for adhesive strength J and safety factor f_S
Q_{MAX}	= maximum circular (C) or racetrack (RT) bond area achievable on the prism mounting surface *

6.3.1 Right-angle prism

Figure 6.1(b) shows the function of this prism in its most common role as a means for deviating a beam by 90° whereas Fig. 6.2 shows its tunnel diagram. Figure 6.7 shows three views, while the caption provides design equations for this prism. A typical bonded interface to a circular mounting pad is indicated. Variations of this prism are used as the Porro prism, the Dove prism, and the double-Dove prism. Each of these designs is considered later.

6.3.2 Beamsplitter (or beamcombiner) cube prism

Two right-angle prisms cemented together at their hypotenuse surfaces with a

---

* NOTE: As discussed in Section 12.10, the stresses induced by temperature changes may set upper limits on bond sizes.

partially reflective coating at the interface form a cube-shaped beamsplitter or beam-combiner. This type of prism is shown in Fig. 6.8. If this prism (or any multiple-component prism) is to be bonded to a mechanical mounting, the adhesive joint should be limited to one component; the bond would then not bridge the cemented joint. This is because the two glass surfaces may not be accurately coplanar and the strength of the bond may be degraded by differences in adhesive thickness. If the adjacent surfaces are reground after cementing, bonding across the joint may be acceptable.

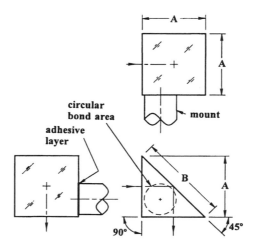

Fig. 6.7 Right-angle prism. (For design and analysis, use File 16.1 of the CD-ROM)

$t_A = A$; $B = 1.414A$; $V = 0.500A^3$; $Q_{MIN} = V\rho a_G f_s/J$; $Q_{MAX\,(C)} = 0.230A^2$

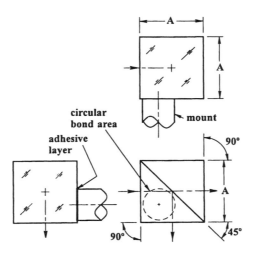

Fig. 6.8 Beamsplitter cube prism. (For design and analysis, use File 16.2 of the CD-ROM)

$t_A = A$; $V = A^3$; $Q_{MIN} = V\rho a_G f_s/J$; $Q_{MAX\,(C)} = 0.230A^2$

Most of the design equations for the beamsplitter cube apply also to a monolithic cube such as might be used as a rotating prism in a high-speed camera. With a solid cube, the bond area, Q, can be as large as $Q_{MAX} = 0.785A^2$.

6.3.3 Amici prism

The Amici prism (see Fig. 6.9) is essentially a right-angle prism with its hypotenuse configured as a 90° "roof" so a transmitted beam makes two reflections instead of just one. A right-handed image is produced. The prism can be used in such a manner that the transmitted beam is split by the dihedral edge between the roof surfaces or (with a larger prism for constant beam size) so the beam hits the roof surfaces in sequence. These possibilities are illustrated in Figs. 6.10(a) and 6.10(b), respectively. In the former case, the dihedral angle must be accurately 90° (i.e., within a few arc-seconds) in order not to produce a noticeable double image. This makes the smaller component's cost higher because of the added labor or fixturing required to correct the roof angle. The prisms of Fig. 6.10 are shown to be of equal size so the beam transmitted without splitting must be smaller than that transmitted with splitting [Fig. 6.10(b)] cannot be larger than A/2. The beam axis is displaced laterally by A/2 in this case.

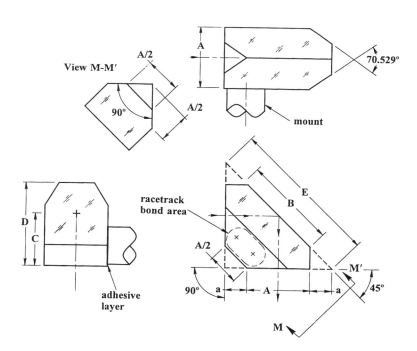

Fig. 6.9 Amici prism. (For design and analysis, use File 16.3 of the CD-ROM)
t_A = 2.707A; a = 0.354A; B = 1.414A; C = 0.854A
D = 1.354A; E = B + 2.828a; V = 0.777A³
Q_{MIN} = $V\rho a_G f_s /J$; $Q_{MAX\,(C)}$= 0.164A²; $Q_{MAX\,(RT)}$ = 0.306A²

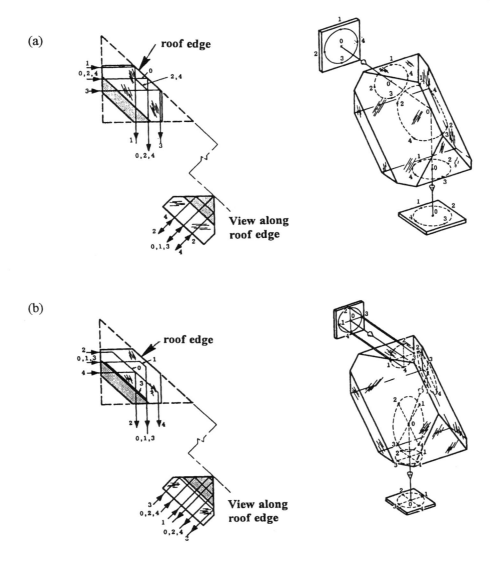

Fig. 6.10 The Amici prism used (a) symmetrically as a split-beam reflector and (b) off-center as a full beam reflector. (From MIL-HDBK-141.[3])

6.3.4 Porro prism

A right-angle prism arranged so the beam enters and exits the hypotenuse surface, as shown in Fig. 6.11(a), is called a "Porro prism." Ray a-a' travels parallel to the axis while rays b-b' and c-c' enter at different field angles. Note that rays a-a' and b-b' turn around and exit parallel to the entering rays; this shows that the prism is retrodirective in the plane of refraction. Path c-c' represents a field ray entering near the edge of the prism. It intercepts the hypotenuse A-C internally and hence has three reflections and produces an inverted image. Such a ray is called a "ghost" ray since it does not contribute useful information to the main image. It does add stray light and thus should be eliminated. The groove cut into the center of the hypotenuse does just that, so it is a usual feature of the Porro design. The tunnel diagram of Fig. 6.11(b) shows all these rays and the groove. The caption for Fig. 6.12 gives the design equations for this prism.

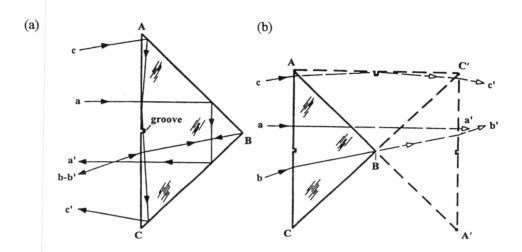

Fig. 6.11 (a) Typical ray paths through a Porro prism. (b) Its tunnel diagram.

Another useful feature of this (and several other types of prisms) is that it produces the same beam deviation (180° for the Porro) even if it is rotated about an axis perpendicular to the plane of refraction. Such a prism is said to be a "constant deviation" prism. Note that the Porro prism produces constant deviation only in one plane.

6.3.5 Abbe version of the Porro prism

Ernst Abbe modified the design of the Porro prism by rotating one half of the prism about the optic axis by 90° with respect to the other half. Figure 6.13 illustrates this prism and provides its design equations in the caption. Note that the aperture A of this prism is shown at the same scale as in Fig. 6.12. The prism appears slightly larger than the standard version because it includes larger bevels. The presence of these bevels and their sizes are design options.

6.3.6 Rhomboid prism

The rhomboid prism shown in Fig. 6.14 is essentially the integration of two right-angle prisms with their reflecting surfaces parallel. It is used to displace the axis laterally without changing the axis direction. The prism is insensitive to tilt in the plane of refraction so it provides constant deviation in that plane. Rotations about the long axis of the prism result in the usual relationship of 2:1 beam deviation vs. reflecting surface rotation.

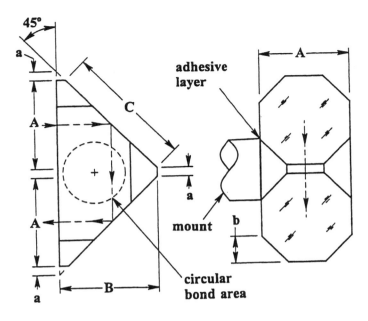

Fig. 6.12 Porro prism. (For design and analysis, use File 16.4 of the CD-ROM)
$t_A = 2A + 3a$; $a = 0.1A$; $b = 0.293A$; $B = A + a$; $C = 1.414A$;
$V = 1.286A^3$; $Q_{MIN} = V\rho a_G f_s /J$; $Q_{MAX (C)} = 0.608A^2$

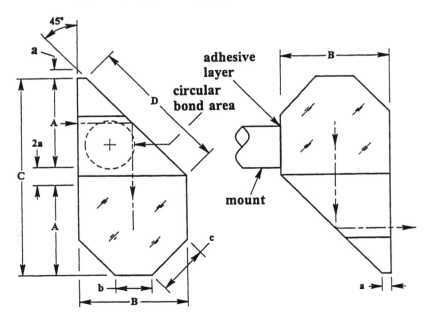

Fig. 6.13 Abbe version of the Porro prism. (For design and analysis, use File 16.5 of the CD-ROM)
$t_A = 2A + 4a$; $a = 0.1A$; $b = 0.414A$; $B = A + 2a$; $C = 2.200A$
$D = 1.556A$; $V = 1.832A^3$
$Q_{MIN} = V\rho a_G f_s /J$; $Q_{MAX (C)} = 0.388A^2$

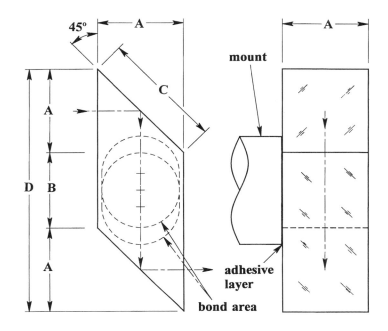

Fig. 6.14 Rhomboid prism. (For design and analysis, use File 16.6 of the CD-ROM)

$t_A = 2A + B$; $B = $ variable; $C = 1.414A$; $D = 2A + B$; $V = A^2 (A + B)$
$Q_{MIN} = V\rho a_G f_s /J$
For $B = 0$: $Q_{MAX (C)} = 0.393A^2$; $Q_{MAX (RT)} = 0.686A^2$
For $B > 0.414A$: $Q_{MAX (C)} = 0.785A^2$; $Q_{MAX (RT)} = 0.578A^2 + 0.500AB$

6.3.7 Porro erecting system

Two Porro prisms oriented at a right angle and connected together, as shown in Fig. 6.3, constitute a Porro erecting system. The axis is displaced laterally in each direction by 2A plus the width of the bevel on the apex of each prism. This system is most frequently used in binoculars and telescopes to erect the image. A design in which the prisms are cemented together is shown in Fig. 6.15. An air space between the prisms does not alter their function. This is not a constant deviation configuration.

6.3.8 Abbe erecting system

The combination of two prisms of the type described in Sect. 6.3.5 creates an erecting prism subassembly (see Fig. 6.16) that functions like a Porro erecting system. For a given prism aperture, A, and with equal bevels, the lateral offset of this configuration is approximately 77% of that with the Porro arrangement. The Abbe erector is not a constant-deviation prism.

A variation on the design has two right-angle prisms cemented side by side, but facing in opposite directions, on the hypotenuse of a Porro prism, (see Fig. 6.16).

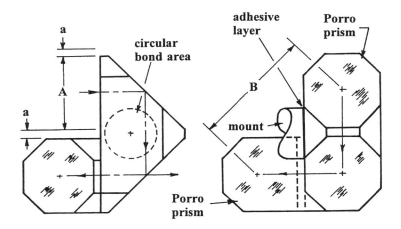

Fig. 6.15 Porro erecting system (cemented). (For design and analysis, use File 16.7 of the CD-ROM)
$t_A = 4A + 6a;\ a = 0.1A;\ B = 1.556A;\ V = 2.573A^3$
$Q_{MIN} = V\rho a_G f_s /J;\ Q_{MAX\ (C)} = 0.459A^2$

6.3.9 Penta prism

The penta prism neither reverts nor inverts the image; it merely turns the axis by exactly 90°. The design is defined in Fig. 6.17. A useful characteristic of this prism is that it provides constant deviation in the plane of refraction. For this reason, it is used in such applications as optical range finders and surveying equipment where an exact right-angle deviation is needed.

6.3.10 Roof penta prism

If we convert one reflecting surface of the penta prism into a 90° roof, the component inverts the image in the direction normal to the plane of refraction. For a given aperture and material, the roof penta is about 17% larger and 19% heavier than the standard penta. Adding the roof does not change the penta's constant deviation characteristic. The roof penta is shown in Fig. 6.18 and its design equations are given in the caption.

6.3.11 Amici/penta erecting system

A combination of the Amici prism with a penta prism provides two reflections in each direction perpendicular to the axis so it can be used as an erecting system. Usually the prisms are cemented together as illustrated in Fig. 6.19(a). This design has been used in some binoculars. A functionally similar erecting system can be obtained by combining a right-angle prism with a roof penta prism [see Fig. 6.19(b)]. For a particular aperture A, the indicated height dimensions differ by about 4%. This system has primarily been used in military periscopes. An easily manufactured variation of this design was used in an experimental compact military binocular.[6] This prism is illustrated in Fig. 6.20.

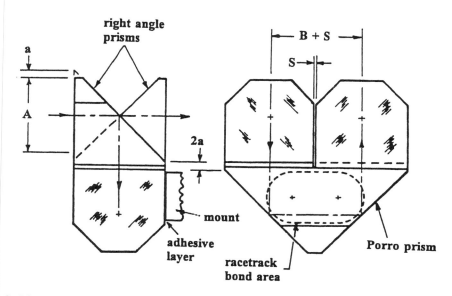

Fig. 6.16 Abbe erecting system (cemented). (For design and analysis, use File 16.8 of the CD-ROM)
$t_A = 4A + 6a + S$; $a = 0.1A$; $B = 2(A + a) + S$
$V = 3.686A^3 + SB[A + (3a/2)]$
$Q_{MIN} = Vpa_G f_S /J$; $Q_{MAX\ (C)} = 0.503A^2$; $Q_{MAX\ (RT)} = 0.957A^2$

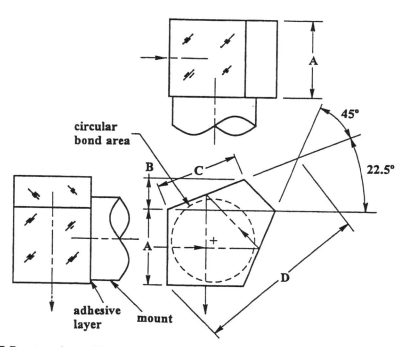

Fig. 6.17 Penta prism. (For design and analysis, use File 16.9 of the CD-ROM)
$t_A = 2A + B + 0.707(A + B) = 3.414A$; $B = 0.414A$; $C = 1.082A$
$D = 2.414A$; $V = 1.500A^3$; $Q_{MIN} = Vpa_G f_S /J$; $Q_{MAX\ (C)} = 1.129A^2$

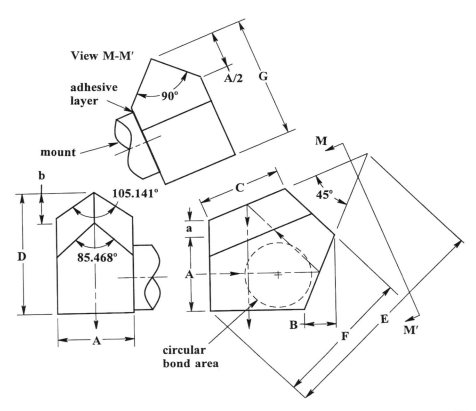

Fig. 6.18 Roof penta prism. (For design and analysis, use File 16.10 of the CD-ROM)

t_A = 4.223A; a = 0.237A; b = 0.383A; B = 0.414A; C = 1.082A
D = 1.651A; E = 2.986A; F = 1.874A; G = 1.621A; V = 1.795A^3
Q_{MIN} = V$\rho a_G f_S$ /J; $Q_{MAX (C)}$ = 0.824A^2

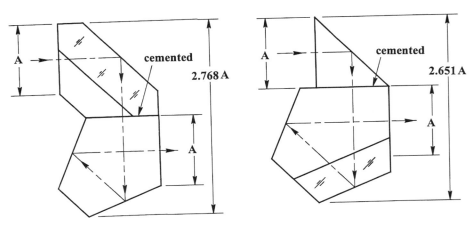

Fig. 6.19 Erecting prism assemblies. (a) Amici/penta system (b) Right-angle/roof penta system.

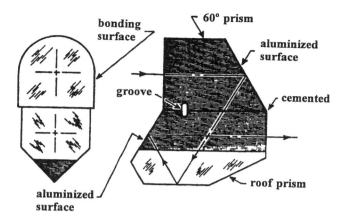

Fig. 6.20 Compact erecting prism assembly used in an experimental military binocular. (From Yoder.[6])

6.3.12 Dove prism

The Dove prism is a right-angle prism with the top section removed and the optical axis parallel to the hypotenuse face as shown in Fig. 6.21. This single-reflection prism inverts the image only in the plane of refraction. It is most commonly used to rotate the image by turning the prism about its optical axis; the image then rotates at twice the speed of the prism. Because of the oblique incidence of the axis at the entrance and exit faces, the prism can be used only in a collimated beam. Alternative versions can have faces tilted at other angles, but here we limit consideration to the 45° incidence case because it is the most common.

The prism dimensions depend upon the prism's refractive index because of deviation of the optical axis at the tilted faces. Table 6.1 shows how the dimensions of a typical Dove prism vary with changes in refractive index. These values were all obtained with the equations given in the caption of Fig. 6.21.

6.3.13 Double-Dove prism

This prism cosists of two Dove prisms, each of aperture A/2 by A, attached at their hypotenuse faces. Figure 6.22 shows the configuration. It is commonly used as an image rotator. The prisms can be air spaced by a small distance and held mechanically. TIR then will occur. They also can be cemented together. In that case, a reflective coating such as aluminum or silver is placed on one prism face before the prisms are cemented to keep the light from passing through the interface. For a given aperture, A, the double-Dove prism is one-half the length of the corresponding standard Dove prism. To minimize light loss, the leading and trailing edges of both prisms are given only minimal protective bevels.

As shown in the end view of Fig. 6.22, the shape of a circular beam entering a double-Dove prism is converted into a pair of "D-shaped" beams with curved edges

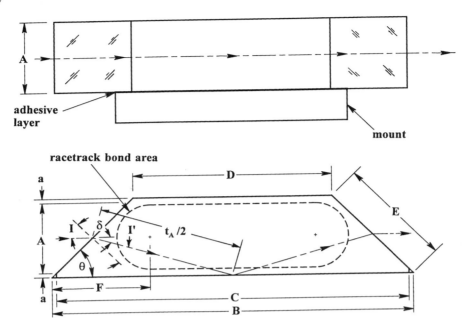

Fig. 6.21 Dove prism. (For design and analysis, use File 16.11 of the CD-ROM)
$\theta = 45°$; $t = (A + 2a)/\sin \delta$; $I = 90° - \theta$; $I' = \arcsin [(\sin I)/n]$; $\delta = I - I'$
$a = 0.050A$; $B = (A + 2a)[(1/\tan \gamma) + (1/\tan \theta)]$
$C = B - 2a$; $D = B - 2(A + 2a)$; $E = (A + a)/\cos \theta$
$F = (A + 2a)/(2\tan (\theta/2))$; $V = (A)(A + 2a)(B) - (A)(A + 2a)^2 - a^2A$
$Q_{MIN} = V\rho a_G f_s /J$; $Q_{MAX (C)} = \pi[(A + a)/2]^2$
$Q_{MAX (RT)} = Q_{MAX (C)} + (A + 2a)(B - 2F)$

Table 6.1 Changes in Dove prism dimensions with refractive index (n)

n	1.5170	1.6170	1.7215	1.8052
A (cm)	3.8100	3.8100	3.8100	3.8100
B (cm)	17.7156	16.3154	15.2541	14.5958
C (cm)	17.3346	15.9344	14.8731	14.2148
D (cm)	9.3336	7.9334	6.8721	6.2138
E (cm)	5.6576	5.6576	5.6576	5.6576
t_A (cm)	14.159	12.8283	11.8303	11.2171

adjacent as it exits. If vignetting is to be avoided, the apertures of subsequent optics must be large enough to accept the divided beam of diameter 1.414A. The modulation transfer function (MTF) of the optical system in which the prism is used is somewhat degraded by the divided aperture. The 45° angles of the prisms must be quite accurate in order to minimize image doubling.

A cemented "cube-shaped" version of the double-Dove prism is sometimes used as a means for scanning the line of sight (LOS) of an optical system in the plane of refraction. In such a prism, the faces with dimensions "C" shown in Fig. 6.22 are extended so the faces marked "D" are reduced to almost zero. The prism is rotated about an axis normal to that plane (parallel to the hypotenuse faces) and passing through the prism's geometric center. When it is located in front of a camera, periscope, or other optical instrument with a collimated beam entering from the object, such a prism can scan the system LOS well over 180° in object space.

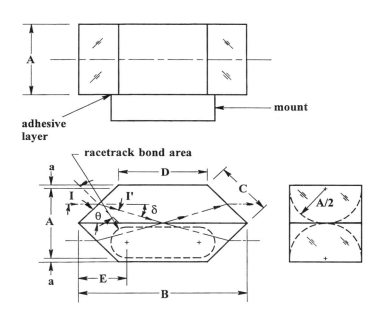

Fig. 6.22 Double-Dove prism (cemented). (For design and analysis, use File 16.12 of the CD-ROM)

$\theta = 45°$; $I = 90° - \theta$; $I' = \arcsin [(\sin I)/n]$; $\delta = I - I'$

$t_A = A/(2\sin \delta)$; $a = 0.05A$

$B = (A + 2a)[(1/\tan \gamma) + (1/\tan \theta)]/2$

$C = A + 2a$; $D = B - 2[(A/2) + a]$; $E = [(A/2) + a]/[2 \tan (\theta/2)]$

$V = (A)(B)(A + 2a) - (2)(A)[(A/2) + a]^2$

$Q_{MIN} = V\rho a_G f_s /J$; $Q_{MAX (C)} = (\pi)[(A/2) + a]^2$

$Q_{MAX (RT)} = Q_{MAX (C)} + (B - 2E)[(A/2) + a]$

6.3.14 Reversion prism

This two-component (cemented) prism is shown in Fig. 6.23. It functions as an image rotator, but it can be used in converging or diverging beams. The central reflecting face, marked "C" in the figure, must have a reflective coating to prevent refraction through it. This surface usually is then covered by a protective coating such as electroplated copper and paint like a "back surface" mirror, (see Sect. 8.1). Another version of this prism has the central reflecting surface C replaced by a 90° roof to invert the image in the direction perpendicular to the plane of refraction.

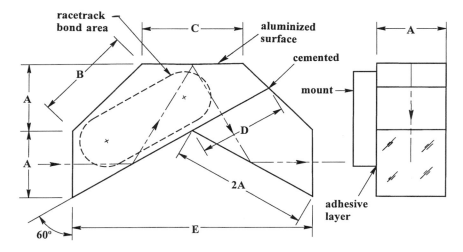

Fig. 6.23 Reversion prism. (For design and analysis, use File 16.13 of the CD-ROM)

t_A = 5.196A; B = 1.414A; C = 1.464A; D = 1.268A

E = 3.464A; V = 4.196A^3

Q_{MIN} = $V\rho a_G f_s /J$; $Q_{MAX (C)}$ = 1.093A^2; $Q_{MAX (RT)}$ = 1.989A^2

6.3.15 Pechan prism

The Pechan prism has an odd number (5) of reflections and is frequently used as a compact image rotator in place of the Dove or double-Dove prisms because it can be used in convergent or divergent beams. The design is shown in Fig. 6.24. The optical

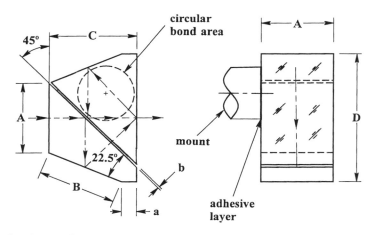

Fig. 6.24 Pechan prism. (For design and analysis, use File 16.14 of the CD-ROM)

t_A = 4.621A; a = 0.207A; b = 0.1 mm (typ.)

B = 1.082A; C = 1.207A; D = 1.707A

V = 1.801A^3, Q_{MIN} = $V\rho a_G f_s /J$; $Q_{MAX (C)}$= 0.599A^2

axis of the nominal design is displaced very slightly owing to the small central air space, but it is not deviated. The two outer reflecting surfaces must have reflective coatings and protective overcoat and/or paint, while the internal reflections occur by TIR so those surfaces are not coated.

The two prisms are usually held mechanically or bonded to a common mounting plate to create a narrow air space between them. A spacing b in the order of 0.1 mm (0.004 in.) is typical. Thin shims of the proper thickness can be placed near the edges of these reflecting surfaces in a clamped mounting. The edges of the air space should be covered by a narrow ribbon of sealant such as RTV to prevent entry of moisture or dust.

6.3.16 Delta prism

Figure 6.25 shows the path of an axial ray through this triangular prism. TIR occurs in sequence at the exit and entrance faces. The intermediate face must be silvered to make it reflect. With the proper choice of index of refraction, apex angle, and prism height, the internal path can be made symmetrical about the vertical axis of the prism; the exiting axial ray then is colinear with the entering axial ray.

With an odd number of reflections (3), the delta prism can be used as an image rotator. Since it has tilted entrance and exit faces, it can be used only in a collimated beam. For a given aperture, the overall size of the delta prism rotator is smaller than the Dove prism.[7] It has fewer lossy reflections and a shorter glass path than the Pechan prism, so it should have better light transmission than the latter.

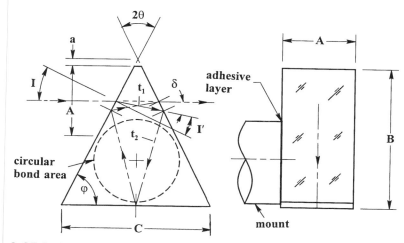

Fig. 6.25 Delta prism. (For design and analysis, use File 16.15 of the CD-ROM)
Given: n and θ calculated as explained in the text
$a = 0.1A$; $B = \{(A + 2a)(\sin (180° - 4\theta)/[(2)(\cos \theta)(\sin \theta)]\} - a$
$C = 2(B + A) \tan \theta$; $\varphi = 90° - \theta$; $I = \theta$; $I' = \arc \sin [(\sin I)/n]$
$t_1 = [(A / 2) + a](\sin 2\theta)/[\cos \theta \sin (90° - 2\theta + I')]$
$t_2 = [B - (A/2) - a - t_1 \sin \delta]/\cos \theta$; $t_A = 2(t_1 + t_2)$
$V = A [(B + a)^2 - a^2] \tan \theta$
$Q = V\rho a_G f_s /J$; $Q_{MAX} = \pi [(C^2 /4) \tan^2 (\varphi/2)]$

Design of this prism starts with choice of the index of refraction, n. A value for one-half the apex angle θ is then assumed. The angle of incidence, I_1, at the first surface equals θ. We vary n and θ until the same value for I_1' is obtained by Eqs. (6.11) and (6.12).

$$I_1' = \theta = \arcsin(I_1/n) \qquad (6.11)$$

$$I_1' = 4\theta - 90 \qquad (6.12)$$

We then calculate $I_2 = (90 - I_2')/2$ and check, using Eq. (6.10), to see if TIR occurs at the second surface, i.e., $I_2 > I_C$, for the chosen glass. If not, a new glass with a higher index must be chosen. Once these conditions are satisfied, we apply the equations from the caption of Fig. 6.25 to complete the design.

6.3.17 Schmidt prism

The Schmidt roof prism will invert and revert an image, so it is usually used as an erecting system in telescopes. It also deviates the axis by 45°, which allows an eyepiece axis orientation with respect to the objective axis that is convenient for some applications. The entrance and exit faces are normal to the axis. Figure 6.26 applies. The prism's refractive index must be high enough for TIR to occur at the entrance and exit faces. If a roof is added to the delta prism described earlier, an image-erecting system with coaxial input and output optical axes will result. This prism would resemble the Schmidt prism, but the entrance and exit faces would be tilted with respect to the axis, so the roof delta prism must be used in a collimated beam.

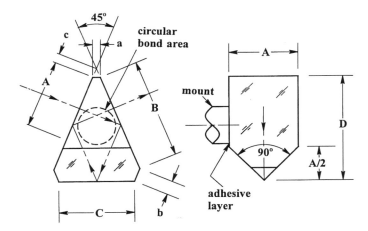

Fig. 6.26 Schmidt prism. (For design and analysis, use File 16.16 of the CD-ROM)
a = 0.1A; b = 0.185A; c = 0.131A
B = 1.468A; C = 1.082A; D = 1.527A; t_A = 3.045A; V = 0.863A³
$Q_{MIN} = V\rho a_G f_S/J$; $Q_{MAX (C)} = 0.318A^2$

6.3.18 45° Bauernfeind prism

The Bauernfeind prism provides a 45° deviation of the axis using two internal reflections. The first reflection is by TIR while the second takes place at a coated reflecting surface. The smaller element of the Pechan prism is of this type. Figure 6.27 shows the design. A 60° deviation version of this prism has also been used in many applications.

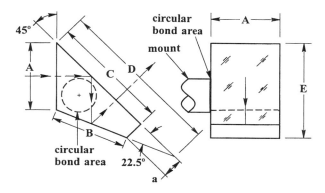

Fig. 6.27 45° Bauernfeind prism. (For design and analysis, use File 16.17 of the CD-ROM)

$a = 0.293A$; $B = 1.082A$; $C = 1.707A$; $D = 2.414A$; $E = 1.414A$

$t_A = 1.707A$; $V = 0.75A^3$; $Q_{MIN} = V\rho a_G f_s / J$; $Q_{MAX (c)} = 0.331A^2$

The combination of a Schmidt prism with a 45° Bauernfeind prism forms a popular erecting system for binoculars because of its compact design. It sometimes is called the Schmidt-Pechan roof prism. An example of a mounting for such a prism is shown in Sect. 7.3.3.

6.3.19 Internally reflecting axicon prism

With conical surfaces as their active optical surfaces, axicons are frequently used to change a small circular laser beam into an annular beam with a larger outside diameter. The version shown in Fig. 6.28 has a coated reflecting surface to return the beam to and through the conical surface. Because of its rotational symmetry, this axicon is made with a circular cross-section and usually is elastomerically secured in a tubular mount. The apex is sharp or carries a very small protective bevel. A centrally perforated flat mirror at 45° can provide a convenient way to separate the coaxial beams if it is located in front of this prism.

An in-line refracting version of this axicon with identical conical surfaces at either end has been used to accomplish the same function, but without the reversal of beam direction. It is twice as long and is more expensive to fabricate because of the additional conical surface.

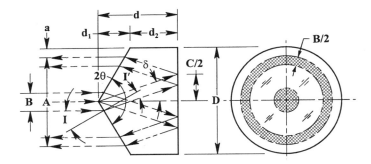

Fig. 6.28 Internally reflecting axicon prism. (For design and analysis, use File 16.18 of the CD-ROM)

A = annulus OD; B = input beam OD; annulus width = B/2; a = 0.1A

$I = 90° - \theta$; $I' = \arcsin (\sin I_1 /n)$; $\delta = I - I'$; $C = (2d)\tan \delta$; $D = A + 2a$

$d = (A/4)[(1/\tan \theta) + (1/\tan \delta)]$; $d_1 = [(A/2) + a]/\tan \theta$; $d_2 = d - d_1$

$t_A = A/(2\sin \delta)$; $V = (0.785d_2 + 0.262d_1)A^2$

6.3.20 Cube-corner prism

A corner cut symmetrically and diagonally from a solid glass cube creates a prism in the geometrical form of a tetrahedron (four-sided polyhedron). It has been referred to as a cube-corner, corner- cube, or tetrahedral prism. Light entering the diagonal face reflects internally from the other three faces and exits through the diagonal face. TIR usually occurs at each internal surface for commonly used refractive index values. The return beam contains six segments, one from each of the pie-shaped areas within the circular aperture shown in Fig. 6.29. If the three dihedral angles between the adjacent reflecting surfaces are exactly 90°, the prism is retrodirective, even if the prism is

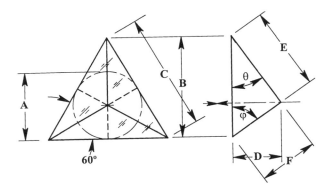

Fig. 6.29 Cube-corner prism. (For design and analysis, use File 16.19 of the CD-ROM)

A = aperture; $B = [(A/2)/\sin 30°] + (A/2) = 1.500A$

$C = 2B\tan 30° = 1.732A$; $D = 0.707A$; $E = 1.225A$; $F = 0.866A$

$\varphi = 54.736°$; $\theta = 35.264°$ $t_A = 2D = 1.414A$

significantly tilted. If one or more of these dihedral angles differs from 90° by an error ε, the deviation differs from 180° by as much as 3.26ε and the reflected beams diverge.[8] This feature is used to advantage in such applications as laser tracking of cooperative targets in space or those involving widely separated transmitter and receiver optical systems used for large-baseline ranging by triangulation.

The generic cube-corner prism of Fig. 6.29 has a triangular form with sharp dihedral edges. Usually its rim is ground to a circular shape circumscribing the aperture (the dashed line). Figure 6.30 shows an example. This is one of the 426 fused silica prisms used on the Laser Geodynamic Satellite (LAGEOS) launched by NASA in 1976 to provide scientists with extremely accurate measurements of movements of the Earth's

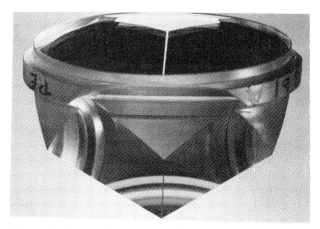

Fig. 6.30 A fused silica cube-corner prism with a 3.81-cm (1.50- in.) circular aperture. (Courtesy of Raytheon Optical Systems Corp., Danbury, CT.)

crust as a possible aid to understanding earthquakes, continental movement, and polar motion. The dihedral angles of the prisms were each 1.25 arcsec greater than 90°. A laser beam transmitted to the satellite was returned with sufficient divergence to reach a receiver telescope even though the satellite moved significantly during the beam's round-trip transit time.

Another possible cube-corner prism configuration has the rim cut to a hexagonal shape circumscribing the prism's circular clear aperture. This allows several of the prisms to be tightly grouped together to form a mosaic of closely packed retrodirective prisms, thereby increasing the effective aperture of the group. Mirror versions of the cube-corner prism frequently are used when operation outside the transmission range of normal refracting materials is needed, (see Sect. 9.2). This so called "hollow cube-corner" has reduced weight for a given aperture.[9]

6.3.21 Biocular prism system

Attributed to Carl Zeiss, the prism system shown in Fig. 6.31 can be used in telescopes and microscopes when both eyes are to observe the same image presented by the objective. It does not provide stereoscopic vision; hence is called "biocular." From Fig. 6.31(a), it can be seen to consist of four prisms: a right-angle prism, P_1, cemented to a rhomboid prism, P_2, with a partially reflective coating at the diagonal interface; an optical path equalizing block, P_3; and a second rhomboid prism, P_4. The observer's interpupillary distance is designated as "IPD". By rotating the prisms about the input axis, the IPD is changed to suit the individual using the instrument. Typically, the IPD is adjustable from at least 56 to 72 mm (2.20 to 2.83 in.). An external scale usually is provided to allow easy reference for setting this IPD.

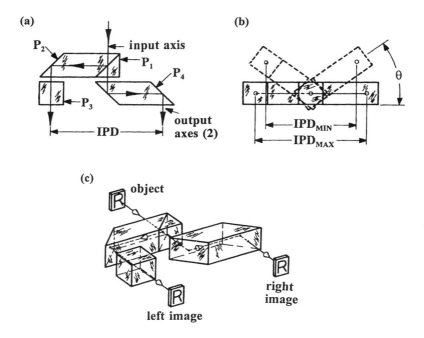

Fig. 6.31 Biocular prism system. (a) Top view, (b) end view, and (c) isometric view. IPD is interpupillary distance. Individual prism dimensions for a uniform aperture A may be obtained from the equations in Figs. 6.7 and 6.14.

6.3.22 Dispersing prisms

Prisms are commonly used to disperse polychromatic light beams into their constituent colors in instruments such as spectrometers and monochromators. The index of refraction, n, of the optical material varies with wavelength, so the deviation (measured with respect to the initial incident ray direction) of any ray transmitted at other than normal incidence to the prism's entrance and exit surfaces will depend upon n_λ, the angle of incidence at the entrance face, and the prism's apex angle, θ. Figure 6.32 illustrates two typical dispersing prisms. In each case, a single ray of "white" light is incident at I_1. Inside each prism, this ray splits into a spectrum of various colored rays. For clarity, the angles between rays are exaggerated in the figures. After refraction at the exit faces, rays of blue, yellow, and red wavelengths emerge with different deviation angles, δ_λ. The blue ray is deviated the most because $n_{BLUE} > n_{RED}$. If the emerging rays are imaged onto a film or a screen by a lens, a multiplicity of images of different colors will be formed at slightly different lateral locations. While we refer here to colors as blue, yellow, and red, it should be understood that the phenomenon of dispersion applies to all wavelengths, so we really mean the shorter, intermediate, and longer wavelength radiation under consideration in any given application. In the design shown in Fig. 6.32(b), the deviation is unchanged for small rotations of the prism about an axis perpendicular to the plane of refraction; hence the name "constant deviation." The refractive index in this case usually is chosen to be large enough to cause TIR at the intermediate surface.

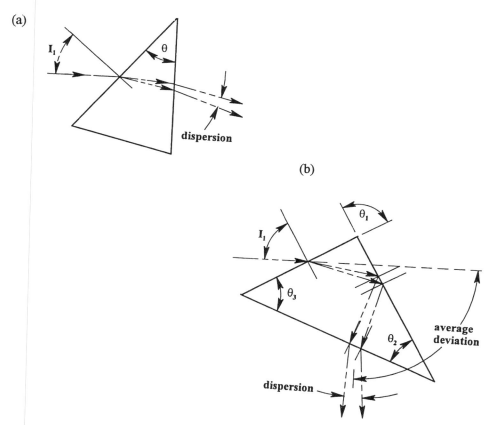

Fig. 6.32 Dispersion of a white light ray by (a) a simple prism and (b) a constant-deviation prism involving TIR.

Example 6.4: Dispersion through a single prism.
(For design and analysis, use File 16.20 of the CD-ROM)
A BK7 prism with apex angle, θ, of 30° disperses a white light collimated beam generally as shown in Fig. 6.32(a). Let the incident angle be $I_1 = 15°$. (a) Applying

Eq. (6.1) (Snell's law), what are the angular separations between the exiting blue (F), yellow (d), and red (C) beams? (b) If focused by an aberration free 105 mm focal length lens onto a screen, what are the linear separations of the blue, yellow, and red images at the screen?

(a)

wavelength	(μm)	0.486 (F)	0.588 (d)	0.656 (C)
apex angle, θ	(°)	30	30	30
I_1	(°)	15	15	15
sin I_1		0.25882	0.25882	0.25882
n_λ		1.52238	1.51680	1.51432
sin I_1'		0.17001	0.17063	0.17091
I_1'	(°)	9.7884	9.8247	9.8410
$I_2 = I_1' - \theta$	(°)	-20.2116	-20.1753	-20.1590
sin I_2		-0.34549	-0.34489	-0.34463
sin I_2'		-0.52597	-0.52313	-0.52188
I_2'	(°)	-31.7332	-31.5427	-31.4581
$\delta = I_1 - I_2' - \theta$	(°)	16.7332	16.5427	16.4581

The angles between the: blue and yellow beams = 16.7332° - 16.5427° = 0.1905°

yellow and red beams = 16.5427° - 16.4581° = 0.0846°

red and blue beams is 16.7332° - 16.4581° = 0.2751°

(b)

Image separation: blue to yellow = 105 tan 0.1905° = 0.3491 mm

yellow to red = 105 tan 0.0846° = 0.1550 mm

red to blue = 105 tan 0.2751° = 0.5041 mm

If a ray or collimated beam of light of wavelength λ passes symmetrically through a prism so that $I_1 = -I_2'$ and $I_1' = -I_2$, the deviation of the prism for that wavelength is a minimum and $\delta_{MIN} = 2I_1 - \theta$. This condition is the basis of one means for experimental measurement of the index of refraction of a transparent medium in which the minimum deviation angle, δ_{MIN}, of a prism made of that material is measured by successive approximations and the following equation is applied:

$$n_{PRISM} = \sin[(\theta + \delta)/2]/\sin(\theta/2) \qquad (6.13)$$

If we want any two of the various colored rays to emerge from the prism parallel to each other, we must use a combination of at least two prisms made of different glasses. Usually, these prisms are cemented together. Such a prism is called an "achromatic prism." Figure 6.33 shows one configuration for an achromatic prism. All such prisms can be designed by choosing refractive indices and the first prism's apex angle, then repeatedly applying Snell's law to find the appropriate incident angle and second prism apex angle that gives the desired deviation for a chosen wavelength and the desired dispersion for two other wavelengths that bracket the chosen one. The angle between the exiting rays with the shortest and longest wavelengths is called the "primary chromatic aberration"; here it should be essentially zero. The angle between either of these extreme wavelength rays and that with an intermediate wavelength is called the "secondary chromatic aberration" of the prism.

To illustrate a typical design procedure, in a two-element prism of the type shown in Fig. 6.33, we might specify that a yellow ray should enter the first prism at I_1, which should be equal to the value for the minimum deviation condition if that prism

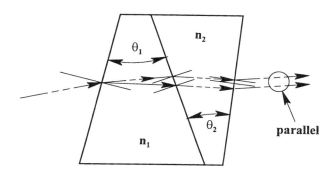

Fig. 6.33 A typical achromatic dispersing prism.

were immersed in air. The blue and red rays would then be dispersed. We would assume a value for θ_1, calculate $I_1' = -I_2 = \theta_1/2$, and obtain I_1 from Snell's law (Eq. 6.1). We would then add the second prism and redetermine I_2'. The following equation could then be used to find θ_2:

$$\cotan\theta_2 = -\left[\frac{\Delta n_2}{2\Delta n_1 \sin(\theta_1/2)\cos I_2'}\right] + \tan I_2' \qquad (6.14)$$

Other than determining the prism glasses and angles required to produce the desired chromatic effect, first-order design of a dispersing prism requires calculation of only the required apertures. Usually we assume a collimated input beam and make the apertures of the prism large enough to not vignette any of the dispersed beams. There are so many dispersing prism types that space here does not allow a comprehensive listing of the pertinent equations for computing these apertures. The techniques discussed earlier for the more often used prism types serve as guidelines for establishing these equations. This task is left to the ingenuity of the reader.

6.3.23 Thin-wedge prisms

Prisms with small apex angles and (usually) axial thicknesses that are small compared with the component apertures are called "optical wedges." One such wedge is shown in Fig. 6.34. Since the apex angle is small, we can assume that the angle expressed in radians equals its sine, and, rewriting Eq. (6.12), we obtain the following simple equation for the wedge deviation:

$$\delta_\lambda = (n_\lambda - 1)\theta \tag{6.15}$$

Differentiating this equation, we obtain the following expression for the dispersion, i.e., chromatic aberration, of the wedge:

$$d\delta_\lambda = dn_\lambda \theta \tag{6.16}$$

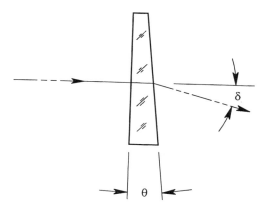

Fig. 6.34 A typical thin wedge.

A wedge so designed is one of minimum deviation. A common arrangement in optical instruments has the incident beam normal to the entrance face. Then $I_2 = \theta$, $I_2' = \arcsin(n \sin I_2)$, and $\delta = I_2' - \theta$. If not otherwise specified, we would assume n to apply to the center wavelength of the spectral bandwidth of interest. The deviation angle will differ from that given by Eq. (6.14) only slightly.

Example 6.5: Calculate deviation of an optical wedge. (For design and analysis, use File 16.21 of the CD-ROM)
Assume a thin wedge has an apex angle of 1.9458°. What is its deviation if the glass index is 1.51680? What is its chromatic aberration for wavelengths corresponding to indices of 1.51432 and 1.52238?

By Eq. (6.14), $\delta = (1.51680 - 1)(1.9458) = 1.0056°$
By Eq. (6.15), $d\delta = (1.52238 - 1.51432)(1.9458) = 0.0157°$

6.3.24 Risley wedge system

Two identical optical wedges arranged in series and rotated equally in opposite directions about the optical axis form an adjustable wedge. They are used in collimated beams to provide variable pointing of laser beams, to angularly align the axis of one portion of an optical system to that of another portion of that system, as the means for measuring distance in some optical range finders, etc. They frequently are referred to as Risley wedges.

The action of a Risley wedge system will be understood from Fig. 6.35. Usually the wedges are circular in shape; here their apertures are shown as small and large rectangles for clarity. In Fig. 6.35(a) and 6.35(c), the wedges are shown in their two positions for maximum deviation. The apexes are adjacent and $\delta_{SYSTEM} = \pm 2\delta$, where δ is the deviation of one wedge. If the wedges are turned from either maximum deviation position in opposite directions by β [see Fig. 6.35(d)], the deviation becomes $\delta_{SYSTEM} = \pm 2\delta\cos\beta$ and the change in deviation from the maximum achievable value is $2\delta(1 - 2\cos\beta)$. If we continue to turn the wedges until $\beta = 90°$, we obtain the condition shown in Fig. 6.35(b) where the apexes are opposite, the system acts as a plane parallel plate, and the deviation is zero.

Since counter rotation of the wedges in a Risley wedge system provides variable deviation in one axis, a second such system, usually identical to the first, is sometimes added to provide independent variation in the orthogonal axis. The deviations from the two systems add vectorially in a rectangular coordinate system. Another arrangement has a single Risley wedge system mounted so both wedges can be rotated together about the optical axis as well as counter rotated. This provides variation of deviation in a polar coordinate system.

6.3.25 Sliding wedge

A wedge prism located in a converging beam will deviate the beam so the image is displaced laterally by an amount proportional to the wedge deviation and the distance from the wedge to the image plane. See Fig. 6.36 for a schematic of the device. If the prism is moved axially by $D_2 - D_1$, the image displacement varies from $D_1\delta$ to $D_2\delta$. This device most frequently was used in military optical range finders before the advent of the laser range finder. The principle can be used in other more contemporary applications in which an image needs to be variably displaced laterally by a small distance. If used with a long focal length lens, the wedge should be achromatic.

6.3.26 Focus-adjusting wedge system

Two identical optical wedges arranged with their bases opposite and mechanized so each can be translated laterally by equal amounts relative to the optical axis provide a variable optical path through glass. Figure 6.37 shows the principle of operation of the device. At all settings, the two wedges act as a plane parallel plate. If located in a convergent beam, this system allows the image distance to be varied and can be used to bring images of objects at different distances into focus at a fixed image plane. This type of focus-adjusting system is sometimes used in large-aperture aerial cameras and

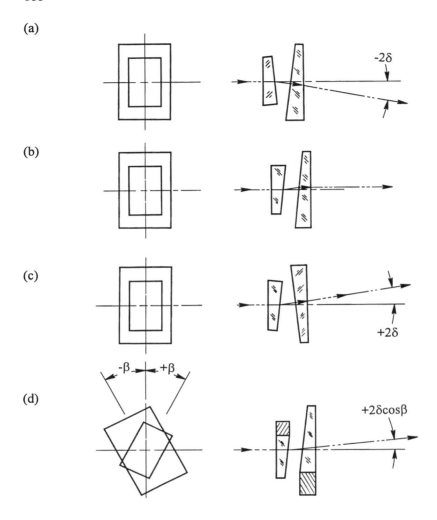

Fig. 6.35 Function of a Risley wedge prism system. (a) Bases down, (b) bases opposed, (c) bases up, wedges counter rotated by $\pm$ β.

telescopes such as those for tracking missiles or spacecraft launch vehicles where target range changes rapidly and the image-forming optics are large and heavy and so cannot be moved rapidly and precisely by small distances. To a first order, $t_i = t_0 \pm \Delta y_i \tan \theta$ and the focus variation is $\pm 2ti[(n - 1)/n]$. Here t_0 is the axial thickness of each wedge at its center. Figure 6.38 shows the optical schematic for a typical application featuring a focus-adjusting wedge system. The changes in glass path as the wedges are moved may cause the aberration balance of the optical system to change. This would limit the focus adjustment range in high-performance applications.

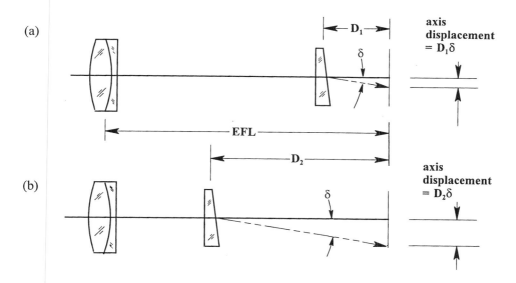

Fig. 6.36 A sliding wedge beam deviating system.

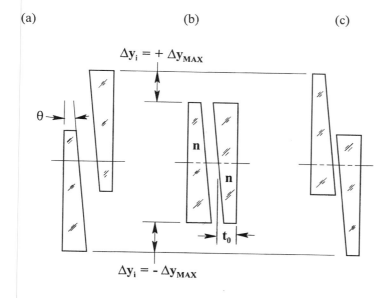

Fig. 6.37 A focus-adjusting wedge system. (a) Minimum path, (b) nominal path, (c) maximum path.

6.3.27 Anamorphic prism systems

A refracting prism, used at other than minimum deviation, changes the width of a transmitted collimated beam in the plane of refraction [see Fig. 6.39(a)]. The beam

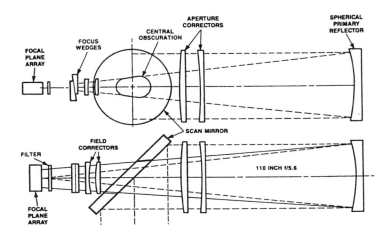

Fig. 6.38 Top and side views of the optical system for a 110-in. focal length, f/5.6 aerial camera lens with a wedge focus adjustment. (From Ulmes.[10])

width in the orthogonal meridian is unchanged, so anamorphic magnification results. Beam angular deviation and chromatic aberration are introduced. Both of these defects can be eliminated if two identical prisms are arranged in opposition as shown in Fig. 6.39(b). Lateral displacement of the axis then occurs, but the angular deviation and chromatic aberration are zero. The beam compression depends upon the prism apex angles, the refractive indices, and the orientations of the two prisms relative to the input axis. The configuration of Fig. 6.39(b) is a telescope in one meridian since the degree of collimation of the beam is unchanged while it is passing through the optics.

(a)

(b)

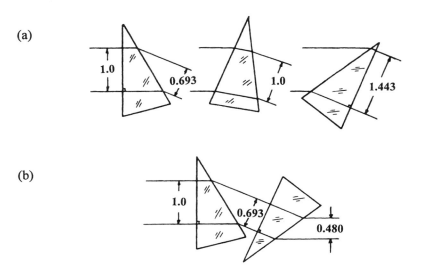

Fig. 6.39 Function of anamorphic prisms. (a) Individual prisms at various incident angles. (b) An anamorphic telescope. (From Kingslake.[11])

Two-prism anamorphic telescopes are attributed to Brewster in about 1835 as a replacement for the cylindrical lenses then used for the purpose.[11] They are commonly used today to change diode laser beam size and angular divergence differentially in orthogonal directions. The telescope shown in Fig. 6.40(a) has achromatic prisms to allow a broad spectral range to be covered.[12] Anamorphic telescopes with many cascaded prisms to produce higher magnification have been described. An extreme example with 10 prisms is shown in Fig. 6.40(b). This configuration is reported to be optimal for single-

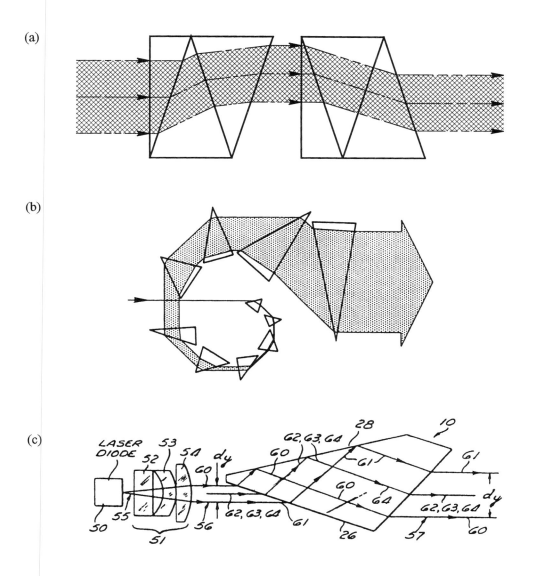

Fig. 6.40 Three anamorphic prism telescope designs. (a) Achromatic prism assembly (From Lohmann and Stork.[12]) (b) Cascaded assembly. (From Trebino.[13]) (c) Single-prism telescope. (From Forkner.[15])

material achromatic expanders of moderate to large magnifications.[13,14] A telescope example consisting of only one prism is shown in Fig. 6.40(c).[15] It has three active faces, one of which functions by TIR. The entrance and exit faces can be oriented at Brewster's angle, so the surface reflection (Fresnel) losses are eliminated for polarized beams.

Anamorphic prism pairs have been used quite successfully to convert rectangular Excimer laser beams into more suitable square ones for materials processing and surgical applications.

References

1. Yoder, P. R., Jr., *Opto-Mechanical Systems Design,* 2nd ed., Marcel Dekker, New York, 1993.
2. Smith, W.J., *Modern Optical Engineering*, 3rd ed., McGraw-Hill, New York, 1999.
3. MIL-HDBK-141*, Optical Design*, U.S. Defense Supply Agency, Washington, 1962.
4. Walles, S., and Hopkins, R.E., "The orientation of the image formed by a series of plane mirrors," *Appl. Opt.* Vol. 3, 1447, 1964.
5. Smith, W.J., Sect. 2 in *Handbook of Optics*, Optical Society of America, Washington, 1978.
6. Yoder, P.R., Jr., "Two new lightweight military binoculars," *J. Opt. Soc. Am.* Vol. 50, 491, 1960.
7. Durie, D.S.L., "A compact derotator design," *Opt. Eng.* Vol. 13, 19, 1974.
8. Yoder, P.R., Jr., "Study of light deviation errors in triple mirrors and tetrahedral prisms," *J. Opt. Soc. Am.* Vol. 48, 496, 1958.
9. PLX, Inc. sales literature, Hard-Mounted Hollow Retroreflector, PLX, Deer Park, NY.
10. Ulmes, J.J., "Design of a catadioptric lens for long-range oblique aerial reconnaissance," *SPIE Proceedings* Vol. 1113, 116, 1989.
11. Kingslake, R., *Optical System Design*, Academic Press, Orlando, 1983.
12. Lohmann, A.W., and Stork, W., "Modified Brewster telescopes," *Appl. Opt.* Vol. 28, 1318, 1989.
13. Trebino, R., "Achromatic N-prism beam expanders: optimal configurations," *Appl.Opt.* Vol. 24, 1130, 1985.
14. Trebino, R., Barker, C.E., and Siegman, A.E., "Achromatic N-prism beam expanders: optimal configurations II," *SPIE Proceedings* Vol. 540, 104, 1985.
15. Forkner, J.F., "Anamorphic prism for beam shaping," U. S. Patent No. 4,623,225, 1986.

CHAPTER 7
Techniques for Mounting Prisms

In this chapter, we consider several techniques for mounting individual prisms in optical instruments by semikinematic or nonkinematic clamping and bonding them to mechanical structures. Techniques for mounting larger prisms on flexures are also described. Although most of the discussions deal with glass prisms interfacing with metal mountings, the designs are generally applicable to prisms made of optical crystals and plastics and to attaching prisms to nonmetallic cells, brackets, and housings. Numerous examples are included to illustrate the use of given design principles.

7.1 Semikinematic mountings

The position (translations) and orientation (tilts) of a prism generally must be established during assembly and then carefully controlled to tolerances that are dependent upon its location and function in the optical system. Control is accomplished through the prism's interfaces with its mechanical surround. If possible, the optical material should always be placed in compression at all temperatures. Kinematic mounting avoids overconstraints that might distort the optical surfaces. The point contacts with potentially high stresses inherent in true kinematic mounts can be avoided by providing semikinematic mounting with small-area contacts at the interfaces. Properly designed spring forces applied over these finite areas allow expansion and contraction with temperature changes while adequately protecting the prism against worst-case acceleration forces.

Contact within the clear apertures of optically active surfaces implies obscuration as well as the possibility of surface distortion. Hence, such contact should be avoided. Since reflecting surfaces are much more sensitive to deformation than refracting ones, they are especially critical. Note that TIR surfaces must not touch anything that will frustrate the refractive index mismatch that causes the internal reflection to take place. If periodic cleaning of a TIR surface is required, the design should provide the necessary convenient access.

Figure 7.1(a) schematically illustrates a semikinematic mounting for a cube-shaped beamsplitter prism described by Lipshutz.[1] Here five springs at the points labeled "K_i" preload the cemented prism against directly opposite coplanar (i.e., lapped) raised pads indicated as "K_∞." Although the contacts occur on refracting surfaces, they are located outside the used aperture, thereby avoiding obscurations and minimizing the effects of surface distortions. The structure supporting the fixed points and the springs is assumed to be rigid; a more realistic case would take the structure design into account. Constraint of the sixth degree of freedom (Z) is provided only by friction in the interfaces.

As shown in Fig. 7.1(b), this beamsplitter is used to divide a beam converging toward an image plane; each beam then forms an image on a separate detector. In order for these images to maintain their proper alignment relative to each other, to the detectors, and to the structure of the optical instrument with temperature changes, the prism must not translate in the XY plane of the figure or rotate about any of the three orthogonal axes. Translation in the Z direction has no optical effect here. This motion is limited to a small value by mechanical stops (not shown). Once aligned, the springs ensure that

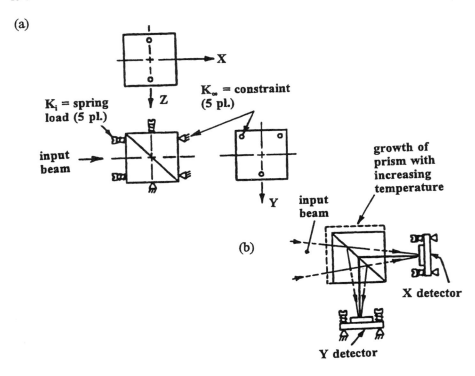

Fig. 7.1 (a) Three views of a semikinematic mount for a cube-shaped beamsplitter prism. (b) Sschematic of a typical optical function showing the effect of temperature rise. (Adapted from Lipshutz.[1])

a small value by mechanical stops (not shown). Once aligned, the springs ensure that the prism always presses against the five pads. The dashed outlines in the figures indicate how the prism will expand if the temperature increases. Registry of the prism surfaces against the pads does not change and the light paths to the detectors do not deviate. This is also true when the temperature decreases.

The preload force, P_i (in pounds), to be exerted by one spring on the prism with the mounting just described may be calculated with the aid of Eq. (7.1). This equation is a minor modification of Eq. (3.18).

$$P = Wa_G/N \qquad\qquad (7.1)$$

where W is the weight of the prism, a_G is the maximum anticipated acceleration expressed as a multiple of ambient gravity, and N is the number of springs active in the direction of the preload force. Note that if the prism weight is expressed in kilograms, Eq. (7.1) must include an additional multiplicative factor of 4.448 to convert units. The preload is then in newtons (N). Friction and moments at the contacts are ignored in the equation.

When the prism configuration is other than a cube, the mounting design can be

Example 7.1: Clamping force needed to hold a beamsplitter cube prism semikinematically.

A beamsplitter cube weighing 0.518 lb is constrained as indicated in Fig. 7.1 and is to withstand 25G accelerations in any direction. What force is needed at each spring?

We apply Eq. (7.1) to each case:

Force per spring on the 3-contact face = (0.518)(25)/(3) = 4.317 lb (19.203 N)
Force per spring on the 2-contact face = (0.518)(25)/(2) = 6.475 lb (28.802 N)

more complex since it may be difficult or perhaps impossible to apply forces directly opposite support pads. Figures 7.2(a) and 7.2(b), adapted from Durie,[2] show one example.

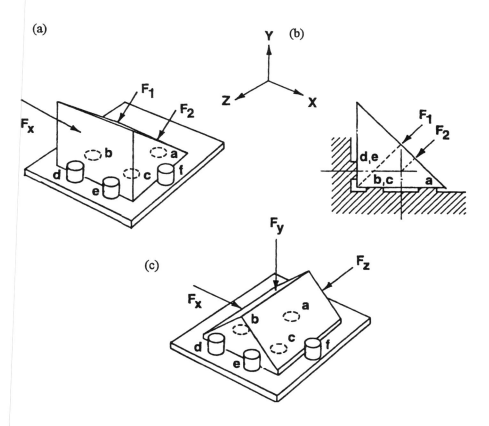

Fig. 7.2 Schematics of semikinematic mounts for (a) and (b) a right-angle prism referenced to one refracting face, and (c) a Porro prism referenced to its hypotenuse face. (Adapted from Durie.[2])

Figure 7.2(a) shows a right-angle prism semikinematically mounted on one of its refracting faces. These faces are square. Three coplanar pads on the baseplate provide constraints in the Y direction while three horizontally oriented locating pins pressed into the base plate add three more (X-Y) constraints. Note that the required perforations (i.e., apertures) in the plate are not shown in Figs. 7.2(a) and 7.2(b). Ideally, all pads and pins contact the prism outside its optically active apertures (not shown). In Fig.(b), the same prism is shown in side view. The preload forces F_2 and F_2 are oriented perpendicular to the hypotenuse face and touch the prism near the longer edges of the hypotenuse. F_1 is aimed symmetrically between the nearest pad (b) and the nearest pin (d) while F_2 is aimed symmetrically between pads a and c and pin e. Horizontal force F_X holds the prism against pin f and horizontal and vertical components of F_1 and F_2 hold the prism against the three pads and remaining two locating pins. Although it is not optimum in terms of freedom from bending tendencies (i.e., moments) because the forces are not directed toward the pads, this arrangement is adequate since the prism is relatively stiff.

In Fig. 7.2(c), the hypotenuse face of a Porro prism is positioned against three coplanar raised pads on a perforated plate (perforations again not shown) while one edge touches two pins and one edge touches a third pin. The pins are perpendicular to the plate surface. Optical clear apertures are not shown. A force, F_Z, directed parallel to and slightly above the plate holds the prism against two pins (d and e) while force F_X, also just above the plate, holds it against the the third pin (f). A third force, F_Y, holds the prism against the three pads (a, b, and c). This force acts against the dihedral edge of the prism at its center. Once again, the prism is stiff enough that surface distortion is minimal.

Example 7.2: Clamping force needed to hold a Porro prism semi-kinematically.

A Porro prism is constrained as indicated in Fig. 7.2(c). It is made of SF8 glass and has an aperture A of 2.875 cm (1.132 in.). It is to withstand 10G accelerations in any of the three axis directions. What should be each of the total forces P_X, P_Y, and P_Z? Ignore friction.

From Fig. 6.12, the prism volume = $V = 1.29A^3 = 30.569$ cm^3
From Table B1, the glass density = $\rho = 4.22$ g/cm^3
Hence, $W = (30.569)(4.22) = 129.001$ g $= 0.129$ kg

From Eq. (7.1): $P_X = P_Y = P_Z = (0.129)(9.8066)(10)/1 = 12.650$ N (2.84 lb)

Figure 7.3 shows a right-angle prism referenced to one triangular ground face. Here also, the prism is pressed against three coplanar raised pads and three locating pins, all on the baseplate. The top plate presses the prism through a resilient (elastomeric) pad under the clamping action of three long screws. A leaf spring anchored at both ends (here we define this as a "straddling" spring) presses the prism against the locating pins. Other spring types could, of course, be used for the latter purpose. An attractive feature of this mounting is that it can be configured so the circular clear apertures of optically active surfaces are not obscured and are not likely to be distorted by the imposed forces.

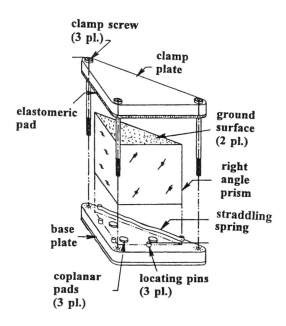

clamp screw
(3 pl.)

clamp
plate

elastomeric
pad

ground
surface
(2 pl.)

right
angle
prism

straddling
spring

base
plate

coplanar
pads
(3 pl.)

locating pins
(3 pl.)

Fig. 7.3 Semikinematic mounting for a right-angle prism with preload provided by a compressed elastomeric pad. (Adapted from Vukobratovich.[3])

The resilient pad provides the spring force (preload) necessary to hold the prism in place under shock and vibration, so we can design the subassembly only if the elastic characteristic of the pad material is known. The pertinent material property is the "spring constant," C_P, defined as the load that must be applied normal to the pad surface to produce a unit deflection [see Eq. (7.2)].

$$C_P = P_i/\Delta y \qquad\qquad (7.2)$$

Most resilient materials have a limited elastic range, tend to creep over time, and typically take a permanent set under sustained high compressive load, i.e., one greater than that for which the material acts elastically. For these reasons, these materials might be considered unreliable for use in the manner suggested here. However, since they are sometimes used, we consider a typical type of material as it might be used here.

Typically, a material such as Sorbothane™, a viscoelastic, thermoset, polyether base polyurethane behaves as indicated in Fig. 7.4 for different durometers and three deflections as percentages of the pad thickness. The material depicted is commonly used in vibration isolators and behaves elastically if the change in thickness is between 10% and 25% of the total thickness.[4] Obviously, a softer material deflects more per unit load. Since we should design the interface for the maximum applied force (which would occur at maximum acceleration), we might well choose the 20% deflection curve of Fig. 7.4 so

C_S (psi)

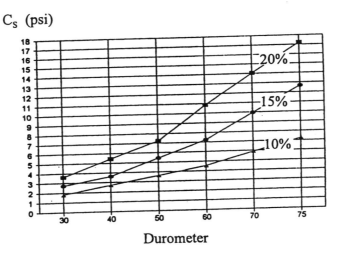

Durometer

Fig. 7.4 Compressive stress (C_S) vs. durometer for a viscoelastic material with deflections of various percentages of pad thickness. (Courtesy of Sorbothane, Inc., Kent, OH.)

deflections under conditions of lesser severity would lie well within the linear range of the material. The manufacturer's literature suggests that deflection, Δy, is related to load, P_i, (in the USC system) as follows:

$$\Delta y = (0.15)(P_i)(t_p)/[(C_S)(1 + 2\gamma^2)(A_p)] \tag{7.3}$$

where:

P_i = required force per pad (in N or lb)
t_p = pad thickness (in mm or in.)
$\gamma = D_p/4t_p$, a "shape factor" for a square or circular pad   (7.4)
D_p = pad width or diameter (in mm^2 or in.^{2})
$A_p = D_p^2$ for a square pad (in mm^2 or in.)   (7.5a)
    $= \pi D_p^2/4$ for a circular pad (in mm^2 or in.^{2})   (7.5b)
C_S = compressive stress in the pad per Fig. 7.4

Example 7.3 illustrates a typical design for a resilient interface. Similar calculations apply to other resilient materials if their elastic properties are available and their force vs. deflection characteristics are appropriate over a reasonable range of deflections.

Another semikinematic mounting is illustrated schematically in Fig. 7.5. Here, a penta prism is pressed against three circular coplanar pads on a baseplate. Three cantilevered springs provide the necessary preload directly through the prism against

Example 7.3: Penta prism clamped through a circular resilient pad. (For design and analysis, use File 17 of the CD-ROM)

A SF6 penta prism with aperture A = 2.000 in. (50.800 mm) is to be clamped against three pads on a baseplate by a rigid plate in a manner similar to that shown in Fig. 7.3. A circular pad with thickness 0.375 in. (9.525 mm) made of material characterized by Fig. 7.4 is placed between the clamping plate and the prism. (a) Using 30 durometer material, what size pad is required if a 20% deflection is to occur at a maximum acceleration of 10 times gravity? (b) What is C_P for the pad?

(a) From Fig. 6.17, we find that the penta prism volume is $1.5A^3$ and from Table B1, we determine that the density of SF6 glass is 0.187 lb/in.^{3} (5.18 g/cm^3). Hence, the prism weight = (volume)(density) = $(1.5)(2.000^3)(0.187)$ = 2.244 lb. (1.018 kg). From Eq. (7.1), the preload required = P_i = (2.44)(10)/1 = 22.440 lb (99.818 N).

From Fig. 7.4, the compressive stress, C_S, in the pad at 30 durometer and 20% deflection is approximately 3.7 lb/in.^{2} (2.55×10^4 Pa).
From Eq. (7.4), $\gamma = D_P/4t_P = D_P/(4)(0.375) = 0.6667D_P$
From Eq. (7.5b), $A_P = \pi D_P^2/4 = 0.7854D_P^2$

From Eq. (7.3), $\Delta y = (0.15)(22.440)(0.375)/[(3.7)(1 + (2)(0.667D_P)^2)(0.785D_P^2)]$.

This deflection also is to be 20% of 0.375 in. or 0.075 in. Equating and applying algebra, we obtain the quadratic equation: $0.194D_P^4 + 0.218D_P^2 - 1.262 = 0$.
Solving for D_P^2 and taking the square root, we obtain D_P = 1.431 in. (3.635 cm).

We need to see if the pad will fit onto the side of the prism. From Fig. 6.17, the largest circular area that can be inscribed within the pentagonal face of the prism is found to be $Q_{MAX(C)} = 1.13A^2 = (1.13)(2.000)^2 = 4.520$ in.^{2}. From this we derive $D_{P\,MAX} = [(4)(4.520)/\pi]^{1/2} = 2.399$ in. (6.094 cm). This shows that the pad will easily fit on the prism face.

(b) The pad's spring constant is C_P = 22.440 / 0.075 = 299.2 lb/in. (528.1 N/cm)

A smaller pad would be used if it were a stiffer material (such as 70 durometer) or if the thickness t_P were reduced.

the pads. This provides three constraints: one translation and two tilts. The remaining translations and one tilt are constrained by three locating pins with a straddling leaf spring to provide preload of the prism against the pins.

Equations (3.28) and (3.29) are used to design the cantilevered springs for this application and to check the bending stress in each spring clip just as they were used in Sect. 3.5 in designing similar constraints for lenses. For convenience of the reader, they are repeated here.

(a)

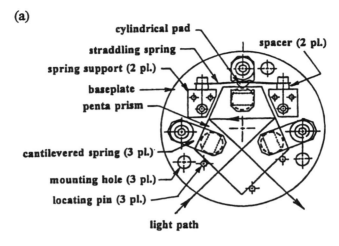

(b)

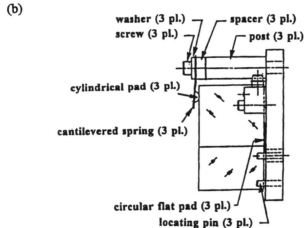

Fig. 7.5 Semi-kinematic mounting for a penta prism with cantilevered and straddling spring constraints: (a) plan view, (b) elevation view.

$$\Delta = (1 - \nu_M^2)(4PL^3)/(E_M bt^3 N) \qquad (3.28)$$

$$S_B = 6PL/(bt^2 N) \qquad (3.29)$$

where:

ν_M = Poisson's ratio for the clip material
P = nominal total preload
L = free (cantilevered) length of the clip
E_M = Young's modulus for the clip material

> b   = width of the clip
> t   = thickness of the clip
> N   = number of clips employed

     Another useful equation pertinent to cantilevered spring design is the angle at which the end of the cantilevered portion of the spring is bent relative to the fixed portion of the spring. This equation (adapted from Roark[5]) is

$$\phi = (1 - v_M^2)(6L^2P_i)/(E_Mbt^3) \qquad\qquad (7.6)$$

Example 7.4: Analysis of a cantilevered spring clip design for clamping a prism. (For design and analysis, use File 18.1 of the CD-ROM)

Assume the following dimensions and material properties for the prism mounting of Fig. 7.5(b): W = prism weight = 0.267 lb (0.121 kg), a_G = acceleration factor = 12, N = number of springs = 3 (BeCu), yield strength of BeCu = 155,000 lb/in.^{2} (1.069×10^3 MPa), P_i = nominal preload per spring = Wa_G/N = 1.068 lb (4.751 N), E_M = spring Young's modulus =18.5×10^6 lb/in. (1.27×10^5 Pa), L = cantilevered length of spring = 0.375 in. (9.525 mm), υ_M = spring Poisson's ratio = 0.35, b = spring width = 0.250 in. (6.350 mm), t = spring thickness = 0.020 in. (0.508 mm). (a) What is the spring deflection needed? (b) What bending stress results in the spring? (c) What is the safety factor for the spring? (d) What is the angle through which the spring is bent?

(a) From Eq. (3.28):
Δ = spring deflection = $(1 - 0.35^2)(4)(0.375^3)(1.068)/[(18.5\times10^6)(0.250)(0.020^3)]$
            = 0.0053 in.

(b) From Eq. (3.29):
S_B = spring stress = $(6)(0.375)(1.068)/[(0.250)(0.020^2)]$
           = 24,030 lb/in.^{2} (165.7 MPa)

(c) The safety factor then is f_S = yield stress/spring stress = 155,000/24,030 = 6.6

(d) From Eq. (7.6):

   ϕ = spring tip angle = $(1 - 0.35^2)(6)(0.375^2)(1.068)/[(18.5\times10^6)(0.250)(0.020^3)]$
             = 0.021 rad = 1.22°

Note: Δy is smaller than might be desired and f_S is too large. We could decrease t to make both more reasonable. This is the subject of Example 7.5.

Example 7.5: Optimize the cantilevered spring deflection for a prism mounting. (For design and analysis, use File 18.2 of the CD-ROM)

In order to demonstrate one logical approach to finding the "optimum" deflection for the spring in the last example, rewrite Eq. (3.29) in parametric form relating S_B to spring thickness t; set that equal to one-half the yield stress for BeCu, and solve for Δy and ϕ:

$S_B = (6)(0.375)(1.068)/(0.250)(t^2) = 9.5940/t^2 = 155,000/2$

Solving for t^2 and taking the square root, we obtain t = 0.011 in. (0.279 mm)

Now we substitute that value into Eq. (3.28) and obtain:
$\Delta y = (1 - 0.35^2)(4)(0.375^3)(1.068)/[(18.5\times10^6)(0.250)(0.011^3)]$
    $= 0.032$ in. (0.813 mm).

From Eq. (7.6):
$\phi = (1 - 0.35^2)(6)(0.375^2)(1.068)/[(18.5\times10^6)(0.250)(0.011^3)]$
    $= 0.128$ rad $= 7.360°$

The deflection can be measured quite accurately and the spring stress is appropriate, so the cantilevered spring design is considered acceptable.

We next consider the straddling-spring constraint shown in Fig. 7.5. The spring dimensions are width b, thickness t, and total free spring length L (not including any portion occupied by a rigid pad). The deflection from the relaxed spring shape and the bending stress in the spring are

$$\Delta y = (0.0625)(1 - v_M^2)(P_i L^3)/(E_M b t^3) \qquad (7.7)$$

$$S_B = (0.75)(P_i L)/(b t^2) \qquad (7.8)$$

Example 7.6: Analysis of a straddling spring design for clamping a prism. (For design and analysis, use File 19 of the CD-ROM)

Consider the prism mounting shown in Fig. 7.5. The dimensions and material properties listed in Example 7.4 apply, as well as the following parameters that pertain to the straddling spring constraint in the plane of reflection: N = number of springs = 1 (BeCu), P_i = preload per spring = Wa_G/N = 3.204 lb (1.452 N), L = spring total free length = 1.040 in. (26.416 mm), b = spring width = 0.250 in. (6.350 mm), t = spring thickness = 0.0115 in. (0.292 mm). (a) What is the spring deflection? (b) What bending stress results in the spring? (c) What is the safety factor for the spring?

From Eq. (7.7):
$$\Delta y = (0.0625)(1 - 0.35^2)(3.204)(1.040^3)/[(18.5 \times 10^6)(0.250)(0.0115^3)]$$
$$= 0.0281 \text{ in. } (0.714 \text{ mm})$$

From Eq. (7.8): $S_B = (0.75)(3.204)(1.040)/[(0.25)(0.014^2)]$
$$= 75,590 \text{ lb/in.}^2 \text{ (521.2 MPa)}$$

From Table B12: S_Y for BeCu = 155,000 lb/in.^{2}
Hence, $f_S = 155,000/75,590 = 2.05$

These results seem acceptable.

The use of cylindrical pads between the springs and the prism surfaces in the design of Figs. 7.5(a) and 7.5(b) ensures that line contact will occur in a reliable manner at each interface. In the absence of a pad, a deflected cantilevered spring could touch the prism at the edge of its protective bevel as shown in Fig. 7.6(a). This is highly undesirable since that edge is sharp and, as will be shown in Sect. 11.4, the stresses at a sharp corner interface typically are large, so the prism is vulnerable to damage from the force exerted by the spring. An alternative interface, again without a pad, is illustrated in Fig. 7.6(b). Here the deflected spring nominally lies flat against the top prism surface by virtue of the wedge-shaped washers placed above and below the spring on the post. The angles of the wedges are set by Eq. (7.4). While this is good from the viewpoint of stress imparted to the prism if the spring is in close contact with an appreciable area on the prism, a potential problem with the latter design is that the angle might be wrong because of a minor manufacturing error or unfavorable tolerance buildup that could cause the end of the spring to touch the prism surface (if the angle is too steep) or the spring to touch the bevel (if the angle is too shallow). Either of these conditions could lead to prism damage from a concentration of stress.

Another version of the area interface of Fig. 7.6(b) is shown in Fig. 7.7. Here a flat surface on a wedged pad attached to the end of the spring provides the angular adjustment needed to bring the pad into close contact with the prism surface. Once again, the design is susceptible to angular errors causing it deteriorate into sharp corner contact at the inner or outer edge of the pad, resulting in undue stress.

Line contact at a rounded portion of the spring occurs if the end of the spring is bent to a convex cylindrical shape as indicated in Fig. 7.8(a). Since it may be difficult to form the spring into a smooth cylinder of a particular radius, a better interface results if a pad is machined directly into the spring as indicated in Fig. 7.8(b). Note that a machined cylindrical pad can also be attached to the spring by screws, welding, or adhesive and achieve the same function. In either case, stress introduced at the interface between the convex cylinder and the flat prism surface can be estimated and adjusted to an acceptable level by careful design. We explain how to do this in Sect. 11.4.

(a)

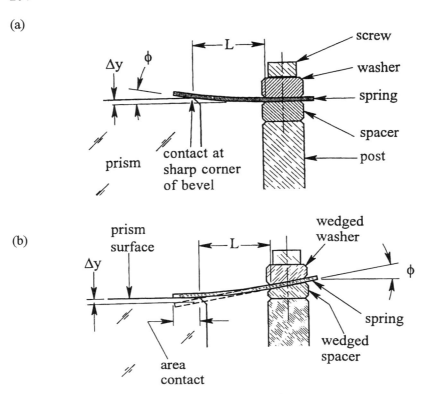

(b)

Fig. 7.6 Two configurations of the cantilevered spring-to-prism interface. (a)
Spring touching prism bevel, (b) spring lying flat on the prism.

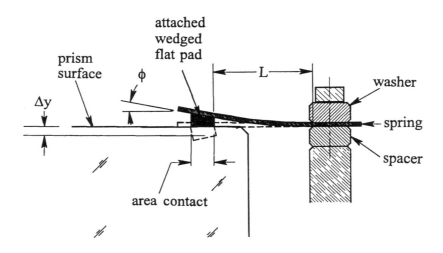

Fig. 7.7 Configuration of a cantilevered spring-to-prism interface with a flat pad
pressing against a flat surface of the prism .

(a)

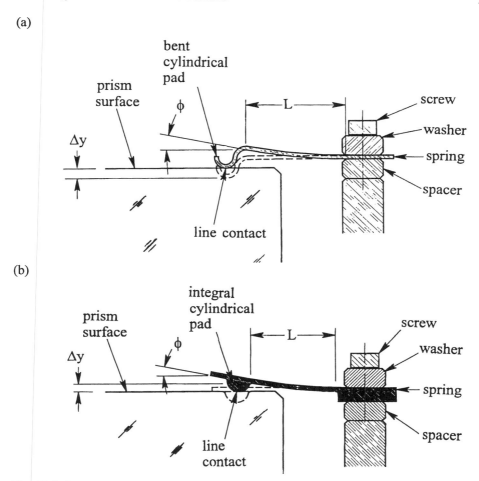

(b)

Fig. 7.8 Configurations for a cantilevered spring-to-prism interface with. (a) the spring bent into a convex curve and (b) an integrally machined cylindrical pad.

Figure 7.9 shows how a straddling spring can be substituted for the three cantilevered spring clips of Fig. 7.5(a) to hold a prism in place. A flat pad is shown in Fig. 7.9(a) as a means for distributing the force over a small area on the prism. This would be acceptable if we could be sure that the spring action is symmetrical and that the pad lies flat on the prism. Dimensional errors or tolerance buildup could tilt the pad at the wrong angle and cause stress concentration at a pad edge. Curving the pad as shown in Fig. 7.9(b) eliminates this possibility. Additional springs can be used if one is not sufficient to provide the required preload or to reduce stress at each interface.

To further illustrate the use of straddling springs to constrain prisms, consider the hardware design for Porro prism mountings in a commercial binocular as shown in Fig. 7.10. The springs press against the apexes of the prisms and hold those prisms against reference surfaces provided in the housings. One end of each spring is secured with a screw while the other end simply slips into a slot machined into the housing wall. No pads are used on the springs.

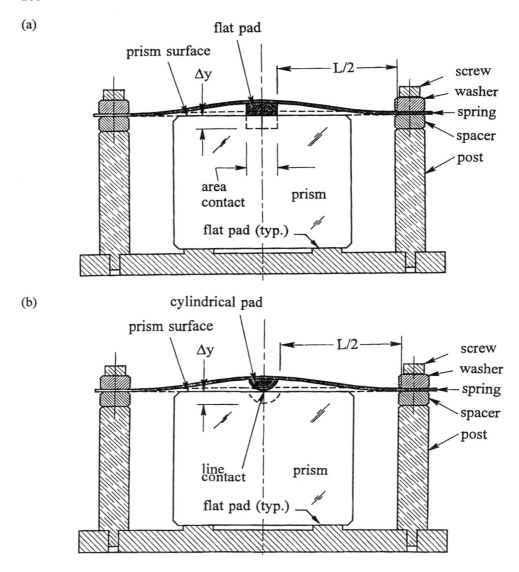

Fig. 7.9 Straddling spring constraints for a prism. (a) With a flat pad, (b) with a cylindrical pad.

Yet another version of the straddling spring prism mounting is illustrated in Fig. 7.11. Here an Amici prism is held against flat pads in a military telescope housing by a spring with bent ends. The screw pressing against the center of the spring forces its ends against the prism. It is very important that the screw not protrude far enough into the housing for the spring to touch the roof edge of the prism. Careful design would specify the correct screw length, while explicit instructions in the manufacturing procedures to check the actual clearance would help avoid damage at assembly or during exposure to shock or vibration, especially at extreme temperatures. Constraint perpendicular to the

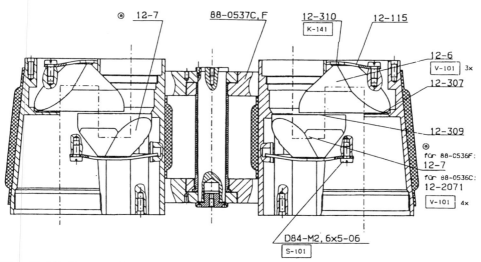

Fig. 7.10 Porro prism mounting in a contemporary commercial binocular. (Courtesy of Swarovski Optik KG, Absam/Tyrol, Austria.)

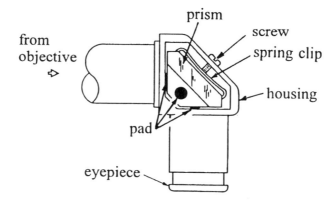

Fig. 7.11 Schematic of a small military elbow telescope with an Amici prism spring loaded against reference pads. (Adapted from Yoder.[6])

plane of the figure is provided by resilient pads attached to the inside surfaces of triangular-shaped covers that are attached with screws to the cast housing.

The author has examined a telescope with this type of mounting and found a fracture in the prism at one spring-to-prism sharp-corner interface; this is believed to have resulted from excess stress that developed during use of the instrument. While it is simple, this type mounting is not recommended for future applications. An improvement that might make the design acceptable would be to add cylindrical pads at each end of the spring and shape that spring so the pads touch the ends of the prism farther from the roof edge.

The designs of the cylindrical pads for use on cantilevered or straddling springs should include consideration of the angular extent of the curved surfaces. Figure 7.12 shows the pertinent geometrical relationships. R_{CYL} is the pad's radius, d_p is the width of the pad, and α is one-half the angular extent of the cylindrical surface measured at its center of curvature. In Fig. 7.12(a), the pad is tangent to the prism surface before the spring is bent. In Fig. 7.12(b), the spring is bent to exert preload P_i, tilting the pad by the angle ϕ per Eq. (7.6). If the worst-case α is greater than ϕ, no sharp edge contact will occur. Once α is determined, we calculate the minimum value for d_p as $2R_{CYL} \sin \alpha$.

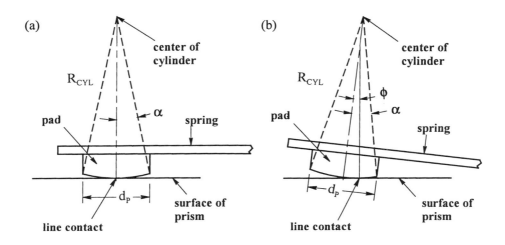

Fig. 7.12 Geometric relationships applied in the design of cylindrical pads for springs. The same geometry applies to spherical pads.

7.2 Mechanically Clamped Nonkinematic Mountings

Springs or straps are frequently used to hold prisms in place against extended flat interfaces in optical instruments. These techniques are not kinematic. One is the Porro prism erecting prism assembly shown schematically in Fig. 7.13. This is typical of prism mountings in many military and consumer binoculars and telescopes.[7] Spring straps (typically made of spring steel) hold each prism against a machined surface in a perforated aluminum mounting shelf that is in turn fastened with screws and locating pins to the instrument housing. The straps are a variation of the straddling spring discussed earlier.

Area contacts occur over annular areas on the racetrack-shaped hypotenuse faces of the prisms, while lateral constraints are provided by recessing those faces slightly into opposite sides of the shelf. An elastomeric-type adhesive (called cement in the figure) is used to keep the prism from sliding in the necessary clearances around the recessed faces. In this design, the prisms are made of high-index (flint) glass so TIR occurs at the four reflecting surfaces. Thin aluminum light shields help prevent stray light from reaching the image plane. These shields have bent tabs that touch the edges of the prism faces to

(a)

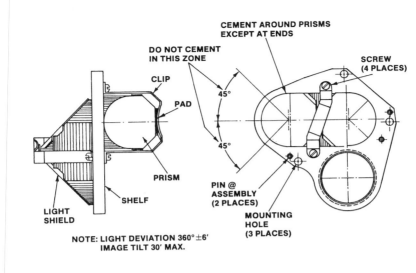

CEMENT AROUND PRISMS
EXCEPT AT ENDS

DO NOT CEMENT
IN THIS ZONE

CLIP

PAD

45°

45°

PRISM

SHELF

LIGHT
SHIELD

SCREW
(4 PLACES)

PIN @
ASSEMBLY
(2 PLACES)

MOUNTING
HOLE
(3 PLACES)

NOTE: LIGHT DEVIATION 360°±6'
IMAGE TILT 30' MAX.

(b)

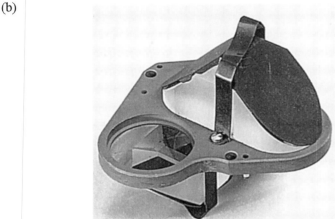

Fig. 7.13 (a) Schematic view and (b) photograph of a typical strap mounting for a Porro prism erecting subassembly. (Adapted from Yoder.[7])

space the shields a short distance away from the reflecting surfaces. Prisms with silvered or aluminized reflecting surfaces do not need these shields.

Figure 7.14 shows the scanning head assembly from a military periscope. It uses a single prism that resembles a Dove prism with angles between faces of 35°, 35°, and 110°. The prism can be tilted about the horizontal transverse axis to scan the periscope's line of sight, in elevation, from the zenith to about 20° below the horizon. The prism is held in place in its cast aluminum mounting by four spring clips, each attached with two screws to the mount adjacent to the entrance and exit faces of the prism. The edges of the reflecting surface (hypotenuse) of the prism rest on narrow lands machined and lapped into the casting. The lands do not extend into the optical aperture. The prism faces protrude slightly [about 0.5 mm (0.02 in.)] from the mount so that preload is obtained

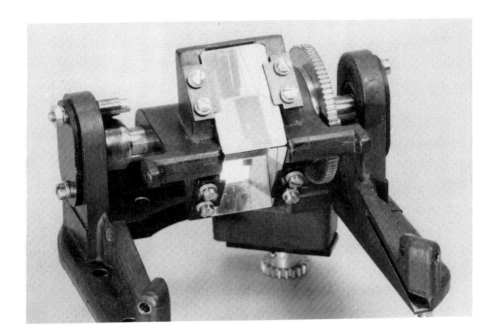

Fig. 7.14 A clamped Dove-type prism used in the elevation scanning head subassembly of a military periscope. (From Yoder.[8])

when the clips are clamped flush against the mount. Once centered, the prism cannot slide parallel to the long edge of its hypotenuse because of the convergence of the clamping forces. The vector sum of these forces is nominally perpendicular to the mounting surface and the tangential force components cancel each other. Lateral motion is constrained by friction and limited by a close fit in the mount.

Figure 7.15 illustrates the scanning function of the prism in Fig. 7.14. This motion is usually limited optically by vignetting of the refracted beam at its top or bottom. Mechanical stops are usually built into the instrument to limit physical motion so that the vignetting at the end-point is acceptable for the application.

The most popular types of derotation prisms are the Dove, double-Dove, Pechan, and delta. In order to function successfully, all these prisms must be mounted securely yet be capable of adjustment at the time of assembly to minimize image motion during operation. A design for an adjustable derotation prism mounting is discussed next.

In Fig. 7.16, we see a sectional view of a representative Pechan prism mounting.[9] If it is used in a collimated beam, it requres only angular adjustment of the optical axis relative to the rotation axis. Here it was to be used in an uncollimated beam, so both angular and lateral adjustments were needed. Bearing wobble would cause angular errors. To minimize this in the design considered here, class 5 angular contact bearings, mounted back to back, were oriented with factory-identified high spots matched and then preloaded. Runout over 180° motion was measured as about 0.0003 in. (7.6 μm). The bearing axis

(a)   (b)   (c)

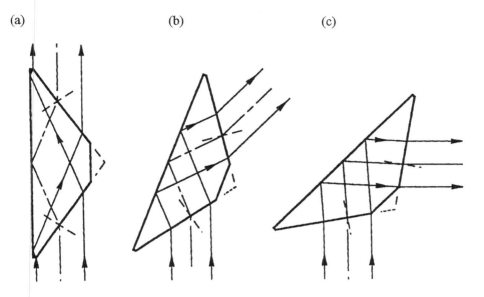

Fig. 7.15 Typical elevation scanning function of a Dove prism.

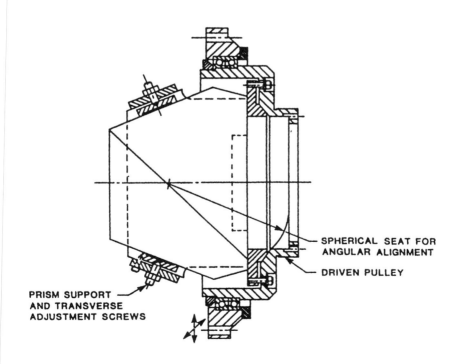

Fig. 7.16 A Pechan prism derotation assembly. (From Delgado.[9])

was adjusted laterally by fine-thread screws (not shown) that permitted centration with respect to the optical system axis to better than 0.0005 in. (12.7 μm). The prism was adjusted laterally within the bearing housing in the plane of refraction by sliding it against a flat vertical reference surface with fine-thread screws pressing against the reflecting surfaces through pressure pads. A spherical seat with its center of rotation at the intersection of the hypotenuse face with the optic axis (to minimize axis cross-coupling) was provided for angular adjustment. This movement was controlled by the adjustment screws indicated.

In each of the last four prism design examples — the Porro, the Amici, the Dove-type, and the Pechan — are loaded against machined surfaces on the mounts. Since it is virtually impossible for the metal surfaces to be as flat as the interfacing glass surfaces, contact will occur first on the three highest points on the mount. Usually these points are not directly opposite the springs that hold the prism in place. Moments are then applied to the glass, and surface deformations may occur. If the spring loading is large, the metal or the glass may bend enough for more point contacts to form. We then have a condition of uncontrolled overconstraint. Since the prisms are stiff and the instruments into which these designs have been incorporated have demonstrated long service life in relatively adverse environments, we conclude that these problems are usually tolerable. Adding small-area pads that can be lapped flat and coplanar and located opposite or nearly opposite the force points, such as those used in the designs shown in Figs. 7.1, 7.2, and 7.5, reduces the likelihood of prism distortion from the applied constraints.

A potential problem occurs if, under shock or vibration, the prism loses contact with some of its interfacing positional references (i.e., the lapped pads). When the driving force is dissipated, the prism may land in a new orientation. It remains there until it is disturbed again. This action introduces uncertainty into the location and/or orientation of the optical component, which may affect performance. If the springs are strong enough that the optic always maintains contact with the references, even at extreme temperatures, this problem should not exist.

7.3 Bonded Prism Mountings

7.3.1 General considerations

Many prisms are mounted by bonding their ground faces to mechanical pads using epoxy or similar adhesives. An example from a military periscope used in armored vehicles is shown in Fig. 7.17. Contact areas large enough to render strong joints can usually be provided in designs with minimum complexity. The mechanical strength of a carefully designed and manufactured bond is adequate to withstand the severe shock and vibration as well as other adverse environmental conditions characteristic of military and aerospace applications. This technique is also used in many less rigorous applications because of its inherent simplicity and reliability.

The critical aspects of the design are the characteristics of the adhesive, the thickness of the adhesive layer, the cleanliness of the surfaces to be bonded, the dissimilarity of coefficients of expansion of the materials, the area of the bond, environmental conditions, and the care with which the parts are assembled. Several typical

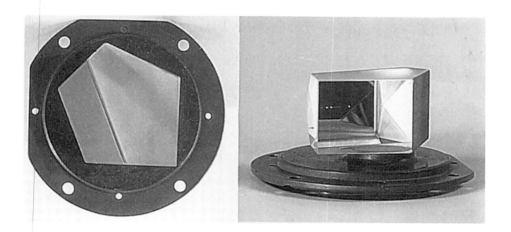

Fig. 7.17 Photographs of a typical roof penta prism bonded to a flange. (From Yoder.[8])

adhesives used for this purpose are listed in Table B14. While the adhesive manufacturer's recommendations should be consulted, experimental verification of the adequacy of the design, the materials to be used, the method of application, and curing temperature and duration are advisable in critical applications.

Guidelines for determining the appropriate bonding area have appeared in the literature.[10] In general, the minimum area of the bond, Q_{MIN}, is determined by Eq. (7.9).

$$Q_{MIN} = W a_G f_s / J \qquad (7.9)$$

where:

W = prism weight
a_G = maximum expected acceleration factor
f_s = safety factor
J = the adhesive shear or tensile strength (usually approximately equal)

The safety factor should be at least 2 and possibly as large as 4 or 5 to allow for some unplanned, nonoptimum conditions, such as inadequate cleaning during processing. Most prism designs considered in Sect. 6.3 list equations for calculating the minimum circular or racetrack shaped bonding area and the maximum bonding area achievable ($Q_{MAX (C)}$ or $Q_{MAX (RT)}$, as appropriate) to simplify the interface design task.

For maximum glass-to-metal bonding strength, the adhesive layer should have a particular thickness. If 3M EC2216-B/A epoxy is used, experience indicates that a thickness of 0.075 to 0.125 mm (0.003 to 0.005 in.) is best. Some adhesive manufacturers recommend thicknesses as large as 0.4 mm (0.016 in.) for their products. A thin bond is stiffer than a thick one (see Miller's analytical results for elastomeric lens mountings discussed in Sect. 3.7). One means for achieving a bond of a particular thickness is to place small shims of the specified thickness at three locations in the interface between the glass and the metal. If possible, these should be arranged in a triangular pattern and lie outside the bonded area. The glass, mount, and shims must be held together to ensure contact and fixtured to prevent lateral and/or rotational motion. Adhesive should not be allowed to get onto the shims. Another way to obtain a layer of a specific thickness is to mix a few percent by volume of small glass beads into the ahesive before applying it to the surfaces to be bonded. When the surfaces are held together, the beads contact both faces and hold them apart. Since such beads can be purchased with closely controlled diameters, achievement of a correct bond thickness is relatively easy.[11] The glass beads have essentially no effect on bonding strength.

Adhesives and metals typically have CTEs larger than those of glasses, so differential dimensional changes at extreme temperatures can be large. Many mounting designs have the required bonding area subdivided into three (or more) smaller areas. These are preferably arranged in a triangular pattern (see Fig. 7.18). This reduces the changes in differential dimensions over the width of the bonds and allows the support to be spread over a larger geometrical pattern for increased stability.

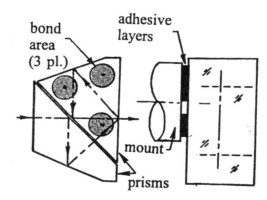

Fig. 7.18 An example of a triangular bond distribution on one prism of a Pechan prism subassembly.

Note that the bonds in Fig. 7.18 are on the larger prism only. Obviously, bonding adhesive should be kept away from the air space between separated prisms such as the Pechan shown here. In fact, even with components cemented together rather than air spaced, bridging the cemented joint with bonding adhesive can cause glass breakage at extreme temperatures, owing to differential shrinkage or expansion of the adhesive trapped within the V-groove formed by bevels on the edges of the optics. An additional reason for not bonding across cemented joints is that the adjacent surfaces are rarely coplanar; they may be skewed or may have a step in height. Either defect would tend to make the adhesive thickness different on the two prisms, and that affects the bond's strength.

Fillets of excess adhesive at the edges of glass-to-metal bonds should be avoided. This is because low-temperature shrinkage along the hypotenuse of a fillet at low temperature is greater than that along the glass or metal surfaces. This shrinkage may be sufficent to fracture the glass. Softer adhesives are better than the harder types if fillets are inevitable, owing, for example, to inaccessibility of the bonded region for inspection and removal of excess material.

Figure 7.19 shows a fused silica cube-shaped prism (beamsplitter) with A = 35 mm (1.375 in.) that was bonded with epoxy over its entire square base to a titanium mount. The prism base had been ground flat after cementing to remove any step. When the unit was cooled to -30°C, the shrinkages of the metal and of the adhesive relative to the prism each applied bending moments to the glass and stressed the glass. It fractured as shown as a result of this differential contraction. Analysis indicated that the bonded area was considerably larger than necessary for the dynamic conditions expected. The bond was changed to three smaller areas to solve the problem.

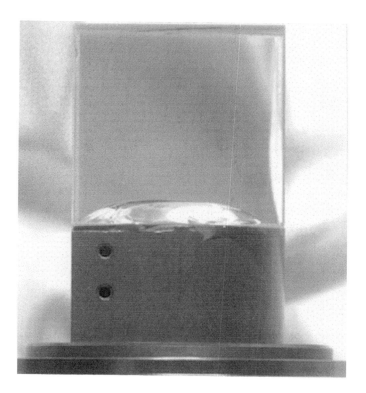

Fig. 7.19 Photograph of a 35-mm fused silica cube beamsplitter bonded across it's face to a titanium mount with an epoxy. Failure occurred at a low temperature because of differential expansion of the glass, adhesive, and metal.

Example 7.7: Dimensional changes in the bonded interface of a beamsplitter cube shown in Fig. 7.19. (For design and analysis, use File 20 of the CD-ROM)

The faces of the cube prism shown in Fig. 7.19 are A = 35 mm (1.370 in.) wide.
The pertinent material properties are

fused silica prism, CTE = 0.52×10^{-6} /°C

titanium mount, CTE = 8.8×10^{-6} /°C

3M 2216B/A adhesive, CTE = 102×10^{-6} /°C

If bonded across the entire prism face, what total and relative dimensional changes occur in the three materials when the temperature drops to -30° C?

$\Delta T = -30 - 20 = -50°$ C

$\Delta L_{GLASS} = (0.52 \times 10^{-6})(35)(-50) = -0.00091$ mm

$\Delta L_{METAL} = (8.8 \times 10^{-6})(35)(-50) = -0.01540$ mm

$\Delta L_{ADHESIVE} = (102 \times 10^{-6})(35)(-50) = -0.17850$ mm

relative $\Delta L_{GLASS-ADHESIVE} = -0.17850 - (-0.00091) = -0.17795$ mm

relative $\Delta L_{METAL-GLASS} = -0.01540 - (-0.00091) = -0.01449$ mm

relative $\Delta L_{METAL-ADHESIVE} = -0.178850 - (-0.01540) = -0.16345$ mm

These are all large relative dimensional changes. Shear stresses in the joint would be expected. This topic is considered in Section 12.10.

A design feature that increases the reliability of glass-to-metal bonds is to specify that the bonding surface on the glass component be fine ground and that the grinding operations consist of three or four steps with progressively finer abrasives. The depth of material removed in each step is at least three times the prior grit size. This process removes subsurface damage from each prior step. Commonly referred to as "controlled grinding," this process produces a surface relatively free of invisible cracks and significantly increases the material's tensile strength at the ground surface.[12] Bonding on polished glass surfaces may not be as successful as bonding on fine-ground surfaces.

7.3.2 Cantilevered bonding techniques

Figures 7.17 through 7.19 have shown a variety of prisms bonded on one ground surface in cantilevered fashion with respect to a mechanical mounting surface. Experience indicates that such mountings provide adequate support for severe shock and vibration conditions.[8] Figure 7.20 shows a design that is known to have withstood shocks of approximately 1200 times gravity without damage. Figure 7.21 shows the same prism assembly mounted in its mechanical support. This assembly is the subject of Example 7.8.

Since during shipment or use the mounting surface could be oriented in any direction with respect to gravity, and environmental acceleration forces could be applied in any direction, the cantilevered prism mounting may not be adequate under extreme conditions. Additional support may be desired. This leads us to the design variations described in Sect. 7.3.3.

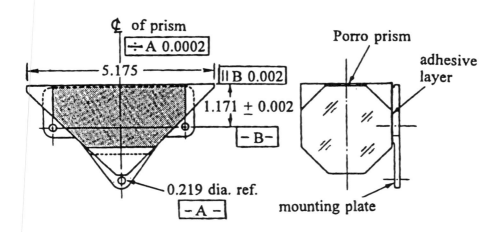

of prism
┌─┴ A 0.0002┐

5.175 ──────►│ ║ B 0.002│

1.171 ± 0.002

│ - B-│

0.219 dia. ref.
│ - A -│

Porro prism

adhesive layer

mounting plate

Fig. 7.20 Mounting design for a Porro prism bonded on one side. Dimensions are in inches. Bonding area shown shaded. (Adapted from Yoder.[8])

Example 7.8: Acceleration capability of a large Porro prism assembly bonded in cantilevered fashion.
(For design and analysis, use File 21 of the CD-ROM)
A Porro prism made of SK16 glass is bonded with EC2216-B/A epoxy to a 416 stainless steel bracket. The bond area Q is 5.6 in.² and the prism weight W is 2.2 lb. What acceleration a_G would the assembly be expected to withstand with a safety factor f_S of 2? Assume the bonding strength J of the cured joint is 2500 lb/in.².

Rewriting and applying Eq. (7.9) we obtain:
   $a_G = JQ/Wf_S = (2500)(5.6)/(2.2)(2) = 3182$ times gravity

This indicates that the prism should withstand acceleration of 1200 times gravity in any direction with a safety factor > 2.

7.3.3 Double-sided bonded support techniques

Some designs for bonding prisms utilize multiple adhesive joints between the prism and structure (see, for example, Fig. 7.22). Here increased bonding area and support from both sides are provided to a right-angle prism by bonding it to the ends of two metal stub shafts. The bonded subassembly rests in and is firmly clamped by two precision-machined pillow blocks of conventional split design. Ease of adjustment of the prism's alignment about the transverse axis is a key feature of this design. Once installed in the

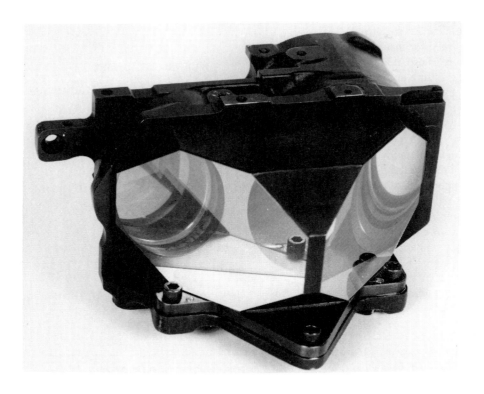

Fig. 7.21 Photograph of the Porro prism of Fig. 7.20 mounted on its bracket. (Courtesy of Raytheon Optical Systems Corp., Danbury, CT.)

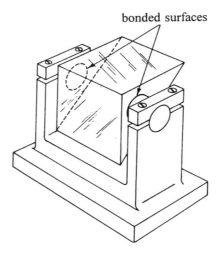

Fig. 7.22 Schematic of a right-angle prism bonded to both sides of a U-shaped mount. (From Durie.[2])

optical instrument and adjusted, the shafts are securely clamped.[2] It is necessary in such designs that the surfaces to be bonded be nearly parallel and that the proper clearances be provided for insertion of the adhesive layers. Tolerances must be held closely enough to ensure these relationships. Furthermore, the bearing surfaces for the shafts in the bonding fixture and in the instrument must be extremely straight and parallel. Otherwise, forces exerted during clamping at assembly or during exposure to vibration, shock, or extreme temperatures could strain the bonds and perhaps cause damage. Fixtures are typically used with this design to position the prism during adhesive curing.

Problems with differential expansion between glass and metal that may occur at extreme temperatures in the design of Fig. 7.22 can be avoided by building flexibility into one support arm of a double-sided prism mounting as indicated in Fig. 7.23. Units made to an earlier design without this flexure were damaged at low temperatures when the aluminum mounting contracted more than than the prism, causing the arms to pivot about the bottom edge of the prism and pull away from the prism at the tops of the bonds. Allowing one arm to bend slightly prevented such damage.[13] Holes were provided in each support arm to allow epoxy to be injected into the spaces between the prism and mounting surfaces after the prism was aligned. One such hole is designated as "P" in Fig. 7.23.

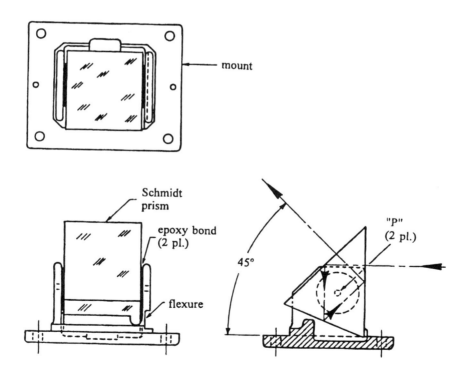

Fig. 7.23 A Schmidt prism bonded on both sides to a U-shaped mount. (Courtesy of Opto Mechanik, Inc., Melbourne, FL.)

A potential problem in any design in which epoxy is injected through access holes to a bond cavity is that the "plug" of adhesive in the hole can shrink significantly at low temperature and perhaps pull the adjacent glass sufficiently to fracture it.[14] Minimizing the length of the hole and hence of the plug would help avoid this problem.

Two versions of another design concept with support provided from two sides by arms forming a U-shaped mount are shown schematically in Fig. 7.24.[14] In Fig. 7.24(a), the crown glass prism is bonded to the ends of two cylindrical stainless steel plates passing through clearance holes in the arms. The entire mount is made of stainless steel so a mismatch of glass-to-metal thermal expansion is not a big problem. The

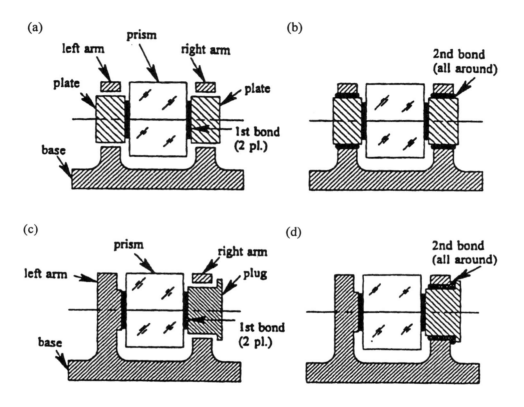

Fig. 7.24 Two concepts for double-sided bonding of a prism to a U-shaped mount. (Adapted from Beckmann.[14])

prism and the plates relative to the mount must be aligned using mechanical references or optical fixturing prior to this first bonding step. After the first bonds have cured, the plates are epoxied to the arms as indicated in Fig. 7.24(b). With this approach, tolerances on location and tilt of the surfaces to be bonded are relaxed since the plates align themselves to the prism in the clearance holes before they are bonded to the arms.

In Fig. 7.24(c), the prism is aligned to the mount and then is bonded to a raised pad on one support arm (left) and to the metal plug shown protruding through, but not attached to the second (right) arm. After these bonds have cured, the plug is bonded to the right arm to provide the required dual support [see Fig. 7.24(d)]. Once again, tolerances on the bonding surface locations and orientations are relatively loose.

Either of the last two design concepts can be extended to allow multiple plates or plugs of selected shapes (not necessarily round) to be passed through clearance holes in the support arms and bonded to opposite sides of the prism. After curing of the first bonds, these plates or plugs would be bonded to the support arms. This assembly process is essentially the same as the "liquid pinning" process described in Sect. 4.5 as a means for locking aligned metal parts together in structures without the dangers associated with drilling and reaming for metal pinning. The beauty of the idea presented here in connection with constraining optical components is that precise fitting of parts is not required, yet the alignment established optically or by fixturing is retained after bonding.

A different optomechanical design involving bonding of prisms is illustrated in Fig. 7.25. Here a Schmidt-Pechan roof prism (cemented subassembly) is inserted into a close-fitting seat molded in the filled-plastic housing of a commercial binocular. The prism subassembly is then provisionally secured in place with dabs of UV-curing adhesive applied through openings in the housing walls.[15,16] After proper alignment is confirmed, the prisms are secured by adding several beads of polyurethane adhesive through the same wall openings. The slight resiliencies of the housing and the adhesive accommodate the differential thermal expansion characteristics of the adjacent materials. With precision-molded structural members and built-in reference surfaces, adjustments are not required. Figure 7.26 shows some details of the internal configuration of such a prism mounting.

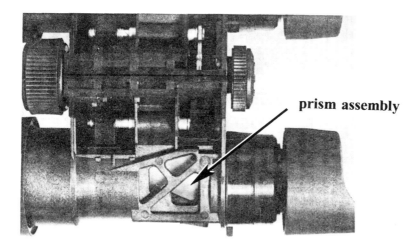

prism assembly

Fig. 7.25 A Schmidt-Pechan erecting prism subassembly mounted in a plastic binocular housing. (Adapted from Seil.[15])

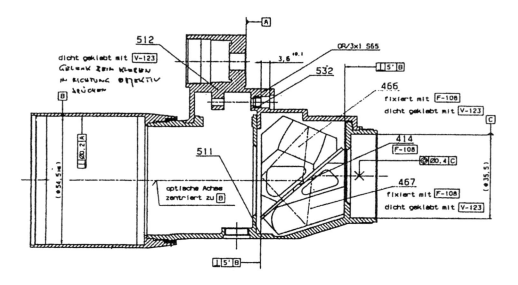

Fig. 7.26 Drawing of a roof prism mounted in the manner of Fig. 7.25. (Courtesy of Swarovski Optik KG, Austria.)

Figure 7.27 is a photograph of an assembly consisting of a Porro prism erecting system and a rhomboid prism mounted by the same general technique described for constraining roof prisms.[16] In this design, one Porro prism is attached with adhesive to its plastic bracket. This bracket then slides on two parallel metal rods to provide axial movement of the prism relative to the second Porro prism for adjusting focus of an optical instrument. The adhesive beads are more clearly shown in Fig. 7.28. Minimization of the number of components and ease of assembly are prime features of this design. Customer experience and acceptance of products made by this technique have demonstrated the durability and adequacy of the optomechanical performance achievable with this type of assembly.

7.4 Flexure Mountings for Prisms

Some prisms (particularly large ones or ones with critical positioning requirements) are mounted with flexures. A generic example is shown in Fig. 7.29. Three compound flexures are bonded with adhesive directly to the prism base and attached by threaded joints to a baseplate (not shown). To reduce strain from differential expansion between the prism material and the baseplate resulting from temperature changes, all three flexures are designed to bend in several directions. They are very stiff axially. Flexure 1 locates the prism horizontally at a fixed point. It has a "universal joint" at its top to allow for angular misalignment at the bonded joint. The second flexure constrains rotation about the fixed point (first flexure), but allows relative expansion along a line connecting the first and second flexures because of its universal joints at the top and at the bottom. The third flexure has a universal joint at the top and a single flexure at the bottom; it supports

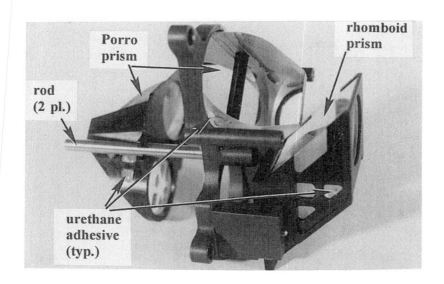

Fig. 7.27 Photograph of a Porro prism image-erecting system and a rhomboid prism mounted by adhesive bonding to plastic structural members for use as an optomechanical subassembly in a commercial telescope. (Courtesy of Swarovski Optik KG, Austria.)

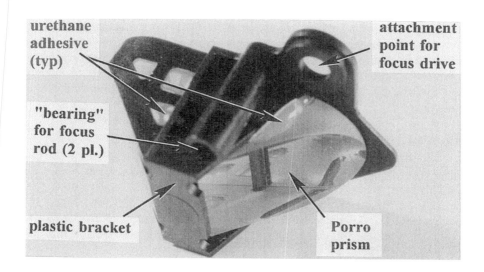

Fig. 7.28 Closeup photograph of the movable Porro prism from the subassembly of Fig. 7.27. The prism is mounted by adhesive bonding to a plastic structural bracket. (Courtesy of Swarovski Optik KG, Austria.)

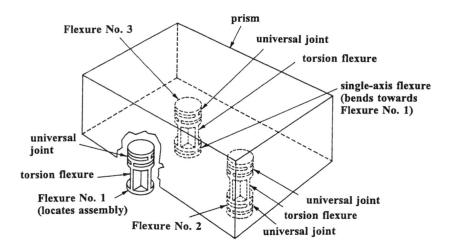

Fig. 7.29 Conceptual sketch of a flexure mounting for a large prism. (Adapted from Yoder.[8])

its share of the prism's weight and prevents rotation about the line connecting the other two flexures. The third flexure does not constrain the prism transversely. All three flexures have torsional compliance. Small differences in the lengths of the flexures and/or the parallelism of their top surfaces are accommodated through compliance of the three top universal joints. Because of the flexures, the prism remains fixed in space without being distorted or disturbing the structure to which it is attached, even in the presence of significant temperature changes and differential expansion of the prism and the mounting structure.[8] Specific examples of flexure mountings for large prisms are discussed in Sects. 13.24 and 13.25.

References

1. Lipshutz, M.L., "Optomechanical considerations for optical beam splitters," *Appl. Opt.* Vol. 7, 2326, 1968.
2. Durie, D.S.L., "Stability of optical mounts," *Machine Des.* Vol. 40, 184, 1968.
3. Vukobratovich, D., "Optomechanical Systems Design," Chapt. 3 in *The Infrared & Electro-Optical Systems Handbook,* Vol. 4, ERIM, Ann Arbor and SPIE, Bellingham, 1993.
4. Sorbothane, Inc., *Engineering Design Guide,* Kent, OH.
5. Roark, R.J., *Formulas for Stress and Strain,* 3rd ed., McGraw-Hill, New York, 1954. See also Young, W.C., *Roark's Formulas for Stress & Strain,* 6th ed., McGraw-Hill, New York, 1989.
6. Yoder, P.R., Jr., "Optical Mounts: Lenses, Windows, Small Mirrors, and Prisms," Chapt. 6 in *Handbook of Optomechanical Engineering",* CRC Press, Boca Raton, 1997.

7. Yoder, P.R., Jr., "Non-image-forming optical components," *SPIE Proceedings* Vol.531, 206, 1985.

8. Yoder, P.R., Jr., *Opto-Mechanical Systems Design*, 2nd ed., Marcel Dekker, New York, 1993.

9. Delgado, R.F., "The multidiscipline demands of a high performance dual channel projector," *SPIE Proceedings* Vol.389, 75, 1983.

10. Yoder, P.R., Jr., "Design guidelines for bonding prisms to mounts," *SPIE Proceedings* Vol. 1013, 112, 1988.

11. Stoll, R., Forman, P.F., and Edleman, J. "The effect of different grinding procedures on the strength of scratched and unscratched fused silica," *Proceedings of Symposium on the Strength of Glass and Ways to Improve It*, Union Scientifique Continentale du Verre, Charleroi, Belgium, 1, 1961.

12. See, for example, certified particle products made by Duke Scientific Corp., (@www.dukescientific.com).

13. Willey, R., private communication, 1991.

14. Beckmann, L.H.J.F., private communication, 1990.

15. Seil, K., "Progress in binocular design," *SPIE Proceedings* Vol. 1533, 48, 1991.

16. Seil, K., private communication, 1997.

CHAPTER 8
Mirror Design

As in the case of prisms, a clear understanding of certain important aspects of mirror design is believed to be necessary before we consider different techniques for mounting those mirrors. This chapter therefore deals primarily with the mirror's geometric configuration. Because mirror size is a prime driver of design and of material choice, we consider sizes ranging from small ones with diameters of a few millimeters to about 0.5 m (1.6 ft) to large, astronomical telescope-sized ones with diameters as large as about 8.4 m (27.6 ft). We begin by defining the relative advantages of first- and second-surface mirror types and show how to determine the appropriate aperture dimensions for a tilted reflecting surface located in a collimated or noncollimated beam. We then illustrate various substrate configurations that might be employed to minimize mirror weight and/or self-weight deflection. Typical designs for metallic mirrors are then considered. The chapter closes with a few observations about the design and use of pellicles.

8.1 First- and Second-Surface Mirrors

Most mirrors used in optical instruments have light-reflective coatings made of metallic and/or nonmetallic thin films on their first optically polished surfaces. These are quite logically called "first-surface" mirrors. The metals commonly used as coatings are aluminum, silver, and gold because of their high reflectivities in the UV, visible, and/or IR spectral regions. Protective coatings such as silicon monoxide or magnesium fluoride are placed over metallic coatings to increase their durability. Nonmetallic films consist of single layers or multilayer stacks of dielectric films. The stacks are combinations of materials with high and low indices of refraction. Dielectric reflecting films function over narrower spectral bands than the metals, but have very high reflectivity at specific wavelengths. They are especially helpful in monochromatic systems such as those using laser radiation. The state of polarization of the reflected beam is modified by all-dielectric stacks or dielectric overcoats when the beam angle of incidence differs from zero. Figures 8.1 and 8.2 show typical reflectance vs. wavelength curves for different first-surface reflective coatings at normal and/or 45° incidence.

Figure 8.3(a) shows reflectance vs. wavelength for a typical multilayer dielectric film, while Fig. 8.3(b) shows reflectance vs. wavelength for a second-surface coating of silver. The latter type of reflective coating is applied to the back, i.e., second surface, of a mirror or prism. This can be an advantage from a durability viewpoint because the film then is protected from the outside environment and physical damage that is due to handling or use. The back of the thin-film coating typically is given a protective coating such as electroplated copper plus enamel for this purpose.

Figure 8.4 illustrates a concave second-surface (or Mangin) mirror and its function in forming a normal image of a distant object. Since the light to be reflected by a second-surface mirror must pass through a refracting surface to get to the reflecting surface, a ghost image is formed by the first surface. This ghost image of the object is superimposed upon the normal image as stray light and tends to reduce the contrast of

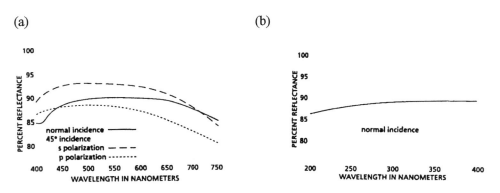

Fig. 8.1 Reflectance vs. wavelength for first-surface metallic coatings of (a) protected aluminum and (b) UV-enhanced aluminum.

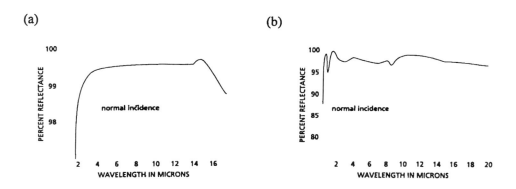

Fig. 8.2 Reflectance vs. wavelength for first-surface thin films of (a) protected gold and (b) protected silver.

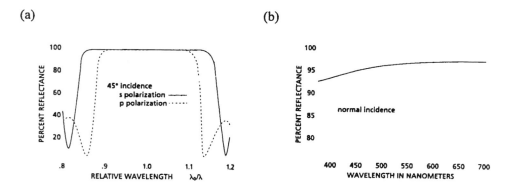

Fig. 8.3 Reflectance vs. wavelength for (a) a first-surface multilayer dielectric thin film and (b) a second-surface thin film of silver.

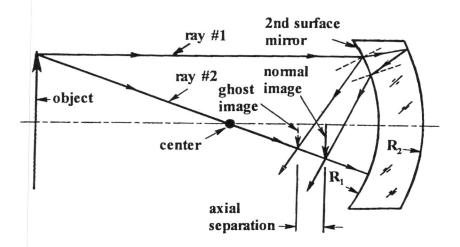

Fig. 8.4 Ghost image formation from the first surface of a second-surface mirror with concentric spherical surfaces. (Adapted from Kaspereit.[3])

the latter image. The axial separation of the two images can be increased or decreased by careful choice of radii and mirror thickness.

The intensity of the ghost image is calculated from the index of refraction of the substrate using Fresnel's equations.[1,2] At normal incidence, the reflectance, R_λ, of an uncoated interface between two materials with refractive indices n_1 and n_2 is

$$R_\lambda = (n_2 - n_1)^2/(n_2 + n_1)^2 \tag{8.1}$$

The transmittance of this interface, also at normal incidence, is given by:

$$T_\lambda = 1 - R_\lambda \tag{8.2}$$

Example 8.1 illustrates an application of these equations.

Example 8.1: Intensity of the ghost reflection from an uncoated first surface of a second-surface mirror.
(For design and analysis, use File 22.1 of the CD-COM)
A second-surface silvered mirror is made of BaK2 optical glass with $n_\lambda = 1.542$ in green light ($\lambda = 0.5461$ μm). The index of air is assumed to be 1.000. What is the intensity of the ghost image relative to that of the normal image if the first surface is uncoated? Neglect absorption.

Assume an incident beam with an intensity of unity.

Applying Eq. (8.1) at the first surface, $R_1 = (1.542 - 1.000)^2 / (1.542 + 1.000)^2$ = 0.045. Multiplying this factor by the intensity of the incident beam, we obtain the intensity of the ghost beam, which is 0.045.

Applying Eq. (8.2), the transmission of the first surface is $T_1 = 1 - 0.045 = 0.955$.

From Fig. 8.3(b), the green-light reflectance R_2 of the silvered surface is 0.97.

The light beam reflected from the mirror's second surface passes twice through the front surface. Hence its intensity upon exiting the mirror is $(0.955)^2 (0.97) = 0.885$ times the intensity of the incident beam or 0.885.

The intensity of the ghost image relative to that of the image reflected from the mirror's second surface is then 0.045/0.884 = 0.051 or 5.1%.

To reduce the intensity of beams reflected from uncoated surfaces, we apply a thin-film coating or a stack of coatings [called an "antireflection" (A/R) coating] to that surface. The fundamental purpose of the simplest case (a single-layer coating) is to cause destructive interference between a first beam reflecting from the air/film interface and a second beam reflecting from the film/glass interface. Destructive interference occurs when these beams are exactly 180° or one-half wavelength out of phase. Since the second beam passes through the film twice, the desired $\lambda/2$ phase shift results if the optical thickness $(n\lambda)$ of the film is $\lambda/4$. The combined intensity of the two reflected beams then is zero because their wave amplitudes subtract.[1,2] The amplitude of a reflected beam is $(R_\lambda)^{1/2}$.

Note that complete destructive interference occurs only at a specific wavelength λ and then only if the beam amplitudes are equal. The latter condition occurs if the following equation is satisfied:

$$n_2 = (n_1 n_3)^{1/2} \qquad\qquad (8.3)$$

where:

$\quad n_2$ = index of refraction of the thin film at wavelength λ
$\quad n_1$ = index of refraction of the surrounding medium (typically air with n = 1)
$\quad n_3$ = index of refraction of the glass at wavelength λ.

If a thin-film material with exactly the right index to A/R coat a given type of glass is not available, imperfect cancellation of the two reflected beams occurs. We calculate the resultant surface reflectance R_S as:

$$R_S = (R_{1,2}^{1/2} - R_{2,3}^{1/2})^2 \tag{8.4}$$

where:

$R_{1,2}$ = reflectance of the air/film interface
$R_{2,3}$ = reflectance of the film/glass interface

Example 2.2 quantifies the advantage of one such coating.

Example No. 8.2: Relative intensity of the ghost reflection from a second-surface mirror with an A/R coating on the first surface. (For design and analysis, use File 22.2)
A single-film A/R coating of MgF_2 with $n_2 = 1.380$ is applied to the first surface of the Mangin mirror from Example 8.1. Its optical thickness in green light is $\lambda/4 = 0.5461/4 = 0.136$ µm. What is the intensity of the ghost image from the coated surface relative to the intensity of the main image?

From Eq. (8.3), the film index n_2 should be $[(1.000)(1.542)]^{1/2} = 1.242$ for a perfect antireflection function. This is not the case here, so the coating is imperfect.

From Eq. (8.1):
  $R_{1,2}$ of the air/film interface is $(1.380 - 1.000)^2/(1.380 + 1.000)^2 = 0.0255$
  $R_{2,3}$ of the film/glass interface is $(1.542 - 1.380)^2/(1.542 + 1.380)^2 = 0.0031$

From Eq. (8.4), the intensity of the ghost imange is
  $R_S = [(0.0255)^{1/2} - (0.0031)^{1/2}] = 0.0108$

From Eq. (8.2), $T_S = 1 - 0.0108 = 0.9892$

The intensity of the main image reflected from the mirror's second surface is $(0.9892)^2 (0.97) = 0.9492$

The relative intensity of the ghost image is then $0.0108/0.9492 = 0.0114 = 1.1\%$.

Even though the thin-film index is not optimum for the given substrate material, it does reduce the relative intensity of the ghost image to about one-fifth that of an uncoated surface (which is 5.1% per Example 8.1).

Figure 8.5 shows formation of a ghost reflection from a flat second-surface mirror of thickness t oriented at an angle of 45° to the axis of an imaging system (lens). With the mirror at 45° in air, the ghost is displaced axially relative to the normal image by a distance $d_A = (2t/n) + d_A$. The ghost reflection is also displaced laterally by a distance

$d_L = 2t/[(2)(2n^2 - 1)]^{1/2}$. Once again, superimposition of the ghost image onto the second-surface reflected image tends to reduce the contrast of the latter image. By A/R coating the first surface, the ghost can be reduced in intensity, as quantified earlier. Fresnel's equation (Eq. (8.1)) must be modified to accommodate the oblique incidence of the beam at the ghost-forming surface.[1,2]

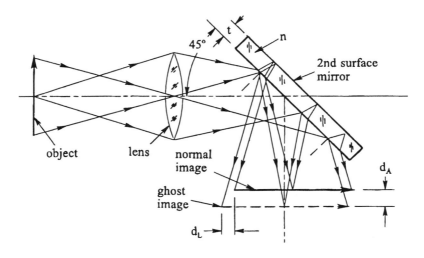

Fig. 8.5 Formation of a ghost image at a second-surface mirror inclined 45° to the axis. (Adapted from Kaspereit.[3])

High-efficiency, multilayer A/R coatings can be designed to have zero reflectivity at a specific wavelength or reduced variations of reflectivity with wavelength. Figure 8.6 shows plots of reflectance vs. wavelength for a single-layer (MgF_2) coating, a "broad

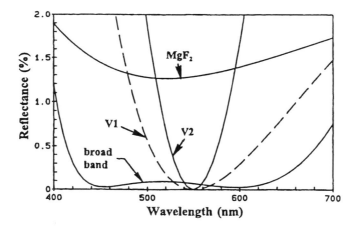

Fig. 8.6 Spectral variations of reflectance for several A/R coatings as identified in the text.

band" multilayer coating with low reflectivity over the entire visible spectrum, and two multilayer coatings with zero reflectivity at $\lambda = 550$ nm. All these coatings are applied to crown glass. Coatings V1 and V2 are called "V-coats" because of their characteristic downward-pointing triangular shapes.

An obvious difference between first- and second-surface mirrors is that a transparent substrate is needed for the latter, but not for the former. Tables B8 and B9 list the mechanical properties and "figures of merit" for the common non-metallic and metallic mirror substrate materials. Of these, only fused silica has good refractive properties. Hence, second-surface mirrors must be made of that material, one of the optical glasses (see Tables B1 and B2), an optical plastic (see Table B3), or a crystal (see Tables B4 through B7). A related advantage of the second-surface mirror is that an additional surface radius and asphericity, an axial thickness, and an index are available for controlling aberrations as well as for controlling the locations of a ghost image as mentioned earlier. The second-surface mirror configuration is most frequently used in Mangin-type primary or secondary mirrors in catadioptric systems for photographic and moderate-sized astronomical telescope applications. Second-surface designs obviously do not work in mirrors with tapered or arched back surfaces or in built-up mirror substrates, such as those discussed in Sect. 8.3.

8.2 Determination of Mirror Aperture

The size of a mirror is set primarily by the size and shape of the optical beam as it intercepts the reflecting surface, plus any allowances that need to be made for mounting provisions, misalignment, and/or beam motion during operation. The so-called "beamprint" can be approximated from a scaled layout of the optical system showing extreme rays of the light beam in at least two orthogonal meridians. This method is time-consuming to use and may be inaccurate as a result of compounded drafting errors. Modern computer-aided design methods have alleviated both these problems, especially with software that interfaces ray-tracing capability with the creation of drawings or graphic renditions to any scale and in any perspective. In spite of these advances, some of us rely upon hand calculations, at least at early stages of system design. We include here a set of equations, adapted from Schubert,[4] that allow minimum elliptical beamprint dimensions for a circular beam intersecting a tilted flat mirror. The geometry is shown in Fig. 8.7. The ellipse is assumed to be centered on the mirror in the minor-axis direction.

$$W = D + 2L\tan\alpha \tag{8.5}$$

$$E = \frac{W\cos\alpha}{2\sin(\theta - \alpha)} \tag{8.6}$$

$$F = \frac{W\cos\alpha}{2\sin(\theta + \alpha)} \tag{8.7}$$

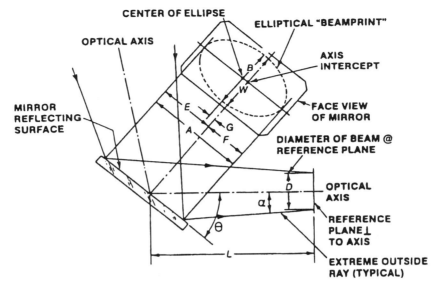

Fig. 8.7 Geometric relationships used to defing the beamprint of a rotationally symmetric beam on a tilted flat mirror. (Adapted from Schubert.[4])

$$A = E + F \qquad\qquad (8.8)$$

$$G = (A/2) - F \qquad\qquad (8.9)$$

$$B = \frac{AW}{(A^2 - 4G^2)^{1/2}} \qquad\qquad (8.10)$$

where:

W = width of beamprint at the mirror/axis intercept
D = beam diameter at a reference plane perpendicular to the axis and located an axial distance L from the mirror/axis intercept
α = beam divergence angle of the extreme off-axis reflected ray
E = distance from the top edge of the beamprint to the mirror/axis intercept
θ = mirror surface tilt relative to the axis = 90° minus the tilt of the mirror normal
F = distance from the bottom edge of the beamprint to the mirror/axis intercept
A = major axis of the beamprint
G = offset of the beamprint center from the mirror/axis intercept
B = minor axis of the beamprint

These equations apply regardless of the direction in which the beam is propagating as long as the reference plane is located where D is smaller than W. For a collimated beam propagating parallel to the axis, α and G are zero and the above equations reduce to the symmetrical case where:

$$B = W = D \tag{8.10a}$$

$$E = F = D/(2\sin\theta) \tag{8.6a}$$

$$A = D/\sin\theta \tag{8.8a}$$

Example 8.3: Beam footprint on a tilted mirror.
(For design and analysis, use File 23 of the CD-ROM)
Calculate the beamprint dimensions for a circular beam of $D = 25.4$ mm incident at $L = 50$ mm on a flat mirror tilted at an angle $\theta = 30°$ to the axis. Assume the beam divergence α to be (a) 0.5° and (b) zero (i.e., collimated).

(a) From Eq. (8.5), $W = 25.4 + (2)(50)(\tan 0.5°) = 26.273$ mm
From Eq. (8.6), $E = (26.273)(\cos 0.5°)/[2 \sin (30° - 0.5°)] = 26.677$ mm
From Eq. (8.7), $F = (26.273)(\cos 0.5°)/[2 \sin (30° + 0.5°)] = 25.881$ mm
From Eq. (8.8), $A = 26.677 + 25.881 = 52.558$ mm
From Eq. (8.9), $G = (52.558/2) - 25.882 = 0.397$ mm
From Eq. (8.10), $B = (52.558)(26.273)/[52.558^2 - (4)(0.397^2)]^{1/2} = 26.276$ mm

(b) From Eq. (8.10a), $B = W = D = 25.400$ mm
From Eq. (8.6a), $E = F = 25.4/(2)(\sin 30°) = 25.400$ mm
From Eq. (8.8a), $A = 25.4/\sin 30° = 50.800$ mm.

As expected, the elliptical beamprint in part (a) is slightly decentered upward with respect to the axis in the plane of reflection, but is symmetrical to the axis in the orthogonal plane. In part (b), the beamprint is symmetrical in both directions.

The dimensions of the reflecting surface should be increased somewhat from those calculated with Eqs. (8.5) through (8.10) and (8.6a), (8.8a), and (8.10a) to allow for the factors mentioned earlier (mechanical mounting clearances, beam motion, etc.) and for reasonable manufacturing tolerances on all dimensions.

8.3 Weight Rreduction Techniques

The most common substrate shapes for small mirrors are the solid cylindrical disk and the solid rectangular or square plate. If possible, they should have thicknesses about one-fifth or one-sixth the largest in-plane dimension to ensure adequate mechanical stiffness. Thinner or thicker substrates are used as the application allows or demands. All mirrors should have protective bevels; some are heavily chamfered to remove unnecessary material. Very small mirrors typically have considerably larger relative thicknesses to allow for mounting.

In large mirrors and even in some small and most modest-sized mirrors, weight minimization can prove advantageous or, in some cases, absolutely necessary. Given a chosen substrate material, a reduction in mirror weight from that of the regular solid can be made only by changing the configuration. The usual ways of doing this are to remove unnecessary material from a solid substrate or to combine separate pieces to create a built-up structure with a lot of empty spaces inside. No matter what technique is used to minimize mirror weight, the end product must be of high quality and capable of economical fabrication and testing. Rodkevich and Robachevskaya correctly stated the fundamental requirements for precision mirrors and lightweight versions of them.[5] These statements are paraphrased here as follows:

1. The mirror material must be highly immune to outside mechanical and temperature influences; it must be isotropic and possess stable properties and dimensions.
2. The mirror material must accept a high-quality polished surface and a coating having the required reflection coefficient.
3. The mirror construction must be capable of being shaped to a specified optical surface contour and must retain this shape under operating conditions.
4. Lightweight mirrors must have a lower mass than those made to traditional designs while maintaining adequate stiffness and homogeneity of properties.
5. Similar techniques should be used for fabricating conventional and lightweight mirrors.
6. If possible, mounting and load relief during testing and use should employ conventional techniques and should not increase the mass of the mirror and/or the complexity of the mechanisms involved.

These idealized principles would serve as useful guidelines for the design of any size of mirror. Material selection, fabrication methods, dimensional stability, and configuration design are key to meeting these guidelines. Tables B8a and B8b list material properties such as coefficient of thermal expansion, thermal conductivity, and Young's modulus, which relate to inherent behavior under changing environmental conditions. Dimensional stability and homogeneity of properties differ from one material type to another. Further information on these topics may be found in other publications, such as those by Englehaupt[6] and by Paquin.[7] Comparisons of mechanical and thermal material figures of merit especially pertinent to mirror design are given in Table B9. Table B10a lists the characteristics of different types of aluminum alloys that are candidates for making metallic mirrors. Typical fabrication methods, surface finishes, and coatings for mirrors made of various materials are listed in Table B11. Mounting methods for smaller mirrors are considered in Chapter 9 of this book, while those typically used to mount larger mirrors are discussed in Chapter 10. The following sections deal with configurations for reducing the weight of mirrors (lightweighting).

8.3.1 Contoured-back configurations

The baseline configuration for mirrors with flat, concave, and convex first (reflecting) surfaces is the regular solid having a flat second surface. We concentrate on circular-aperture mirrors since they are the most common. In general, the following discussion applies also to rectangular or nonsymmetrical designs. Reduction of weight by thinning the baseline substrate also reduces stiffness and increases self-weight deflection and susceptibility to acceleration forces. Hence that technique can be used only within limits. The simplest means for lightweighting front-surface mirrors is to contour the second (back) surface. Figure 8.8 illustrates this approach for a series of six concave mirrors with the same diameter $D_G = 2r_2$ and radius of curvature of the reflecting surface (R_1). Fabrication complexity increases from left to right in Fig. 8.8(a) through 8.8(f). Figure 8.8(g) shows, for comparison, a double concave version that is <u>not</u> lightweighted.

We discuss each variation in turn and show how to calculate mirror volume, which when multiplied by the appropriate density, gives the mirror weight. We also work out typical examples in which the mirror diameters, the radius of curvature of the reflecting surfaces, the material types, and the axial thicknesses are the same, but their R_2 surfaces are variously contoured. This allows direct comparison of relative weights for the different designs. For information about the effect of contouring on optomechanical performance, including variations of axis orientation with respect to the gravity vector, the reader is referred to the detailed treatment by Cho et al.[8]

Figure 8.8(a) shows the baseline planoconcave type of mirror. Its axial and edge thicknesses are t_A and t_E respectively. The sagittal depth, S_1, is given by Eq. (8.11) while the mirror volume is given by Eq. (8.12).

$$S_1 = R_1 - (R_1^2 - r_2^2)^{1/2} \tag{8.11}$$

$$V_{baseline} = \pi r_2^2 t_E - (\pi/3)(S_1^2)(3R_1 - S_1) \tag{8.12}$$

Example 8.4: Baseline solid flat-back concave mirror.
(For design and analysis, use File 24 of the CD-ROM)
A concave mirror made of Corning ULE as in Fig. 8.8(a) of diameter $D_G = 18.0$ in. (457.2 mm) and axial thickness $t_A = 18.0/6 = 3.0$ in. (76.2 mm) has a radius of curvature R_1 of 72.0 in. (1828.8 mm). Calculate (a) the volume and (b) the weight of the mirror.

Per Fig. 8.8(a), $\quad r_2 = 18.0/2 = 9.0$ in. (228.6 mm)
By Eq. (8.11), $\quad S_1 = 72 - (72^2 - 9^2)^{1/2} = 0.565$ in. (14.351 mm)
$\quad\quad\quad\quad\quad t_E = 3.0 + 0.565 = 3.565$ in. (90.551 mm)
By Eq. (8.12), $\quad$ Volume $= (\pi)(9^2)(3.565) - (\pi/3)(0.565^2)[(3)(72) - 0.565]$
$\quad\quad\quad\quad\quad\quad = 907.18 - 72.018 = 835.16$ in.^{3} (13,685.82 cm^3)

238

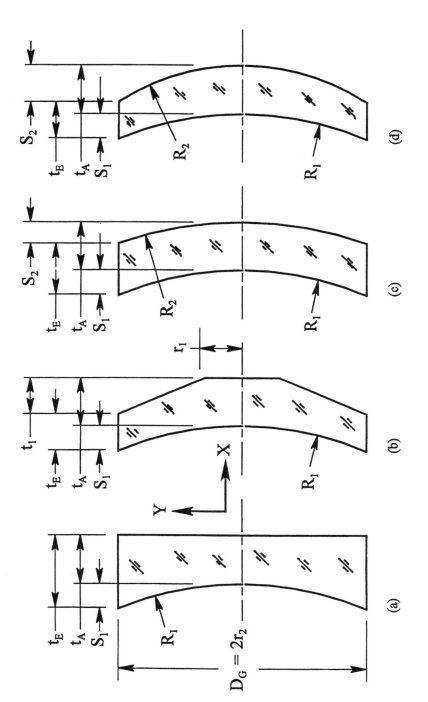

Fig. 8.8 Examples of concave mirrors with weight reduced by contouring the rear surface. (a) Baseline with flat rear surface, (b) Tapered (conical) rear surface, (c) Concentric spherical front and rear surfaces with $R_2 = R_1$ + t_1, (d) Spherical rear surface with $R_2 < R_1$ (continued on next page).

239

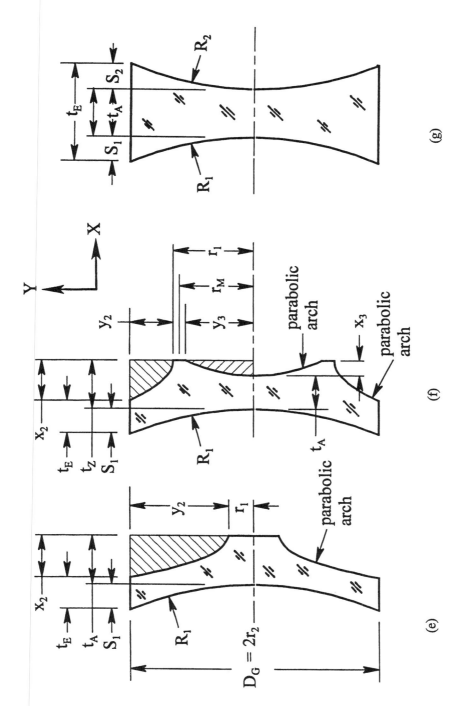

Fig. 8.8 (continued) Examples of concave mirrors with weight reduced by contouring the rear surface. (e) Single-arch configuration, (f) Double-arch configuration. (g) Double concave configuration (not lightweighted) for comparison.

From Table B8a, ρ for ULE is 0.0797 lb/in.^{3} (2.205 g/cm^3)

Mirror weight = (0.0797)(835.16) = 66.562 lb (30.193 kg)

Note: This weight serves as the baseline for comparison in the following examples.

The simplest back-surface contour is tapered (or conical), as indicated in Fig. 8.8(b). Thickness varies linearly between some selected radius, r_1, and the rim. The flat region on the back surface within r_1 might be used to mount the mirror if the thin edge is thought to be too fragile. Equation (8.13) is used to calculate the mirror volume.

$$V_{tapered} = V_{baseline} - (\pi t_1/2)(r_2^2 - r_1^2) \tag{8.13}$$

Example 8.5: Solid tapered-back concave mirror.
(For design and analysis, use File 25 of the CD-ROM)

Assume that the back surface of the mirror in Example 8.4 is contoured as shown in Fig. 8.8(b) starting at a radius r_1 = 1.5 in. (38.1 mm) and tapering to an edge thickness, t_E, of 0.5 in. (12.7 mm). What is the mirror weight and how does it compare with the baseline mirror weight?

From Example 8.4, S_1 = 0.565 in. (14.351 mm)

$t_1 = t_A + S_1 - t_E = 3.000 + 0.565 - 0.500 = 3.065$ in. (77.851 mm)

From Eq. (8.13), $V_{TAPERED}$ = 835.16 - [(π)(3.065)/2)(9^2 - 1.5^2)]

= 835.16 - 379.14 = 456.02 in.^{3} (7472.845 cm^3)

Mirror weight = (0.0797)(456.02) = 36.345 lb. (16.4860 kg)

The mirror weight has been reduced to (36.345/66.562)(100) = 55% of the baseline mirror weight.

In Fig. 8.8(c) and 8.8(d), we see meniscus-shaped mirrors with radii $R_2 = R_1 + t_1$ and $R_2 < R_1$, respectively. The first case has concentric spherical surfaces and a uniform thickness over the aperture, so only a slight reduction in weight from the planoconcave case [Fig. 8.8(a)] is possible. The second case allows greater weight reduction because the rim is significantly thinner. The latter type of mirror is usually mounted on a hub passing through a central perforation.

Equation (8.14) is used to estimate the volume of the meniscus-shaped mirror.

$$V_{concentric} = V_{baseline} - \pi r_2^2 S_2 + (\pi/3)(S_2^2)(3R_2 - S_2)$$ (8.14)

We now consider examples of concentric and non-concentric meniscus mirrors.

Example 8.6: Solid concentric meniscus mirror.
(For design and analysis, use File 26 of the CD-ROM)

Assume that the mirror from Example 8.4 has a spherical back surface with radius $R_2 = R_1 + t_A = 72.0 + 3.0 = 75.0$ in. (1905.0 mm). Figure 8.8(c) applies. What are t_E and the mirror weight and how does the latter compare with the baseline mirror weight?

From Eq. (8.11), $S_2 = 75^2 - (75^2 - 9^2) = 0.542$ in. (13.767 mm)
From example 8.4, $S_1 = 0.565$ in. (14.351 mm)
$$t_E = 3.0 + 0.565 - 0.542 = 3.023 \text{ in. (76.784 mm)}$$

From Eq. (8.14),
$$V_{concentric} = 835.16 - (\pi)(9^2)(0.542) + (\pi/3)(0.542^2)[(3)(75) - 0.542]$$
$$= 835.16 - 137.92 + 69.05 = 766.29 \text{ in.}^3 \text{ (12,557.3 cm}^3\text{)}$$

Mirror weight = $(0.0797)(766.29) = 61.073$ lb (27.703 kg)

The mirror weight has been reduced to $(61.073/66.562)(100) = 92\%$ of the baseline mirror weight.

Example 8.7: Solid meniscus mirror with $R_2 < R_1$.
(For design and analysis, use File 27 of the CD-ROM)

Assume that the mirror from Example 8.4 has a spherical back surface as in Fig. 8.8(d) with radius $R_2 = 14.746$ in. (374.548 mm). What are t_E and the mirror weight and how does the latter compare with the baseline mirror weight?

From Eq. (8.11), $S_2 = 14.746 - (14.746^2 - 9^2)^{1/2} = 3.065$ in. (77.851 mm)
From Example 8.4, $S_1 = 0.565$ in. (14.351 mm)
$$t_E = 3.000 + 0.565 - 3.065 = 0.500 \text{ in. (12.700 mm)}$$

From Eq. (8.14),
$$V_{concentric} = 835.16 - (\pi)(9^2)(3.065) + (\pi/3)(3.065^2)[(3)(14.746) - 3.065]$$
$$= 835.16 - 779.95 + 405.05 = 460.26 \text{ in.}^3 \text{ (7542.33 cm}^3\text{)}$$

Mirror weight $= (0.0797)(460.26) = 36.683$ lb (16.639 kg)

The mirror weight has been reduced to $(36.683/66.562)(100) = 55\%$ of the baseline mirror weight. This shows the advantage of reducing the back surface radius from the concentric value.

The mirror design in Fig. 8.8(e) is called the "single-arch" configuration. The best way to mount such a mirror is on a central hub. The back surface could have a parabolic or circular contour. In the former case, the axis of the parabola may be oriented parallel to the mirror axis (X) and decentered to locate the vertex at P_1 on the rim of the mirror (X-axis parabola) or oriented radially with the vertex at P_2 on the mirror's back (Y-axis parabola). The circle might well be parallel to the reflecting surface at the mirror's rim. It must pass through P_1 and P_2. These possibilities are drawn approximately to scale in Fig. 8.9 for the mirror considered in the examples. The volume of material removed by contouring the back surface with either a parabolic or a circular contour can be calculated by finding the sectional area to the right of the appropriate curve in Fig. 8.9 and bound at the right by the vertical line A-B, then revolving that area around the mirror's axis at the radius of the area's centroid. It may be seen that the sectional area is smaller for the chosen circular contour than for either parabolic contour. This means that the mirror's weight with that circular back contour will be greater than the same mirror with a parabolic contour.

The sectional area, A_P, for each half-parabola is given by Eq. (8.15) where x_2 and y_2 are as illustrated in Fig. 8.9. The greatest volume is removed with the X-axis parabola because it has a slightly larger radius of revolution. The mirror volume for the X-axis and Y-axis cases are given by Eq. (8.16).

$$A_p = (2/3)(x_2)(y_2) \tag{8.15}$$

$$V_{S\text{-}arch} = V_{baseline} - (A_p)(2\pi)(y_{centroid}) \tag{8.16}$$

where:

$$y_{centroid\ Y} = r_1 + (3/5)(y_2) \tag{8.17}$$

$$y_{centroid\ X} = r_1 + y_2 - (3/8)(y_2) \tag{8.18}$$

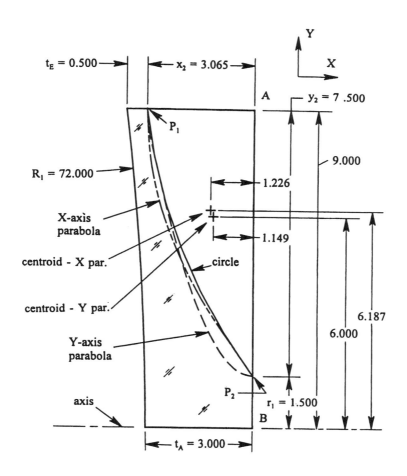

Fig. 8.9 Three possible contours (X-axis parabola, Y-axis parabola, and circle) for the single-arch mirror plotted to the same scale. Dimensions are in inches and apply to Examples 8.8 and 8.9.

The parabola with symmetry about the Y-axis might be preferred since the thickness then decreases monotonically with increasing distance from the axis. This is not necessarily the case for the X-axis parabola; this is indicated in Fig. 8.9, where the minimum mirror thickness occurs well inside the rim.

Example 8.8: Solid single-arch mirror with Y-axis parabolic back. (For design and analysis, use File 28 of the CD-ROM)
Change the back surface of the mirror from Example 8.4 to the single-arch, parabolic form with the vertex of the parabola at the back surface of the mirror, i.e.,

a Y-axis parabola. Assume t_E is 0.500 in. and r_2 = 1.500 in. Figures 8.8(e) and 8.9 apply. What is the mirror weight and how does the latter compare with the baseline mirror weight?

By observation, x_2 = 3.000 + 0.565 - 0.500 = 3.065 in. (77.851 mm)
y_2 = 9.000 -- 1.5 = 7.500 in. (190.500 mm)

From Eq. (8.15), A_P = (2/3)(3.065)(7.5) = 15.325 in.^{2} (9887.08 cm^2)

From Eq. (8.17), $y_{\text{centroid Y}}$ = 1.5 + (3/5)(7.5) = 6.000 in. (152.400 mm)

From Eq. (8.16), $V_{\text{S-arch}}$ = V_{baseline} - (15.325)(2π)(6.000)
= 835.16 - 577.739 = 257.42 in.^{3} (4218.37 cm^3)

Mirror weight = (0.0797)(257.42) = 20.516 lb (9.306 kg)

The mirror weight has been reduced to (20.516/65.562)(100) = 31% of the baseline mirror weight.

Example 8.9: Solid single-arch mirror with X-axis parabolic back. (For design and analysis, use File 29 of the CD-ROM)

Change the back surface of the mirror from Example No. 8.4 to a single-arch, X-axis parabola. Assume t_E is 0.500 in. Figure 8.8(e) applies. What is the mirror weight and how does the latter compare with the baseline mirror weight?

By observation, x_2 = 3.000 + 0.565 - 0.500 = 3.065 in. (77.851 mm)
y_2 = 9.000 - 1.5 = 7.500 in. (190.500 mm)

From Eq. (8.15), A_P = (2/3)(3.065)(7.5) = 15.325 in.^{2} (9887.08 mm^2)

From Eq. (8.17), $y_{\text{centroid X}}$ = 1.5 + 7.5 - (3/8)(7.5) = 6.187 in. (157.150 mm)

From Eq. (8.16), $V_{\text{S-arch}}$ = V_{baseline} - (15.325)(2π)(6.187)
= 835.16 - 595.74 = 239.41 in.^{3}

Mirror weight = (0.0797)(239.41) = 19.081 lb (8.655 kg)

The mirror weight has been reduced to (19.081/66.562)(100) = 29% of the baseline mirror weight. Comparison with the result for Example No. 8.8 confirms that this design with an X-axis parabola gives a slightly lower total mirror weight than the corresponding Y-axis parabola case.

Cho et al[8] showed that a single arch mirror with a Y-axis parabolic back surface gives the best compromise between self-weight deflections when the mirror axis is oriented at the zenith and the horizon.

The double-arch mirror of Fig. 8.8(f) is thickest at a zone chosen as about 55% of the mirror's diameter.[8] It typically is supported at three or more points within this zone. The rear surface is shaped as two parabolic curves with minimum (and perhaps equal) thickness at the rim and axis. The outer arch might well be a Y-axis parabola, while the inner arch might be an X-axis parabola. The latter choice is made to avoid an inflection point in the inner arch surface at the axis. The sectional areas of the inner and outer arches can be calculated from Eqs. (8.15) [we set $A_{P-outer} = A_P$] and (8.19), respectively.

$$A_{P-inner} = (2/3)(x_3)(y_3) \tag{8.19}$$

where the x and y dimensions are as shown in Fig. 8.9.

The radius of revolution for the outer arch ($y_{centroid\,Y}$) and the volume of that arch of the mirror are given by Eqs. (8.20) and (8.21), while those parameters for the inner arch are given by Eqs. (8.22) and (8.23).

$$y_{centroid\,Y} = r_1 + (3/5)(y_2) \tag{8.20}$$

$$V_{outer\,arch} = (A_{P-outer})(2\pi)(y_{centroid\,Y}) \tag{8.21}$$

$$y_{centroid\,X} = (3/8)(y_3) \tag{8.22}$$

$$V_{inner\,arch} = (A_{P-inner})(2\pi)(y_{centroid\,X}) \tag{8.23}$$

The mirror volume is then:

$$V_{D-arch} = V_{baseline} - V_{outer\,arch} - V_{inner\,arch} \tag{8.24}$$

Example 8.10: Solid double-arch mirror.
(For design and analyis, use File 30 of the CD-ROM)

Recontour the back surface of the mirror in Example 8.4 to a double-arch configuration with Y-axis and X-axis parabolas for the outer and inner arches, respectively. Figure 8.8(f) applies. Assume $t_E = t_A = 0.5$ in. Let $t_Z = 3.0$ in., $S_1 = 0.565$ in., $r_M = 0.55r_2 = 4.950$ in., and the annular zone width = 0.6 in. What is the mirror weight and how does it compare with the baseline mirror weight?

$$r_1 = 4.950 + (0.6/2) = 5.250 \text{ in. } (133.350 \text{ mm})$$
$$y_3 = 4.95 - (0.6/2) = 4.650 \text{ in. } (118.110 \text{ mm})$$
$$y_2 = r_2 - r_1 = 9.0 - 5.250 = 3.750 \text{ in. } (92.250 \text{ mm})$$

By observation, $t_A = 0.5$ in. $= t_Z - x_3 = 3.0 - x_3$, so $x_3 = 2.5$ in. (63.500 mm)
$$t_E = 0.5 \text{ in. } = t_Z + S_1 - x_2 = 3.0 + 0.565 - x_2,$$
so $x_2 = 3.565 - 0.5 = 3.065$ in. (77.851 mm)

By Eq. (8.15), $A_{P\text{-outer}} = (2/3)(3.065)(3.750) = 7.662 \text{ in.}^2 (49.432 \text{ cm}^2)$

By Eq. (8.19), $A_{P\text{-inner}} = (2/3)(2.5)(4.650) = 7.750 \text{ in.}^2 (50.000 \text{ cm}^2)$

By Eq. (8.20), $y_{\text{centroid Y}} = 5.250 + (3/5)(3.750) = 7.500 \text{ in. } (190.599 \text{ mm})$

By Eq. (8.21), $y_{\text{centroid X}} = (3/8)(4.650) = 1.744 \text{ in. } (44.291 \text{ mm})$

By Eq. (8.22), $V_{\text{outer arch}} = (7.662)(2\pi)(7.500) = 361.063 \text{ in.}^3 (5916.766 \text{ cm}^3)$

By Eq. (8.23), $V_{\text{inner arch}} = (7.750)(2\pi)(1.744) = 84.923 \text{ in.}^3 (1391.647 \text{ cm}^3)$

By Eq. (8.24),
$$V_{\text{D-arch}} = 835.16 - 361.063 - 84.923 = 389.174 \text{ in.}^3 (6377.419 \text{ cm}^3)$$

Mirror weight $= (0.0797)(389.174) = 31.017$ lb. (14.069 kg)

The mirror weight has been reduced to $(31.017/66.562)(100) = 47\%$ of the baseline mirror weight.

It should be noted that others have configured double-arch mirrors with a weight relative to the equivalent flat-back version as low as about 30%.[9]

The symmetrical doubleconcave (DCC) mirror configuration shown in Fig. 8.8(g) does not reduce substrate weight, but is included here for comparison. It is generally used only when the axis is horizontal, or nearly so, because gravity deflections then are symmetrical about the midplane and are smaller than with nonsymmetrical configurations. This mirror suffers excessively from surface deformation when the axis is vertical.[9] This situation also applies to the symmetrical convex-surfaced mirror.

The volume of this type mirror is:

$$V_{\text{DCC}} = (\pi)(r_2^2)(t_E) - (\pi/3)(S_1^2)(3R_1 - S_1) - (\pi/3)(S_2^2)(3R_2 - S_2) \qquad (8.25)$$

Example 8.11: Solid double concave mirror.
(For design and analysis, use File 31 of the CD-ROM)
Change the back surface of the mirror in Example 8.3 to the symmetrical concave form. Maintain the axial thickness at 3.000 in. (7.62 cm). What is the resulting mirror weight and how does it compare with that of the baseline version?

By Eq. (8.11), $S_2 = S = 72 - (72^2)^{1/2} = 0.565$ in. (14.351 mm)
$$t_E = 3.0 + S_1 + S_2 = 3.0 + 0.565 + 0.565 = 4.130 \text{ in (104.902 mm)}$$

From Eq. (8.25), since $R_1 = R_2$ and $S_1 = S_2$:
$$\text{Volume} = (\pi)(9^2)(4.130) - (2)\{(\pi/3)(0.565^2)[(3)(72) - 0.565]\}$$
$$= 1050.957 - (2)(72.018) = 906.921 \text{ in.}^3 \ (14,861.772 \text{ cm}^3)$$

The mirror weight is then $(0.0797)(906.921) = 72.282$ lb (32.787 kg)

The mirror weight has been <u>increased</u> by a factor of $(72.282/66.562)(100) = 109\%$ as compared to the baseline design.

8.3.2 Cast ribbed substrate configurations

Historically, early attempts to reduce the weight of large mirrors for astronomical telescopes involved casting pockets into the back surface of the substrate to eliminate material that contributed little or nothing to the strength or stiffness of the mirror. Notable in these early efforts was the casting by the Corning Glass Works of two blanks for the 200-in. (5.1-m)-diameter Hale telescope that has been operational on Mt. Palomar in California since 1949. These blanks, which were cast before World War II, were made of a then new borosilicate crown glass (Pyrex) with CTE of $2.5 \times 10^{-6}/°C$. To accelerate temperature stabilization, the structures cast into the substrates have ribs of approximately 4 in. (10.2 cm) maximum thickness. The overall edge thickness of the mirror used in the telescope is about 24 in. (61 cm); the central hole for light passage is about 40 in. (102 cm) in diameter. The weight of the mirror is about 20 tons (1.8×10^4 kg), representing a saving of about 50% over that of a solid disk with an equivalent self-weight deflection.[10]

A vast amount of material was removed from the blank for the Hale primary as it was ground to a f/3.3 parabola. More modern techniques for making even larger cast mirrors involve spin casting the glass in a mold containing numerous hexagonal-shaped ceramic voidformers (cores) arranged as the negative of the desired structure. The mold is located within a furnace that is slowly rotating about a vertical axis. After the raw glass is melted on top of the cores, centrifugal force creates a near net shape parabolic surface, thereby minimizing subsequent material removal. Several large mirrors have been made by this basic process from Ohara E6 glass and Zerodur at the Steward Observatory Mirror Laboratory in Arizona and at Schott Glaswerke in Mainz, Germany, respectively.

The largest monolithic mirror substrates made so far are two that have diameters of 8.42 m (27.62 ft), central holes of 0.889 m (2.92 ft) diameter, edge thicknesses of 0.894 m (2.93 ft), and weights of 16,000 kg (35,274 lb). These blanks, which are to be used in the Large Binocular Telescope (LBT) on Mt. Graham in Arizona, were cast at the Steward Observatory Mirror Laboratory in 1997 and 2000. Figure 8.10 shows the first blank, while Fig. 8.11 shows a partial section view through the mold and furnace.[11,12] The E6 glass was slowly heated to and then melted at 1180 °C. Cooling and annealing took about 1 month thereafter. This particular blank had a small defect that was due to an inadvertent leak in the wall of the mold. This was repaired successfully by fusing additional glass onto the blank and reannealing it.

8.3.3 Machined-back and built-up structural configurations

Figure 8.12 shows various construction configurations for machined and built-up lightweight mirrors.[13] These include symmetrical and nonsymmetrical sandwiches, partly and fully open ("waffle") back designs, and fused-fiber or foam-filled sandwich constructions. Each of these would have a characteristic areal density in pounds per square foot or kilograms per square meter depending on material type, material distribution, thickness of members (faceplate, backplate, and core webs), etc. In some designs, the core is integral with the front and back facesheets of the structure, while in others the parts are separate and partially attached together. The attachment means include thermal fusing, adhesive and frit bonding, and, for metal mirrors, brazing or welding. The pattern of cells in the core has a strong influence on the mirror's weight and stiffness. Triangular, square, circular, and hexagonal shapes are most commonly used in cells.

| (a) | (b) | (c) | (d) | (e) |

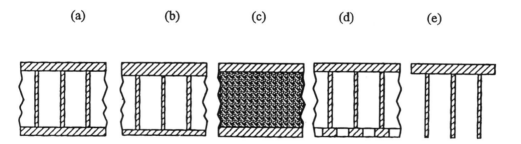

Fig. 8.12 Cross-sections for machined and built-up mirror substrates. (a) Symmetrical sandwich, (b) nonsymmetrical sandwich, (c) foam or fused-fiber core sandwich, (d) partially open back, and (e) open back. (From Seibert. [13] **)**

As noted earlier, a mirror lightweighted by removing nonessential material from within the substrate envelope is structurally more efficient than an equivalent-sized solid mirror. Since the material near the neutral plane contributes little to bending stiffness, it can safely be eliminated. This reduces weight so a desirably high stiffness-to-weight ratio can be provided. This results in some reduction of shear resistance. The manner in which the mirror is supported contributes strongly to the effects of gravity and externally applied accelerations.

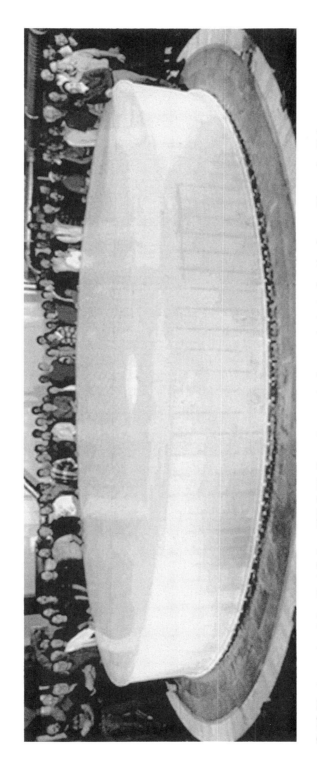

Fig. 8.10 Photograph of the first 8.4-m (27.6-ft)-diameter cast mirror substrate for the Large Binocular Telescope. (From Hill et al.[11])

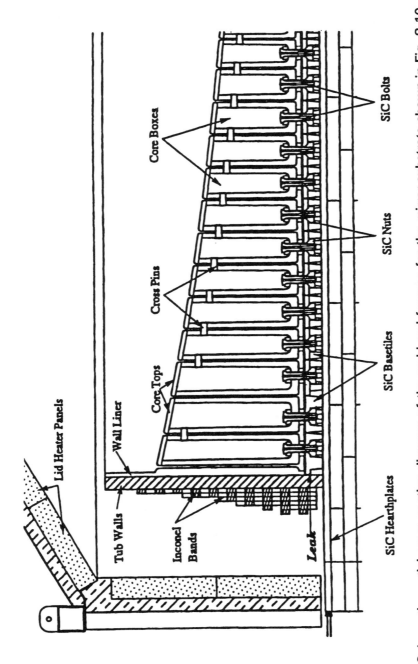

Fig. 8.11 Schematic partial cross-section diagram of the mold and furnace for the mirror substrate shown in Fig. 8.10. (From Hill et al.[12])

Figure 8.13 shows one classic type of built-up construction; it is called an "egg-crate" configuration. The core is created as cellular "webs" made of thin slotted strips that interlock, but are not attached to each other. Front and back faceplates are fused to the top and bottom edges of the core to form the mirror substrate. The diameter-to-thickness ratio of such a mirror is typically about 7:1, so a 20-in. (50.8-cm) diameter mirror would be about 2.85 in. (7.239 cm) thick. Since not all parts of the core are connected, it is not as stiff as some of the more modern types, such as the fused monolithic structure.[14]

A fusing process developed by Corning Glass Works entails building the core by attaching together "ell-shaped" strips of the mirror material as indicated in Fig. 8.14 using multiple torches to locally soften the material so adjacent regions fuse.[15] In some designs, cylindrical rings are fused to the outer rim of the core to enclose it and to increase its stiffness. If the mirror is perforated, a ring may be fused into the central hole for the same reasons (see, for example, Fig. 8.15). When the entire core has been created, its top and bottom ends are usually ground flat and parallel. In some cases they may be generated or ground spherical to form a meniscus shape. In either case, facesheets are located on the core and the entirety is heated in a furnace until it is fused together. If it is fused on a curved mandrel, the structure can be sagged to the meniscus shape desired for minimum

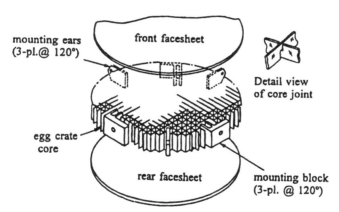

Fig. 8.13 Parts of a typical "egg-crate" mirror. (Adapted from Yoder.[14])

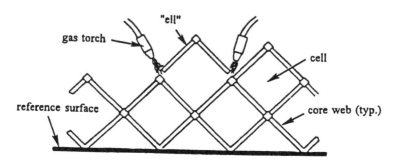

Fig. 8.14 Corning's process for attaching 90° "ells" by torch welding to form a monolithic fused mirror core. (Adapted from Lewis.[15])

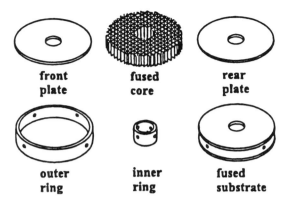

Fig. 8.15 Basic parts of a typical perforated fused monolithic mirror substrate. (Adapted from Lewis.[15])

glass removal. The substrate so created is monolithic and has the characteristics of the bulk material throughout. During the fusing operation, the softened material usually distorts, resulting in shape defects, as indicated schematically in Fig. 8.16(a). The annealed blank is carefully inspected to find the region nearest the front surface of the front fcesheet with minimum internal defects (bubbles and included impurities). Manufacture proceeds by grinding away the unwanted material as indicated in Fig. 8.16(b) to locate the optical surface within this so-called critical zone.

Another type of mirror blank can be formed by making a core and attaching it to the facesheets using an assembly process similar to brazing in which all parts are attached to each other by "frit." Frit is an "adhesive" made of an organic vehicle and powdered glass that melts well with ULE. The CTE of the frit is controlled so as not to introduce excessive stress into the blank during or subsequent to application. The resulting blank is free of the defects shown in Fig. 8.16(a) because the mirror's previously annealed structural elements never reach their softening temperature. Figure 8.17 shows a typical configuration for a planoconcave, closed sandwich substrate designed for this type of assembly. Mirror blanks made by this process can have thinner webs and a higher diameter-to-thickness ratio (typically by 167%) than monolithic fused blanks. Tighter dimensional tolerances can be held in a frit-bonded substrate because the structural members do not distort. The frit-bonded mirror will weigh significantly less (typically by 27%), yet have greater rigidity (typically by 164%) than the conventional fused monolithic type.[16] A comparison of design characteristics adapted from Edwards[17] for fused monolithic and frit-bonded mirrors is given in Table 8.1.

A fused silica lightweight mirror substrate with a core machined from a solid disk is illustrated in Fig. 8.18. This has a symmetrical concave form. Its core was machined from a solid blank by boring through holes of various shapes and grinding a concave surface on both sides. This core was fused to preformed meniscus-shaped facesheets. The 20-in. (50.8-cm) diameter mirror weighed about 16 lb (7.3 kg).[18] Figure 8.19 shows the pattern of holes produced by drilling and grinding with annular diamond-bonded core and end-mill tools. The cusps remaining after core drilling were removed

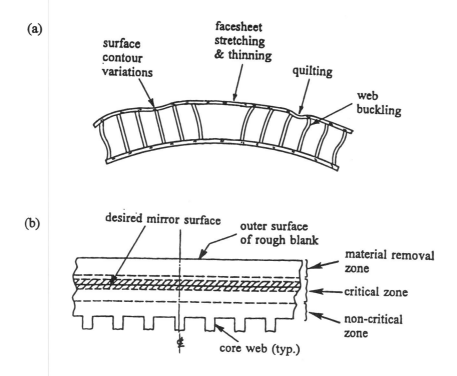

Fig. 8.16 Details of the monolithic fused mirror blank. (a) Typical defects caused by heating ULE above the annealing point. (b) Location of the mirror surface within the best region of the front sheet. (Adapted from Yoder.[14])

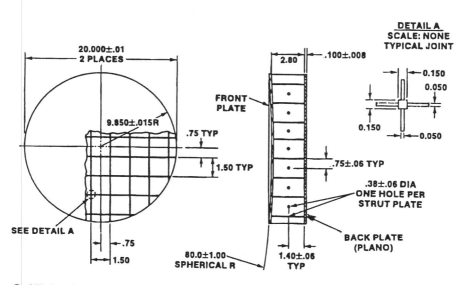

Fig. 8.17 A mirror design suitable for frit bonding. (Adapted from Fitzsimmons and Crowe.[16])

Table 8.1 Design characteristics of fused and frit-bonded mirrors.

Characteristic	Fusion bonded	Frit bonded
Minimum core density	10%	3%
Mean bond stength	2500 lb/in.^{2} (17.2 MPa)	5000 lb/in.^{2} (34.5 MPa)
Mounting blocks	Fused in place	Fused or frit bonded in place
Maximum cell size	4 in. (10.2 cm)	(6 in. (15.2 cm)
Minimum rib thickness	0.150 in. (3.81 mm)	(0.050 in. (1.27 mm)
Average plate thickness for a given mirror diameter D:		
D < 30 in.	0.160 in. 4.06 mm)	0.100 in. (2.54 mm)
30 in. < D < 90 in.	0.38 in. (9.65 mm)	0.30 in. (7.62 mm)
D > 90 in.	0.60 in. (15.24 mm)	0.40 in. (10.16 mm)

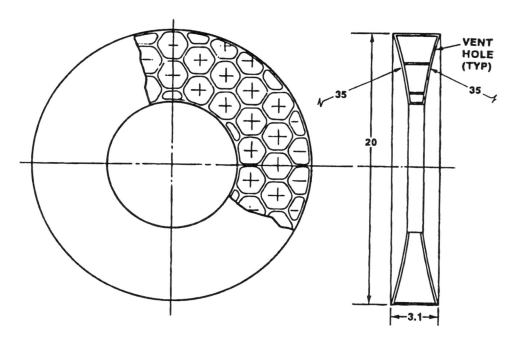

Fig. 8.18 Configuration of a symmetrical concave mirror with core machined from a solid blank. The front and rear plates were preshaped (sagged over a convex mold) to meniscus form and fused to the core. Dimensions are in inches. (From Pepi and Wollensak.[18])

with diamond cutters. The wall thicknesses after machining were 1 to 3 mm. After fusing, the substrate was monolithic. Mirrors of this shape are best used with their axes horizontal since self-weight deflections with vertical axes are relatively large.

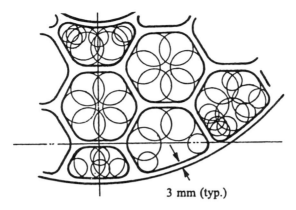

3 mm (typ.)

Fig. 8.19 Typical core machining pattern for a mirror such as that shown in Fig. 8.18. (From Pepi and Wollensak.[18])

A more recent technique for making a lightweight core from a solid blank uses an abrasive water jet (AWJ) cutting process perfected by Corning Glass Works. Edwards[17] described the technique and apparatus used (see Fig. 8.20) as follows:

The system is powered by two 250 horsepower motors driving hydraulic pumps, which in turn feed intensifiers that output over 60,000 psi water pressure. Passing through a 0.040 in. (1.02 mm) diameter sapphire jewel orifice, the waterjet creates a vacuum, pulling abrasive garnet into the stream. After fully entraining the abrasive in a mixing tube, the water exits the nozzle at over Mach 2, capable of cutting through 30 cm thick glass. A tool check station provides alignment and process parameter calibration. The five-axis head can compensate for slight changes in the shape of the cut due to wear of the jewel and mixing tube during jet-on time as well as any slight part movement. The system manipulator positions the nozzle in the 150 in. × 250 in. × 48 in. workspace to an accuracy of better than ± 0.0025 in., repeatable to within ± 0.001 in. Each day the operator makes test cuts which are measured to determine the health and contour of the jet. Ongoing verification throughout the waterjet process ensures tight dimensional tolerances are maintained in the resultant lightweight cores. (Ref. 17, p. 705)

Figure 8.21 shows a typical product made by the Corning AWJ process. This is a 1.1-m (43.3-in.) diameter core to be incorporated into one of the tertiary mirrors for the 6.5-m (255.9-in.) aperture Magellan Telescopes. This particular design incorporated thicker webs at the outer edge and central mounting hub, a hexagonal pattern superimposed on an elliptically shaped blank, and a circular central through-hole.[17] The machine shown in Fig. 8.20 is capable of handling substrates up to about 3 m (118 in.) in diameter.

Lightweighting a mirror substrate from a solid plate by machining cell pockets into the blank through small access holes bored into its back surface results in a monolithic structure without fusing. An example is shown in Fig. 8.22.[19,20] This is a

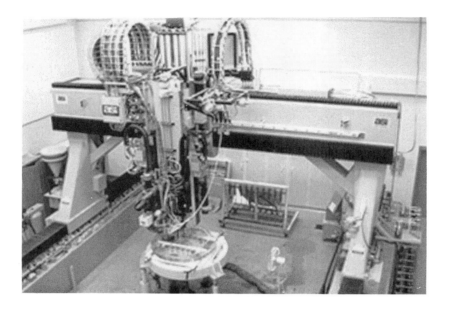

Fig. 8.20 Photograph of the Corning abrasive water jet machine used to make lightweight cores for mirror substrates. (From Edwards.[17])

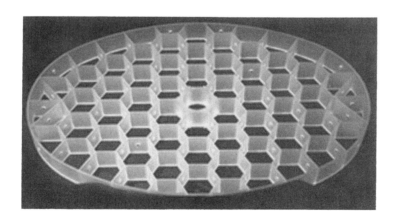

Fig. 8.21 Typical example of a mirror core lightweighted by the Corning AWJ process. (From Edwards.[17])

diagram of the back side of the 2.7-m (106-in.) diameter primary mirror for the Stratospheric Observatory for Infrared Astronomy (SOFIA) telescope that is soon to replace NASA's Kuiper Airborne Observatory (KAO) telescope discussed in Sect. 8.4. The mirror design is a planoconcave structure with a heavily beveled rim formed into "flying buttress" lateral supports and a circular central hole. Hexagonal cells with thin webs

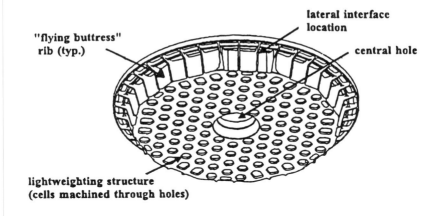

"flying buttress" rib (typ.)

lateral interface location

central hole

lightweighting structure (cells machined through holes)

Fig. 8.22 The back side of the SOFIA primary mirror lightweighted by machining pockets through holes in the back. (Adapted from Erdman et al.[19])

were machined into the Zerodur blank using diamond tools to undercut material and leave a nearly complete backplate. After machining, the substrate was acid etched to further reduce weight and to remove microscopic cracks created during the grinding operation. The weight of the resulting structure was about 880 kg (1940 lb). This is about 20% of the weight of a corresponding solid mirror. The supports for this mirror are described in Sect. 10.1.1.3.

In yet another technique for forming small- to moderate-sized lightweight mirrors (the Hextek process), short tubes of glass are placed on end between glass facesheets to form a sandwich configuration. The rear facesheet is perforated with one hole per tube. The assembly is heated to the softening point in a furnace while air or other gas is pumped into the holes to pneumatically force the softened tubes into intimate contact and to fuse together to form a square or hexagonal cell pattern. Tube placement prior to fusing is illustrated in Fig. 8.23. The result is a monolithic structure. Examples are shown in Fig. 8.24.

The materials typically used in the Hextek mirrors are Corning Pyrex 7740, Schott Tempax, Vycor, and fused silica. Weight is considerably reduced from that of the built-up fused monolith because the pressure support allows thinner walls and facesheets to be used.[21]

8.3.4 Thin facesheet configurations

If the substrate for a mirror is reduced drastically with respect to its diameter, inherent rigidity is impossible. Success in supporting the substrate during manufacture, establishing and maintaining high-quality performance (i.e., optical figure) during use, and protecting the substrate from damage caused by extreme vibration and shock depends upon the ability of a companion structure to support the mirror adequately at all times. During use, this structure plays a strong role in controlling mirror shape. The latter

(a)   (b)

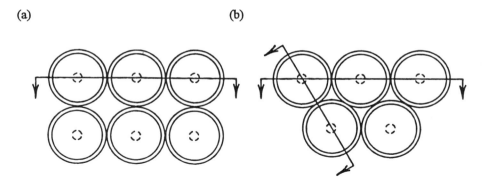

Fig. 8.23 Tube placement prior to heating and pneumatic expansion in the Hextek manufacturing process. (a) Square cells, (b) hexagonal cells. (Courtesy of Hextek Corp., Tucson, AZ.)

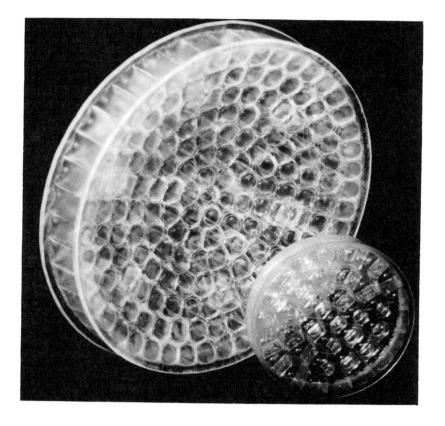

Fig. 8.24 Photographs of two fused monolithic mirror blanks made by the Hextek process. (Courtesy of Hextek Corp., Tucson, AZ.)

requirement makes the optical component only one part of a much more complex system that can sense errors in the mirror's shape and apply the appropriate forces to correct those errors. The need for such "adaptive optics" technology results from a desire to improve the performance of increasingly large ground-based astronomical telescopes that cannot be built with the above-discussed technology because weight and cost would increase beyond reasonable limits and because adaptive capability allows compensation for atmospheric effects on "seeing." It also would allow much larger astronomical optical systems to be carried into space and operated from that vantage point. Other aerospace applications as well as military ones can also benefit from the availability of this technology.

To illustrate this new technology, we summarize one of several approaches being considered for the primary mirror of the next-generation space telescope (NGST) which may be at least 6 m (236 in.) in diameter; should have a low mass per unit area (< 15 kg/m^2), including the reaction structure; must provide long-term, diffraction-limited performance in the near-IR spectral region at cryogenic temperature (40 K); and must be affordable.

Burge et al.[22] proposed to build this mirror as a 2-mm (0.078-in.) thick glass membrane supported on numerous (perhaps 50) actuators per square meter. The actuators would be screwdriven, capable of 6 nm rms resolution, and would require no power to hold their position. The assembly would be attached to a structure made from composite carbon fiber with a mass density of <5 kg/m^2. The adjustment of the mirror shape would be under the control of a closed-loop system functioning by sensing the quality of the image of a bright star within the telescope's field of view and applying phase retrieval algorithms to derive commands to be sent to the actuators. Control of the mirror figure during operation would be needed only occasionally since the membrane plus support structure would be rigid enough and the external disturbances on orbit benign enough to alleviate the need for real-time adjustment.

The key to achieving a successful design is the use of proven methods for fabricating the mirror membrane. The approach advocated by Burge et al.[22] is sketched in Fig. 8.25. Here the membrane starts as a thick meniscus that is attached with pitch to a much thicker blocking body that provides stress-free support for the membrane. The upper surface of the membrane is reduced in thickness and eventually polished using the "stressed lap" technique under computer control.[23] Once polished to the required quality, the membrane would be removed (by heating the pitch slightly) and attached to the actuators. The proposed interface between the membrane and each actuator is described in Sect. 10.5. Tests of a simulated membrane mirror have indicated that the real mirror will survive the launch environment, the worst exposure coming from acoustic loading.

Other designs for the NGST currently being considered include ones with a segmented primary mirror consisting of perhaps eight "petals" surrounding an octagonally shaped annular central mirror.[24] The petals would be deployed on orbit and aligned using active control driven by a figure sensor. Some design concepts feature as many as 32 deployable mirrors made, perhaps, of beryllium.[25] Others consider glass-type materials and/or composite optics and structures. Some segment designs might be sufficiently rigid to not need active figure control, while others would employ adaptive figure control

Fabricate thick substrate
for membrane

Fabricate blocking body

Attach matching structure

Generate membrane to
thickness & polish

De-block membrane

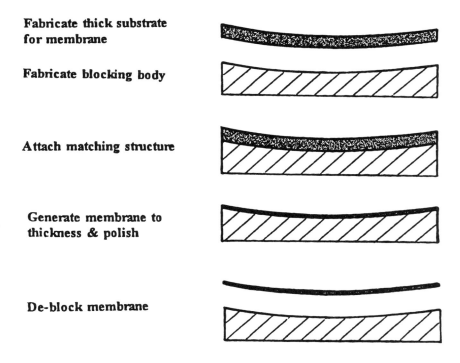

Fig. 8.25 A concept for fabricating a thin glass membrane mirror for the next-generation space telescope. (Adapted from Burge et al.[22])

basically similar to the concept described earlier. Segment alignment to form a usable total optical surface will be essential in all cases. It will be interesting to see which concept is chosen and then to watch the design materialize in the years to come.

8.4 Metallic Mirrors

The metals commonly used to make mirrors are listed with their key mechanical properties in Table B8b. The most common are wrought aluminum and beryllium, the latter being most popular in cryogenic space applications. Mirrors for use in high-energy laser applications or with high-power light sources need to be cooled. This frequently is done by circulating coolant through tubular passages machined into the mirror substrate. These usually are made of oxygen-free high-conductivity (OFHC) copper or TZM, an alloy of titanium, zirconium, and molybdenum. Fabrication of metallic mirrors typically involves the following steps: formation of the blank, geometric shaping, stress relieving, plating (usually with electroless nickel), optical finishing, and optical coating. Many materials can be cast; others are welded or brazed from components. Single-point diamond turning has found great application in creating fine-quality optical surfaces in metals such as aluminum, brass, copper, gold, silver, electroless nickel (coating), and beryllium copper. The purity of the material is very important.[26] The surface finish of metal surfaces is inferior to glass-type materials, but is adequate for infrared systems and some visible-light applications. Figure 8.26 shows a variety of metal mirrors made by one maufacturer using SPDT methods.

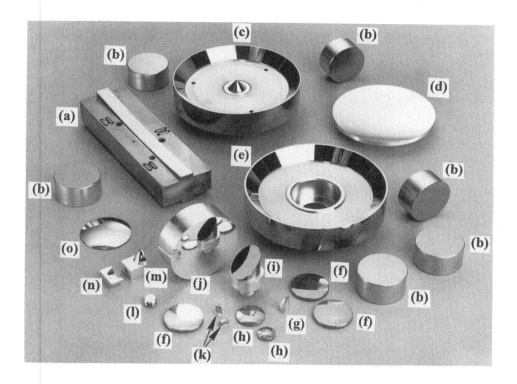

Fig. 8.26 Photograph of a variety of optical components made by the SPDT process. Shown are (a) CO_2 slab laser mirror, (b) water-cooled CO_2 laser mirror, (c) Cu waxicon, (d) on-axis parabolic mirror, (e) copper axicon, (f) ZnSe aspheric windows, (g) parabolic reflector, (h) aspheric ZnSe lens, (i) Ni-plated Be mirror, (j) spherical Al mirror, (k) ZnSe aspheric retroreflector, (l) Cu "button" mirror, (m) parabloic replica mold, (n) electron microscope collimating mirror, and (o) aspheric Ge lens. (Courtesy of II-VI, Inc., Saxonburg, PA.)

Figure 8.27 shows the back side of a typical metal mirror. It is the 7.3-in. (18.5-cm)-diameter by 0.7-in. (1.78-cm)-thick secondary mirror used in the infrared telescope of NASA's Kuiper Airborne Observatory.[27] Lightness of weight and low inertia are essential to the success of this equipment since the mirror moves mechanically in oscillatory tipping fashion to rapidly switch the field of view of the telescope from the target of interest to the sky background for calibration purposes.

The 7:1 diameter-to-thickness type 5083-O aluminum substrate was lightened by machining open pockets into a solid blank. The total weight was 1.1 lb (0.5 kg), representing a 70% reduction from a solid. The convex hyperboloidal optical surface (which was not electroless nickel plated) was created by SPDT machining to the final figure. The quality of the surface was about $\lambda/1.5$ p-v at a 633-nm wavelength over 90% of the aperture. The final surface was coated with aluminum and silicon monoxide films. The mounting surfaces at the center of the mirror were diamond turned to facilitate accurate turning of the optical surface when the blank was reversed later. The surface figure achieved at the -40°C operating temperature was $\lambda/2$ at a 633-nm wavelength.

The mirror is shown mounted on its drive mechanism in Fig. 8.28. The square-wave response of the mirror and its drive mechanism for beam tilt angles up to $\pm$ 23 arcmin was about 40 Hz. It was driven in orthogonal tilts by four electromagnetic actuators located symmetrically at the back of the mirror. The moving assembly [weight about 2 lb (4.4 kg)] tilted about its center of gravity on two-axis flex pivot gimbals. The actuator coils were mounted to a stationary baseplate that provided a conductive path for temperature control. The entire moving assembly could be moved axially by a motor-driven ball screw through a range of $\pm$ 1.3 cm (0.51 in.) for focus adjustment during flight.

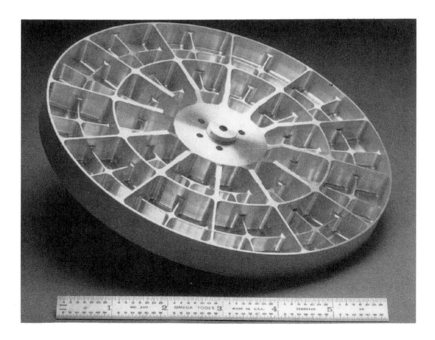

Fig. 8.27 Photograph of the lightweighted aluminum scanning secondary mirror used in the Kuiper Airborne Observatory. (From Downey et al.[27])

Many other lightweight beryllium mirrors have been fabricated by techniques similar to those just discussed. Usually these were used in space applications, although some have been used in high-speed scanning applications where high stiffness and low

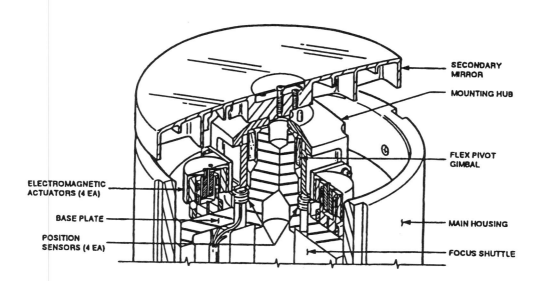

SECONDARY MIRROR

MOUNTING HUB

FLEX PIVOT GIMBAL

ELECTROMAGNETIC ACTUATORS (4 EA)

BASE PLATE

POSITION SENSORS (4 EA)

MAIN HOUSING

FOCUS SHUTTLE

Fig. 8.28 Mirror from Fig. 8.27 mounted on its drive mechanism. (From Downey et al.[27])

weight are required to prevent surface distortion by centrifugal force. For wavelengths beyond about 3 μm in the infrared, polished bare beryllium has high reflectance so it is not necessary to apply electroless nickel plating. This avoids thermal problems caused by bimetallic effects from a CTE mismatch.[28]

One very successful means for making beryllium mirrors is an improved powder metallurgy technique patented by Gould[29] and described by Paquin et al.[30] and Paquin.[31] In this process, high-purity beryllium powder is subjected to hot isostatic pressing (HIP) under high temperature and pressure. This yields blanks of near net shape with low porosity and few inclusions. The process improvement included forming internal lightweighting pockets by compressing the material around void formers made of leachable material (copper) that could be removed after compacting. Figure 8.29 shows such mirrors. They were 9.5-in. (24.1-cm) diameter by 1.2-in. (2.8-cm) monolithic closed sandwiches weighing 2.16 lb (0.98 kg). Hexagonal cells measuring 1 in. (2.5 cm) and webs 0.05 in. (1.3 mm) thick were formed in these mirrors. In the foreground of the figure, the back face of one mirror shows access holes for supporting the void formers and removing them later. After polishing, the front facesheets typically had figures of λ/25 p-v at a 633-nm wavelength.

These experimental mirrors were extremely stiff, with first resonance at about 8700 Hz. The manufacturing process is scalable to larger mirror sizes. At a 17-in. (43.2-cm) diameter, the mirror's weight would be 7.1 lb (3.3 kg) and the structure would be stiff enough for mounting on a three-point support.

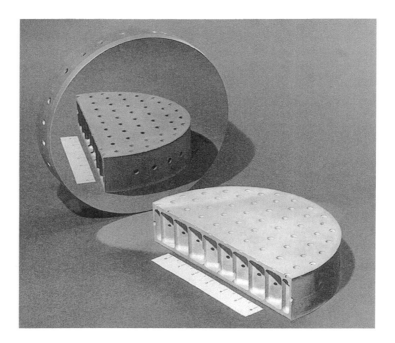

Fig. 8.29 Photograph of 9.5-in. (24.1-cm) diameter monolithic, closed sandwich beryllium mirrors made by the HIP process. (From Paquin.[31])

8.5 Pellicles

Very thin mirrors, beamsplitters, and beamcombiners can be made from films of material such as nitrocellulose, polyester, or polyethylene. Their thicknesses typically are 5 μm (0.0002 in.) ± 10%, although 2 μm (0.00008 in.) ± 10% thick films and special ones up to 20 μm (0.0008 in.) thick also are available. The surface quality of standard varieties typically is better than 40/20 scratch and dig while figure typically is 0.5 to 2λ per inch. The base material transmits well (>90%) from 0.35 to 2.4 μm, but has numerous deep absorbing regions beyond 2.4 μm.[32] See Fig. 8.30 for a simplified representation of the transmission characteristics of a typical standard type pellicle. Pellicles can be coated to reflect, split, or combine light beams in the visible to near IR region with conventional or custom-designed coatings. Standard A/R coatings can be applied to the back side of the films. Figure 8.31 shows mounted pellicle products as supplied by one manufacturer.

A prime feature of the pellicle is the absence of ghost imaging since the first and second surface reflections at 45° incidence (see Fig. 8.5) are so close together they appear superimposed. Interference effects are frequently seen. A pellicle with uncoated front and A/R coated back surfaces at 45° incidence serves as a 4% beam sampler. If both surfaces are uncoated, it has about 8% total reflectance and transmittance of about (0.92)(0.90) = 83% in the visible spectral pass-band. Beamsplitters and combiners achieve the same ghost-free advantage over thicker conventional glass components.

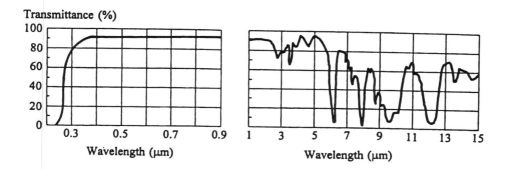

Transmittance (%)

Wavelength (μm)   Wavelength (μm)

Fig. 8.30 Simplified transmission characteristics of a standard nitrocellulose pellicle in the visible and infrared regions. (Courtesy of National Photocolor Corp., Mamaroneck, NY.)

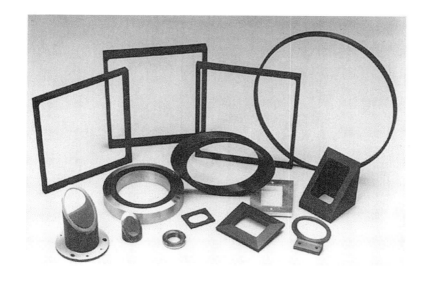

Fig. 8.31 A variety of standard mounted pellicles as supplied by one manufacturer. (Courtesy of National Photocolor Corp., Mamaroneck, NY.)

Pellicles are supported by circular, square, or rectangular frames with beveled and lapped front surfaces to which the stretched film is attached. Frames typically are black anodized aluminum and have threaded holes for mounting. Special units can be made of stainless steel or ceramic. Figure 8.32 shows the configurations and dimensions of standard pellicle frames as supplied by one manufacturer.

Since pellicles are thin, they are more fragile than conventional plane parallel optics. They are susceptible to the acoustic vibration of adjacent air columns, but work

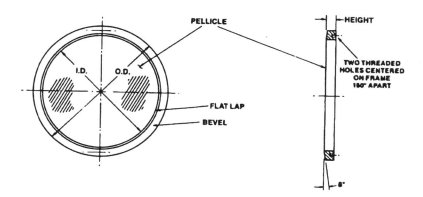

Size	I.D.	O.D.	Height	Mounting Holes
1″	1″ (25.4mm)	1³/₈″ (34.9mm)	³/₁₆″ (4.8mm)	#2-56 thd. x ¹/₈″ dp.
2″	2″ (50.8mm)	2³/₈″ (60.3mm)	³/₁₆″ (4.8mm)	#2-56 thd. x ¹/₈″ dp.
3″	3″ (76.2mm)	3¹/₂″ (88.9mm)	¹/₄″ (6.4mm)	#6-32 thd. x ¹/₈″ dp.
4″	4″ (101.6mm)	4¹/₂″ (114.3mm)	¹/₄″ (6.4mm)	#6-32 thd. x ¹/₈″ dp.
5″	5″ (127.0mm)	5¹/₂″ (139.7mm)	⁵/₁₆″ (7.9mm)	#6-32 thd. x ¹/₈″ dp.
6″	6″ (152.4mm)	6¹/₂″ (165.1mm)	³/₈″ (9.5mm)	#6-32 thd. x ³/₁₆″ dp.

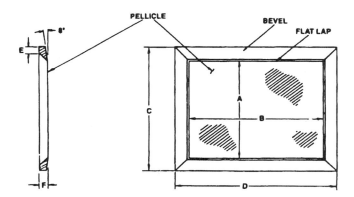

Nominal Dimensions

	Inches	Millimeters
A	5	127.0
B	7	177.8
C	6⁵/₈	168.3
D	8³/₈	212.7
E	⁵/₁₆	7.9
F	⁷/₁₆	11.1

Fig. 8.32 Some standard pellicle frame designs and dimensions. (Courtesy of National Photocolor Corp., Mamaroneck, NY.)

well in a vacuum. Some thicker varieties (notably, ones made of polyester films) can be used under water. The temperature range of usefulness is about -40° to +90° C. They can tolerate relative humidity to 95%. Pellicles must be mounted so that the frames are not distorted because that would distort the optical surfaces. Custom frames can be designed in stiffer configurations to withstand significant mounting forces.

References

1. Jenkins, F.A., and White, H.E., *Fundamentals of Optics*, McGraw-Hill, New York, 1957.
2. Smith, W.J., *Modern Optical Engineering,* 3rd ed., McGraw-Hill, New York, 2000.
3. Kaspereit, O.K., ORDM 2-1, *Design of Fire Control Optics*, U.S. Army Ordnance (out of print).
4. Schubert, F., "Determining optical mirror size," *Machine Des.* Vol. 51, 128, 1979.
5. Rodkevich, G.V., and Robachevskaya, V.I., "Possibilities of reducing the mass of large precision mirrors," *Sov. J. Opt. Technol.* Vol. 44, 515, 1977.
6. Englehaupt, D., Chapt. 10 in *Handbook of Optomechanical Engineering*, CRC Press, Boca Raton, 1997.
7. Paquin, R., Chapt. 3 in *Handbook of Optomechanical Engineering*, CRC Press, Boca Raton, FL, 1997.
8. Cho, M.K., Richard, R., and Vukobratovich, D., "Optimum mirror shapes and supports for light weight mirrors subjected to self-weight," *SPIE Proceedings* Vol. 1167, 2, 1989.
9. Vukobratovich, D., Chapt. 3, "Optomechanical Systems Design," in *The Infrared & Electro-Optical Systems Handbook,* Vol. 4, ERIM, Ann Arbor, and SPIE, Bellingham, 1993.
10. Loytty, E.Y., and DeVoe, C.F., "Ultralightweight mirror blanks", *IEEE Trans. Aerospace Electron. Syst., AES-5,* 300, 1969.
11. Hill, J.M., Angel, J.R.P., Lutz, R.D., Olbert, B.H., and Strittmatter, P.A., "Casting the first 8.4 meter borosilicate honeycomb mirror for the Large Binocular Telescope", *SPIE Proceedings* Vol. 3352, 172, 1998.
12. Hill, J.M. and Salinari, P., "The Large Binocular Telescope Project", *SPIE Proceedings* Vol. 3352, 23, 1998.
13. Seibert, G.E., "Design of Lightweight Mirrors," *SPIE Short Course Notes*, SPIE Press, Bellingham1990.
14. Yoder, P. R., Jr., *Opto-Mechanical Systems Design,* 2nd ed., Marcel Dekker, New York, 1993.
15. Lewis, W.C., "Space telescope mirror substrate," *OSA Optical Fabrication and Testing Workshop, Tucson,* Optical Society of America, Washington, 1979.
16. Fitzsimmons, T.C., and Crowe, D.A., "Ultra-lightweight mirror manufacturing and radiation response study," RADC-TR-81-226, Rome Air Development Ctr., Rome, 1981.
17. Edwards, M.J., "Current fabrication techniques for ULE™ and fused silica lightweight mirrors," *SPIE Proceedings* Vol. 3356, 702, 1998.
18. Pepi, J.W., and Wollensak, R.J., "Ultra-lightweight fused silica mirrors for cryogenic space optical system," *SPIE Proceedings* Vol. 183, 131, 1979.
19. Erdman, M., Bittner, H., and Haberler, P., "Development and construction of the optical system for the airborne observatory SOFIA", *SPIE Proceedings* Vol. 4014, 309, 2000.

20. Espiard, J., Tarreau, M., Bernier, J., Billet, J., and Paseri, J., "S.O.F.I.A. lightweighted primary mirror," *SPIE Proceedings* Vol. 3352, 354, 1998.

21. Cannon, J.E., and Wortley, R.W., "Gas fusion center-plane-mounted secondary mirror," *SPIE Proceedings* Vol. 966, 309, 1988.

22. Burge, J.H., Angel, J.R.P., Cuerden, B., Martin, H.M., Miller, S.M., and Sandler, D.G., "Lightweight mirror technology using a thin facesheet with active rigid support", *SPIE Proceedings* Vol. 3356, 690, 1998.

23. Martin, H.M, Anderson, D.S., Angel, J.R.P., Burge, J.H., Davison, W.B., DeRigne, S.T., Hille, B.B., Ketelsen, D.A., Kittrell, W.C., McMillan, R., Nagel, R.H., Trebisky, T.J., West, S.C., and Young, R.S., "Stressed-lap polishing of 1.8-m f/1 and 3.5-m f/1.5 primary mirrors," *Proc. ESO Conference on Progress in Telescope and Instrumentation Technologies*, 169, European Optical Society, Hannover, Germany, 1992.

24. Jacobson, D.N., Nein, M., Craig, L., Schunk, G., Rakoczy, J., Cloyd, D., Ricks. E., Hadaway, J., Redding, D., and Bely, P., "Design of a large lightweight space telescope optical system for the next generation space telescope," *SPIE Proceedings* Vol. 3356, 74, 1998.

25. Woodruff, R.A., Meyer, W.W., Reinert, R.P., and the Ball NGST Team, "System design trades for the next generation space telescope (NGST)," *SPIE Proceedings* Vol. 3356, 46, 1998.

26. Dahlgren, R., and Gerchman, M., "The use of aluminum alloy castings as diamond machining substrates for optical surfaces," *SPIE Proceedings* Vol. 890, 68, 1988.

27 Downey, C.H., Abbott, R.S., Arter, P.I., Hope, D.A., Payne, D.A., Roybal, E.A., Lester, D.F., and McClenahan, J.O., "The chopping secondary mirror for the Kuiper airborne observatory," *SPIE Proceedings* Vol. 1167, 329, 1989.

28. Vukobratovich, D., Gerzoff, A., and Cho, M.K., "Therm-optic analysis of bi-metallic mirrors," *SPIE Proceedings* Vol. 3132, 12, 1997.

29. Gould, G., "Method and means for making a beryllium mirror," U.S. Patent No. 4,492,669, 1985.

30. Paquin, R.A., Levenstein, H., Altadonna, L., and Gould, G., "Advanced lightweight beryllium optics," *Opt. Eng* Vol. 23, 157, 1984.

31. Paquin, R.A., "Hot isostatic pressed beryllium for large optics," *Opt. Eng.* Vol. 25, 2003, 1986.

32. Stern, A.K., private communication, 1998.

CHAPTER 9
Techniques for Mounting Small Mirrors

The appropriateness of a mechanical mounting for a mirror depends on a variety of factors, including:

- the inherent rigidity of the optic;
- the tolerable movement and distortion of the reflecting surface or surfaces;
- the magnitudes, locations, and orientations of the steady-state forces holding the optic against its mounting surfaces during operation;
- the transient forces driving the optic against, away from, or transversely to the mounting surfaces during exposure to extreme shock and vibration;
- the effects of steady-state and changing temperatures;
- the number, shapes, sizes, and orientations of mounting interfaces between the optic and mount;
- the rigidity and long-term stability of the mount;
- assembly, adjustment, maintenance, package size, weight, and configuration constraints; and
- affordability in the context of cost of the entire instrument.

In this chapter we address a variety of techniques commonly used to constrain mirrors in the size range from about 0.5 in. (1.2 cm) to about 24 in. (61 cm). At the small end of this range, where the mounts tend to be very simple, techniques used for mounting lenses may suffice. As would be expected, complexity increases with mirror size. The general techniques considered include mechanical clamping, elastomeric bonding, optical contacting, and mounting on flexures. Mountings appropriate for nonmetallic and metallic mirror substrates are included. In general, we progress from smaller to larger-sized optics. Mountings for mirrors to be used in astronomical telescope applications are discussed in the next chapter. It is pointed out that many mounting problems sometimes thought to exist only with the largest mirrors also exist with small mirrors; the difference is one of scale. In some contemporary designs involving "small" size, but high performance, these same problems are of sufficient magnitude to warrant special consideration.

9.1 Mechanically Clamped Mirror Mountings

Circular, rectangular, or nonsymmetrically shaped mirrors can often be mounted in the same manner as a lens. Circular mirrors up to perhaps 4 in. (10.2 cm) in diameter can be held with threaded retaining rings. Circular or noncircular ones can be held with flanges or cantilevered springs. The OD limit for a threaded mount is set primarily by the increasing difficulty of machining thin circular retaining rings with sufficient quality in larger diameters.

Figure 9.1 shows the retaining ring concept. The mirror is shown as a convex sphere although a mirror with an aspheric, or concave surface could be mounted similarly. The reflecting surface is registered (i.e., aligned) against a shoulder in the mount by an axial preload exerted by tightening the retainer. The ring typically has a loose fit (Class 1 or 2 per ANSI publication B1.1-1982) in the mount's ID. Contact occurs on the polished surface of the mirror to encourage precise centering of the curved-surfaced optic on the mechanical axis of the mount as a result of balancing of the radial components of the

269

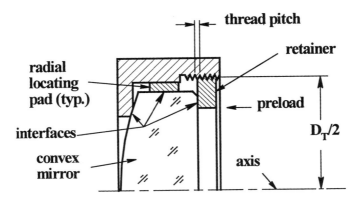

Fig. 9.1 Conceptual configuration of a convex mirror secured in its mount with a threaded retaining ring

axial force [see Fig. 2.2(b)].

Precise edging or close tolerances on the OD of the mirror are not required if custom-fitted spacers are used as radial locating pads. Although it is not indicated in the figure, contact on the convex surface should occur at the same height from the axis as the center of the opposite contact area to minimize bending of the mirror. Sharp-corner contact on the polished surface is shown. To minimize contact stress in the mirror (see Sect. 11.2), a tangential (conical) or toroidal (donut-shaped) interface would be preferred. Section 3.6 gives the details of various shapes of mechanical interfaces for lenses that are equally applicable to small mirrors.

As in the case for lens retainers, two or more holes are sometimes drilled into the exposed face of the retainer to accept pins on the end of a cylindrical wrench used to tighten the ring. Alternatively, a diametrical slot may be cut across the face of the retainer for this purpose. A flat plate that spans the retainer can be used as the wrench in the latter case. If a retaining force is applied to the back of the mirror and the fixed interface is at the front surface, the possibility of damaging the reflecting surface is reduced.

As in lens mounting, the magnitude of the total preload (P) developed in a threaded retainer lens mounting design with a specific torque (Q) applied to the ring at a fixed temperature can be estimated by the following equation:

$$P = 5Q/D_T \tag{3.19a}$$

where D_T is the pitch diameter of the thread as shown in Fig. 9.1.

Note that the accuracy of this equation is subject to the same limitations discussed in Sect. 3.4.1 and depends primarily upon the coefficient of friction in the threaded joint, which is quite uncertain in real life. This means that the torque applied to a threaded retainer cannot be relied upon to produce a specific preload.

Another mounting for a small circular mirror, in this case a Mangin (second surface) type, is shown in Fig. 9.2. Here the mirror surface registers against a tangential interface while the flat bevel on the front of the mirror touches a toroidal interface on the retainer. Contacts occur at the same height on both sides. The choice of these interface shapes, the dimensions, and a "loose" fit in the retainer threads ensure minimal contact stress as well as minimal tendency to bend the mirror by mount-induced moments.

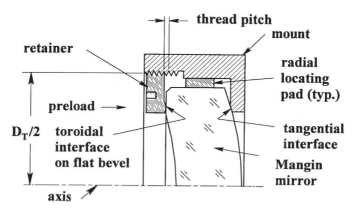

Fig. 9.2 Conceptual configuration of a threaded retaining ring mounting for a Mangin mirror.

A typical design for a circular mirror mounting involving a continuous-type flange is shown in Fig. 9.3. This type of retainer is most frequently used with mirrors larger than typically could be held with threaded rings or if a more precise axial preload is needed in the application. Several close-fitting locating pads around the rim of the mirror help to center it to the mechanical axis of the mount. An annular locating land on the shoulder localizes contact on the mirror's flat back directly opposite the clamping (preload) force. The land surface should be lapped flat to minimize distortion of the mirror's reflecting surface by overconstraint.

The interface between the flange and the flat bevel on the mirror is shown as toroidal to minimize contact stress. A flat surface on the flange would work well if it could always be aligned exactly to the bevel, but a sharp-corner contact and thus increased stress in the optic could result from machining errors or temperature changes.

Temperature changes also can create problems with regard to the fit of the radial locating pads and the constancy of axial preload in this and all the other mirror mounts discussed here because of differential expansion or contraction of the optical and mechanical parts. This topic is considered and corrective measures outlined in Chapter 12.

The function of the clamping flange in the Fig. 9.3 design is the same as that of the threaded retainer described earlier. The magnitude of the preload exerted in this way

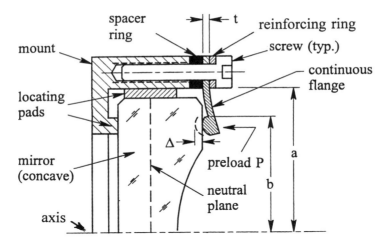

Fig. 9.3 Schematic configuration of a circular flange-type retainer axially constraining a concave mirror in a mount.

can be determined fairly closely using Eqs. (3.23) through (3.25) which acording to Roark,[1] apply to a perforated circular plate with the outer edge fixed and an axially directed load applied uniformly along the inner edge to deflect that edge:

$$\Delta = (K_A - K_B)(P/t^3) \tag{3.23}$$

where:

$$K_A = \frac{3(m^2 - 1)[a^4 - b^4 - 4a^2b^2\ln(a/b)]}{4\pi m^2 E_M a^2} \tag{3.24}$$

$$K_B = \frac{3(m^2 - 1)(m + 1)[2\ln(a/b) + (b^2/a^2) - 1][b^2 + 2a^2b^2\ln(a/b) - a^2b^2]}{(4\pi m^2 E_M)[b^2(m + 1) + a^2(m - 1)]}$$

and   P = total preload
        t   = thickness of flange cantilevered section
        a   = outer radius of cantilevered section
        b   = inner radius of cantilevered section
        m = reciprocal of Poisson's ratio (υ_M) of the flange material
        E_M = Young's modulus of the flange material

The spacer under the flange can be ground at assembly to the particular axial thickness that produces the predetermined flange deflection when firm metal-to-metal contact is achieved by tightening the clamping screws. Variations in as-manufactured mirror thicknesses are accommodated by customizing the spacer. The flange material and thickness are the prime design variables. The dimensions a and b, and hence the annular width (a - b), can also be varied, but these are usually set primarily by the mirror aperture, mount wall thickness, and overall dimensional limitations.

The stress, S_B, built up in the bent portion of the flange must not exceed the yield strength of the material. This equation applies:

$$S_B = K_C P / t^2 \tag{3.26}$$

where:

$$K_C = (\frac{3}{2\pi})[1 - \frac{2mb^2 - 2b^2(m + 1)\ln(a/b)}{a^2(m - 1) + b^2(m + 1)}] \tag{3.27}$$

The reader is referred to Sect. 3.4.2 for discussions of the use of these equations and for worked-out numerical examples illustrating their applications.

As in the previously considered case of flange constraint for refracting optics, the deflections Δ measured between the attachment points (screws) should be essentially the same as those existing at those points. This ensures uniform contact at the desired zonal height from the axis. This can be accomplished by machining the flexing portion of the flange as a thinned annular region in a thicker ring, thereby providing extra thickness at the clamped annular zone of the flange. It also could be done by reinforcing the flange with a backup ring as shown schematically in Fig. 9.3.

Increasing the number of screws also tends to reduce the possibility of non-uniform preload around the mirror's edge. If we adopt the advice of Shigley and Mischke[2] with regard to spacing of screw constraints on a gasketed flange for a high-pressure chamber and apply it to the mirror mounting case, the number of screws, N, should be:

$$3 \le \frac{\pi D_B}{Nd} \le 6 \tag{9.1}$$

where:
D_B = diameter of the circle passing through the centers of the screws
d = diameter of the screw head

This criterion may be overly conservative in an optical application, especially if a stiff backup ring is employed or the flange is thickened in the region where it is clamped. Engineering judgment and possibly experimentation might well be applied here.

Figure 9.4 shows a simple means for attaching a nonmetallic- or metallic-type mirror configured as a plane parallel plate to a metal surface. The reflecting surface is pressed against three flat machined (lapped) pads by three spring clips. The spring

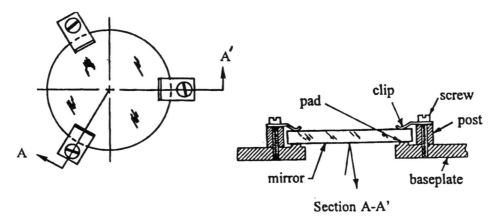

Fig. 9.4 A simple spring-clamped mirror mounting. (Adapted from Durie.[3])

contacts are directly opposite the pads to minimize imposed bending moments. This design constrains one translation and two tilts. The spacers that position the clips are machined to the proper length for the clips to exert clamping forces (preload) of a controlled magnitude normal to the mirror's surface. The spring clips should be strong enough to hold the mirror against the shock and vibration to which it may be subjected.

The ends of the spring clips shown as bearing on the mirror in Fig. 9.4 are shaped as cylindrical pads. They are similar to those shown in Fig. 7.8 for a prism constraint. Line contact occurs. Stress generation along these lines is discussed in Chapter 11. Other spring-end shapes are possible, of course. The discussion of the effects of contact shape and geometric errors in orientation and/or location of contacts in Sect. 7.1 applies here too.

It is highly desirable for the rim of the mirror's reflecting surface to contact fixed reference pads rather than for the back side of the mirror to do so. This is because any wedge in the mirror substrate will then not affect pointing of the reflected beam. Obviously, the reference pads and the portion of the mirror contacting them must be clean; dirt between those surfaces could tilt the mirror. The pads must be coplanar and located directly opposite the applied forces so the clamping preload will not exert bending moments on the optic. Figure 9.5 shows the possible moment-generating effect of an irregularity on a pad surface or of a bit of dust or other particulate matter located in the interface. Orientation and/or the figure of the reflecting surface could change if that defect were to change size or if the particle were to shift location during vibration or shock.

In Fig. 9.6 we show a variation on this design in which the spring force is supplied by compressed resilient pads.[4] The reflecting surface bears against rigid clips that are in contact with the main portion of the mount. The chief objection to this design is that the soft material may compress and lose its resilience with time if it is not carefully chosen. Preload then is not necessarily constant in the long term. A design of this type of constraint using a compressed resilient material for spring loading might well follow the method explained in conjunction with Fig. 7.3 in Sect. 7.1.

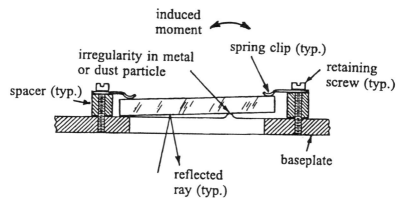

Fig. 9.5 Representation of pad irregularity or dirt particle in a mirror-to-mount interface. (Adapted from Durie.[3])

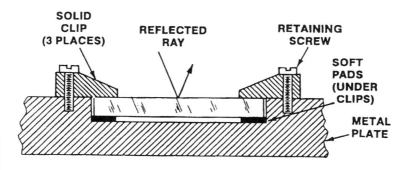

Fig. 9.6 Mirror constraint using resilient pads as springs. (From Yoder.[4])

A mounting for a partially reflecting mirror used as a beamsplitter plate is illustrated in Fig. 9.7. As in the discussion of a cube-shaped beamsplitter in connection with Fig. 7.1, this plate registers against fixed "points" and is spring loaded directly opposite these points. Here, and in any design with hard contacts against the reflecting side of the mirror, the location and orientation of that surface do not change with the temperature of the optic. Displacements of the mounting points caused by temperature changes may, of course, affect the location and orientation of that surface.

The optic is not constrained laterally other than by friction in the designs represented in Figs. 9.4 through 9.7. This may be acceptable because the performance of a flat mirror is generally insensitive to these motions. Excessive lateral movement of the optic can be prevented by spring loading it against stops. CTE differences must be considered if the mirror touches hard stops without springs.

A design concept that includes spring-loaded constraints in the plane of the reflecting surface is illustrated in Fig. 9.8.[6] While compression coil springs are shown, cantilevered clips could be employed. This mount is semikinematic since all six degrees of freedom are constrained by spring loads and the contacts are small areas instead of points.

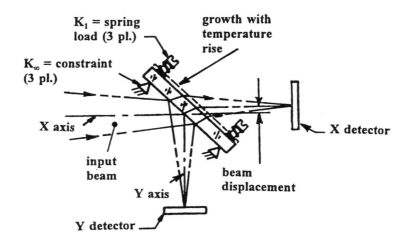

Fig. 9.7 A mounting for a beamsplitter plate. (Adapted from Lipshutz.[5])

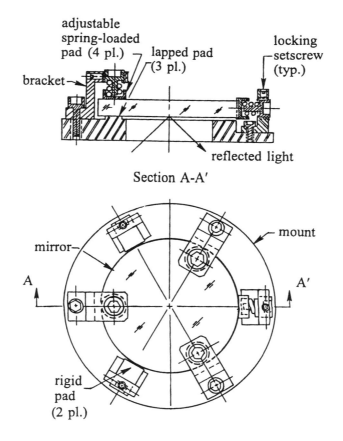

Fig. 9.8 Concept for a spring-loaded mirror mounting. (From Yoder.[6])

Example 9.1: Clamping force required to constrain a mirror. (For design and analysis, use File 32 of the CD-ROM)

Neglecting friction, what normal axial force is required of each of three springs to constrain a flat round mirror weighing 0.090 lb (0.041 kg) in the manner of Fig. 9.8 with a safety factor of 2 under acceleration of 15 times gravity?

From Eq. (7.1) $P_i = Wa_Gf_S/N = (0.090)(15)(2)/3 = 0.900$ lb (4.003 N)

A nonkinematic mounting for a 16-in. (40.6-cm)-diameter fused silica spherical primary mirror that John Strong used in a Schmidt telescope is shown in Fig. 9.9.[7] The mirror rim was ground with a spherical contour, centered at the mirror's face, to avoid chipping when installed or removed for recoating. A narrow [0.25 in. (6.35 mm) annular width] flat bevel ground on the mirror's face was pressed against three steel pads (called "lugs" in the figure) inside an Invar mirror cell. The pads had previously been filed coplanar and perpendicular to the axis of the telescope tube. The cell was attached to a perforated Invar telescope tube. Three shims with an aggregate thickness of about 0.09 in. (2.3 mm) were inserted between the spherical ground rim of the mirror and the ID of the cell. These shims caused the cell to spring very slightly out of round. By successive adjustments of the thicknesses and locations of the shims, the mirror's central normal was brought parallel to the telescope axis. The decentration thus produced was equivalent to tipping the mirror.

This mirror was restrained axially by three retaining spring clips that clamped the mirror against the three axial constraining pads. Friction prevented it from rotating about the telescope axis. One layer of thin plastic tape (Scotch tape) was used to isolate the mirror from the pads. This increased the mount's resistance to mechanical shock and provided some thermal isolation.

A mounting for a meniscus-shaped mirror using spring clips that hold the mirror so its back surface interfaces axially with spherical pads is discussed in Sect. 13.17.

9.2 Bonded Mirror Mountings

First-surface mirrors with diameters typically about 6 in. (15.2 cm) or smaller can be bonded directly to a mechanical support in much the same manner as described earlier for prisms. The ratio of the largest face dimension to the thickness should be less than 10:1 and preferably no more than 6:1 in order for dimensional changes in the adhesive during curing or under temperature changes not to distort the mirror surface excessively. Figure 9.10 illustrates such a design. The mirror is made of Schott BK7 glass, is 2.0 in. (5.1 cm) in diameter, and is 0.33 in. (0.84 cm) thick (6:1 ratio). It weighs 0.09 lb (0.04 kg). The mounting base is type 416 stainless steel. The bonding pad is circular and has an area of 0.50 in.^{2}. The adhesive is EC2216B/A epoxy made by 3M (see Table B14). The determination of the required total bonding area, Q_{MIN}, follows the methods that were explained in Sect. 7.3. Equation 7.9 applies here.

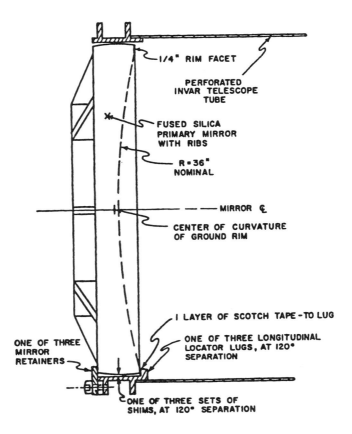

Fig. 9.9 Nonkinematic rim mounting for a Schmidt telescope primary mirror. (From Strong.[7])

$$Q_{MIN} = W\,a_G\,f_S/J \qquad\qquad (7.9)$$

where:

    W = the mirror's weight
    a_G = the worst-case acceleration factor (times gravity)
    f_S = the desired safety factor (typically 2 to 5)
    J = the adhesive's shear or tensile strength (usually approximately equal)

As pointed out earlier in discussions of bonded prisms, for maximum glass-to-metal bond strength, the adhesive layer should have a particular thickness. Experience has indicated that 3M EC2216-B/A epoxy should have a thickness of 0.075 to 0.125 mm (0.003 to 0.005 in.). Some adhesive manufacturers recommend thicknesses as large as 0.4 mm (0.016 in.) for their products, while some users have found success with 0.05-mm (0.002-in.) thicknesses. A thin bond is stiffer than a thick one (see Miller's analytical results for elastomeric lens mountings discussed in Sect. 3.7). A means for ensuring that

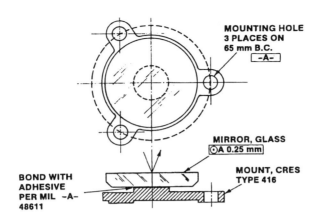

Fig. 9.10 A typical bonded first-surface mirror assembly. (From Yoder.[4])

a particular bond thickness is achieved is to place shims of the specified thickness at three locations in the interface between the glass and the metal. If possible, these should be arranged in a triangular pattern and lie outside the bonded area. The glass, mount, and shims must be held together securely during curing to ensure contact. Adhesive should not be allowed to get onto the surfaces of the shims. Another technique for obtaining a layer of uniform thickness is to mix a few percent by volume of small glass beads into the ahesive before applying it to the surfaces to be bonded. When the surfaces are clamped together, the beads contact both faces and hold them apart. Since such beads can be purchased with closely controlled diameters, achievement of correct bond thickness is relatively easy.[9] The glass beads have essentially no effect on bond strength.

Because adhesives and metals typically have CTEs larger than those of glasses and mirror substrate materials, differential dimensional changes at extreme temperatures can be significant. It is advisable to keep bond areas as small as possible while providing adequate strength. As in the case of prism bonding (see Sect. 7.3), the adhesive should, if possible, be distributed in small separated areas with the total area equal to the calculated minimum value for the anticipated shock and vibration loadings. This minimizes thermal expansion problems and helps secure the mirror in a more kinematic fashion. A pattern of three small bonds arranged in a triangle has been found to work well. A ring of small bonds has been used successfully with circular optics. The ring diameter should be about 70% of the mirror diameter in that case.

Another quite different technique for bonding a mirror to a mechanical support is sketched in Fig. 9.11. Here a round mirror is bonded to three flexure blades that are in turn attached by screws, rivets, or adhesive to a circular mount of essentially the same diameter as the mirror. The flexures are flat so they can flex radially to accommodate differences in thermal expansion. They have the same free length and are of the same material so that thermally induced tilts are minimized. The local areas on both the mirror and mount where the flexures are attached are flattened in order to obtain adequate contact area for bonding and to prevent cupping of the springs. The blades should be as light and flexible as is consistent with vibration and shock requirements. Høg discussed a design of this type.[10] Other flexure mountings for mirrors are discussed in Sect. 9.4.

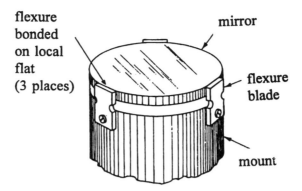

Fig. 9.11 Sketch of a mirror mount with radially compliant flexures. (Adapted from Høg.[10])

Although it is discussed here in the context of mountings for nonimage-forming optics, the mounting arrangement of Fig. 9.11 can also be used to support image-forming mirrors since the design serves to keep the optic centered in spite of temperature changes.

Example 9.2: Acceleration resistance of a bonded mirror.
(For design and analysis, use File 33 of the CD-ROM)

What acceleration should the bonded mirror shown in Fig. 9.10 be able to withstand with a safety factor f_s of 5? Assume the mirror weight W is 0.090 lb (0.041 kg), the bond strength J is 2500 lb/in.^{2} (17.2 MPa), and the bond area Q is 0.500 in.^{2} (322.7 mm^2).

Rearranging Eq. (7.9): $a_G = JQ/Wf_s = (2500)(0.5)/(0.09)(5) = 2778$ times gravity

We conclude that this design should be adequate for most applications.

Example 9.3: Distributed bond size required to constrain a mirror under acceleration.
(For design and analysis, use File 34 of the CD-ROM)

A circular Zerodur mirror with a diameter D_G of 4.250 in. (107.950 mm) and thickness 0.708 in. (17.983 mm) is to withstand 200 times gravity accelerations with a safety factor of 4 when bonded with epoxy of strength 2500 lb/in.^{2} (17.24 MPa) arranged in (a) a single circular area or (b) a triangular pattern of three equal circular areas on the mirror's back. What should be the individual bond diameters in each case?

From Table B8a, the density of Zerodur is 0.091 lb/in.^{2} The mirror weight is then:
$$W = \pi(D_G/2)^2t\rho = (\pi)(4.250/2)^2(0.708)(0.091) = 0.914 \text{ lb } (0.414 \text{ kg})$$

From Eq. (7.9), the minimum total bond area required is
$$Q_{MIN} = (0.914)(200)(4)/2500 = 0.292 \text{ in.}^2 (1.884 \text{ cm}^2)$$

(a) If a single circular bond is used, the diameter = $2\sqrt{(Q_{MIN}/\pi)}$
$$= (2)(0.292/\pi)^{1/2} = 0.610 \text{ in. } (15.494 \text{ mm})$$

(b) The minimum diameter of each of the three bonds is
$$2\sqrt{(Q_{MIN}/3\pi)} = (2)[0.292/(3\pi)]^{1/2}$$
$$= 0.352 \text{ in. } (8.941 \text{ mm})$$

The single and multiple areas would then appear
as shown at the right (drawn to actual scale).

9.3 Multiple Mirror Mountings

Although mirrors are generally thought of as single optical elements, it is occasionally advantageous to use two or more such optics in optomechanical assemblies in order to serve some particular function. For example, two flat mirrors oriented at 45° to each other can be used to deviate a light beam by 90°. If rigidly attached together, they will serve the same function as a penta prism (i.e., as a constant deviation reflector), but transmission of the beam through glass is not required. This allows the penta mirror to be used in the UV or IR, assuming appropriate coatings are applied. Furthermore, the weight of the penta mirror is generally lower than that of a penta prism of equivalent aperture.

The problem in the design and fabrication of the penta mirror is how to hold the mirrors in the proper relative orientation to maintain long-term alignment stability and not distort the optical surfaces. One approach that was used successfully was to clamp the mirrors individually to a precision-machined metal block or built-up structure providing the 45° dihedral angle (see Fig. 9.12). Here two rounded-end rectangular gold-coated mirrors were held by three screws to coplanar lapped pads on either side of an aluminum casting. The screws passed through clearance holes in the mirrors and each compressed two Belleville washers that provided preload against the lapped pads. This hardware was used as part of an automatic theodolite system for prelaunch azimuth alignment of the Saturn space vehicles, so it was used in a generally stable environment inside a concrete bunker at Cape Canaveral.[11]

A penta mirror used successfully in military optical range finders had the glass mirrors bonded on edge to a glass baseplate, which was in turn attached to the optical bar of the range finder.[12] Figure 9.13 shows an assembly of this general type made by PLX Corp. The baseplate in this example is metal. The aperture exceeds 50 mm (1.97 in.).

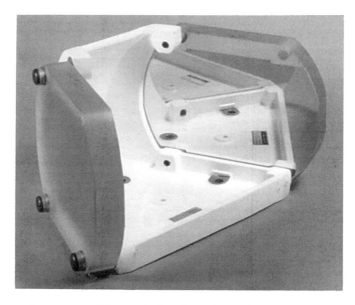

Fig. 9.12 Penta mirror assembly made by clamping mirrors to a precision metal casting. (Courtesy of **NASA Marshall Space Flight Center.**)

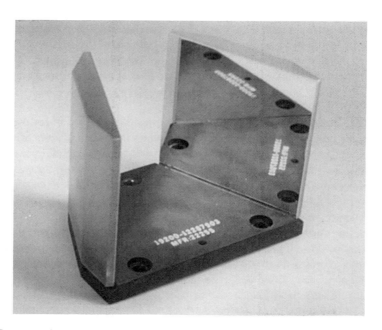

Fig. 9.13 Penta mirror made by bonding glass mirrors on edge to a metal bracket. (Courtesy of **PLX Corporation, Deer Park, NY.**)

Figure 9.14 shows another approach for creating a penta mirror assembly. Here the polished faces of two very flat Cer-Vit* mirrors were optically contacted along their innermost edges to a Cer-Vit angle block that had been ground and polished to within 1 arcsec of the nominal 45°. The angle block was hollowed out to reduce weight without reducing strength. The mirror plates measured approximately 11 by 16 by 1.3 cm (4.33 by 6.30 by 0.51 in.); the assembly had a clear optical aperture of 10 cm (3.94 in.). Triangular Cer-Vit cover plates were attached with optical cement to both the top and bottom of the assembly as shown in the figure and a rectangular Cer-Vit cover plate was cemented across its back. These three plates served not only as mechanical braces, but also to seal the exposed edges of the contacted joints against intrusion of moisture. An Invar plate was bonded to one of the cover plates to serve as a mechanical mounting interface. This penta mirror assembly and a roof penta mirror assembly of similar construction and size (shown in Fig. 9.15) have been described in the literature.[13]

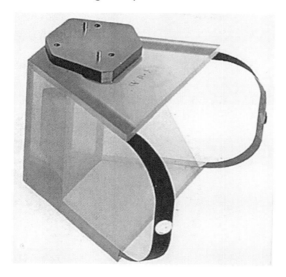

Fig. 9.14 A 10-cm (3.94-in.)-aperture penta mirror assembly made by optically contacting Cer-Vit components. (From Yoder.[13])

To verify these optically contacted designs, a prototype of the penta mirror and mounting assembly (see Fig. 9.16) was subjected to adverse thermal, vibration, and shock environments. It was temperature cycled several times from -2 to +68°C (28 to 154°F) while the reflected wave front was monitored interferometrically. The test setup was capable of detecting changes of $\lambda/30$ for $\lambda = 633$ nm and had an instrumental error of less than $\lambda/15$. The maximum thermally induced peak-to-valley reflected wave-front distortion was measured as $\lambda/4$. The assembly was vibrated without failure at loadings of up to 5 times gravity and frequencies of 5 to 500 Hz along each of three orthogonal axes. Shock testing at up to 28 times gravity peak loading delivered in 8 ms in two directions caused no damage to the test item.

---

* Cer-Vit is an obsolete low-expansion optical material formerly made by Owens-Illinois.

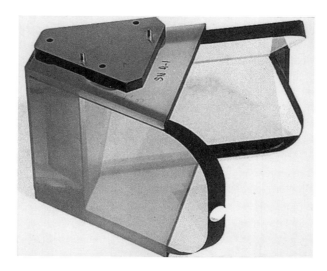

Fig. 9.15 A 10-cm (3.94-in.)-aperture roof penta mirror assembly made by optically contacting Cer-Vit components. (From Yoder.[13])

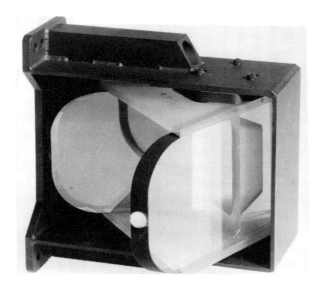

Fig. 9.16 Photograph of the penta mirror assembly of Fig. 9.14 mounted in its Invar housing. (From Yoder.[13])

A roof mirror functionally equivalent to a Porro prism is shown in Fig. 9.17. This assembly has an aperture of slightly over 1.75 by 4.0 in. (4.4 by 10.2 cm). Its mirrors are 0.5-in. (12.7-mm)-thick Pyrex. These mirrors are epoxied on one long edge to a Pyrex keel that is in turn bonded to a 0.125-in. (3.2-mm)-thick stainless steel mounting plate. The end plates are made with nominal 90° angles. Each plate is cemented to the top of one mirror and the end of the other mirror. Cementing is done in a jig that aligns the

one mirror and the end of the other mirror. Cementing is done in a jig that aligns the mirrors to 90° within tolerances as small as 0.5 arcsec. The mirror figure tolerance is as small as 0.1 wave at 633 nm.

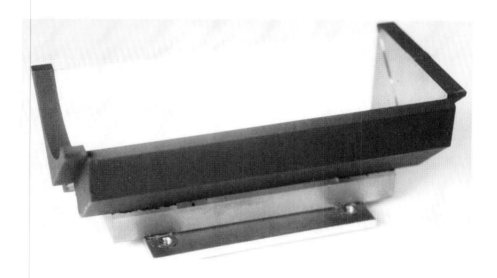

Fig. 9.17 Photograph of a Porro-type roof mirror made by bonding two flat mirrors at 90°. (Courtesy of PLX Corp., Deer Park, NY.)

Figure 9.18 shows front and back views of a hollow cube corner reflector comprising three square-faced Pyrex mirrors. The aperture of this unit is approximately 4.5 cm (1.77 in.). The mirrors are cemented together then "potted" into an aluminum housing using an elastomeric material (shown in white) surrounding three rubbery inserts (shown in gray). Accuracy of the nominally 180° light deviation (typically between 0.5 arcsec and 5 arcmin) is achieved by jigging during curing of the elastomer. Apertures as large as about 127 mm (5 in.) have been made.

A variation of the hollow retroreflector is the so-called lateral-transfer hollow cube corner retroreflector. An example of one such unit is shown in Fig. 9.19. It has one flat mirror mounted at 45° at the end of an elongated box housing and a roof mirror at the other end of that box. The three mirrors are nominally mutually perpendicular, so the assembly functions as a transverse section through a lateral-transfer retroreflector. Devices of this type with apertures of up to 2 in. (5.1 cm) and lateral offsets of the axis of more than 30 in. (76 cm) are commercially available. A similar device with 6-in. (15.2-cm) offset made entirely of beryllium has also been described.[14] That unit had a beamsplitter at one end instead of a conventional mirror. The Be unit was lighter than the equivalent glass and metal version would be.

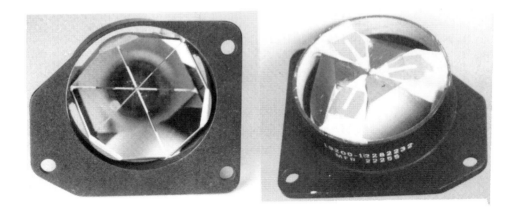

Fig. 9.18 Front (a) and back (b) photographs of a hollow corner retroreflector made by bonding three flat square mirrors in mutually-perpendicular fashion. (Courtesy of PLX Corp., Deer Park, NY.)

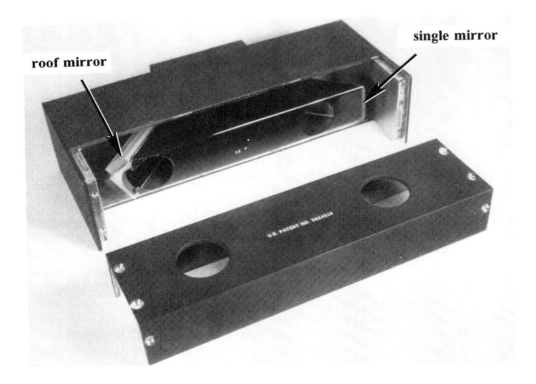

Fig. 9.19 Photograph of a partially disassembled lateral-transfer hollow retroreflector. (Courtesy of PLX Corp., Deer Park, NY.)

9.4 Flexure Mountings for Mirrors

In optical instrument applications, flexures are passive mechanical devices that are used to isolate optical components from mechanical and thermally induced forces acting on the structual support system and thereby minimize the effects of those forces on optical performance. Flexures are free of stick-slip and friction effects that hamper the use of spherical ball joints and hinges in optical instruments. In most cases, flexures are designed with compliance in one direction, but stiffness in the two orthogonal directions.

The principle underlying one type of flexure mounting for mirrors is illustrated by Fig. 9.20. The mirror is circular and mounted in a cell. That cell is suspended from three thin flexure blades. The single direction of allowable motion for each flexure acting alone is indicated by a curved arrow. For small deflections, these curved motion paths closely approximate straight lines. Ideally, these lines of freedom should intersect at a

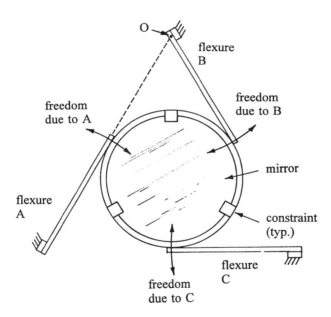

Fig. 9.20 Concept for a flexure mounting for a circular mirror. (From Yoder.[4])

point; this point should coincide with the center of gravity of the mirror. The flexures should be made of the same material and their free lengths should be equal; the fixed ends fixed ends of the three flexures should form an equilateral triangle. The function of this system of flexures may be explained as follows. In the absence of flexure C, the combination of flexures A and B will permit rotation only about point O, which is the intersection of flexure B with a line extending flexure A. With flexure C in place, rotation about O is prevented, since flexure C is stiff in that direction. Although it is not apparent in the figure, the flexure blades have sufficient depth perpendicular to the mirror face to prevent the mirror from translating axially.

When temperature changes cause differential thermal expansion of the structure to which the flexures are attached relative to the mirror and cell assembly, radial motion of the mirror will be impeded without stressing the mirror. The only motion permitted as a result of expansion or contraction is a small rotation about the normal through the intersection of the lines of freedom. This occurs because of small changes in lengths of the flexures. The magnitude of this rotation, θ, in radians, may be approximated as:

$$\theta = 3\alpha\Delta T \qquad\qquad (9.2)$$

where:

α = flexure material CTE
ΔT = temperature change

Example 9.4: Rotation of a flexure-mounted mirror about its axis as a result of a temperature change.
(For design and analysis, use File 35 of the CD-ROM)
If the flexures of Fig. 9.20 are beryllium copper and ΔT is 100°F (55°C), what is the mirror rotation, θ? Assume the CTE of BeCu is 9.9×10^{-6}/°F (17.8×10^{-6}/°C)

From Eq. (9.2), $\theta = (3)(9.9 \times 10^{-6})(100) = 0.0030$ rad = 10.2 arcmin

This rotation probably is inconsequential in most applications.

Figure 9.21 shows a variation of the above flexure mounting concept in which the rim of a circular mirror is bonded centrally to three flexures oriented tangentially to that rim and anchored to the structure at both ends. Conceptually, this follows the same

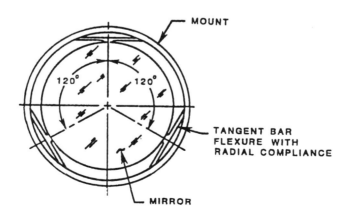

Fig. 9.21 Mounting for a circular mirror employing three tangential flexures supported at both ends. (Adapted from Vukobratovich.[15])

principle underlying the design for a flexure mounting for a lens discussed in Sect. 3.9 and illustrated in Fig. 3.42. The flexure configuration of the detail view (b) in that figure applies. Some compliance must be provided in the interface to the mount at one end of each flexure to allow for temperature changes if the flexure is not made of the same material as the mount. Alignment of the flexures at the time of bonding would be facilitated by the use of appropriate fixturing.

Figure 9.22 schematically shows a possible interface between a cantilevered flexure and the rim of a mirror. Here a square boss is attached (i.e., bonded) to the rim of the mirror. The free end of the blade is bonded to this boss. In order to accommodate small misalignments between the bosses and the seats caused by manufacturing or assembly errors, sub-flexures are provided at four places in each flexure as indicated. The bonded interfaces to the bosses are at the squared-off ends of the subflexures.

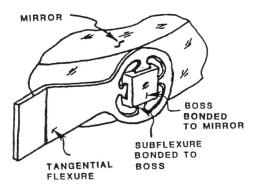

Fig. 9.22 A possible interface between the free end of a cantilevered flexure blade and a boss bonded to the rim of a circular mirror. (Adapted from Vukobratovich.[15])

Figure 9.23 shows the mechanical design of a boss intended to be bonded to the rim of a 15.0-in. (38.1-cm)-diameter mirror. The material of such a boss should be selected to match its CTE with that of the mirror as closely as possible. For example, a boss made of Invar 36 might well be used with a ULE or Zerodur mirror. An adhesive such as EC2216B/A might be chosen for use with those materials. The adhesive would be injected through the 0.045-in. (1.14-mm)-diameter access hole at the center of each boss. The adhesive thickness could be fixed by the use of shims or microspheres added to the adhesive. Flexures of the type shown in Fig. 9.22 might be interfaced with this boss.

Another configuration for a flexure that would interface with the boss of Fig. 9.23 is illustrated schematically in Fig. 9.24. This flexure might be made of 6Al4V titanium. The through hole at the left allows the flexure to be attached to the structure. A small amount of rotation about the axis of that hole may be needed to align the square recess with the boss on the mirror. The square hole would be sized slightly larger than the mating boss to allow space for the appropriate thickness of adhesive to be inserted. Dimensions of the boss and the hole would need to be closely toleranced for this to

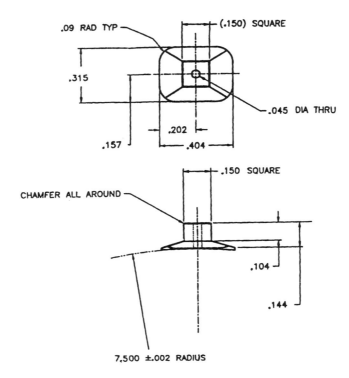

Fig. 9.23 Design of a boss suitable for bonding to the rim of a 15.0-in. (38.1-cm)-diameter mirror for mounting in the fashion depicted in Fig. 9.22.

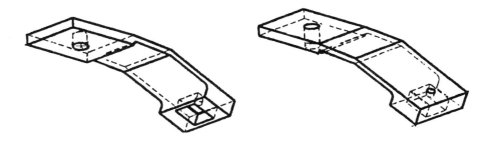

Fig. 9.24 Schematic configuration of a cantilevered flexure shaped to interface with the boss of Fig. 9.23 and the cylindrical mounting for a circular mirror.

happen. A locating pin can be passed temporarily through the holes in the boss and at the center of the square recess to align the mating parts and to provide equal gaps on all sides of the boss. This pin would then be removed so the adhesive can be injected into the joint.

A mirror of rectangular shape might be supported in a cell attached to three deep cantilevered flexure blades as shown in Fig. 9.25. The dashed lines indicate the directions of freedom (approximated as straight lines). In this case, the intersection of these lines, which is stationary, does not coincide with the geometric center of the mirror or the center of gravity of this particular mirror and cell combination. By changing the angles of the corner bevels and relocating the flexures, the intersection point could be centralized and the design improved from a dynamic viewpoint. Differential thermal expansion across the mount-to-structure interface can then occur without stressing the mirror. Axial movement of the mirror is prevented by the high stiffness of the blades in that direction.

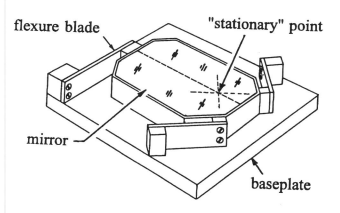

Fig. 9.25 Concept for a flexure mounting for a cell-mounted rectangular mirror. (From Yoder.[4])

If the rectangular mirror is to be mounted without a cell, bosses such as that shown in Fig. 9.26 might be bonded directly onto the rim of the mirror. They would be attached in the same manner described for the circular mirror with bosses. Figure 9.27 shows a flexure concept that might be used to interface with such a mounting boss.

Figure 9.28 schematically shows some other types of bosses, threaded studs, and flexures that have been successfully bonded to mirrors to allow them to be attached to the optical instrument structure. Those in Fig. 9.28(a) are bonded into recesses or notches ground into the mirror substrate, while those in Fig. 9.28(b) are bonded externally to the mirror surfaces.

Another concept for mounting a circular mirror with cantilevered tangential flexures is depicted in Fig. 9.29. Here the flexures are integral with the body of the ring-shaped mounting. The flexures typically would be created by machining narrow slots using an electric discharge machining process. This mirror mounting is an extension of a design concept advanced for lens mounting in the literature[16] and was discussed in Sect. 3.9. Once again, the blades are stiff in the tangential and axial directions and compliant radially as would be appropriate to negate decentrations that are due to temperature changes.

Modest-sized mirrors [say, those in the 15- to 24-in. (38.1- to 61-cm)-diameter range] or smaller mirrors used in high-precision, high-performance applications may benefit from being mounted in the manner shown in Fig. 9.30. Here a circular mirror with

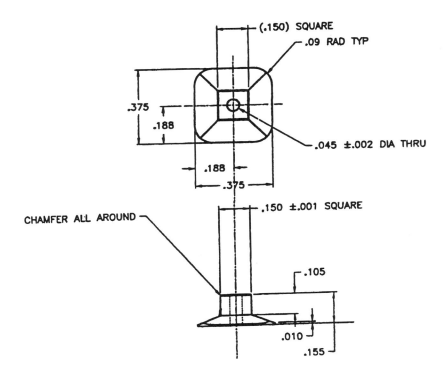

Fig. 9.26 Design of a boss suitable for bonding directly to the rim of a rectangular mirror for mounting in the manner shown in Fig. 9.25.

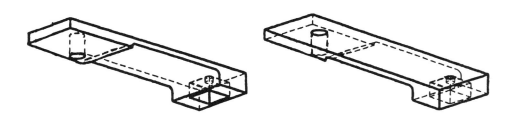

Fig. 9.27 Schematic configuration of a cantilevered flexure shaped to interface with the boss of Fig. 9.26 and the mounting for a rectangular mirror.

(a)

(b)

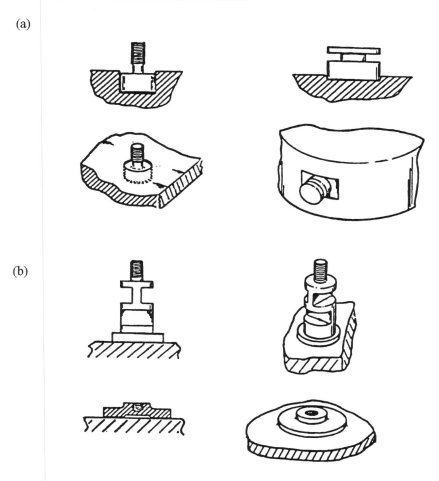

Fig. 9.28 Illustrations of some different types of bosses, threaded studs, and flexures that can be bonded to mirrors for attachment to structure.

three bonded-on bosses is attached to tangentially oriented arms containing dual sets of universal joint-type flexures. Three axial metering rod-type supports that include flexures are also attached to the bosses. Such a mounting is essentially radially insensitive to temperature changes because of the action of the tangent arm flexures. The thermal compensation mechanisms shown in the axial supports make the design less sensitive in that direction to temperature changes. The latter mechanism consists of selected lengths of dissimilar metals arranged in a reentrant manner. The function of this type of mechanism is explained in Sect. 12.3. Differential screws might be employed to advantage as the means for attaching the fixed ends of the tangent arms to the brackets in some applications. This would provide fine adjustment of the lengths of the tangent flexures. The "turnbuckle" mechanisms shown in the metering rods would facilitate axial adjustment. These could also be differential screws. Two-axis tilts of the mirror can be adjusted with these axial mechanisms.

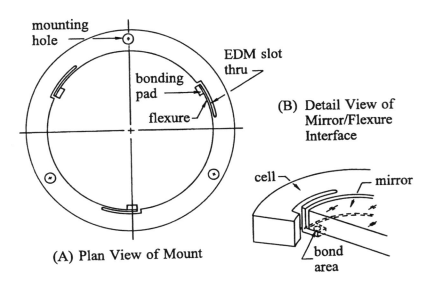

Fig. 9.29 Concept for a mirror mounting with integral flexures. (Adapted from Bacich.[16])

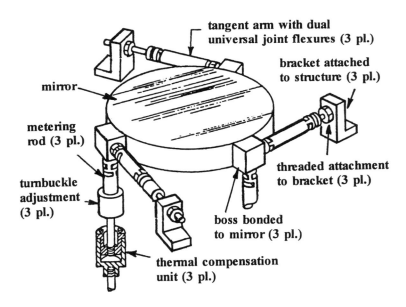

Fig. 9.30 A system of flexures configured to minimize displacement and/or distortion of the optical surface of a modest-sized mirror caused by temperature changes and mounting forces.

9.5 Center Mountings for Circular-Aperture Mirrors

Some lightweighted mirrors are mounted on a hub that protrudes through a central perforation in the mirror substrate. An example is shown in Fig. 9.31. This is the back end of a 150-in. (3.81-m)-focal length (EFL), f/10 catadioptric objective that was used in a photographic application for tracking missiles.[4] The system is discussed in Sect. 13.18. Both surfaces of the primary mirror are spherical, the first being the reflecting surface while the second is shaped to reduce weight. Figure 8.8(d) applies. The first surface registers against a convex spherical seat on an integral shoulder of the hub. The seat radius is ground to match that of the mirror in the manner illustrated by Fig. 3.30. A toroidal land is provided on the cylindrical hub. The OD of this land is lapped to closely match the ID of the hole in the mirror. A threaded retaining ring bearing against the flat bevel at the back of the mirror provides axial preload. In the original design of this instrument, Mylar shims were inserted into all axial glass-to-metal interfaces to help achieve close contact between the optical component surfaces and the less perfect mechanical surfaces. In Sect. 13.18, alternative ways to interface these optics to their mounts are explained.

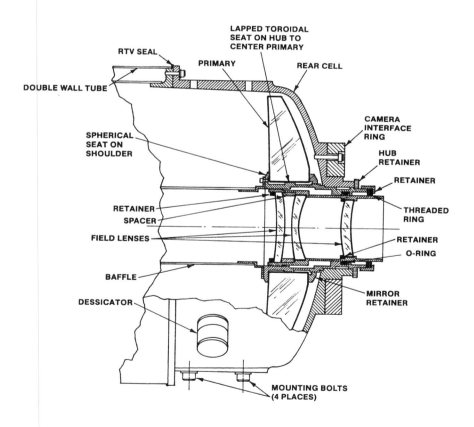

Fig. 9.31 Sectional view of the back cell portion of a catadioptric lens featuring a hub-mounted 15-in. (38.1-cm)-aperture mirror. (From Yoder.[4])

Small- to modest-sized single-arch lightweighted mirrors also are center mounted on hubs since their rims typically are very thin and so lack adequate strength to support the mirror. Designs typically follow the general lines of the mounting shown in Fig. 9.31. More sophisticated, athermal designs, such as that described by Sarver et al.[17] and involving a conical interface, might be used with larger mirrors since the mirrors usually are more flexible and hence more susceptible to gravitational effects. This mounting concept is shown in Fig. 9.32. The clamp constrains the mirror in all six degrees of freedom at its thickest and strongest region with large area contacts. This minimizes stress from clamping forces. A flat surface is provided on the back of the mirror: the axis of the conical surface is perpendicular to this surface and the apex of the cone lies in the plane of this surface. Slippage occurs between the conical surfaces when the temperature changes, but expansion or contraction of the mounting materials does not alter the apex location relative to the flat plane. The arrangement is athermal because all the materials used in the metal parts are the same.

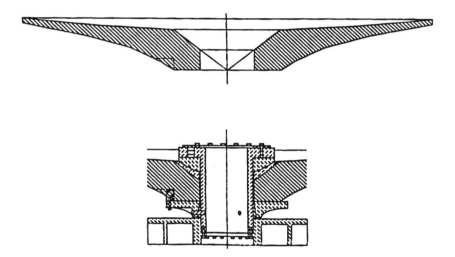

Fig. 9.32 Schematic of an athermal hub mounting for a single-arch mirror featuring a conical optomechanical interface. (Adapted from Sarver et al.[17])

Double-arch lightweighted mirrors are typically mounted on three or more supports attached to the back surface of the substrate at its thickest point. Figure 9.33 shows such a design. This design was created to support a 20-in. (50.8-cm)-diameter double-arch mirror with three equally spaced clamp and flexure assemblies oriented so the flexures were compliant in the radial direction, but stiff in all other directions. This allowed the aluminum mounting plate to contract differentially with respect to the fused silica mirror as the temperature was lowered to about 10 K. Each clamp was a "tee"-shaped Invar 36 piece that engaged a conical hole in the strong annulus of the mirror's back surface. The twin parallel flexures were 91 mm (3.6 in.) long by 15 mm (0.6 in.) wide and were made of 0.04-in. (1.0-mm)-thick 6Al4V-ELI titanium. The blades were separated by 25 mm (1 in.). This mounting design was analyzed extensively and found to provide acceptable thermal performance and to withstand launch loads typical of the Space Shuttle as well as to survive (with some damage) a crash landing of the Shuttle.[18]

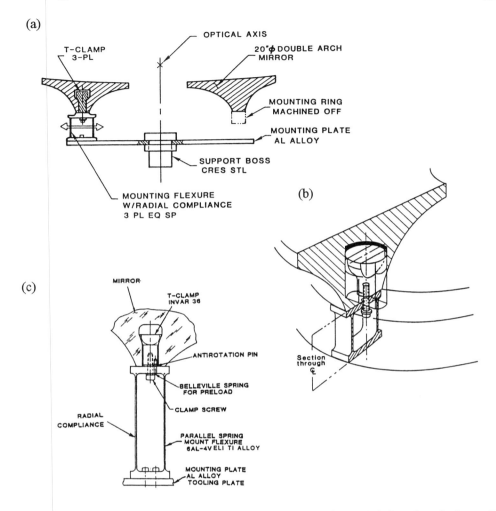

Fig. 9.33 A mounting design for a double-arch mirror. (a) Sectional view, (b) isometric view of one clamp and flexure mechanism, and (c) sectional view through the latter mechanism. (From Iraninejad et al.[18])

9.6 Mounting Metal Mirrors

Small- and moderate-sized metal mirrors can often be mounted using the same techniques discussed for nonmetallic mirrors if there are no unusual requirements inherent in the application, such as extreme temperatures (e.g., cryogenic applications), exposure to high-energy thermal radiation (such as that from lasers or solar simulators), or extreme shock or vibration. The prime differences between metallic and nonmetallic mirror types have to do with differences in key mechanical properties, such as density, Young's modulus, Poisson's ratio, thermal conductivity, CTE, and specific heat. We can take advantage of these differences by using metals whose unique properties allow significant improvements in performance, weight, environmental resistance, etc.

The preferred methods for supporting these metal mirrors involve mounting provisions built into the mirrors themselves. We illustrate a simple case in Fig. 9.34, which shows a section through a mirror with machined slots that isolate the mounting ears from the main part of the mirror so forces exerted when attaching the mirror to the mount shown at the bottom of the figure are not transmitted to the optical surface.[19] Figure 9.35

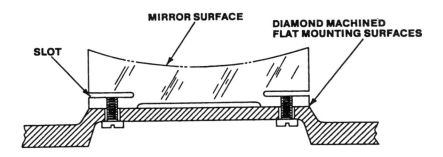

Fig. 9.34 Diagram of a strain-free mounting for a small metal mirror. (From Zimmerman.[19])

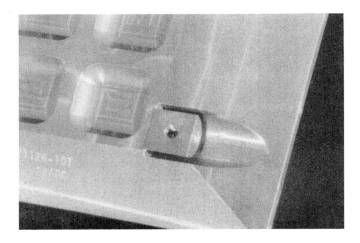

Fig. 9.35 Closeup view of a mounting ear (flexure) machined into a metal mirror. (From Zimmerman.[19])

shows a closeup photograph of the back side of a rectangular metal mirror having the same type of feature. In this case, it is apparent that the mounting ears have been machined into the mirror by core-cutting parallel to the mirror back surface at three locations. The hole in the ear is threaded for the mounting screw. This feature is repeated at three places on the back of the mirror.

One major advantage of metallic mirrors is their compatibility with single-point diamond turning, which produces precision surfaces with minimal force exerted by the cutting tool on the surface being machined. This technique also results in accurate relationships between surfaces, especially when they can all be created without removing the part from the machine. When this is not feasible, key mounting surfaces can be machined first and then used as the references for turning the optical surfaces and other mounting interfaces. The optical and mounting surfaces of the mirror of Fig. 9.34 were finished in a SPDT machine.

Figure 9.36 shows another mirror made in this manner. Here a circular mirror face was SPDT machined on the front side of the mirror blank, the slot for an O-ring seal and a pilot diameter for centration were cut, and finally the reference surface -A- was cut. All these operations were done without disturbing the alignment of the part to the spindle axis. Hence they all have minimum relative errors.[20]

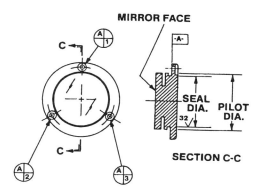

Fig. 9.36 A metal mirror with optical and interface surfaces cut without removing the part from the SPDT machine. (From Addis.[20])

Another hardware example showing the advantage of metal mirrors for some applications is the multicomponent telescope shown in Fig. 9.37.[21] The primary mirror diameter was 8 in. (20.3 cm); the entire assembly was made of 6061 aluminum. The individual components were SPDT machined with integral interface surfaces so they fit together to create an assembly with built-in precise alignment. The primary and secondary mirrors were designed to have spherical reference surfaces whose nominal optical centers coincided with the intersection of the axis and the system focal plane. The order of machining operations was chosen to allow alignment of the part on the turning machine using the interface and reference surfaces as the metrology features. This maximized accuracy of surface interrelationships, even when the part had to be turned over and reattached to the spindle. Once all parts were machined, they all fit together without adjustment to produce the required optical performance. With a single material used in its construction, the system remained aligned, at least to liquid nitrogen temperature.

In Sect. 8.4 we discussed a 7.3-in. (18.5-cm)-diameter aluminum secondary mirror used in NASA's Kuiper Airborne Observatory. That mirror, shown in Fig. 8.27, has a central mechanical interface with three coplanar pads and a central pilot diameter

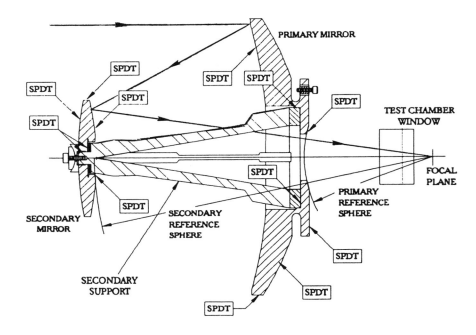

Fig. 9.37 Schematic of all-aluminum telescope system machined for easy and precise assembly by SPDT methods. (From Erickson et al.[21])

stud SPDT machined to facilitate mounting. Figure 8.28 shows the mirror, in section, attached to the scanning mechanism. Attachment is with three stainless steel bolts using Belleville washers to accommodate differential expansion. Minimal localized distortion of the optical surface that occurs as a result of clamping forces lies within the central obscuration of the system and thus has no effect on performance.

9.7 Gravitational Effects on Small Mirrors

So far in this chapter we have ignored the effects of external forces such as gravity and operational accelerations on mirror surface figure. When the aperture is modest, the thickness and material choice conducive to stiffness, and the performance requirements not too high, the optic can be considered a rigid body and mounted semi-kinematically or even nonkinematically without excessive performance problems. If, however, any or all of these attributes do not prevail, we must consider the effects of external forces. Gravity is the most prevalent, so we will limit our discussion to that force, frequently called "self-weight deflection." A special case is gravity release in space and the related problems of making and mounting a mirror so it does not become distorted when normal gravitational force is missing. That aspect of the problem will be considered in the next chapter.

The largest gravitational disturbances occur when the mirror axis is vertical. The way the mirror is held then affects the magnitude of surface deformation and the resulting surface contour. Let us consider two cases: (a) a circular mirror simply supported around its rim and (b) a rectangular mirror simply supported at its rim. Using Roark's theory for flexure of simple unclamped plates under uniform gravitational load normal to the plate's surface,[1] we can derive the following equations for the deflections:

$$\Delta y_C = 3W(m-1)(5m+1)(a^2)/(16\pi E_G m^2 t_A^3) \tag{9.3}$$

$$\Delta y_R = 0.1422 w b^4/[E_G t_A^3(1+2.21\xi^3)] \tag{9.4}$$

where:

W = total mirror weight   w = weight/area
m = 1/Poisson's ratio E_G = Young's modulus
a = semidiameter or longest dimension   b = shortest dimension
t_A = mirror thickness ξ = b/a.
area = πa^2 (circular) or ab (rectangular)

The induced sags (Δy_i) are measured at the mirror center and, for small deflections, represent changes in sagittal depth if the mirror is not flat. Figure 9.38 shows the geometry. Example 9.3 may help the reader assess typical self-weight mirror deflection magnitudes.

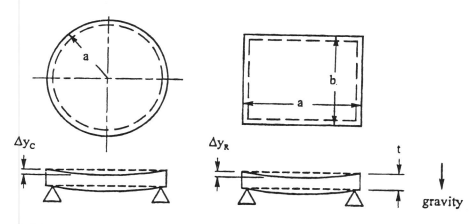

Fig. 9.38 Geometry of rim-supported circular and rectangular mirrors.

Example 9.5: Gravity-induced deflections of vertical-axis circular and rectangular mirrors.
(For design and analysis, use Files 36.1 & 36.2 of the CD-ROM)
(a) A 20.000-in. (50.800-cm)-diameter plane parallel, fused silica mirror is uniformly supported around its rim with its axis vertical. Assume $D_G/t_A = 6$. Calculate its self-weight deflection in waves of red light [$\lambda = 2.49\times10^{-5}$ in. (0.6328 µm)].

(b) Repeat these calculations for a rectangular mirror assuming a = 20.000 in. (50.800 cm) and b = 12.500 in. (31.750 cm). Let $a/t_A = 6$.

For fused silica, from Table B5: $\rho = 0.0796$ lb/in.^{3} (2.202 g/cm^3)
$E_G = 10.6 \times 10^6$ lb/in.^{2} (7.3× 10^{10} Pa)
$\upsilon_G = 0.17$ $m = 1/\upsilon_G = 5.882$

(a)   a = $D_G/2$ = 10.000 in. (25.400 cm),
W = $\pi a^2 t_A \rho$ = $(\pi)(10.000^2)(20.000/6)(0.0796)$ = 83.356 lb (37.810 kg)

From Eq. (9.3),

$$\Delta y_C = \frac{(3)(83.356)(5.882 - 1)[(5)(5.882) + 1](10.000^2)}{16\pi(10.6 \times 10^6)(5.882^2)(20.000/6)^3}$$

= 5.44 × 10^{-6} in. = 0.22 λ_{RED}

(b) ξ = b/a = 12.500/20.000 = 0.625, t_A = a/6 = 3.333 in. (8.466 cm)
W = $abt_A \rho$ = (20.000)(12.500)(3.333)(0.0796) = 66.327 lb (30.085 kg)
w = W/ab = 66.327/[(20.000)(12.500)] = 0.265 lb/in.^{2}

From Eq. (9.4),
Δy_R = (0.1422)(0.265)(12.500^4)/{(10.6 × 10^6)(3.333^3)[1 + (2.21)(0.625^3)]}
= 1.52 × 10^{-6} in. = 0.06 λ $_{RED}$

We see that the circular mirror sags the most.

If the mirrors are nominally flat, we would expect that contour lines of an equal change in sag on the deflected circular mirror's reflecting surface would be circles while those for the rectangular mirror would be generally elliptical. If the same circular mirror were supported at three points rather than all around the rim, and if those points were located at different radial zones of the mirror's aperture, the shapes of the surfaces would appear somewhat as indicated in Fig. 9.39. The support points are indicated by crosses. Although originally drawn for a large perforated mirror, the same patterns would be expected in smaller mirrors; only the scale would change. The same general effects would be expected if the mirror were rectangular. The surface deformation contours would then be modified elliptical lines.

There is an optimum zonal radius for a three-point support of a circular mirror of constant thickness, t, that gives minimum surface deflection [see Fig. 9.40(a)]. A minor rewriting of an equation by Vukobratovich[23] gives the following approximation for this deflection. He indicated that this applies at R_E = 0.68 times the mirror radius, R_{MAX}. Supporting the back of an upward-looking vertical-axis mirror on a circle of this radius produces a "hole and downward rolled edge" contour under the influence of gravity. The surface also is deformed in a six-lobed figure, as indicated in Fig. 9.39(b).

(a) (b) (c)

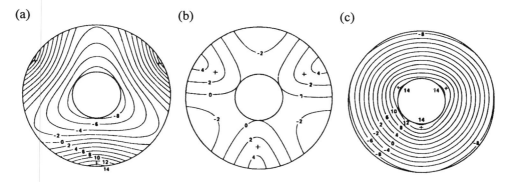

Fig. 9.39 Contour patterns for a circular mirror supported on three points at different zonal radii. (a) At 96%, (b) at 73%, and (c) at 38%. Contour intervals apply to a 4-m (158-in.)-diameter solid mirror. (From Malvick and Pearson.[22])

$$\Delta y_{MIN} = 0.343\,\rho\,R_{MAX}^4(1 - \nu^2)/(Et^2) \qquad (9.5)$$

If the three equally spaced zonal supports are moved to the edge of the mirror, the deflection at the mirror's center is increased from the minimum value derived from Eq. (9.5) by a factor of about 3.9. The shape of a nominally flat mirror would then resemble a dish, i.e., high at the rim and low at the center. The rim would also droop significantly between the supports, as indicated in Fig. 9.39(a).

If the three equally spaced zonal supports were to be moved close to the center of the mirror, its rim would droop nearly equally all around as indicated in Fig. 9.39(c). The almost symmetrical appearance of this pattern leads one to believe that a simple refocusing of the system would tend to compensate for the gravity effect and improve the image. It should be noted that gravity effects on small circular mirrors vary approximately as the cosine of the angle between the local vertical and the axis of symmetry of the mirror.

Adding axial support points would reduce the magnitude of the surface distortion for any mirror. Multipoint supports with six, nine, eighteen, twenty-seven, etc., support points acting through three or more symmetrically located lever mechanisms might be used. These mounts are called "Hindle" mounts in recognition of the 1945 contribution of J.H. Hindle.[24] He started with three support points angularly equidistant on a circle of radius R_S located just outside the radius $R_{E\,2}$ [dashed line in Fig. 9.40(b)] that divides the frontal area of a uniform-thickness circular plate into a central disk of one-third the total area and an annulus of two-thirds that area. Three and six support points lie on circles of radius R_I and R_O, respectively. Equations (9.6) through (9.9) then apply. Each set of three support points is connected by a triangular (or delta) plate that is pivoted at a point one-third of the way up the triangle's altitude from its base. Each contact point then carries equal weight. The mechanism thus formed is usually termed a "whiffletree" from its similarity to the lever configuration used to harness beasts of burden to a load.

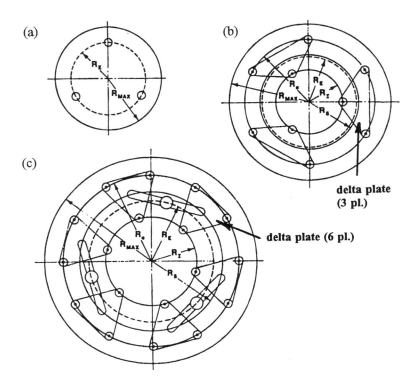

Fig. 9.40 Multipoint mechanical flotation systems for mirrors. (a) 3-point, (b) 9-point, and (c) 18-point configurations.

$$R_E = (\sqrt{3}/3) R_{MAX} \qquad (9.6)$$

$$R_I = (\sqrt{6}/6) R_{MAX} \qquad (9.7)$$

$$R_O = (\sqrt{6}/3) R_{MAX} \qquad (9.8)$$

$$R_S = (0.6075) R_{MAX} \qquad (9.9)$$

Hindle's paper also described an 18-point mounting of the form shown in Fig. 9.40(c). Figure 9.41 shows one support assembly for such a mounting. Equations for designing this mounting and more complex versions have been published by Mehta.[25]

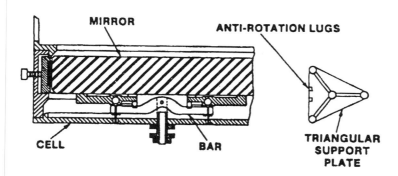

Fig. 9.41 Diagrams of one mirror support mechanism for an 18-point Hindle mirror mount. (Adapted from Hindle.[24])

It should be noted that use of a Hindle mount with more than nine support points probably would be unlikely for mirrors under 24 in. (61 cm) diameter considered here. The more complex versions would be applicable to larger mirrors such as those considered in the next chapter.

When a mirror is supported with its axis horizontal, the magnitude of gravity-induced distortion of the optical surface is reduced. The change in surface contour is, however, always nonsymmetrical. This was explained by Schwesinger in 1954[26] using the geometry of Fig. 9.42. Radially directed forces varying in magnitude around the rim of the mirror and distributed approximately equally axially support the weight of each volume element of the substrate. If the mirror has one or both surfaces curved, elemental bending moments are produced. The resultant of all these moments is proportional to the mirror weight and the distance from the CG to the mirror midplane (dashed line). The resultant moment causes the surface to deform. Schwesinger expressed the rms figure error from a true sphere in the form of Eq. (9.10).

$$\Delta_s = C_K [2\gamma (D_G /2)^2]/(E\lambda) \qquad (9.10)$$

where C_K is a computed constant given by Schwesinger for each of six types of mounts used to support a mirror radially; γ is weight/volume, $D_G /2$ is semi-diameter, E is Young's modulus, and λ is wavelength.

If the rim of a horizontal-axis mirror is supported on two parallel horizontal posts as in the mounting in Fig. 9.43, the value of C_k of Eq. (9.10) is 0.0548 for a flat mirror, 0.0832 for one with K = sagittal depth/axial thickness = 0.1, and 0.1152 for one with K = 0.2. The surface deformation thus grows with curvature of the mirror as well as with diameter. Equation (9.10) can be used to estimate surface deformation or, conversely, to find the maximum mirror diameter or curvature (i.e., EFL) that will suffer a given deformation.

When a mirror is supported on edge on two horizontal posts or in a Vee-block, the surface deforms in a particular manner, depending upon the locations of the

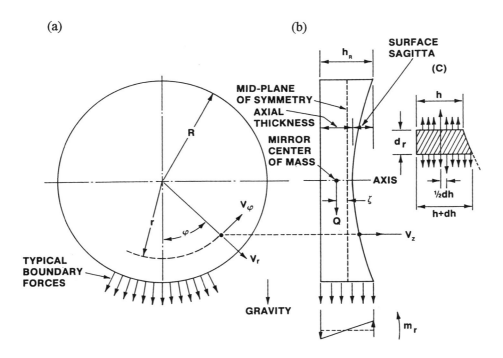

Fig. 9.42 Geometry of gravitational bending of a concave mirror with its axis horizontal. (From Schwesinger.[26])

supports relative to the vertical centerline. Figure 9.44 shows typical contours for a mirror supported at $\pm30°$ and $\pm45°$ from that vertical.[27] In both cases, the mirror becomes astigmatic.

The commercial mounting shown in Fig. 9.43 can be used with mirrors in the 9.0- to 25.0-cm (3.5- to 9.8-in.)-diameter range. Mounts for larger mirrors are custom designs. Small mirrors can be installed in mounts such as Newport Corporation's model P100-A (see Fig. 9.45), which has two parallel plastic rods for the mirror to rest on and a nylon-tipped setscrew at the top to apply a radial preload. Care must be exercised in the use of such a mount to prevent mirror distortion by excessive radial force from the clamping screw. Checking the mirror figure interferometrically after assembly would detect such errors. Once clamped, the orientation of the mirror axis relative to gravity can be varied as long as the imposed accelerations are not severe.

When a mirror is oriented with its axis at an arbitrary angle of elevation, the surface deformation is a combination of the horizontal-axis and vertical-axis conditions just discussed. No simple means are available to determine actual surface contours for the general orientation. Finite element analysis methods can, of course, be used. It may be sufficient to show that the deformation at the two extremes would be acceptable. It then would be assumed to be acceptable for an attitude between these extremes.

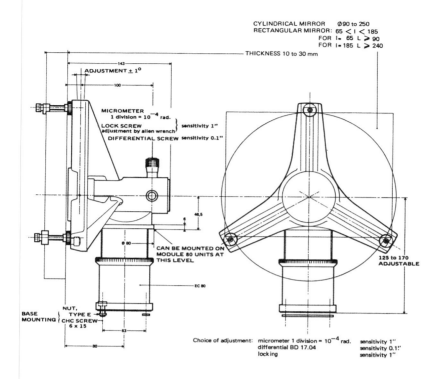

Fig. 9.43 Commercial mirror mount with two horizontal post support. (Courtesy of Newport Corp., Irvine, CA.)

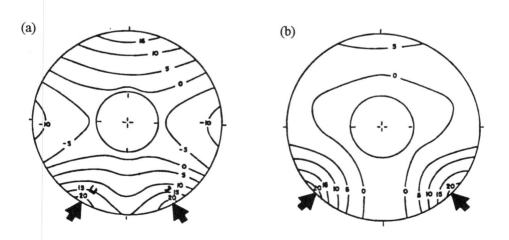

Fig. 9.44 Surface contours for a mirror with its axis horizontal supported on parallel horizontal posts at (a) ±30° and (b) ±45° from the vertical centerline. (From Malvick.[27])

Model P100-A Face

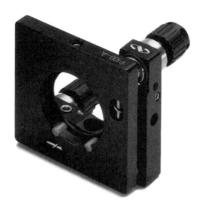
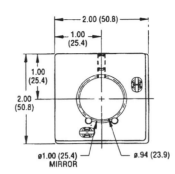

Fig. 9.45 A typical commercially available mount providing parallel rods for rim support of small mirrors. (Courtesy of Newport Corp., Irvine, CA.)

References

1. Roark, R.J., *Formulas for Stress and Strain*, 3rd ed., McGraw-Hill, New York, 1954. See also Young, W.C., *Roark's Formulas for Stress & Strain*, 6th ed., McGraw-Hill, New York, 1989.

2. See Chapt. 8, "The Design of Screws, Fasteners, and Connections," in Shigley, J.E. and Mischke, C.R., *Mechanical Engineering Design*, 5th ed., McGraw-Hill, New York, 1989.

3. Durie, D.S.L., "Stability of optical mounts," *Machine Des.* Vol. 40, 184, 1968.

4. Yoder, P.R., Jr., *Opto-Mechanical Systems Design*, 2nd ed., Marcel Dekker, New York, 1993.

5. Lipshutz, M.L., "Optomechanical considerations for optical beam splitters," *Appl. Opt.* Vol. 7, 2326, 1968.

6. Yoder, P.R., Jr., Chapt. 6 in *Handbook of Optomechanical Engineering*, CRC Press, Boca Raton, 1997.

7. Strong, J., *Procedures in Applied Optics*, Marcel Dekker, New York, 1989.

8. Yoder, P.R., Jr., "Non-image-forming optical components," *SPIE Proceedings* Vol. 531, 206, 1985.

9. See, for example, certified particle products made by Duke Scientific Corp. (www.dukescientific.com).

10. Høg, E., "A kinematic mounting," *Astrom. Astrophys* Vol. 4, 107, 1975.

11. Mrus, G.J., Zukowski, W.S., Kokot, W., Yoder, P.R., Jr., and Wood, J.T., "An automatic theodolite for pre-launch azimuth alignment of the Saturn space vehicles," *Appl. Opt.* Vol. 10, 504, 1971.

12. Patrick, F.B., "Military optical instruments," Chapt. 7 in *Applied Optical and Optical Engineering* Vol. V, Academic Press, New York, 1969.

13. Yoder, P.R., Jr., "High precision 10-cm aperture penta and roof-penta mirror assemblies", *Appl. Opt.* Vol. 10, 2231, 1971.

14. Lipkins, J., and Bleier, Z., "Beryllium retroreflectors expand boresight uses," *Laser Focus World*, Nov. 1996.

15. Vukobratovich, D., "Flexure mounts for high-resolution optical elements", *SPIE Proceedings* Vol. 959, 18, 1988.

16.. Bacich, J., "Precision lens mounting," U.S. Patent No. 4,733,945, Mar. 1988.

17. Sarver, G., Maa, G., and Chang, L., "SIRTF primary mirror design, analysis, and testing," *SPIE Proceedings* Vol. 1340, 35, 1990.

18. Iraninejad, B., Vukobratovich, D., Richard, R., and Melugin, R., "A mirror mount or cryogenic environments," *SPIE Proceedings* Vol. 450, 34, 1983.

19. Zimmerman, J., "Strain-free mounting techniques for metal mirrors," *Opt. Eng.* Vol. 20, 187, 1981.

20. Addis, E.C., "Value engineering additives in optical sighting devices," *SPIE Proceedings* Vol. 389, 36, 1983.

21. Erickson, D.J., Johnston, R.A., and Hull, A.B., "Optimization of the opto-mechanical interface employing diamond machining in a concurrent engineering environment," *SPIE Critical Review* Vol. CR43, 329, 1992.

22. Malvick, A.J. and Pearson, E.T., "Theoretical elastic deformations of a 4-m diameter optical mirror using dynamic relaxation," *Appl. Opt.* Vol. 7, 1207, 1968.

23. Vukobratovich, D., "Lightweight Mirror Design," Chapt. 5 in *Handbook of Optomechanical Engineering*, CRC Press, Boca Raton, 1997.

24. Hindle, J.H., "Mechanical flotation of mirrors," in *Amateur Telescope Making, Book One*, Scientific American, New York, 1945.

25. Mehta, P.K., "Flat circular optical elements on a 9-point Hindle mount in a 1-g force field," *SPIE Proceedings* Vol. 450, 118, 1983.

26. Schwesinger, G., "Optical effect of flexure in vertically mounted precision mirrors," *J. Opt. Soc. Am. Vol. 44*, 417, 1954.

27. Malvick, A.J., "Theoretical elastic deformations of the Steward Observatory 230-cm and the Optical Sciences Center 154-cm mirrors," *Appl. Opt.* Vol. 11, 575, 1972.

CHAPTER 10
Techniques for Mounting Large Mirrors

In this chapter we continue our considerations of mountings for mirrors by discussing techniques that can be used to mount mirrors in the size range from about 0.6 m (24 in.) in diameter to more than 8 m (315 in.). Weight minimization is increasingly important as mirror size increases. With one exception, the mirrors considered here are too flexible for 3-point, rim, or hub mounting and so must be supported at many points. Axial supports, usually applied to the back of the mirror; radial supports, usually applied to the rim of the mirror; and "defining supports" (locating and orienting the mirror) pose major design issues. Some designs have the supporting forces applied within the interior of the substrate at or near the neutral plane where gravitational moments of the localized volumes are balanced. Selected examples of historically important large mirror mounts as well as operational and developmental large mirrors and their mounts are considered here. Thin (membrane) mirrors must be supported by active mechanisms that maintain the optical figure under the command of optical surface figure or image quality sensors and control systems of major complexity. An example of such an "adaptive" mirror (for the Gemini telescopes) is discussed. Most of the large mirrors mentioned here are intended for astronomical applications as scientists begin to reap the benefits of new design, manufacturing, and control technologies that break the boundaries previously imposed on ground-based systems by residual manufacturing errors, gravitational effects, and atmospheric turbulence. Unique features of the mountings for large mirrors in three space-borne telescopes [Infrared Astronomical Satellite (IRAS), Hubble, and Chandra] are discussed.

10.1 Mounts for Variable-Orientation Applications

10.1.1 Counterweighted lever-type mountings

10.1.1.1 General principles

The geometry of a counterweighted lever mirror flotation mechanism as used with a typical solid substrate is illustrated by Fig. 10.1. Arrays of these mechanisms located strategically (usually symmetrically) about the mirror's back and rim provide axial forces proportional to $\sin \theta$ and radial forces proportional to $\cos \theta$ where θ is the inclination angle of the mirror's axis. Counterweights W_1 and W_2 act through levers hinged to the mirror's cell structure at H_1 and H_2, respectively. Each of the N mechanisms supports 1/N times the mirror's weight with lever mechanical advantages of y_2/y_1 and x_2/x_1, respectively. Typically, the latter ratios are 5:1 to 10:1. As the elevation angle changes, the support forces automatically switch from one lever system to the other.

Figure 10.2 shows the lever mechanisms used to support a 2.08-m (82-in.)-diameter solid primary mirror in a telescope at McDonald Observatory.[1] The axial and radial supports have rolling contacts and bearings under significant loads. The rolling contacts accommodate temperature changes.

Some ribbed-back mirrors have both axial and radial supports built into the

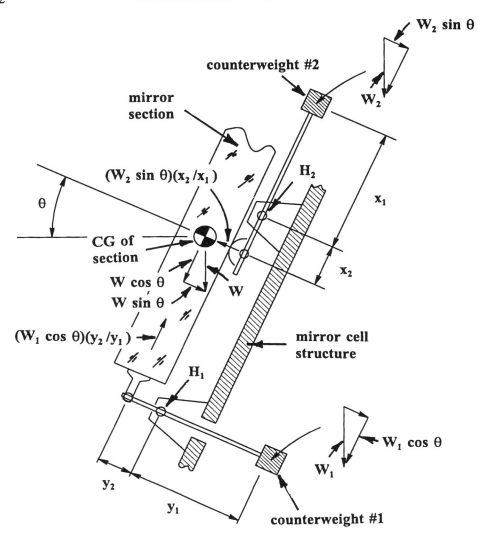

Fig. 10.1 Geometry of typical lever-type axial and radial mirror flotation mechanisms. Force vector diagrams are not to scale.

same lever mechanism. Supports with this configuration were used with a 2.13-m (84-in.)-diameter primary of a telescope on Kitt Peak and with the 5.1-m (200-in.)-diameter primary of the Hale telescope on Mt. Palomar. These designs are described in Sects. 10.1.1.2 and 10.1.1.3. They are included here primarily for their historic value.

Franza and Wilson[2] pointed out that mirror support levers should function as astatic mechanisms; i.e., the force exerted should be essentially constant in the presence of small changes in the location of the lever fulcrum caused by structural or temperature changes. To illustrate, if a fulcrum of a typical axial support moves a distance δy as

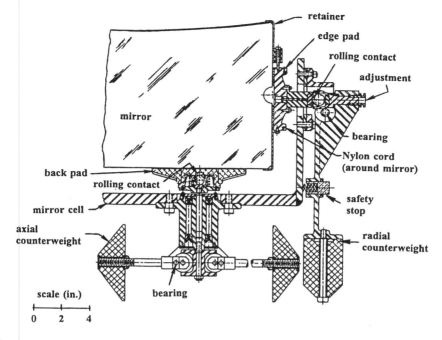

Fig. 10.2 Sectional view of a support mechanism for a 2.08-m (82-in.)-diameter solid mirror used at the McDonald Observatory. (Adapted from Meinel.[1])

indicated in Fig. 10.3, the angular motion $\delta\theta$ of the lever will be arcsin ($\delta y/x_1$). The corresponding change δF in force F will be F(1 - cos θ). For δy = 1 mm (0.0394 in.) and x_1 = 100 mm (3.937 in.), δF will be only 0.005% of F. The delivered force remains essentially fixed.

A potentially serious problem with any lever mechanism is friction and stiction in the hinges. The ball and roller bearings used in early designs caused nonsymmetry and nonrepeatability in the forces applied to the mirrors, primarily because these bearings do not work well for infinitesimal rotations. Astigmatism in mirror surfaces typically results. This problem was significantly reduced when flexure bearings of the type shown in Fig. 10.4 became available. Some early mirror mountings were modified to use this new technology, resulting in improved telescope performance.

The typical flexure bearing sketched in Fig. 10.4 is manufactured by TRW Lucas. It has martensitic stainless steel torsional members connecting concentric cylinders. For load and deflection combinations not exceeding 30% of maximum, these devices provide essentially infinite life. They do show very small amounts of hysteresis and axis shift as results of angular deflections. Various sizes of pivots are available in cantilevered (as shown) and double-ended configurations.

10.1.1.2 The 2.13-m (84-in.) Kitt Peak telescope

Figure 10.5 is a schematic diagram of one of the lever support mechanisms for

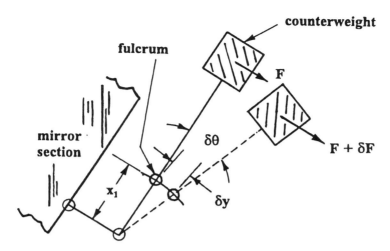

Fig. 10.3 Illustration of geometrical error resulting from an error in location of the fulcrum of a lever mechanism. (Adapted from Franza and Wilson.[2])

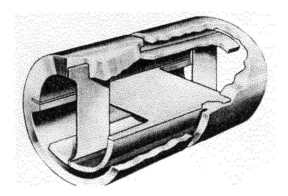

Fig. 10.4 Schematic of a typical flexure pivot that can be used to eliminate friction in bearings for counterweighted lever and other types of mirror mounts. (Courtesy of TRW Lucas Corp., Utica, NY.)

the 2.13-m (84-in.)-diameter primary of a telescope operated some time ago on Kitt Peak. Separate counterweights were used in the axial and radial supports. Figure 10.6 shows a photograph of a similar mechanism used in a different telescope. The function of the latter, and hence of both designs, was described by Baustian[3] as follows:

> The radial components are transmitted through the ball-bearing head located at the upper end of the unit and are carried by a central lever arm whose disc-shaped counterweight is visible at the bottom of the unit. The axial component of the mirror weight is supported on the flange located at the central section,

315

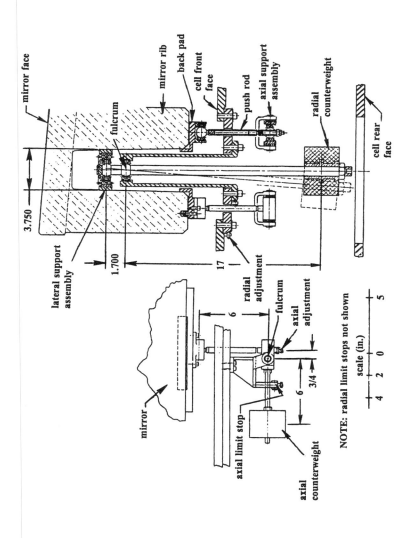

Fig. 10.5 Diagrams of a back support for the 2.13-m (84-in.) ribbed primary mirror for a telescope used at the Kitt Peak National Observatory. (Adapted from Meinel.[1])

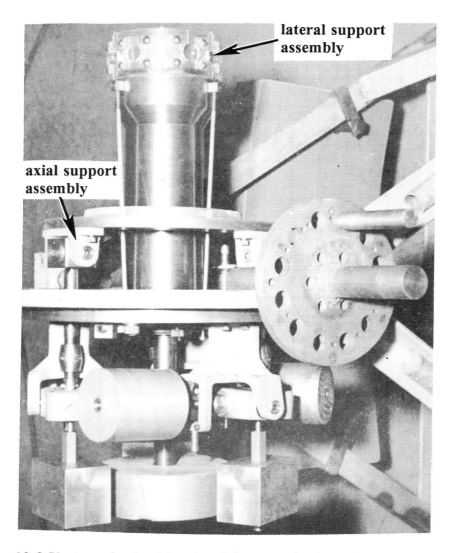

Fig. 10.6 Photograph of axial and radial support hardware functioning in the manner of the mechanism shown in Fig. 10.5. (Adapted from Baustian.[3])

with the load being transmitted through three push rods to their individual counterweight levers, located below the mounting flange of the support unit. The cylindrical counterweight of one of these levers is visible in the central foreground. The rectangular counterweights are auxiliary balance weights to neutralize the weight of the flange bearing the axial load so as to neutralize its tendency to shift the center of gravity of the mirror. (Ref. 3, p. 16)

10.1.1.3 The 5.1-m (200-in.) Hale telescope

When the 5.1-m (200-in.)-diameter Hale telescope was designed prior to World

War II, it was realized that its "lightweight" mirror with D/t = 8.33 would not be stiff enough to be supported at just a few points. The Pyrex mirror blank (see Fig. 10.7) was cast around void formers to create many pockets in the back surface. In this design, radial support would occur deep inside the 36 circular pockets shown in the photograph near the plane of the mirror's center of gravity. Axial support would occur on annular areas on the mirror's back surrounding these holes. Figure 10.8 schematically shows one of the mechanisms used.

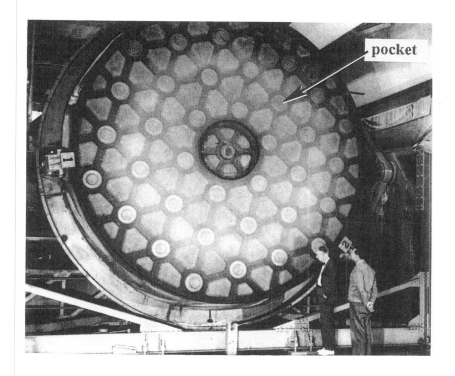

Fig. 10.7 Photograph showing the ribbed structure of the 200-in. (5.08-m)-diameter Hale telescope primary mirror. (Adapted from Bowen.[4])

The mirror here is looking at the zenith. The following is a description of the function of this mechanism paraphrased from Bowen.[4] The support ring, B, makes contact with the mirror in a plane normal to the optic axis through the center of gravity of the mirror. As the telescope turns from the zenith, the lower end of the support system, including the weights, W, attempts to swing about the gimbals, G_1, and thereby exerts a force on the ring B through the gimbals G_2 in a direction normal to the optic axis. The weights and lever arms are adjusted so that the force exerted balances the component in the opposite direction of gravity acting on the section of the mirror assigned to this support. Likewise, the weights W pivot about bearings, P, in such a way as to exert a force along the rod, R, which is transmitted to the ring, S, by the gimbals, G_2. These weights and lever arms are likewise adjusted so that the force exerted balances the

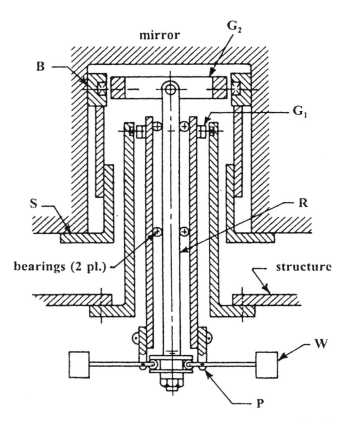

Fig. 10.8 One of 36 combined axial and radial support mechanisms used in the Hale telescope primary mirror mounting. (Adapted from Baustian.[3])

component parallel to the optic axis of the pull of gravity on this same section of the mirror. The mirror is therefore floating on these supports, and no forces are transmitted across the mirror.

To define the orientation of the optic axis of the mirror and the position of the mirror for axial translation, three of the weights located at 120° intervals in the outer ring of supports are locked in a fixed position. For radial translation, the mirror is defined by four pins mounted on the tube that extends through the central hole in the mirror to support the Coudé flat. These pins bear on the inside of the 40-in.-diameter central hole in the mirror. They are constructed of materials to compensate for differences in the thermal expansion of Pyrex and steel and operate through ball bearings to eliminate the transmission of forces parallel to the axis.

In some other mirror support systems, the radial support levers may also be used for locating, i.e., defining, the mirror center. Since these levers are mounted on gimbals, expansion can be compensated for by orthogonal sets of slotted stops surrounding the levers, as indicated schematically in Fig. 10.9. These stops are spring loaded and adjustable by micrometers. Positive locking after adjustment is needed.

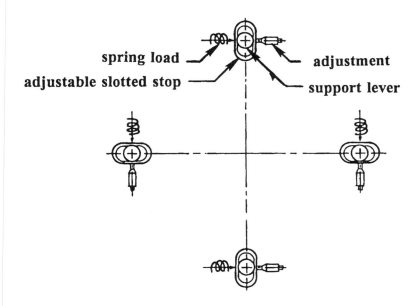

Fig. 10.9 Defining, i.e., locating, the center of the mirror by constraining radial support levers. (Adapted from Baustian.[3])

10.1.2 Hindle mounts

10.1.2.1 10-m (3940-in.) Keck telescope

The general characteristics of the Hindle or whiffletree mount were discussed in Sect. 9.7 in the context of mirror sizes to about 61 cm (24 in.) in diameter. Larger mirrors mounted in the same manner (see Fig. 9.40) need many more supports. For example, the primary mirrors of the two 10-m (394-in.)-aperture Keck telescopes on Mauna Kea contain 36 hexagonal segments, each supported axially by 36-point Hindle mounts. Each segment is Zerodur, 7.5 cm (3 in.) thick, has a 1.8-m (72-in.) point-to-point "diameter," and has a D/t ratio of 24:1. The optical surfaces have concave radii of curvature of approximately 35 m (1378 in.), but the actual shape of each surface is an asphere.

Figure 10.10 shows the mounting layout for one segment [1] while Fig. 10.11 is a photograph of the back of a typical segment. The three whiffletrees interface with the structure at three points and with the mirror at twelve points. The latter interfaces are created by flexure rods that penetrate blind holes bored into the back of the mirror to the neutral plane. Because of the meniscus shape of the mirror, this plane is 9.99 mm (0.39 in.) in front of the midplane of the shell. All bearings linking components of the whiffletrees are flexure pivots that allow small rotations without friction.

The locations of the mount-to-mirror attachment points and the geometry of each whiffletree were optimized for minimum rms mirror deflection under gravity loading in the axial direction.[5] At the bottom of each axial support hole, the flexure rods are attached

(a)   (b)

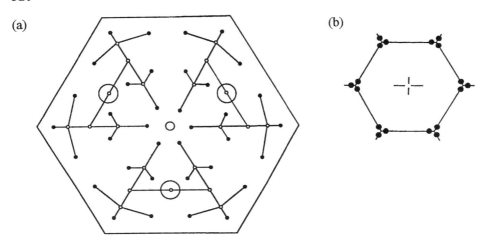

Fig. 10.10 (a) Schematic of axial supports for a segment of the Keck telescope primary mirror. The 3 large circles represent axial actuators; the 42 small open circles represent flexure pivots; and the solid circles represent the 36 supports. (b) Locations of edge sensors on the segment. (From Mast and Nelson.[5])

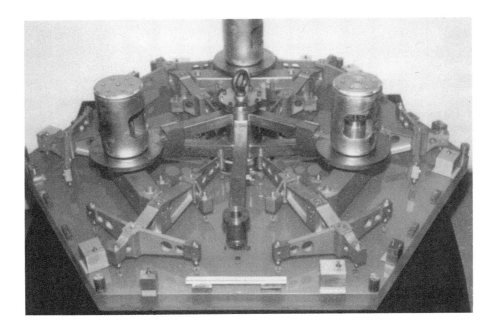

Fig. 10.11 Photograph of the back of one segment of the Keck primary mirror showing the three actuators (cylindrical housings) and levers (radially and tangentially oriented bars). A hoisting structure is attached at the center. Portions of edge sensors may be seen around the edge of the mirror. (Courtesy of Terry Mast, UC Lick Observatory.)

to Invar plugs that in turn are epoxied to the Zerodur mirror (see Fig. 10.12). Iraninejad et al. showed that the thickness of the epoxy layer was critical in terms of minimizing mirror surface deformation and would be optimum at a 0.25-mm (0.010-in.) thickness.[6]

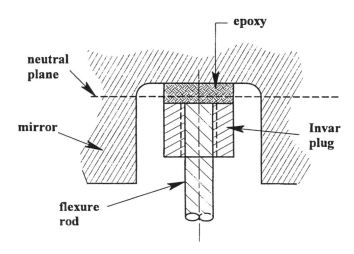

Fig. 10.12 Geometry of the axial support interfaces deep within a Keck primary segment. (Adapted from Iraninejad et al.[6])

During manufacture, the segments start as uniform-thickness, 1.9-m (74.8-in.)-diameter by 7.5-cm (2.95-in.)-thick meniscus-shaped disks. These are ground and polished using stressed mirror techniques developed especially for this purpose.[7,8,9] To contour the optical surface, the blank is supported on its back in the grinding and polishing machine. Lever mechanisms bonded to the rim of the mirror are loaded with weights so as to apply specific moments to the substrate at various locations around the mirror's rim. A cross-section view of the fabrication station is shown in Fig. 10.13. After being polished to a sphere, the mirror is removed from the machine and cut to the required hexagonal aperture shape. The mirror then naturally assumes an aspheric contour closely, but not exactly corresponding to the intended location for that segment in the aperture of the composite mirror as a result of elastic relaxation. Sets of six different nonrotationally symmetrical aspheres are required to fill the telescope's aperture.

Because of residual global stresses within the substrate that are released during cutting, the figure of each hexagonal mirror must be corrected in order to achieve the required performance. Since there is good repeatability in the springback after cutting, localized polishing processes were supplemented by attaching a set of springs called a "warping harness" to elastically correct the residual contour errors of the mirror segment when installed in its 36-support axial mount.[5] Figure 10.14 shows the locations of the set of springs on one whiffletree. Similar sets are attached to the other two whiffletrees in each segment mount. Each spring is an aluminum bar about 4 by 10 by 100 mm (0.158 by 0.394 by 3.94 in.). Moments are applied to each tripod pivot by two springs, and an additional moment is applied by another spring to each secondary beam pivot. These

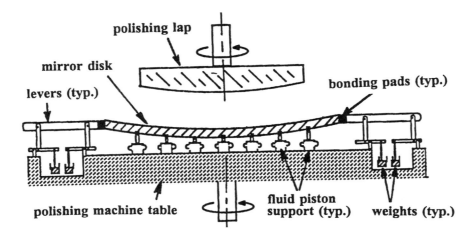

Fig. 10.13 Schematic diagram of the stressed mirror grinding and polishing station used to fabricate the Keck primary mirror segments. (Adapted from Mast and Nelson.[5])

moments are set by manually adjusting screws while measuring the imposed force with a strain gauge bonded to each bar. Each adjustment is locked after setting. The design goal for stability of the adjustment is better than 5% for at least 1 year over the normal temperature range of 2°C $\pm$ 8°C with full gravity direction variation from zenith to horizon. The total time required to adjust the thirty springs on each segment is typically 45 min.[5]

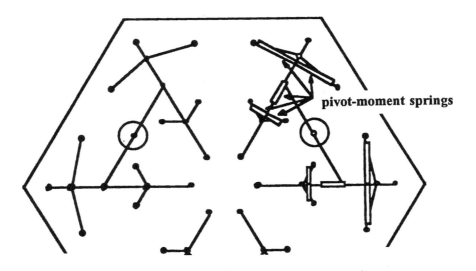

Fig. 10.14 Diagram showing the locations of leaf springs added to the whiffle-trees of Fig. 10.11 to create a warping harness that allows adjustment of the final figure of the polished mirrors after mounting. (From Mast and Nelson.[5])

Since axial supports are designed to be soft in the radial direction so as not to impart moments to the optical surface, separate supports are needed to constrain mirrors in that direction. Iraninejad et al.[6] defined the design of the radial supports for the Keck segments. A conceptual sectional view of one of these supports is shown in Fig. 10.15. With the telescope axis horizontal, the weight of the segment is supported by a 0.25-mm (0.010-in.)-thick flexible stainless steel diaphragm centrally attached to a rigid post extending from the telescope's structure. The edge of the diaphragm is attached to an Invar ring approximately 10 mm (0.4 in.) thick that is bonded into a circular blind hole of 254 mm (10 in.) diameter recessed into the center of the segment. The interface between the cylindrical wall of this recess and the ring is through six 0.4-mm (0.016-in.) thick tangential leaf springs attached to six Invar pads, as indicated in Fig. 10.16. This feature of the design prevents excessive distortion of the mirror by temperature fluctuations. The pads are epoxied to the ID of the hole with thin adhesive joints. The centers of the springs and the diaphragm are necessarily located in the plane of the mirror's center of gravity, which is 2.2 mm (0.087 in.) in front of the mirror's midplane. This location does not exactly coincide with the neutral plane of the mirror so a small (but tolerable) moment is exerted upon the mirror when its axis is horizontal.

The use of a diaphragm to support the segment radially allows it to move axially or tilt in any direction by small amounts as needed to align it with respect to its neighbors and create the required contiguous mirror surface. The orientation and axial position of each segment are measured with twelve edge sensors as illustrated schematically in Fig. 10.17; they are located on the back of the segments as indicated in Fig. 10.10(b). The sensor body is attached to one mirror and the drive paddle is attached to the adjacent mirror. Narrow air spaces on either side of the paddle are carefully controlled by close tolerancing of parts and careful alignment at assembly. Motions of the drive paddle relative to the sensor body are sensed as a change in capacitance. Signals from a preamplifier and analog-to-digital converter are processed into drive commands for the actuators on the adjacent mirror segments. Tests indicated that the measurement errors were about 9 nm rms.[10] This was well below the budgeted error. Since the sensors are mounted to the mirrors, their weights were minimized so as not to significantly affect optical performance as a function of telescope orientation relative to gravity.

One of the actuators used to align the mirror segments to each other so as to form a contiguous full-aperture primary mirror for the telescope is illustrated schematically in Fig. 10.18. A shaft extends from a 10,000-position encoder at left through a dc servomotor and bearing to a 1-mm-pitch threaded interface with a nut that rides on a ball slide. At the right end of this nut is a small piston that presses into a volume of mineral oil encased in a bellows. A larger piston is spring loaded against the right end of the bellows. Rotation of the motor-driven shaft advances the large piston and, hence the output shaft as well as the center of the associated whiffletree at a rate of 4 nm per encoder increment. A relative mirror positional accuracy of better than 7 nm rms is achieved.[11]

10.1.2.2 A laser beam expander

Figure 10.19 shows the conceptual design for a typical 1.52-m (60-in.)-diameter fused and slumped monolithic ULE mirror substrate intended for use as the primary mirror of a high-energy infrared laser beam expander telescope. The basic construction

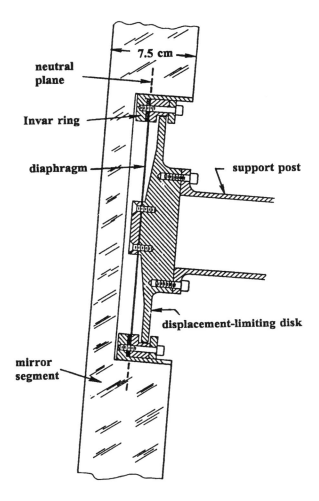

Fig. 10.15 Basic radial support concept for the Keck telescope primary segments. Tangential flexures interfacing the ring to the hole wall are not shown. (Adapted from Iraninejad et al.[6])

is as indicated in Fig. 8.15. The core cells are 7.6-cm (3-in.) squares. The meniscus-shaped mirror is 25.4 cm (10 in.) thick, so the D/t ratio is 6:1. Outer and central rings (or edge bands) are provided to increase stiffness and, in the case of the outer ring, to provide a means for attaching tangent arms as radial supports.

This mirror is much stiffer than the Keck telescope primary segments, and the tolerances for surface figure errors here are much more lenient than those for that astronomical instrument, so a nine-point Hindle axial support is adequate. The configuration of this mount is shown in Fig. 10.20. Invar bosses of the general type shown in Fig. 9.28(b) are epoxied to the back of the mirror at the zonal radii indicated for

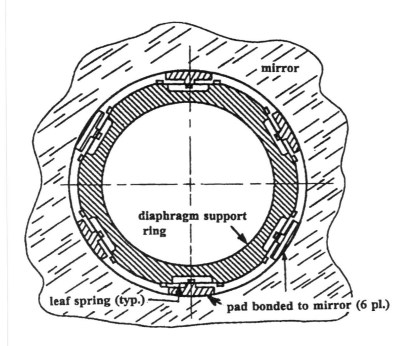

Fig. 10.16 Flexure spring interface between the diaphragm support ring and the central hole ID of the Keck primary segment. (Adapted from Iraninejad et al.[6])

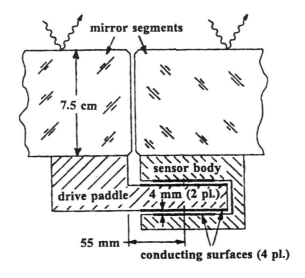

Fig. 10.17 Schematic diagram of one edge sensor used to sense alignment errors between adjacent segments of the Keck primary mirror mosaic. (Adapted from Minor et al.[10])

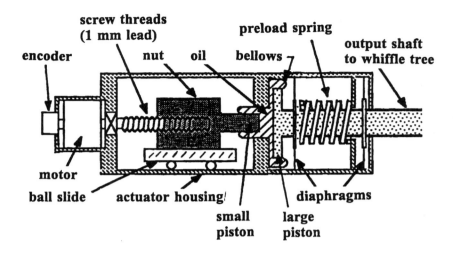

Fig. 10.18 Schematic of one actuator used to align the Keck primary segments. (Adapted from Meng et al.[11])

attachment to the delta plates of the whiffletree mechanisms. Note that the core elements are thickened in the regions surrounding the nine attachment points for added strength. Dual-axis flexures are incorporated into these bosses; one compliant motion is oriented toward the mirror center to accommodate temperature changes while the other bending axis is perpendicular to the first. These flexures act as a "universal joint." A similar dual-axis flexure is located at the other end of a short rod connecting the boss to the delta plate corner. In combination, these flexures accommodate minor misalignment errors and/or displacements caused by externally applied acceleration forces.

This mirror is radially supported by the three tangent arms as shown in Fig. 10.19. These arms have universal-joint flexures of the type indicated in Fig. 9.30 at each end. Titanium is typically used in such flexures because of its very high yield stress and excellent fatigue life characteristics. The tangent arms are attached to the mirror in the plane of the mirror's center of gravity.

10.1.2.3 SOFIA telescope

As a final example of a Hindle mount, we show in Fig. 10.21 a back view of the mounting for the 2.7-m (106.3-in.)-diameter f/1.19 parabolic lightweighted Zerodur primary mirror for the SOFIA telescope (see Fig. 8.22). This mounting is an 18-point axial support system with three whiffletrees as depicted in Fig. 10.22. The support rods attach to bosses (or pads) epoxied to the mirror's back surface in equilateral triangle patterns. Universal joint flexures can be seen at each end of these rods. The far ends of the rods attach to triangular support structures (called "star panels" in the figure) that serve as load spreaders. These structures are attached through flexures, each with two degrees of freedom, to a center panel that in turn is attached at its center of gravity through one-DOF flexures to the centers of three mirror support beams. The latter beams are rigidly attached to a shear box attached to the main structure of the telescope.[13]

327

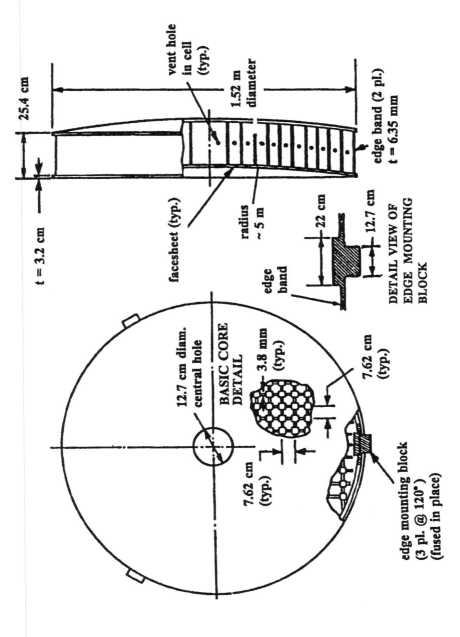

Fig. 10.19 Layout of a typical 1.52-m (60-in.)-diameter, D/t = 6, fused monolithic ULE mirror substrate intended for use in a laser beam expander telescope. (Adapted from Yoder.[12])

328

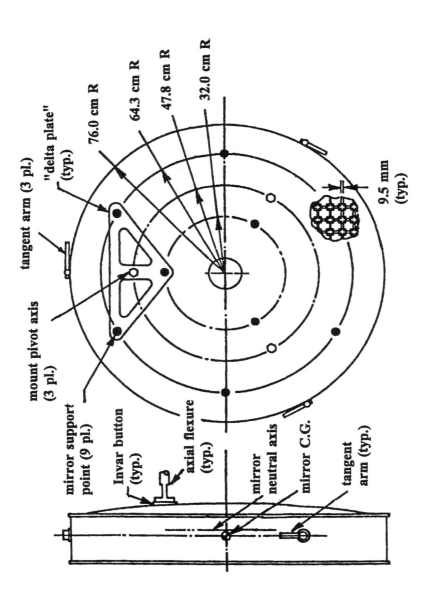

Fig. 10.20 General layout of the nine-point Hindle mount interface with the mirror substrate of Fig. 10.19. (Adapted from Yoder.[12])

Radial support for the mirror is provided by three tangentially oriented beams as indicated in Fig. 10.23. Each beam is attached to the shear box through arrays of parallel steel flexures as indicated in Fig. 10.24. These flexures bend relatively easily in the direction radial to the mirror. Attached to the pad on each arm is a curved stainless steel bipod. The FEA analysis model of Fig. 10.25 shows the bipods attached to the mirror. Each bipod end is attached by four screws to an Invar pad that is bonded to the mirror rim. The configuration of one bipod is indicated in the figure. Necked-down regions provide the desired flexibility in all directions except that tangent to the mirror.[14]

Because the normal mode of operation of the SOFIA telescope is in a Boeing 747SP aircraft with no window, airstream turbulence will cause extreme vibrational disturbance at frequencies up to 100 Hz. The telescope and all its parts must therefore be of high stiffness. This is the reason for the complex designs of both the axial and radial supports for the primary mirror. Analyses indicated the lowest resonance of the mirror in its supports to be about 160 Hz. These results are due to a large degree to the use of a high-stiffness, low-density, low-CTE, carbon fiber-reinforced composite material in the mounting. Other materials used are steel and titanium. The optomechanical design is athermalized by judicious choice of materials, component dimensions, and intercomponent interfaces. Only low outgassing materials are used in the mirror mounting so the mirror can be cleaned and recoated without removing it from the cell. To provide greater performance margin within the tight image quality budget, the final figuring of the mirror surface compensates for the predicted surface deformation at the 45° mean elevation of the telescope during operation.[14]

As a safety precaution, a tubular structure with a flange has been designed into the SOFIA primary mirror cell so as to protrude through the mirror's central hole. This feature of the structure (see Fig. 10.26) does not normally touch the mirror, but provides a mechanical constraint about 0.5 mm (0.020 in.) away that would catch and hold the mirror if the bonded axial and radial supports discussed earlier were to fail during an emergency landing of the aircraft.[13]

10.1.3 Pneumatic and hydraulic mounts

10.1.3.1 General principles

The supports for large mirror substrates described in this section use pneumatic and/or hydraulic actuators to apply force at multiple points on the mirror. Since the mirrors are not stiff and their mass distribution is not uniform, the force delivered by any one actuator will typically be different from the others in a given mount. Each force is usually controlled by monitoring it directly and "closing the loop" of an associated servosystem so the actual force corresponds to the unique value needed at each support point. Means for locating and orienting the mirror are also needed. These usually are independent of the axial and radial supports. The mounts should be astatic so that small temporary or permanent errors in alignment or externally induced dimensional changes, such as thermal ones, do not adversely affect the mount's performance.

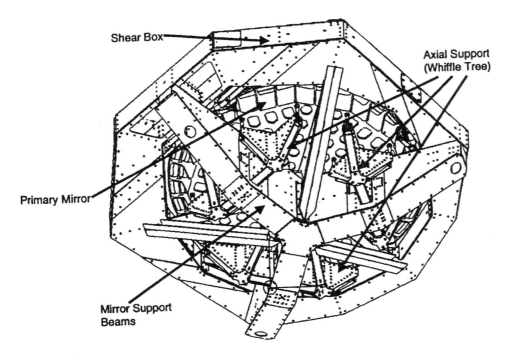

Fig. 10.21 Back view diagram of the SOFIA primary mirror in its 18-point Hindle-type axial mounting. (From Erdmann et al.[13])

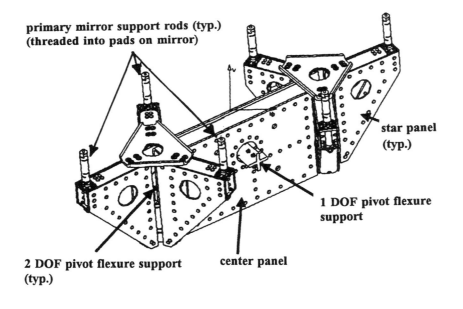

Fig. 10.22 One whiffletree from the SOFIA mirror mounting of Fig. 10.21. (Adapted from Erdmann et al.[13])

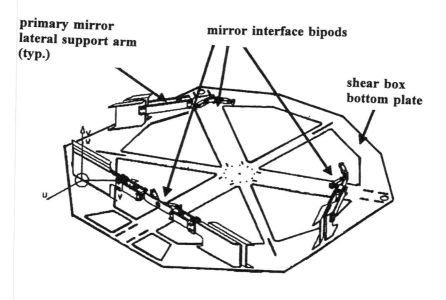

Fig. 10.23 Three radial support arms for the SOFIA primary mirror attached to the shear box. (Adapted from Espiard et al.[14])

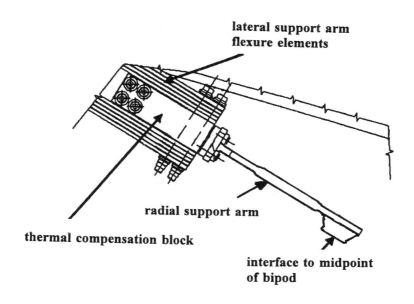

Fig. 10.24 Interface between radial support arms and the shear box by parallel steel flexure plates. (From Erdmann.[13])

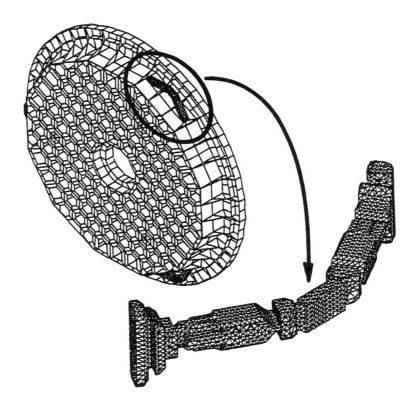

Fig. 10.25 FEA models of the SOFIA primary mirror with three bipods attached for radial support and one of those bipods. Note the multiple flexures in the bipod. (Adapted from Geyl et al.[14])

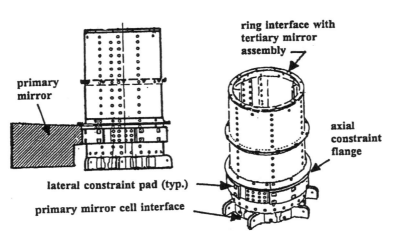

Fig. 10.26 Features built into the SOFIA tertiary mirror support structure to provide an emergency landing safety constraint for the primary mirror. (Adapted from Erdmann et al.[13])

10.1.3.2 A large UK telescope

One of the few pneumatically supported mirrors for which technical information is available in the open literature is the 4.2-m (165.4-in.)-diameter planoconcave solid primary for an astronomical telescope designed in the UK for use at the Spanish International Observatory in the Canary Islands. It also was one of the first mirror mountings designed with the aid of finite-element analysis. With a D/t ratio of 8:1, it was supported axially by a three-ring array of pneumatic actuators and radially by a series of identical counterweighted levers (see Fig. 10.27).[15]

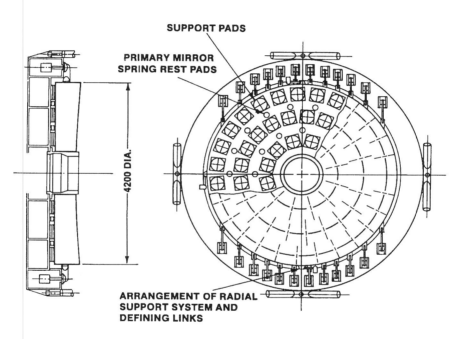

Fig. 10.27 Schematic diagram of the mount for an early 4.2-m (165.4-in.)-diameter UK mirror. (Adapted from Mack.[15])

The axial support system consisted of rings of 12, 21, and 27 supports at radii of 0.798 m (31.4 in.), 1.355 m (53.3 in.), and 1.880 m (74.0 in.), respectively. These supports were circular pads of 298.5 mm (11.75 in.) diameter to distribute the forces over significant areas on the back of the mirror. Analysis predicted the stress distribution that was due to the axial mount through a section of the mirror as shown in Fig. 10.28. Estimates of the peak deviation from the true parabola and the change in focal length were 3 nm and <0.01 μm, respectively. This performance was judged to be satisfactory.

The radial supports were arranged to exert parallel push-pull forces on the mirror's rim as indicated in the FEA model of Fig. 10.29. These forces were all the same in magnitude and supported twelve vertical slices of equal weight. These forces were directed toward the centers of gravity of the individual slices, taking into account the curvature of the optical surface. Analysis showed that the positive gravity-induced

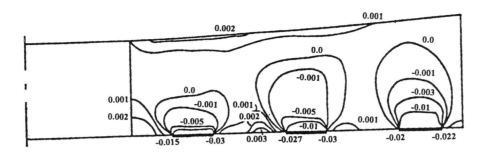

Fig. 10.28 Analytically estimated distribution of stress in the UK mirror in Fig. 10.27 that is due to its ring supports with the axis vertical. (Adapted from Mack.[15])

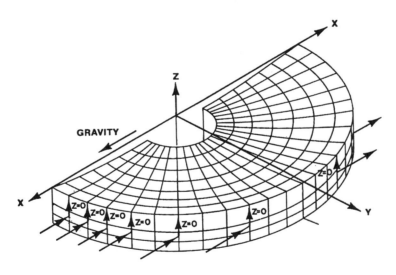

Fig. 10.29 The three-dimensional FEA model used to analyze surface deformations of the UK mirror in Fig. 10.27 that are due to its radial supports with the axis horizontal. (Adapted from Mack.[15])

deformations of the lower half of the mirror were balanced by the equal negative deformations of the upper half. This caused the reflected wave front to be tilted slightly in the vertical plane, but the peak induced departures of the surface from a true parabola would not exceed a tolerable 0.03 μm. Figure 10.30 shows how these were concentrated at the lower extremes of the aperture when the telescope axis was horizontal.

10.1.3.3 The converted "multiple mirror" telescope

The multiple mirror telescope (MMT) on Mt. Hopkins originally had six

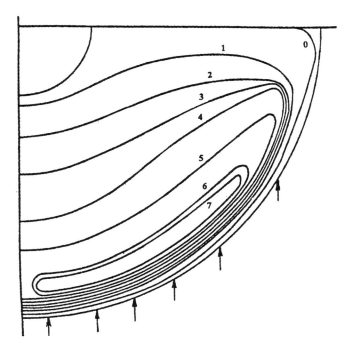

Fig. 10.30 Estimated stress distribution in the UK mirror in Fig. 10.27 that is due to its ring supports with the axis horizontal. (Adapted from Mack[15])

mirrors of 1.8 m (70.9 in.) diameter arranged in a ring to achieve an effective aperture of 4.5 m (177.2 in.). As mirror-making technology improved, it was decided to redesign the telescope to utilize the largest single mirror that would fit inside the existing elevation yoke and a slightly modified observatory building.[16] A 6.5-m (256.5-in.)-diameter borosilicate honeycomb mirror with a relative aperture of f/1.25 was spin cast for this purpose. This mirror was mounted in a cell that served multiple structural purposes as well as holding the mirror.

Figure 10.31 shows the new planoconcave mirror in its cell with the associated components aft of the elevation axis. The mirror is supported axially and radially by 104 pneumatic actuators (called "Belloframs" in the figure). Figure 10.32(a) shows part of the honeycomb structure with actuators acting independently and through double and triple whiffletree load spreaders at the points indicated.[17] Figure 10.32(b) shows (as rectangles) typical locations of the supports for the actuators on the octagonally shaped mirror cell. This cell consists of a top plate reinforced by a grid of 30-in. (762-mm)-high webs that form compartments.[18]

These compartments contain the actuators and other mechanisms and are closed by removable covers, but are interconnected by holes through the webs to form part of the thermal control system.[18] A return plenum for this system is formed by the space between the back of the mirror and the top plate of the cell as shown in Fig. 10.33.

336

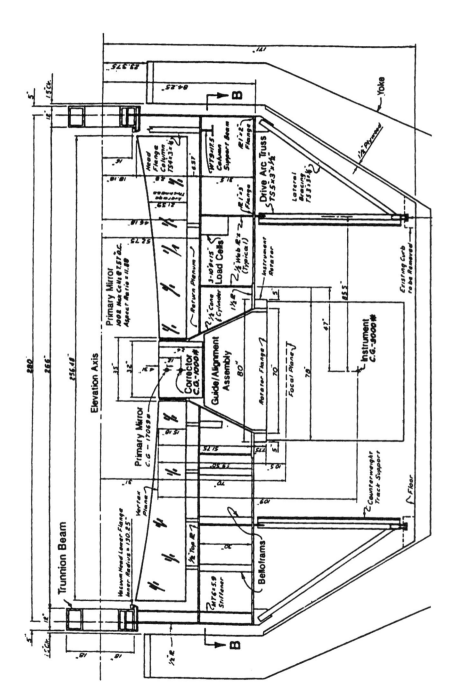

Fig. 10.31 Diagram of the new 6.5-m (256.5-in.)-diameter MMT mirror in its cell. (Adapted from Antebi et al.[16])

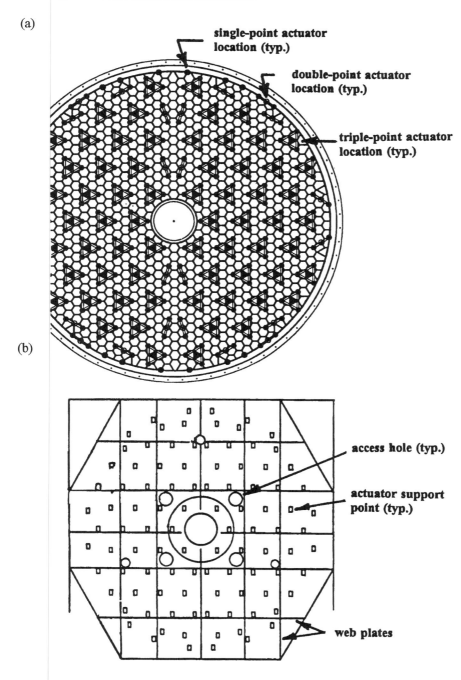

Fig. 10.32 (a) Layout of support points (some single and others acting through double and triple load spreaders) on a portion of the MMT honeycomb mirror substrate. (Adapted from Gray et al.[17]) (b) Section view B-B' from Fig. 10.31 passing through the support mechanisms. (Adapted from Antebi et al.[16])

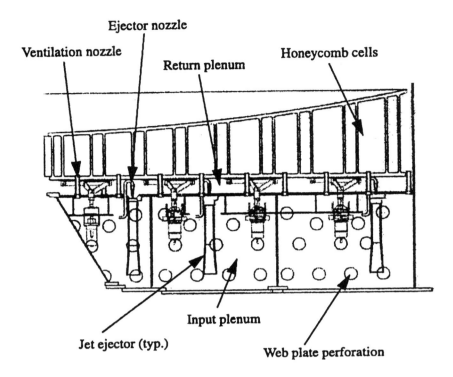

Fig. 10.33 Layout of thermal control system components in the MMT mirror cell. (From West et al.[18])

Pressurized air from an off-board chiller and blower is forced through each of many ejector nozzles and passes through jet ejectors drawing air from the mirror cells and into the input plenum. The mixture of new air and the air from the mirror cells exhausts from that plenum back into the mirror cells via a series of ventilation nozzles, and the cycle repeats. About 10% of the air volume escapes from the cell to allow space for the pressurized air input. This forced-air ventilation through the honeycomb cells of the mirror keeps that optic within 0.15°C of ambient and isothermal to 0.1°C.[19-21] This is consistent with the findings of Pearson et al.[22] and Stepp[23] regarding thermal gradient effects on telescope image quality. Details of the design of the thermal control system and of the temperature-sensing system for the new MMT mirror may be found in Lloyd-Hart[21] and in Dryden and Pearson.[24]

As indicated earlier, most of the actuators contact the mirror through load spreaders that function exactly as their name suggests. Diagrams of these mechanisms are shown in Fig. 10.34. The actuator attachment is at the center of each device. The frames for these load spreaders are made of Invar and steel with dimensions to match thermal deformations of the Ohara E6 glass in the mirror. Contact is through 100-mm (3.94-in.)-diameter pucks made in two parts from the same batch of steel so the CTEs are the same. The lower part is a conical annulus to minimize weight and optimize load-induced distortions. The upper part has a necked rod flexure to decouple the puck from twisting

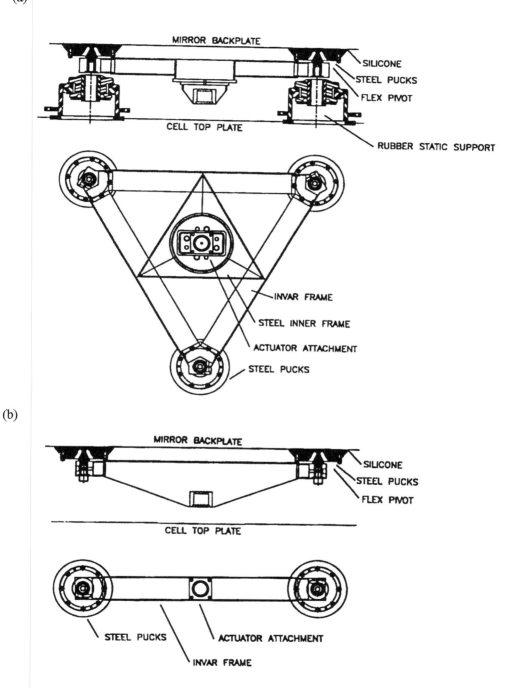

Fig. 10.34 (a) Triple and (b) double load spreaders for the new MMT primary mirror. (Adapted from Gray et al.[17])

of the load spreader frame. Each puck is attached to the mirror with a 2-mm (0.078-in.)-thick layer of silicone rubber adhesive (Dow Corning type 93-076-2) whose compliance absorbs thermally induced stresses and cushions the load.

Also shown in Fig. 10.34 are rubber static stops that are spaced at short distances from the corners of the load spreaders to serve as mirror constraints if the air pressure to the actuators were to fail during operation or when the system is inactive. These are commercial engine mounts; they consist of rubber "donuts" bonded to steel shafts. Shoulder bolts connected to the corners of the load spreaders limit shear and axial tension forces when the stops are in use.

The actuators themselves consist of pneumatic cylinders with pressure regulators, a load cell for force feedback, and a ball decoupler to eliminate transverse forces and moments. Figure 10.35 shows the two basic configurations. At left is a single-axis actuator with a double load spreader. It provides axial force only. The arrangement at right has two actuators, one working axially and the other working at 45° to the mirror's back surface. There are 58 of the latter type of devices. They apply radial forces near the back plate of the mirror and therefore produce moments as well as deflections. An enlarged view of the two-actuator device is shown in Fig. 10.36.

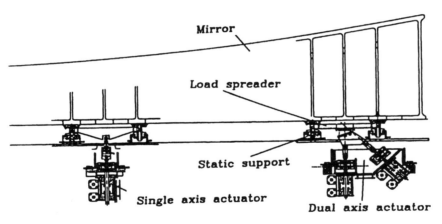

Fig. 10.35 Schematic showing a single-axis actuator and a dual-axis actuator as used to support the new MMT mirror. (From West.[18])

The MMT mirror is constrained in its cell as a rigid body by hard point supports as indicated in Fig. 10.37. Each of these supports is an adjustable, but when clamped, it becomes a very stiff strut that connects the back plate of the cell to the back plate of the mirror. These struts are arranged as three bipods so orientation and location of the mirror is completely determined. Each strut includes a load cell that provides information that is fed back to the actuators. Adjustments are made so that near zero force is exerted at each hard point.

10.1.3.4 The Gemini telescopes

The pneumatic mounting for each of the two 8.1-m (318.9-in.)-diameter ULE

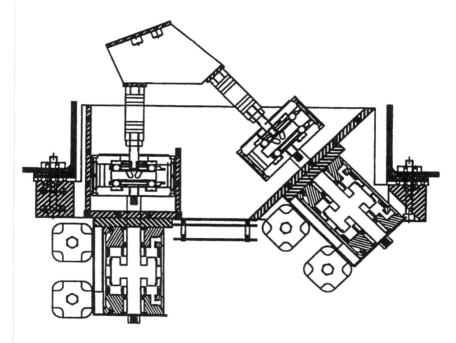

Fig. 10.36 Dual-action actuator used at 58 locations on the new MMT primary mirror. (From Martin et al.[25])

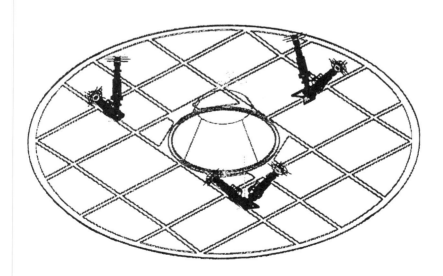

Fig. 10.37 Configuration of six struts in bipod arrangements to provide hard points for determination of location and orientation of the new MMT mirror. (From West et al.[18])

meniscus primary mirrors in the Gemini telescope is of distinctly different design from those previously discussed. The axial support consists of uniform air pressure enclosed by seals at the outer and inner edges of the 220-mm (7.87-in.)-thick mirror plus 120 mechanisms that include a passive hydraulic cylinder and an active pneumatic actuator.[26] The radial support has 72 hydraulic mechanisms located around the rim of the mirror. Both axial and radial supports use hydraulic whiffletree systems to define the position of the mirror. These are adjusted as the telescope changes orientation, introducing small controlled mirror translations and tilts to maintain alignment with the rest of the telescope optics. The mounting system also enables compensation for thermally induced surface deformations; errors in force magnitude, angle, and position; radial support errors; and air pressure errors. In addition, the system can compensate for gravity sag of the secondary mirror and, if needed, change the primary figure from the parabola of the Cassegrain mode to the aspheric of the Ritchey-Chretien mode.[27]

Most of the weight of the mirror is supported axially by a mechanical "air bag" for which the mirror acts as one wall and the cell makes up the other wall. Flexible rubber seals at the inner and outer edges of the mirror complete enclosure of the pressurized region. The pressure required to float most of the mirror's weight is approximately 3460 Pa (0.5 lb/in.^{2}). This air pressure, combined with the force exerted by the seals, produces a small amount (~100 nm rms) of spherical aberration in the mirror's surface. The active support system easily compensates for this error.

About 20% of the mirror's weight is carried by the 120 support and defining mechanisms. This means that the actuators operate in push mode only and do not need to be connected (by bonding) to the mirror. Removal of the mirror from its cell for recoating is significantly simplified by this design choice.

Figure 10.38 shows the 120 support points arranged in five rings of 12, 18, 24, 30, and 36 contacts. The localized forces of magnitudes between 285 N (64 lb) and 386 N (86.7 lb) produce bumps on the surface, as indicated by the contour maps, but their maximum heights are only about 10 nm rms. Since these errors are fixed on the surface, they can be compensated for by localized polishing in the zenith-looking orientation during manufacture so the "print-through" pattern disappears. Throughout the operational inclination range of 0.5° to 75°, the air pressure is controlled, so the errors are tolerable.[27]

The Gemini primary mirror assembly consisting of the cell, mirror, and axial and radial actuators is shown in Fig. 10.39. The welded steel mirror cell was designed in the manner of a honeycomb mirror structure to ensure stiffness without adding excessive weight (see Fig. 10.40). It is supported from the telescope structure on four bipods oriented at 45° to the elevation axis at a radius of about 60% of the cell radius as illustrated in Fig. 10.41. This bipod orientation was chosen because any distortion of the cell from horizon-pointing loading is symmetrical about the Y axis and antisymmetric about the X axis. This minimizes flexure of the mirror. Furthermore, under normal loading conditions, flexure of the telescope will not bend the mirror. Typical worst case distortion contours of the cell's top surface (to which the mirror is attached) at the zenith and horizon are shown in Fig. 10.42. FEA analysis indicated that the expected cell distortions are within the allowable error budget for that portion of the system.[26,27]

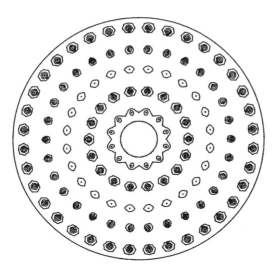

Fig. 10.38 Surface contours of the Gemini primary mirror under 80% uniform pneumatic axial support plus 20% localized axial support at 120 points. The effects of air pressure seals are included. Contour interval = 10 nm, surface figure = 54 nm p-v (10 nm-rms). (From Cho.[27])

The axial actuators are hydraulic cylinders connected as indicated in Fig. 10.43. They are operated under computer control in either of two modes: three-zone semikinematic support and six-zone overconstrained (nonkinematic) support. The mode is chosen by opening or closing valves in the pipelines. Figure 10.44 illustrates the advantage of the latter mode in controlling surface deformation when the telescope is undergoing uneven wind loading. Surface error under typical adverse wind conditions can be reduced by a factor of 6 by changing the mode.[26]

The mirror is supported laterally by 72 actuators applying forces at the locations indicated in Fig. 10.45. Because of the meniscus shape of the mirror, the radial forces have three-dimensional components. The resultant force components are indicated by the directions of the vectors in the figure. Figure 10.46 shows typical mirror deformations from optimized lateral forces and corrective active forces.[26]

10.2 Mounts for Fixed-Orientation Applications

10.2.1 General principles

When a mirror has a fixed orientation relative to the Earth's gravity vector, much simpler mounting designs than those considered in Sect. 10.1 can be used. One does not need to be concerned about changes in orientation causing changes in forces applied to the mirror by the supports. Most fixed-orientation applications also do not entail variable axial or transverse accelerations. Compensation for self-weight deflections during the mirror-polishing process thus becomes a distinct possibility. In this case, it is important to support the mirror during operation as nearly as possible in the same manner as that

344

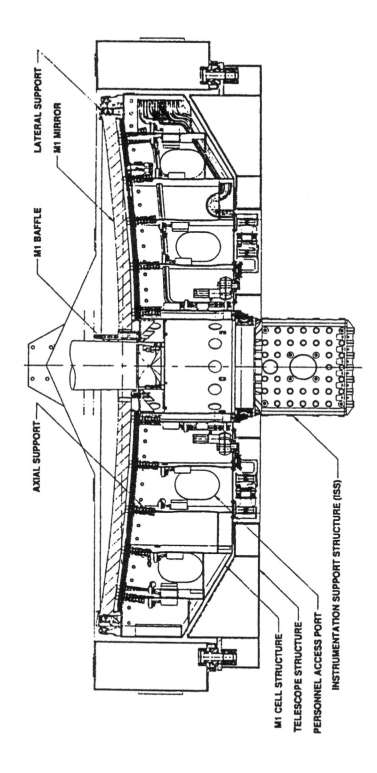

LATERAL SUPPORT

M1 MIRROR

M1 BAFFLE

AXIAL SUPPORT

M1 CELL STRUCTURE

TELESCOPE STRUCTURE

PERSONNEL ACCESS PORT

INSTRUMENTATION SUPPORT STRUCTURE (ISS)

Fig. 10.39 Schematic diagram of the Gemini primary mirror cell showing the mirror and actuators. (From Huang.[28])

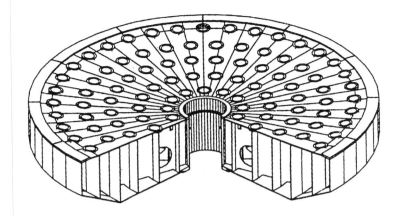

Fig. 10.40 Cut-away sketch of the honeycomb structure of the Gemini mirror cell. (From Stepp et al.[26])

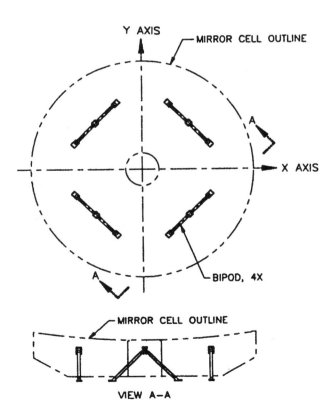

Fig. 10.41 Schematic of the bipod support for the Gemini mirror cell. (From Stepp et al.[26])

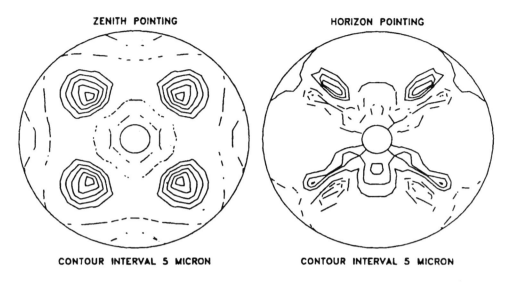

Fig. 10.42 Anticipated extreme gravitational deflections of the top surface of the Gemini mirror cell on the four-bipod mounting. (From Stepp et al.[26])

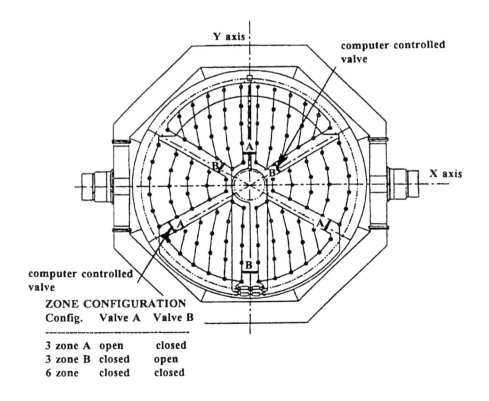

Fig. 10.43 Schematic of the three-zone and six-zone hydraulic system modes in the Gemini primary mount. (From Huang.[28])

(a) (b)

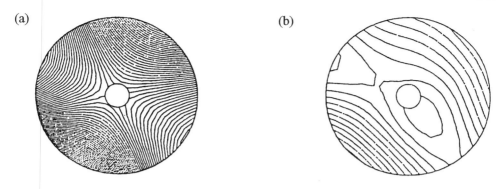

Fig. 10.44 Gemini mirror surface deformation under a typical uneven wind load with axial support operating in (a) three-zone (semikinematic) and (b) six-zone (overconstrained) modes. (From Huang.[28])

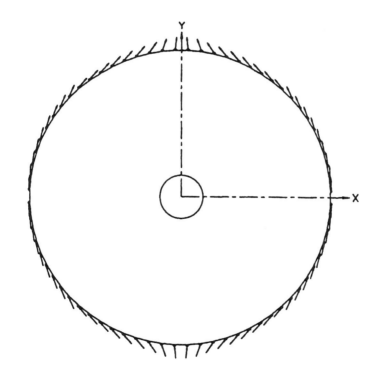

Fig. 10.45 Distribution and resultant directions of radial support forces applied to the rim of the Gemini mirror. (From Cho.[27])

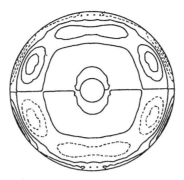

Fig. 10.46 Gemini mirror surface contours with typical radial support optimization. Contour interval = 5 nm, surface figure = 38 nm p-v (5 nm-rms). (From Cho.[27])

used during final figuring and testing. Mounts used during the latter operations frequently are called "metrology" mounts. In this section, we consider a variety of techniques that have been used for mounting fixed-orientation mirrors. Some can be used as variable-orientation operational mountings when the variations are not excessive and when environmentally imposed effects such as temperature changes are relatively benign.

10.2.2 Air bag-type axial supports

Axial supports using air-filled bags or bladders have been installed in many astronomical telescope primary mirror mounts as a means of distributing axial forces over the back surface of the mirror. They are of two general types: those with large area contact provided by circular bladders and those with annular area contacts at two or more selected radial zones. These types are illustrated schematically in Fig. 10.47. Systems in which axial support is provided to a mirror by a series of discrete, usually circular, air bags that act as pistons pressing against localized areas of the mirror's back surface function in the manner of the multiple-point supports discussed earlier.

Air bags typically are made of two sheets of neoprene or neoprene-coated Dacron cemented together at the edges. Vukobratovich indicated that a special variety of ozone-resistant neoprene is needed if the air bag is to be used at a high altitude, such as in mountain-top observatories.[29] The mirror's location and orientation usually are referenced to three or more hard points projecting from the cell backplate through sealed holes through the bag. A low-pressure pump supplies air to the bag through a pressure regulator. The bag typically supports 90% to 95% of the mirror's weight, the remaining weight being supported by the hard points. If the application is not fixed with respect to gravity, the air pressure can be adjusted to compensate, at least partially, for this effect. Safety provisions usually are in the form of nearby multiple soft supports that hold the mirror when air pressure is not supplied and it lowers onto these auxiliary supports.

An air bag can also be constructed in the form of three or more pie-shaped sectors connected in parallel to the air manifold[30] or differentially inflated to support a

(a)   (b)

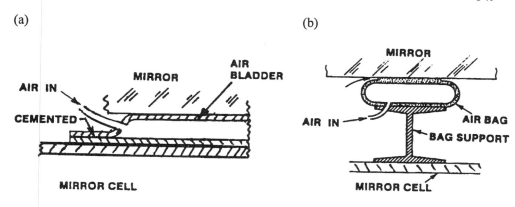

Fig. 10.47 Schematic sectional views through (a) bladder-type and (b) ring-type air bag mirror supports.

mirror with nonuniform weight distribution. In such designs, the hard points can be located at the radial intersections of the sectors. The lack of support at the narrow regions between the sectors can usually be tolerated.

It is difficult to design a single air bag that will produce the required force distribution for uniform support of mirrors with a thickness varying significantly in the radial direction. Multiple annular air bags can have different pressures, thereby accommodating this variation. Control of pressure to the required degree of precision is no small task in any air bag system; the problem is compounded if multiple bags are involved.

A limitation on dynamic performance of an air bag-type support system results from the low air pressure needed to support the mirror. Proper axial support to a mirror cannot be provided during rapid changes in elevation of the mirror's axis because the air pressure within the support(s) cannot be changed fast enough at such low pressure. This problem does not occur in static installations; hence, the air bag support has been used most successfully in fixed orientation applications, such as polishing and testing a mirror with its axis vertical.

During the manufacture of a 1.8-m (70.9-in.)-diameter, f/2.7 paraboloid to be used as a spare mirror for the original MMT telescope, this 1200-lb (544-kg) slumped fused silica egg-crate mirror was supported on its back with approximately 93% of its weight on a full-diameter neoprene air bag and the remaining 7% supported by three swivel defining pads. That bag and the pads are shown in Fig. 10.48. The pressure needed to support the mirror was only about $(0.93)(1200)/(\pi)(35.45)^2 = 0.28$ lb/in.^{2} (1930 Pa). The mirror was first ground and polished to a sphere. This allowed the choice of weight distribution between bag and small-area support to be based on measurement of the effects of varying pressure vs. the surface deformation. The pad "print-through" was also adequately minimized at that weight distribution.[31]

It should be noted that an air bag or bladder in contact with the back of a mirror tends to thermally insulate that mirror from its surround. This might be undesirable for

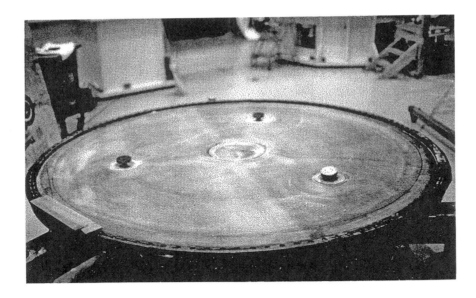

Fig. 10.48 Photograph of the full-diameter air bag support used during polishing and testing of the spare 1.8- m (70.8-in.)-diameter mirror for the original MMT telescope. (Courtesy of the Optical Sciences Center, University of Arizona.)

stability. It is obvious that this effect needs to be considered during the design of the temperature control system for any application where temperature varies significantly.

Figure 10.49 illustrates a generic type of support that can be used beneath a vertical-axis mirror in the manner of a small air bag.[32] It consists of a pneumatic cylinder sealed at the top with a rolling diaphragm that supports a metal pad that in turn supports the mirror. An array of these devices can serve as a metrology mounting for a large mirror. A hydraulic version of this device can also be used for the same purpose. Air or oil pressure can be differentially adjusted to provide the correct force to support local areas of a mirror with nonuniform weight distribution. Figure 10.50 shows an array of supports of this general type having circular diaphragms attached to cylindrical pressurized housings. Metal plates ride on the tops of the diaphragms and interface with the back of the mirror (not shown).[33] Circular air bags could be confined within the cylinders to accomplish the same function.

10.2.3 Spring-type axial supports

Before NASA accepted the planned procedure and apparatus to be used to manufacture the primary mirror for the Hubble space telescope, they decided that a demonstration should be conducted with a subscale version of that mirror. A 1.5-m (60-in.)-diameter scaled version of the full-sized mirror was manufactured and tested by Perkin-Elmer. The mirror was solid, but its thickness [3.82 in. (9.70 cm)] and meniscus shape gave it the same structural flexibility as the lightweighted full-sized version. The

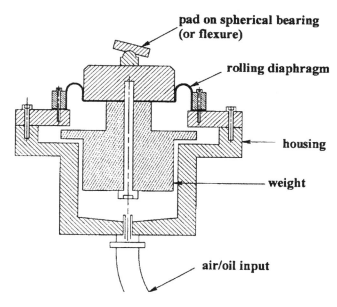

Fig. 10.49 Schematic of a generic rolling-diaphragm-type pneumatic or hydraulic actuator that can be used for axial support of a local area on a large mirror.

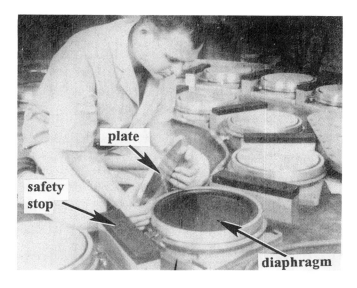

Fig. 10.50 Photograph showing several rolling-diaphragm-type supports used for axial support of a 3.8-m (150-in.)-diameter mirror during manufacture and testing with the axis vertical. (Adapted from Cole.[32])

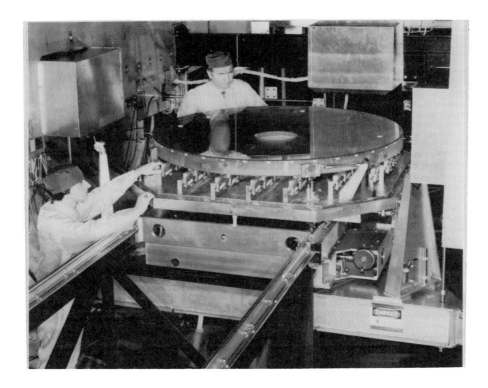

Fig. 10.51 Photograph of the 1.5-m (60-in.)-diameter mirror and multipoint axial and radial support mount used to prove the manufacturing and testing methods for creating the full-sized Hubble space selecope primary mirror. (From Babish and Rigby.[33])

surface figure goal for the demonstration was $\lambda/60$ rms at $\lambda = 633$ nm. The following is a description of the mount (see Fig. 10.51) designed to meet that specification.

The base of the mount was a 152- cm (60-in.)-square by 2.5-cm (1.0-in.)-thick cast and annealed aluminum jig plate. This material was selected for dimensional stability, low cost, and lightness of weight. Several ribs, 10.2 cm (4.2 in.) high on 20.4 cm (8 in.) centers, were attached to the upper surface of the baseplate. These provided mounting surfaces for multiple axial support mechanisms and stiffened the baseplate. Four additional ribs were attached to the bottom surface of the plate orthogonal to the upper ribs to increase the cross-axis stiffness.[33]

The support mechanisms, one of which is shown schematically in Fig. 10.52, were designed to provide a very low spring rate. This ensured that after each mechanism was adjusted to provide a prescribed force, that force would not be altered significantly by a minor change in mirror position or deflection of the baseplate. The low spring rate was achieved by use of a nonlinear linkage loaded by a conventional tension spring. A negative force gradient of the linkage was designed to nearly cancel the positive force

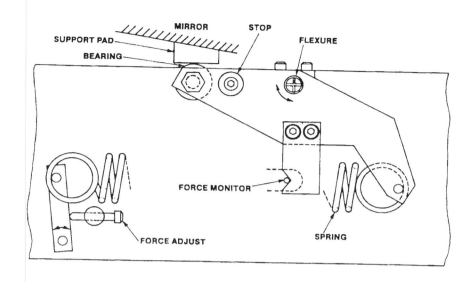

Fig. 10.52 Schematic diagram of one of the axial support mechanisms used in the mirror support shown in Fig. 10.51. (Courtesy of Optical and Space Systems Division, Goodrich Corp., Danbury, CT.)

gradient of the spring. This mechanism could have been designed to have a positive, negative, or zero net spring rate over the normal (small) travel range. In practice, it was determined that a positive spring rate of 2 to 3 lb/in. provided the best performance. This made it possible to control the net force reaction at three axial position-control (hard) points by a slight adjustment in vertical position of the mirror. Each linkage was mounted on a flexure pivot of the general type shown in Fig. 10.4 for minimum friction and hysteresis. The vertical force developed by each support mechanism was transmitted to the mirror by a ball bearing mounted at the end of each lever. Horizontal force components and moments transmitted to the mirror were minimized by this design.[33]

Cer-Vit buttons 1.25 in. (32 mm) in diameter were bonded to the bottom (spherical) surface of the mirror at each support point to provide a horizontal interface surface for the bearing. This was required to avoid lateral force components that would result if the bearing contacted a sloped surface. Cer-Vit was selected to minimize thermal stress at the mirror interface. Since the bond was compression loaded, a soft, room-temperature vulcanizing silicone rubber was used as adhesive to minimize bond curing stress in the mirror and to facilitate removal of the buttons at the completion of the fabrication and testing cycle. A screw adjustment was provided for precise adjustment of spring force. The adjusting screws were located so as to be accessible for adjustment with the mirror installed on the mount.[33]

The axial support mechanisms did not ensure stability of the mirror's lateral position. Three tangent arms were located at 120° intervals around the outer edge of the mirror to serve as hard points. These arms had universal flexures at each end to minimize vertical or lateral force reactions that could affect the mirror figure. One of these arms can be seen at the right foreground of Fig. 10.51. It was necessary to monitor vertical force as well as position at these points. The algebraic sum of the force errors at each of the support force points reacted at the position control points. This required precise calibration of the support forces. The position-monitoring points were instrumented to measure the force reaction. This made it possible to trim local support forces with the mirror in place, thereby limiting figure errors that are due to localized bending of the mirror.[33] The axial and lateral forces imposed by the computer-controlled polishing technique used to figure both the simulated and actual Hubble space telescope primaries were inherently much lower than would occur with conventional polishing techniques so they had little effect upon the forces delivered by the mount.

10.2.4 Mercury tube and strap radial supports

10.2.4.1 Mercury tube supports

A classical type of radial support for the fixed horizontal-axis mirror has the mirror resting inside an annular tube filled with mercury. That tube is constrained by the ID of a rigid cylindrical cell. The width of the tube is chosen so that when it is nearly full of mercury, the mirror will be floated. Typical designs call for flattened neoprene-coated Dacron tubes to hold the mercury. If possible, the axial location of the tube center should coincide with the plane through the center of gravity of the mirror so that overturning moments are avoided. Axially spaced dual mercury tubes have also been used successfully. The mercury tube positions the mirror laterally without the need for hard radial defining point supports. Mirrors as large as 1.5 m (60 in.) in diameter have been held centered within 0.012 mm (0.0005 in.) with mercury tube radial supports.[12]

Figure 10.53 illustrates the forces applied and the resultant surface contour deformations one might expect for a 4-m (157-in.)-diameter solid mirror supported with the axis horizontal in a typical mercury radial support.[34] The contour interval is 1×10^{-6} cm (3.9×10^{-7} in.), so the indicated p-v surface error is $[35 - (-10)][1\times10^{-6}] = 4.5\times10^{-5}$ cm = 0.7 wave at $\lambda = 0.633$ µm. As in the case of the parallel-post or V-block mounting described in Sect. 9.7, this error can be polished out during manufacture if the mirror will always have the same orientation with respect to the gravity vector. A distinct advantage of the mercury radial support is that stress is minimized owing to the relatively large area over which the force is distributed.

A serious limitation on the use of the mercury mounting is the potential health hazard that results from human exposure to mercury and mercury fumes. Since other types of radial mountings for large mirrors that give equivalent performance are available, the risk seems not worth taking.

10.2.4.2 Strap supports

A strap-type mounting supports the lower half of the mirror's periphery by applying compressive forces directed through the mirror's center of gravity. As with the mercury tube mounting, these forces are distributed over large areas, so stress is low. Figure 10.54 shows a once-available commercial version of such a mount. Mounts of this

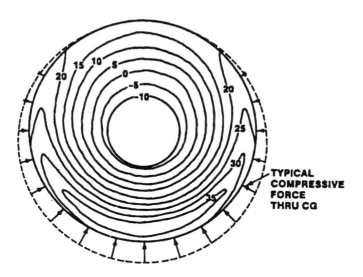

Fig. 10.53 Surface deformation contours for a 4-m (157-in.)-diameter solid mirror supported in a mercury ring support. (From Malvick and Pearson.[34])

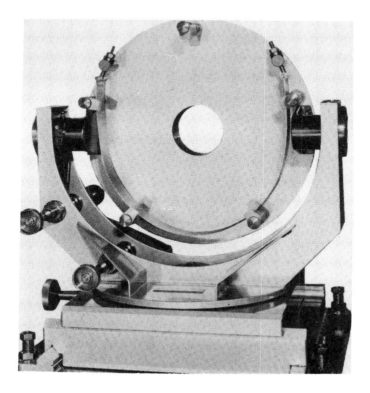

Fig. 10.54 A typical strap mounting for horizontal-axis mirrors. (Courtesy of John Unertl Optical Co., Pittsburgh, PA.)

type made with stainless steel straps have been used with mirrors as large as 1.8 m (72 in.) in diameter. Such mounts are not new; they were first described by Draper in 1864.[35] The analytical basis for their design and meaningful performance prediction methods were not available until at least 90 years later.[34,36,37] Figure 10.55 shows the surface deformations typical of the simple strap mounting.[35]

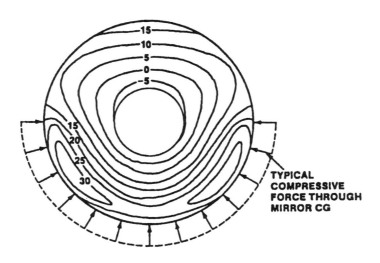

Fig. 10.55 Self-weight surface deformation contours typical of a large solid mirror with the axis horizontal in a strap mounting. (From Malvick and Pearson.[34])

Malvick analyzed the performance of the basic strap mounting supplemented by a variety of judiciously positioned point supports to offload some of the mirror's weight. The advantages of adding the point supports were judged not to be worth the additional complexity in the mount.[34] Malvick also investigated the advantages of this splitting of the strap support into two narrower and separated straps to give more localized support to the mirror's rim. He showed that by adjusting the locations of these two supports in the axial direction, surface roll-off effects at the mirror's edge could be minimized.[37]

Vukobratovich and Richard showed how dual-steel roller chains can be used successfully as a support for mirrors as large as 1.87 m (73.6 in.). Their analysis and later experiments pertained to the lightweighted fused silica primary mirrors for the original MMT. The roller chains were placed around the rims of the front and back faceplates of the honeycomb mirrors. Self-weight deflections of those mirrors were found analytically to be approximately the same as if they were supported in a mercury tube mount.[38] Those authors cited advantages and limitations of the use of the roller chain support as follows.

An important advantage of the roller chain is the commercial availability of roller chain. A wide variety of chain sizes and load capacities are available, and are relatively low in cost. Special chain links are available to permit the attachment of spacers and safeties to the roller chain. Roller chain supports are very compact, taking space around the mirror edge equal to the chain thickness. For optical shop testing, a roller chain permits ease of rotation in its support to test for astigmatism.

Point contact between the rollers and the mirror edge, with resulting high stress and possible local fracture, is a drawback of the roller chain support. Careful installation of the roller chain minimizes potential fracture at the mirror edge. Variable orientation applications, such as an altitude-over-azimuth mounted telescope, requires the use of a counterweight-lever mechanism to unload the chain as the telescope moves toward the zenith. Since a roller chain support functions only in a single plane, a roller chain support is impractical for the primary mirror of an equitorial mounted telescope. Dynamic stability of the mirror in a roller chain support is poor, limiting application to quasi-static systems unless supplementary defining points are used. (Ref. 38, p. 524)

10.3 Supports for Large, Spaceborne Mirrors

10.3.1 General considerations

The major differences in large mirror mounting design for a space application are the large accelerations experienced during launch, release of gravity effects once orbit is achieved, and thermal effects. The first of these generally requires a means for locking or "caging" the mirror mount so that shock and vibrations do not damage the mechanisms or optics, while the second requires that the optics be supported in a different manner during operation than was used during manufacture and testing on Earth. The operational temperature distribution may vary from that predicted in advance. Techniques for accommodating these conditions are discussed in the following three hardware examples.

10.3.2 The Infrared Astronomical Satellite telescope

The Infrared Astronomical Satellite (IRAS) was a cryogenically cooled, Ritchey-Chretien telescope orbited by NASA in January of 1983.[39,40] Its general optomechanical configuration is depicted in Fig. 10.56. The telescope was designed to operate at 2 K and form images in the 8- to 120-μm spectral region.

The 609.6-cm (24-in.)-diameter, beryllium primary mirror was lightweighted to 12.6 kg (27.8 lb) by machining pockets into the rear surface as shown in Fig. 10.57. It was cantilevered from the lightweighted (i.e., pocketed) beryllium baseplate by three flexure links of the T-shaped configuration shown in Fig. 10.58(a). These were located at 120° intervals on a 23.4-cm (9.2-in.) radius [see Fig.10.58(b)]. The flexure design provided stiff and compliant axes as shown in Fig. 10.58(a). The points of attachment of the flexures were in the neutral planes of the baseplate and of the mirror. In the case of the mirror, this plane was 4.42 cm (1.74 in.) from the back surface. The mirror was made of Kawecki-Berylco HP-81 optical grade beryllium with inhomogeneity specified to be no greater than 76 ppm/°C. The flexures were Ti-5Al-2.5Sn ELI* titanium alloy with a

---

*ELI means "extra-low interstitial." See Carman and Katlin.[41]

358

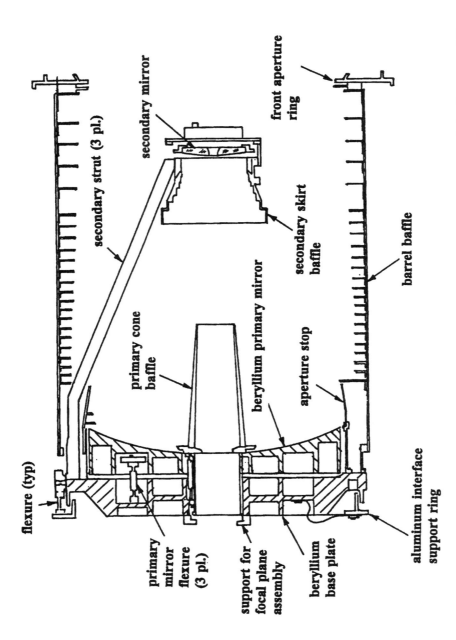

secondary mirror

secondary strut (3 pl.)

front aperture ring

secondary skirt baffle

barrel baffle

primary cone baffle

beryllium primary mirror

aperture stop

flexure (typ)

primary mirror flexure (3 pl.)

support for focal plane assembly

beryllium base plate

aluminum interface support ring

Fig. 10.56 Optomechanical configuration of the IRAS telescope. (Adapted from Schreibman and Young.[39])

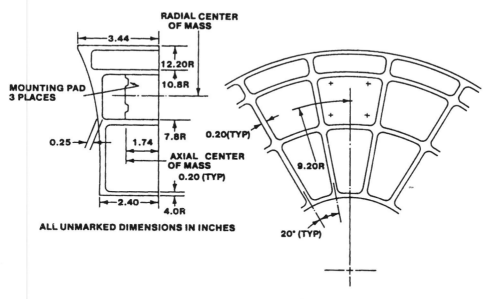

Fig. 10.57 Detail views of the lightweighted beryllium primary mirror for IRAS. (From Young and Schreibman.[40])

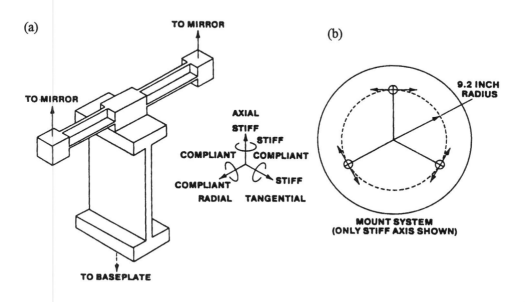

Fig. 10.58 (a) Schematic of one of three flexure links that supported the IRAS primary mirror. (b) Frontal view showing the orientation of the flexures on the mirror. (From Schreibman and Young.[39])

coefficient of thermal expansion closely matching that of beryllium. Vukobratovich et al.[42] indicated that Ti-6A1-4V-ELI would be a better material for such flexures because of the low fracture toughness of the former material as reported by Carman and Katlin[41] and other researchers.

The mirror was flexure mounted on the baseplate throughout the final stages of manufacture and testing to minimize temperature effects from room-temperature polishing and cryogenic testing (done at 40 K). The use of the above-described flexures ensured that temperature changes would not excessively distort the mirror while on Earth or in orbit.

10.3.3 The Hubble telescope

The primary mirror for the Hubble space telescope is a 2.49-m (98-in.)-diameter by 30.5-cm (12-in.)-thick fused monolithic eggcrate structure similar in construction to the mirror shown in Fig. 10.19. It is made of Corning 7941 ULE. The clear aperture of the mirror is 2.4 m (94.5 in.). The central hole is 71.1 cm (28 in.) in diameter. The front and back facesheets are nominally 2.54 cm (1.0 in.) thick and are separated by 25.4-cm (10.0-in.) by 0.64-cm (0.25-in.)-thick ribs on 10.2-cm (4.0-in.) centers. Inner and outer edge bands also 0.64 cm (0.25 in.) thick and equal in depth to the ribs form circumferential reinforcements. Three localized areas within the core where the flight supports discussed below are attached have somewhat thicker ribs for added strength. The mirror weighs 4078 kg (1850 lb); this is approximately 25% of the equivalent solid structure.

The concept for the multipoint mounting arrangement used to support the primary mirror during manufacture and testing with the axis vertical was described in Sect. 10.2.3 in the context of the preparation and testing of a scaled-down version of the flight mirror. Additional details pertaining to the 134-point metrology mounting were given by Krim.[43] Analysis indicated that this number of support points was sufficient to simulate the gravity-free condition of operation. The actual thicknesses of the mirror's components were mapped ultrasonically to an accuracy of ±0.05 mm (±0.002 in.) as required inputs to a detailed FEA model of the substrate that was used to determine the distribution of forces required to support the mirror.

After polishing was completed the mirror was transferred from the metrology mounting to its flight mounting. There the mirror is supported axially by three stainless steel links that penetrate the substrate at the three locations indicated in Fig. 10.59. The cell structure of the mirror can also be seen in this photograph. It is supported radially by three tangent arms attached to Invar saddles bonded to the back of the mirror.

Figure 10.60 schematically shows the rear surface of the mirror. The detail view shows one tangent arm saddle and the clevis that connects it to a bracket, which is in turn attached to a main box ring outside the mirror. This ring is attached with tangent arms and axial links to the spacecraft structure. Figure 10.61 shows a schematic partial section view through one of the mirror axial supports. The relationship between the mirror and the main ring is more apparent in this view. The radial supports (tangent arms) for the main ring are not shown.

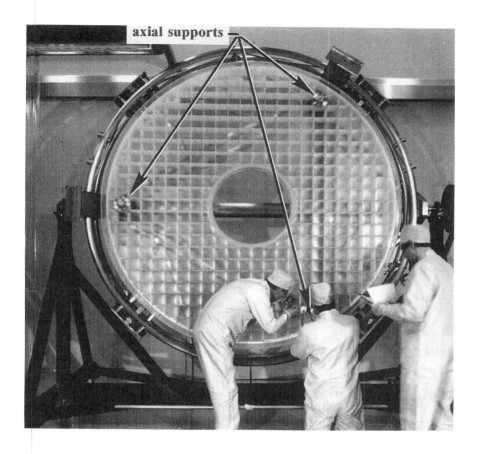

Fig. 10.59 Frontal view of the primary mirror for the Hubble space telescope during preparation for coating. The internal cell structure and the three holes for flight axial supports can be seen. (Courtesy of Optical and Space Systems Division, Goodrich Corp., Danbury, CT.)

Also shown in Fig. 10.60 are the locations of 24 bosses bonded to the back of the mirror to act as interfaces to actuators provided for limited on-orbit reshaping of the optical surface. These actuator mechanisms used stepper motors to drive precision ball-screws to apply localized forces to the mirror. They were not intended for real-time control of the mirror's figure, but were provided as a means to correct minor astigmatism anticipated as a result of gravity release in space. Unfortunately, owing to the square core configuration used in the substrate, it was not possible to correct curvature or spherical aberration with this figure adjustment system. Had means for adjustment of those parameters been provided, on-orbit correction of the asphericity error problem built into the mirror during manufacture might have been possible.

A brief explanation of the concept for attaching the axial supports to the mirror

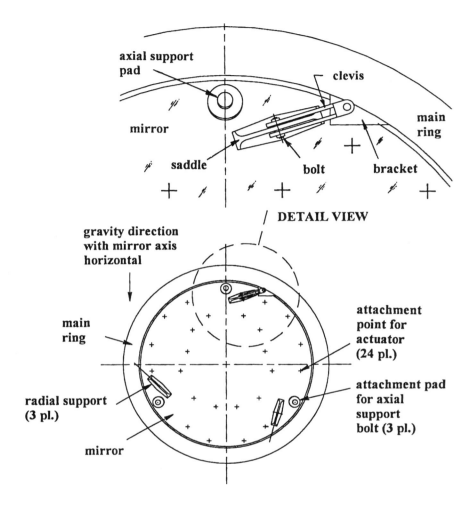

Fig. 10.60 Schematic diagram of the rear surface of the Hubble telescope primary mirror showing axial and radial supports as well as attachment points for actuators. (Adapted from drawings provided by Optical and Space Systems Division, Goodrich Corp., Danbury, CT.)

is in order. Referring again to Fig. 10.61, we see that a flexure link with a cruciform section lies between two spherical bearings. One bearing is attached to the bracket on the main ring and the other to the back of the mirror's rear facesheet. That facesheet is clamped between outer and inner plates that span a cell in the mirror core. Preload is applied by a threaded nut acting through a spring. This mechanism, repeated three places at ~120° intervals on the mirror's surface is all that holds the mirror axially. The design provided sufficient rigidity to hold the mirror during coating, installation in the telescope, shipping, integration into the spacecraft, and launch. It still functions well in space where the environment is quite benign. The design is also capable of supporting

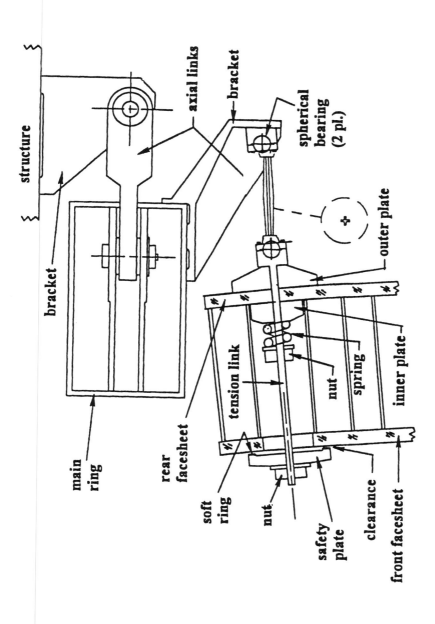

Fig. 10.61 Schematic diagram of one axial support for the Hubble primary mirror. (Adapted from drawings provided by Optical and Space Systems Division, Goodrich Corp., Danbury, CT.)

and protecting the mirror during the rigors of Space Shuttle landing in case return of the telescope to earth is attempted. The safety plate and nut shown in Fig. 10.61 outside the front facesheet of the mirror serve as a stop to hold the miror axially during the rapid axial deceleration during such a landing. Note the small clearance between the safety plate and the mirror surface and the soft ring pad provided to soften the interface. Forward motion of the mirror would be constrained safely, the tension links transferring force to the bracket and thence to the main ring and structure.

10.3.4 The Chandra telescope

The Chandra x-ray telescope [formerly called the advanced x-ray astrophysics facility (AXAF)], launched by NASA in 1999, has two major modular assemblies: the optical bench assembly (OBA) and the high-resolution mirror assembly (HRMA). The OBA contains the main conical structural component supporting the 1588-kg (3500-lb) HRMA at the forward end and the 476-kg (1050-lb) integrated science instrument module (ISIM) at the aft end. The OBA also contains light baffles, strong magnets that deflect electrons away from the x-ray sensors in the ISIM, electronics, heaters, and wiring.[44,45]

The optical system, depicted in Fig. 10.62, has four concentric cylindrical mirror pairs (paraboloids followed by hyperboloids) that intercept incoming x-rays at grazing incidence (between 0.5° and 1.5°) and focus them at the focal surface 10 m (394 in.) away. The configuration is known as Wolter I geometry.[46] The diameter of the smallest mirror is 0.68 m (26.77 in.), while that of the largest mirror is 1.2 m (47.24 in.). The mirrors are 0.84 m (33.1 in.) long. All mirrors were made of Zerodur, chosen for its low

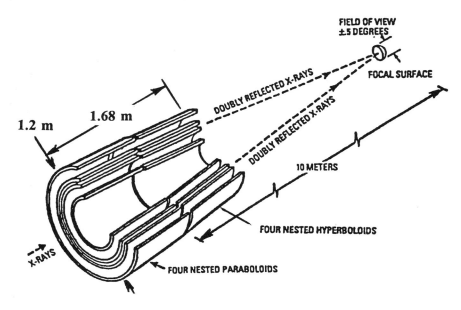

Fig. 10.62 Optical system configuration of the Chandra telescope. (Adapted from Wynn et al.[44])

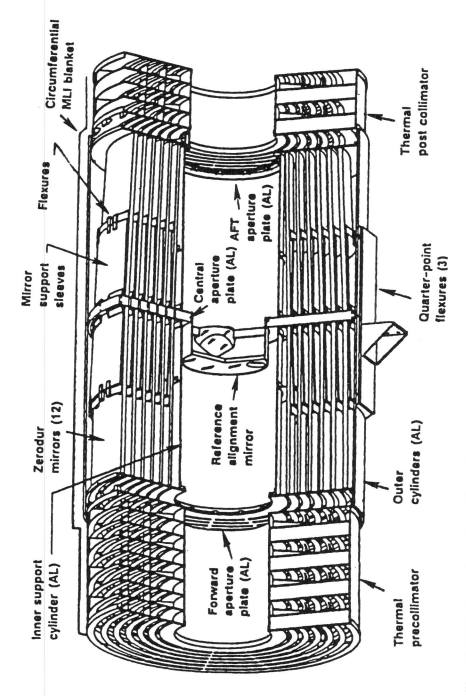

Inner support cylinder (AL)

Zerodur mirrors (12)

Mirror support sleeves

Flexures

Circumferential MLI blanket

Central aperture plate (AL)

AFT aperture plate (AL)

Reference alignment mirror

Outer cylinders (AL)

Quarter-point flexures (3)

Thermal post collimator

Forward aperture plate (AL)

Thermal precollimator

Fig. 10.63 Optomechanical configuration of the Chandra telescope's high resolution mirror assembly (HRMA). (From Cohen et al.[47])

CTE ($0.07 \times 10^{-6}/°C$), high polishability (better than 7 Å rms surface roughness), and compatability with fabrication in the required cylindrical configuration. The mirrors were coated with iridium to enhance reflectance of x-rays.

Each mirror is supported at the plane of its axial centroid by twelve titanium flexures oriented as indicated in Fig. 10.63 and attached to Invar pads bonded to the mirrors with epoxy.[47] It should be noted that this figure shows six nested pairs of mirrors for a total of twelve. The number of mirrors was reduced to four pairs after publication of this figure. The flexures are epoxy bonded to the ends of mirror support sleeves made of graphite epoxy. These sleeves are in turn attached to an aluminum central aperture plate. This plate has multiple rings of annular slots for passage of the x-rays. Aluminum inner and outer cylinders enclose the mirrors after installation. The outer cylinder interfaces with three sets of bipods (not shown) that link the optical assembly to the optical bench.

The assembled telescope was required to image collected x-rays from all four pairs of mirrors at an axial point, with 90% of the energy falling into a circle smaller than 0.05 mm (0.002 in.) in diameter. This demanded that the mirrors be aligned within 0.1 arcsec in tilt and centered to a common axis within 7 μm. To mount the mirrors to the flexures without residual gravity-induced strain, each was first attached to a system of gravity offloaders. These offloaders were attached to a cradle equipped with precision stepper motor-driven actuators capable of moving the mirror in all six degrees of freedom in 0.1-μm increments. When aligned, the mirrors were tack bonded in place with epoxy to prevent motion caused by hydrostatic pressure from the bonding gun, followed by full bonding and curing. The instrumentation used to sense alignment errors was capable of measuring tilt errors smaller than 0.01 arcsec and lateral displacements of 1 μm.[44,48]

The temperature control system for the telescope was designed to actively maintain the internal optical cavity at a constant temperature of 69.8°F (21°C), which duplicates the temperature at assembly. The rest of the telescope is maintained at 50°F (10°C) during observations. Temperature is adjusted by on-board computer controls using radiative heater plates at either end of the optical assembly, and temperature-controlled light baffles. Thermal isolation is provided by an external covering for the HRMA with multilayer insulation (MLI) and the OBA with MLI plus an external layer of silver-coated Teflon film (both for solar radiation rejection). A full-aperture door at the forward end of the HRMA served as a contamination shield during launch and, once opened on orbit, shields the optics from direct sunlight beyond 45° to the line of sight. The ISIM also is insulated and precisely temperature controlled.[49]

The entire telescope was designed to withstand the rigors of Shuttle launch, during which vibrational reaction loads as great as 30,000 lb (133,450 N) can be encountered. Static and dynamic FEA analyses were conducted throughout the design process to ensure stability of the structure. Measurements of the modal dynamic response of simulated critical components of the telescope to external driving forces verified the models for these analyses.

References

1. Meinel, A.B. "Design of Reflecting Telescopes," in *Telescopes*, G. P. Kuiper and B. M. Middlehurst, eds., Univ. of Chicago Press, Chicago, p. 25, 1960.

2. Franza, F., and Wilson, R. N., "Status of the European Southern Observatory new technology telescope project," *SPIE Proceedings* Vol. 332, 90, 1982.

3. Baustian, W.W., "The Lick Observatory 120-Inch Telescope," in *Telescopes*, G.P. Kuiper and B.M. Middlehurst, eds., Univ. of Chicago Press, Chicago, p. 16, 1960.

4. Bowen, I.S., "The 200-inch Hale Telescope," in *Telescopes*, G.P. Kuiper and B.M. Middlehurst, eds., Univ. of Chicago Press, Chicago, p.1, 1960.

5. Mast, T., and Nelson, J., "The fabrication of large optical surfaces using a combination of polishing and mirror bending," *SPIE Proceedings* Vol. 1236, 670, 1990.

6. Iraninejad, B., Lubliner, J., Mast, T., and Nelson, J., "Mirror deformations due to thermal expansion of inserts bonded to glass," *SPIE Proceedings* Vol. 748, 206, 1987.

7. Lubliner, J., and Nelson, J.E., "Stressed mirror polishing: 1. a technique for producing non-axisymmetric mirrors," *Appl. Opt.* Vol. 19, 2332, 1980.

8. Nelson, J.E., Gabor, G., Lubliner, J., and Mast, T.S., "Stressed mirror polishing: 2. fabrication of an off-axis section of a paraboloid," *Appl. Opt.* Vol. 19, 2340, 1980.

9. Pepi, J.W., "Test and theoretical comparisons for bending and springing of the Keck segmented ten meter telescope," *Opt. Eng.* Vol. 29, 1366, 1990.

10. Minor, R., Arthur, A., Gabor, G., Jackson, H., Jared, R., Mast, T., and Schaefer, B. "Displacement sensors for the primary mirror of the W. M. Keck telescope," *SPIE Proceedings* Vol. 1236, 1009, 1990.

11. Meng, J., Franck, J., Gabor, G., Jared, R.; Minor, R., and Schaefer, B., "Position actuators for the primary mirror of the W. M. Keck telescope," *SPIE Proceedings* Vol. 1236, 1018, 1990.

12. Yoder, P.R., Jr., *Opto-Mechanical Systems Design, 2nd ed.*, Marcel Dekker, New York, p. 365, 1993.

13. Erdmann, M., Bittner, H., and Haberler, P., "Development and construction of the optical system for the airborne observatory SOFIA," *SPIE Proceedings* Vol. 4014, 309, 2000.

14. Geyl, R., Tarreau, P., and Plainchamp, P, "SOFIA primary mirror fabrication and testing," *SPIE Proceedings* Vol. 4451, 126, 2001.

15. Mack, B., "Deflection and stress analysis of a 4.2-m diam. primary mirror of an altazimuth-mounted telescope," *Appl. Opt.* Vol. 19, 1000, 1980.

16. Antebi, J., Dusenberry, D.O., and Liepins, A.A., "Conversion of the MMT to a 6.5-m telescope," *SPIE Proceedings* Vol. 1303, 148, 1990.

17. Gray, P.M., Hill, J.M., Davison, W.B., Callahan, S.P., and Williams, J.T., "Support of large borosilicate honeycomb mirrors," *SPIE Proceedings* Vol. 2199, 691, 1994.

18. West, S.C., Callahan, S., Chaffee, F.H., Davison, W., DeRigne, S., Fabricant, D., Foltz, C.B., Hill, J.M., Nagel, R.H., Poyner, A., and Williams, J.T., "Toward first light for the 6.5-m MMT telescope," *SPIE Proceedings* Vol. 2871, 38, 1996.

19. Siegmund, W.A., Stepp, L., and Lauroesch, J., "Temperature control of large honeycomb mirrors," *SPIE Proceedings* Vol.1236, 834, 1990.

20. Cheng, A.Y.S., and Angel, J.R.P., "Steps towards 8 m honeycomb mirrors VIII: design and demonstration of a system of thermal control," *SPIE Proceedings* Vol. 628, 536, 1986.

21. Lloyd-Hart, M, "System for precise thermal control of borosilicate honeycomb mirrors," *SPIE Proceedings* Vol. 1236, 844, 1990.

22. Pearson, E., and Stepp, L., "Response of large optical mirrors to thermal distributions," *SPIE Proceedings* Vol. 748, 215, 1987.

23. Stepp, L., "Thermo-elastic analysis of an 8-meter diameter structured borosilicate mirror," *NOAO 8-meter Telescopes Engineering Design Study Report No. 1*, National Optical Astronomy Observatories, Tucson, 1989.

24. Dryden, D.M. and Pearson, E.T., "Multiplexed precision thermal measurement system for large structured mirrors," *SPIE Proceedings* Vol. 1236, 825, 1990.

25. Martin, H.M., Callahan, S.P., Cuerden, B., Davison, W.B., DeRigne, S.T., Dettmann, L.R., Parodi, G., Trebisky, T.J., West, S.C., and Williams, J.T., "Active supports and force optimization for the MMT primary mirror," *SPIE Proceedings* Vol. 3352, 412, 1998.

26. Stepp, L., Huang, E., and Cho, M., "Gemini primary mirror support system," *SPIE Proceedings* Vol. 2199, 223, 1994.

27. Cho, M.K., "Optimization strategy of axial and lateral supports for large primary mirrors," *SPIE Proceedings* Vol. 2199, 841, 1994.

28. Huang, E.W., "Gemini primary mirror cell design,", *SPIE Proceedings* Vol. 2871, 291, 1996.

29. Vukobratovich, D., private communication, 1992.

30. Chivens, C.C. "Air Bags," in *A Symposium on Support and Testing of Large Astronomical Mirrors*, D.L. Crawford, A.B. Meinel, and M.W. Stockton, Eds., Kitt Peak National Lab. and the Univ. of Arizona, Tucson, 105, 1968.

31. Crawford, R. and Anderson, D. "Polishing and aspherizing a 1.8-m f/2.7 paraboloid," *SPIE Proceedings* Vol. 966, 322, 1988.

32. Cole, N. "Shop supports for the 150-inch Kitt Peak and Cerro Tololo primary mirrors," in *Optical Telescope Technology Workshop,* NASA Rept. SP-233, NASA, Huntsville, p. 307, 1970.

33. Babish, R.C. and Rigby, R.R., "Optical fabrication of a 60-inch mirror," *SPIE Proceedings* Vol. 183, 105, 1979.

34. Malvick, A.J. and Pearson, E.T., "Theoretical elastic deformations of a 4-m diameter optical mirror using dynamic relaxation," *Appl. Opt.* Vol. 7, 1207, 1968.

35. Draper, H., "On the construction of a silvered glass telescope, fifteen and a half inches in aperture and its use in celestial photography", in *Smithsonian Contributions to Knowledge,* 1864.

36. Schwessinger, G., "Optical effects of flexure in vertically mounted precision mirrors," *J. Opt. Soc. Am.,* Vol. 44, 417, 1954.

37. Malvick, A.J., "Theoretical elastic deformations of the Steward Observatory 230-cm and the Optical Sciences Center 154-cm mirrors," *Appl. Opt.* Vol. 11, 575, 1972.

38. Vukobratovich, D. and Richard, R.M., "Roller chain supports for large optics," *SPIE Proceedings* Vol. 1396, 522, 1991.

39. Schreibman, M. and Young, P., "Design of infrared astronomical satellite (IRAS) primary mirror mounts," *SPIE Proceedings* Vol. 250, 50, 1980.

40. Young, P. and Schreibman, M., "Alignment design for a cryogenic telescope," *SPIE Proceedings* Vol. 251, 17 1, 1980.

41. Carman, C.M., and Katlin, J.M., "Plane Strain Fracture Toughness and Mechanical Properties of 5Al-2.5Sn ELI and Commercial Titanium Alloys at Room and Cryogenic Temperature," in *Applications-Related Phenomena in Titanium Alloys,* ASTM STP432, American Society for Testing and Materials, Philadelphia, p. 124, 1968.

42. Vukobratovich, D., Richard, R., Valente, T., and Cho, M., *Final Design Report for NASA Ames/Univ. of Arizona Cooperative Agreement No. NCC2-426 for period April 1, 1989 - April 30, 1990*, Optical Sciences Ctr., Univ. of Arizona, Tucson, 1990.

43. Krim, M.H., "Metrology mount development and verification for a large spaceborne mirror," *SPIE Proceedings* Vol. 332, 440, 1982.

44. Wynn, J.A., Spina, J.A., and Atkinson, C.B., "Configuration, assembly, and test of the X-ray telescope for NASA's advanced x-ray astrophysics facility," *SPIE Proceedings* Vol. 3356, 522, 1998.

45. Olds, C.R., and Reese, R.P., "Composite structures for the advanced x-ray astrophysics facility (AXAF)," *SPIE Proceedings* Vol. 3356, 910, 1998.

46. Wolter, H., *Ann. Phys.* Vol. 10, 94, 1952.

47. Cohen, L.M., Cernock, L., Mathews, G., and Stallcup, M., "Structural considerations for fabrication and mounting of the AXAF HRMA optics," *SPIE Proceedings* Vol. 1303, 162, 1990.

48. Glenn, P., "Centroid detector system for AXAF-I alignment test system," *SPIE Proceedings* Vol. 2515, 352, 1995.

49. Havey, K., Sweitzer, M., and Lynch, N., "Precision thermal control trades for telescope systems," *SPIE Proceedings* Vol. 3356, 10, 1998.

CHAPTER 11
Estimation of Mounting Stresses in Optical Components

Contact stress is created whenever force is applied within small areas on the surface of an optical component. This stress depends upon the magnitude of the force, the shapes of the surfaces in contact, the size of the contact area between the optical and mechanical bodies (both considered to be elastic), and the pertinent mechanical properties of the contacting materials. In this chapter, we summarize a theory based on equations of Roark[1] for estimating the magnitude of contact stress for a variety of commonly used glass-to-metal interface types involving lenses, windows, mirrors, and prisms. The variability of contact stress with material type is demonstrated. The stress resulting from radially unsymmetrical application of axial clamping forces on opposite sides of rotationally symmetrical components is quantified. Tensile stress in the single-sided bonded joint also is discussed The analytical models forming the bases for the stress equations given here are believed be conservative representations of real-life situations. Therefore, the stresses calculated by the methods presented here should be somewhat higher than those that would actually be experienced by hardware under the prescribed conditions. The magnitude of this overestimation is not now known. It is hoped that it will someday be revealed through experimental measurements.

11.1 General Considerations

A compressive force exerted over a small area on an optical surface causes elastic deformation, i.e., strain, of the local region and hence proportional stress within that region. If the stress exceeds the damage threshold of the optical material, failure may occur. Rigorous calculations of damage thresholds for glass-type materials are complex and rely on statistics to determine the probability of failure under specified conditions.[2] As a short cut, we here apply rule-of-thumb values for the stress in glass that might cause damage. In compression, this is 50,000 lb/in.^{2} (345 MPa) while in tension, it is 1000 lb/in.^{2} (6.9 MPa).[3] As a further approximation, we assume that the same tolerances apply to nonmetallic mirror materials and optical crystals. For simplicity, we refer to all optical materials as glass and all mechanical ones as metal.

Stress also builds up within the mechanical members that compress the glass. This usually is compared with the yield strength of that metal (generally taken as that stress resulting in a dimensional change of two parts per thousand) to see if an adequate safety margin exists. In critical applications (such as those demanding extreme long-term stability), stress in mechanical components may be limited to the microyield stress value for the material.

Since operational conditions invariably are less stringent than survival conditions, damage is not a concern, but detrimental effects on performance can occur. Mounting forces then may cause optical surfaces to deform, i.e., become strained. Such deformations may affect performance. No meaningful general tolerances for surface deformations can be given since they depend upon the level of performance required and the location of the surface in the system (they are less sensitive near an image and more sensitive near a pupil). Simple equations for estimating surface deformations as functions of force applied to optical components are not generally available. These calculations are best done by finite-element analysis methods. The stress induced by operational levels of strain can affect the performance of optical components used in applications involving polarized light through the introduction of birefringence. This is a localized change in refractive index of the material that affects the phase of the orthogonal polarized components of the radiation transmitted through the stressed region. The magnitude of the effect depends on the stress level, the stress optic coefficient for the material, and the path length within that material. The tolerable level of stress that does not produce detectable birefringence effects in visual optical systems and many photographic systems is approximately 500 lb/in.[2] (3.4 MPa). Polarimeters and systems involving polarized laser light may suffer noticeably from stress in the optical components of less than 50 lb/in.[2] (0.34 MPa). It should be noted that surface deformations and birefringence effects as seen primarily in the local region where the clamping force is applied.[4] Typically, this is near, but outside the optic's aperture, so the effects may not be significant over most of that aperture.

11.2 Average Compressive Stress

The worst case average stress developed at any optomechanical interface is given by the following simple equation:

$$S_{AVG} = P/A_C \tag{11.1}$$

where:

P = assembly preload holding the components together
A_C = area of contact

Two surfaces in intimate contact over a significant area, such as a flat bevel on a lens touching the flat surface of its mount or a prism spring loaded against a flat locating pad, will produce little stress in the glass under reasonable preload because the contact area is large. As mentioned in Sect. 2.1.3, true intimate contact results only if the interfacing surfaces are accurately flat and parallel. If these conditions are not met, localized contact will occur first at the three highest points, and as preload is increased, the surfaces will deform so that multiple contacts occur and the optic becomes overconstrained. Equation (11.1) ignores bending stresses that might occur in the loaded interface as a result of this overconstraint. To maintain contact between the interfacing surfaces at all temperatures, differential expansion and contraction effects must be considered. This is discussed in Chapt. 12.

The Microsoft Excel spreadsheet provided in the form of a CD-ROM with this book facilitates computation of stresses in the optomechanically interfacing components. Problems similar to the ones employed in this chapter to illustrate analysis of typical situations encountered in the design of optical instruments can be solved easily by substituting new input data in the applicable file. The program then solves those problems. This is especially useful when parameters need to be varied to achieve a favorable design.

Example 11.1: Average contact stress in an axially preloaded flat window. (For design and analysis, use File 37 of the CD-ROM)
Assume that a plane parallel window with diameter D_G = 1.968 in. (50.000 mm) intimately contacts a cell shoulder over an annular width w_a = 0.079 in. (2.000 mm) around the window's edge. Calculate the average stress in the glass at the interface if the axial preload is 16.861 lb (75.000 N).

The annular area of contact $A_C = (\pi D_G^2/4) - [\pi(D_G - w_a)^2/4]$
$= [(\pi)(1.968)^2/4] - [(\pi)(1.968 - 0.079)^2/4] = 0.239$ in.^{2} (154.193 mm^2)

By Eq. (11.1), S_{AVG} = 16.861/0.239 = 70.5 lb/in.^{2} (0.49 MPa)

This compressive stress is negligible in comparison with the rule-of-thumb tolerance for glass of 50,000 lb/in.^{2} (345 MPa).

11.3 Peak Axial Contact Stress in a Lens

The axial stress developed within a single-element lens in a surface-contact mounting configuration from axial force applied around the edge of the polished surface by a threaded retainer (see Fig. 3.12) or a circular flange (see Fig. 3.16) depends on the force, the radius of the optical surface, the geometric shape of the mount's surface, and the physical properties of the materials involved. The force generally varies with temperature (see Sect. 12.2.3). For survival under vibration or shock in the axial direction at assembly temperature, the axial preload P used in stress estimation equals Wa_G.

Since the lens and mounting materials are both elastic, axial stress has a peak value along the centerline of the narrow annular area of contact between the metal and glass. The stress decreases at points within the lens progressively farther away from this centerline; i.e., toward and away from the lens axis. The average contact stress can be calculated using Eq. (11.1) once the annular width of the deformed area is determined.

The peak axial contact stress S_C at the surface of a lens preloaded at a height y_C from the axis can be estimated from the following equation adapted [5,6] from Roark: [1]

$$S_C = 0.798(K_1 p/K_2)^{1/2} \tag{11.2}$$

where K_1 depends on the optomechanical interface design and the lens surface radius, K_2 depends on the elastic properties of the lens and mount materials, and p is the linear preload (or load per unit length) as determined from the total axial preload P by:

$$p = P/(2\pi y_C) \qquad (11.3)$$

The term K_1 is discussed in the following subsections in conjunction with various possible interface types.

For all interface types, the term K_2 is the sum of terms for the glass and for the metal as follows:

$$K_2 = K_G + K_M = [(1 - v_G^2)/E_G] + [(1 - v_M^2)/E_M] \qquad (11.4)$$

where v_G, E_G, v_M, and E_M are Poisson's ratio and Young's modulus for the glass and metal respectively. Computed values of K_G and K_M are listed for selected glasses, crystals, and metals in Tables B1, B4 through B7, and B12.

Figure 11.1 shows a graphical comparison of the magnitudes of K_G for the 68 optical glasses listed in Table B1. The glasses with highest (F4) and lowest (LaSFN30) values within this group are indicated by arrows. Note that K_G varies by no more than a factor of 2.3 for all these glasses. Figure 11.2 shows similar plots of K_M for the six metals most frequently used in optical instruments. The magnitude of K_M varies significantly (by a factor of 5.7) within this group.

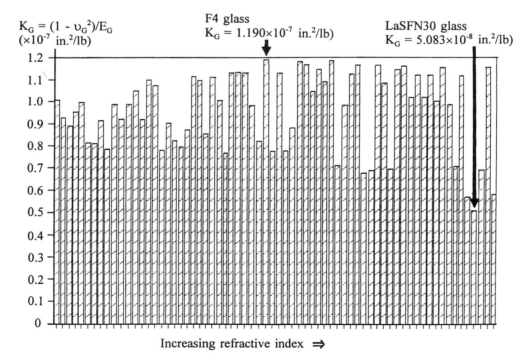

Fig. 11.1 Graphical comparison of K_G for the 68 commonly used optical glasses listed in Table B1. (From Yoder.[7])

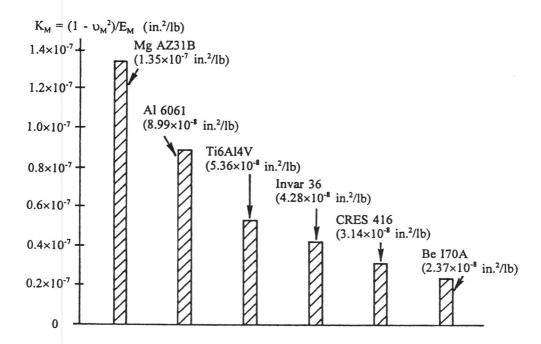

$K_M = (1 - \upsilon_M^2)/E_M$ (in.²/lb)

1.4×10⁻⁷ — Mg AZ31B (1.35×10⁻⁷ in.²/lb)

Al 6061 (8.99×10⁻⁸ in.²/lb)

Ti6Al4V (5.36×10⁻⁸ in.²/lb)

Invar 36 (4.28×10⁻⁸ in.²/lb)

CRES 416 (3.14×10⁻⁸ in.²/lb)

Be I70A (2.37×10⁻⁸ in.²/lb)

Fig. 11.2 Graphical comparison of K_M for the six metals most commonly used in optical instruments (see Table B12). (From Yoder.[7])

A geometric model of the interface between the spherical lens surface and the contacting mechanical surface is shown in Fig. 11.3. The lens here is represented by the larger cylinder of diameter D_1 while the mount is represented by the smaller cylinder of diameter D_2. Both cylinders have lengths equal to the perimeter of a circle of radius y_C or $2\pi y_C$. The cylinders are pressed against each other by the linear preload p as indicated in the figure. The annular width of the elastically deformed region is indicated as Δy.

Again applying an equation from Roark,[1] the value of K_1 in Eqs. (11.2) and (11.6) for an optomechanical interface of any geometric contour is given by

$$K_1 = (D_1 \pm D_2)/(D_1 D_2) \tag{11.5}$$

where:

D_1 = twice the lens surface radius
D_2 = twice the mechanical interface radius

The plus sign in this equation is used for convex lens surfaces [Eq. (11.5a)] and the negative sign is used for concave lens surfaces [Eq.(11.5b)]. Although it is physically

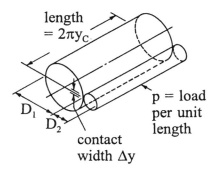

Fig. 11.3 General analytical model of the surface contact lens-to-mount interface. (Adapted from Yoder.[8])

possible in some cases for the mechanical surface to be concave, this contour is not generally used. D_1 and D_2 are both considered positive. K_1 is always positive.

The size of the elastically deformed contact area in the glass-to-metal interface depends on the same parameters as the axial contact stress. Under light preload, the contact is essentially a "line" of length $2\pi y_C$ and infinitesimal width (and area). As the preload increases, the line contact widens. The resulting area is computed as:

$$A_C = 2\pi y_C \Delta y \tag{11.6}$$

where:

$$\Delta y = 1.600 (K_2 p / K_1)^{1/2} \tag{11.7}$$

and all terms except K_1 are as defined.

The combination of Eq. (11.6) with Eq. (11.1) gives the average stress S_{AVG} in the interface. It can easily be shown that $S_C / S_{AVG} = (0.798)(1.600)$, so the peak axial contact stress is always 1.277 times the average value.

11.3.1 The sharp-corner interface

The sharp-corner interface was described in Sect. 3.6.1 as one in which the intersection of the flat and cylindrical machined surfaces on the metal part has been burnished to a radius on the order of 0.002 in. (0.051 mm).[5] This small-radius mechanical surface contacts the glass at height y_C, as shown schematically in Fig. 11.4. The angle between the intersecting machined surfaces can be 90° (as shown) or preferably >90° without affecting the analytical model.

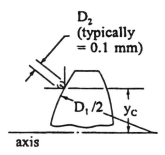

Fig. 11.4 Sectional view through the interface between a sharp corner mechanical surface and a convex lens surface. (Adapted from Yoder. [8])

Assuming D_2 for the sharp corner is always 0.004 in. (0.102 mm), substitution of this value into Eq. (11.7) gives $K_{1\,SC} = (D_1 \pm 0.004)/0.004D_1$ (in U.S. customary units) and $K_{1\,SC} = (D_1 \pm 0.100)/0.100D_1$ (in metric units). Then, for a convex or concave surface radius larger than 0.200 in. (5.080 mm), D_2 can be ignored; the value of $K_{1\,SC}$ is constant at 250/in. (10/mm).[6] The error that is due to this approximation does not exceed 2%.

Example 11.2: Peak and average axial contact stress in a lens with sharp-corner interfaces.

(For design and analysis, use File 38 of the CD-ROM)

Consider a biconvex germanium lens with the following dimensions: $D_G = 3.100$ in. (78.740 mm), $R_1 = 18.000$ in. (457.200 mm), and $R_2 = 72.000$ in. (1828.800 mm). The lens is mounted in a 6061 aluminum cell with sharp-corner interfaces at $y_C = 1.500$ in. (38.100 mm) on both surfaces. (a) What peak contact stresses are developed at each interface if the axial preload is 20.000 lb (88.964 N)? (b) What is the average contact stress in the germanium?

(a) From Table B6, $E_G = 1.504 \times 10^7$ lb/in.^{2} (1.037×10^{11} Pa) and $\upsilon_G = 0.278$.
From Table B12, $E_M = 9.9 \times 10^6$ lb/in.^{2} (6.82×10^{10} Pa) and $\upsilon_M = 0.332$.

From Eq. (11.3), $p = 20.000/[(2\pi)(1.500)] = 2.122$ lb/in. (3.716 N/cm).

From Eq. (11.4),
$$K_2 = [(1 - 0.278^2)/1.504 \times 10^7] + [(1 - 0.332^2)/9.9 \times 10^6]$$
$$= 6.135 \times 10^{-8} + 8.988 \times 10^{-8} = 1.512 \times 10^{-7} \text{ in.}^2/\text{lb } (2.193 \times 10^{-11} \text{ Pa}^{-1})$$

Since R_1 and R_2 both exceed 0.200 in. (5.080 mm), $K_{1\,SC} = 250$/in. (10/mm) for each surface.

From Eq. (11.2), $S_{C\,SC} = 0.798[(250)(2.122)/1.512\times10^{-7}]^{1/2}$
$$= 47{,}268 \text{ lb/in.}^2 \text{ (325.91 MPa) at each surface.}$$

These stress levels almost equal our rule-of-thumb tolerance of 50,000 lb/in.^{2} (345MPa), so the design is not satisfactory. Another type of glass-to-metal interface with lower stress-generating characteristics should be employed here.

(b) From Eq. (11.7), $\Delta y = 1.6[(1.512\times10^{-7})(2.122)/250]^{1/2}$
$$= 5.732\times10^{-5} \text{ in. } (1.456\times10^{-3} \text{ mm})$$

From Eq. (11.6), $A_C = (2\pi)(1.500)(5.732\times10^{-5}) = 5.402\times10^{-4} \text{ in.}^2 \ (0.348 \text{ mm}^2)$

From Eq. (11.1), $S_{AVG} = 20.000/5.402\times10^{-4}$
$$= 37{,}021 \text{ lb/in.}^2 \text{ (255.3 MPa) at each surface.}$$

Note: the ratio of $S_{A\,SC}$ to S_{AVG} is 47,268/37,021 = 1.277 as predicted above.

11.3.2 The tangential interface

The tangential interface is depicted in the sectional view (a) and analytical model (b) of Fig. 11.5. It was described in Sect. 3.6.2 as an interface in which a convex spherical lens surface contacts a conical mechanical surface. It cannot be used with a concave lens surface.

(a)   (b)

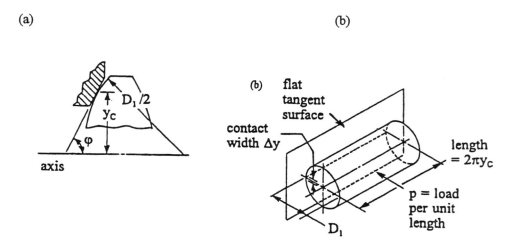

Fig. 11.5 (a) Sectional view through the tangential lens-to-mount interface. (b) Applicable analytical model of that interface. (From Yoder.[8])

The parameter D_2 of Eq. (11.5) is infinite for the conical interface. The value of K_1 for a lens surface of radius R therefore reduces to:

$$K_{1TAN} = 1/D_1 \qquad\qquad (11.8)$$

where D_1 is twice the lens surface radius.

Examination of Eq. (11.2) and Eq. (11.8) reveals that the estimated axial stress developed in a lens of a given surface radius $(D_1/2) > 0.200$ in. (5.080 mm) by a given preload with a tangential interface is smaller by a factor of $(250 D_1)^{1/2}$ than that for a sharp-corner interface.

Example 11.3: Peak and average axial contact stress in a lens with a tangent interface.

(For design and analysis, use File 39 of the CD-ROM)

(a) Repeat the calculations for surface R_1 in Example 11.2(a) with the interface changed to the tangential configuration. (b) What is the average stress in the interface?

(a) From Eq. (11.8), $K_{1\,TAN} = 0.5/18.000 = 0.0278$ in.$^{-1}$ (0.0011 mm^{-1})
From Example 11.2, $K_2 = 1.512\times10^{-7}$ in.^{2}/lb (2.193×10^{-11} Pa^{-1})
$\qquad\qquad$ P = 20.000 lb (88.964 N) $\qquad$ p = 2.122 lb/in. (371.617 Pa)

From Eq. (11.2), $S_{C\,TAN} = 0.798[(0.0278)(2.122)/1.512\times10^{-7}]^{1/2}$
$\qquad\qquad\qquad\qquad = 498$ lb/in.^{2} (3.43 MPa).

In comparison with the result of the stress calculation in Example 11.2, the stress with the tangential interface is found to be significantly reduced. We would expect the ratio $S_{C\,SC}/S_{C\,TAN}$ to be $[(250)(36)]^{1/2} = 94.9$. Not too surprisingly, this is what we obtain from 47,268/498. The advantage of the tangential interface over the sharp-corner interface from the viewpoint of peak contact stress is apparent.

(b) From Eq. (11.7), $\Delta y = 1.600[(1.512\times10^{-7}\,\text{lb/in.}^2)/0.0278]^{1/2}$
$\qquad\qquad\qquad\qquad = 0.0054$ in. (0.138 mm)

From Eq. (11.6), $A_C = (2\pi)(1.500(0.0054) = 0.0509$ in.^{2} (32.838 mm^2)

From Eq. (11.1), $S_{AVG} = 20.000/0.0509 = 392.927$ lb/in.^{2} (2.709 MPa)

The ratio of peak to average stress is 498/393 = 1.267. This is approximately as predicted for all interfaces in which Eq. (11.5) is applicable.

11.3.3 The toroidal interface

In Sect. 3.6.3, toroidal (or donut-shaped) mechanical surfaces contacting spherical lens surfaces were described. Figure 11.3 again applies, and K_1 for interfaces on convex or concave surfaces is given by Eq. (11.5) with D_1 set equal to twice the lens surface radius and D_2 set equal to twice the sectional radius (R_T) of the toroid. The choice of plus or minus sign in the equation depends, as before, on whether the lens surface is convex or concave.

Mechanical toroids contacting lens surfaces are almost always convex. The limiting case for small values of R_T would be equivalent to a sharp corner. If R_T increases to infinity and the lens surface is convex, the limiting case is the same as a tangential interface. Only a convex toroid can contact a concave lens surface. The limiting case for a large R_T then is matching radii. This is equivalent to a spherical interface.

Although it is not commonly done, a concave toroid can be used with a convex lens surface. The lower limiting case for R_T then is the matching radius (i.e., a spherical interface) while the upper limiting case for R_T then is infinity (i.e., a tangential interface).

Example 11.4: Peak axial contact stresses in a lens with toroidal interfaces. (For design and analysis, use File 40 of the CD-ROM)
Let us change the shape of the lens from Example 11.2 to a meniscus with R_1 convex and R_2 concave. The magnitudes of those radii are unchanged. (a) What is $S_{C\,TOR}$ for each surface (b) How do these compare with those for the sharp-corner and toroidal interfaces?

For reasons given in Sect. 11.3.3, we assume $D_2 = (2)(10R_1) = 360.000$ in. (9144.000 mm) at the convex surface, and $D_2 = (2)(0.5R_2) = 72.000$ in. (1828.800 mm) at the concave surface. The linear preload p is 2.122 lb/in. (371.617 Pa) and $K_2 = 1.512\times10^{-7}$ in.$^{-1}$/lb (2.193×10^{-11} Pa^{-1}) as before.

(a) At the convex surface, $D_1 = (2)(18.000) = 36.000$ in. (914.400 mm). Applying Eqs. (11.5) and (11.2):

$K_1 = (36.000 + 360.000)/[(36.000)(360.000)] = 0.0305$ in.$^{-1}$

$S_{C\,TOR} = 0.798[(0.0305)(2.122)/1.512\times10^{-7}]^{1/2} = 522$ lb/in.^{2} (3.60 MPa)

At the concave surface, $D_1 = (2)(72.000) = 144.000$ in. (3657.600 mm).

Applying Eqs. (11.5) and (11.2):

$K_1 = (144.000 - 72.000)/[(144.000)(72.000)] = 6.944\times10^{-3}$ in.$^{-1}$ (2.7340×10^{-4} mm^{-1})

$S_{C\,TOR} = 0.798[(6.944\times10^{-3})(2.122)/1.512\times10^{-7}]^{1/2} = 249$ lb/in.^{2} (1.72 MPa)

(b) We note that the contact stresses at both surfaces are reduced significantly from those with a sharp-corner interface. Here they are the same order of magnitude as that with the tangential interface on the convex surface. Since a toroid also works well with a concave surface, it is seen to be a favorable type of interface.

11.3.4 The spherical interface

Spherical mechanical contact on a convex or concave lens surface (discussed in Sect. 3.6.4) distributes axial preloads over large annular areas and hence can be nearly stress free. If the surfaces match closely (i.e., within a few wavelengths of light) in radius, the contact stress equals the total preload divided by the annular area of contact per Eq. (11.1). Since the area is relatively large, the stress is almost always small and it is usually ignored. If the surfaces do not match closely, the contact can degenerate into a small annular area or even a line (i.e., a sharp-corner interface). Either of these alternatives would be unfavorable because of the high potential for stress generation.

11.3.5 The flat-bevel interface

In Sect. 3.6.5 we considered flat-bevel interfaces. As in the case of the spherical interface, the contact stresses that are due to axial preloads (total preload/contact area) are inherently small because the area of contact is large. Therefore these stresses may be ignored. However, if the contacting surfaces are not truly flat and parallel, the area of contact will decrease and the stress will increase. In the limit, line contact (i.e., a sharp-corner interface) occurs. This could lead to high localized stress.

11.4 Parametric Comparisons of Interface Types

Figure 11.6 shows the variation of axial stress with radius of the contacting mechanical surface for a particular design having a given convex lens surface with R = 1.000 in. (25.400 mm), a given lens diameter of 2.000 in. (50.800 mm), and a given mechanical linear preload p of 1.000 lb/in. (0.175 N/mm). The lens is made of BK7 glass and the mounting is made of 6061 aluminum. Both the stress and the mechanical surface radius are plotted logarithmically to cover large ranges of variability. At the left is the short radius characteristic of the sharp-corner interface (at the dashed vertical line) while at the right, the tangential interface case is approached asymptotically. Between these extremes are an infinite number of toroidal interface designs. The "preferred" minimum toroidal radius (equal to 10R) for which the stress is within 5% of the value that would exist with a tangential interface is indicated by the small circle.[8] This particular value of toroidal radius was used at the convex surface in Example 11.4.

Figure 11.7 shows a similar relationship for a concave lens surface example. All

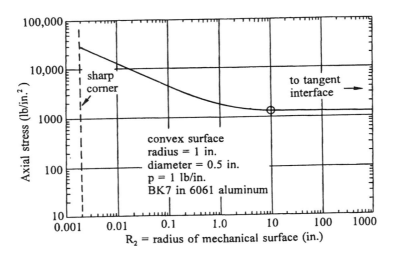

Fig. 11.6 Variation of contact stress in a typical preloaded convex lens surface as a function of sectional radius of the mechanical contacting surface. (Adapted from Yoder.[6])

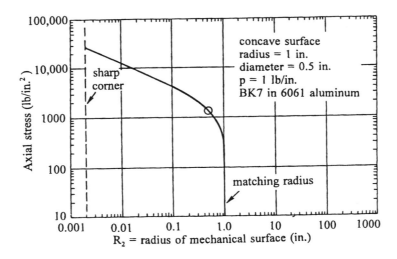

Figure 11.7 Variation of contact stress in a typical preloaded concave lens surface as a function of sectional radius of the mechanical contacting surface. (Adapted from Yoder.[8])

parameters are the same as in Fig. 11.6. The sharp-corner case is again represented by the dashed vertical line at the left. As the toroidal corner radius increases toward the matching radius limit (which is equivalent to the spherical interface), the stress decreases. The circle represents the "preferred" minimum toroidal radius of 0.5R at which the stress will approximate the value that would prevail at the same preload on a convex surface of the same radius using a 10R toroidal interface.[9] This particular value of toroidal radius was used at the interface with the concave surface in Example 11.4.

Figures 11.6 and 11.7 show conclusively that the axial contact stress is always significantly higher with a sharp-corner interface than with any other type of interface. This author recommends that whenever a slightly higher manufacturing cost than that associated with the sharp-corner interface can be tolerated, tangential interfaces be used on all convex lens surfaces, and toroidal interfaces of a radius of approximately 0.5R be used on all concave surfaces.

Figure 11.8 shows what happens to the axial contact stress for a 0.500-in. (12.700-mm)-diameter BK7 lens surface with a convex radius of 1.000 in. (2.540 mm) if the linear preload p is changed by factors of 10 from 0.01 to 10 lb/in. (1.75×10^{-3} to 1.75 N/mm). Figure 11.9 shows a similar relationship for a concave surface with all other parameters unchanged.

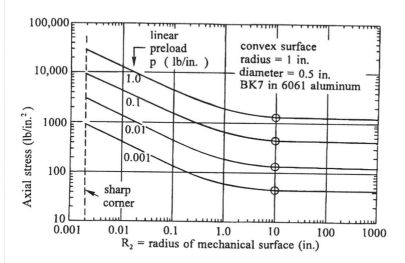

Fig. 11.8 Variation of axial contact stress in a typical preloaded convex lens surface as functions of the mechanical interface radius and linear preload. (Adapted from Yoder.[8])

If the total axial preload P on a lens with any type of interface and any surface radius increases from P_1 to P_2 while all other parameters remain fixed, the resulting axial

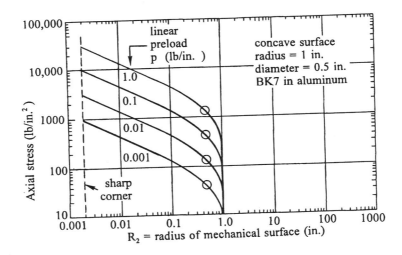

Fig. 11.9 Variation of axial contact stress in a typical preloaded concave lens surface as functions of mechanical interface radius and linear preload. (Adapted from Yoder.[8])

contact stress changes by a factor of $(P_2/P_1)^{1/2}$. A tenfold increase in preload therefore increases the stress by a factor of 3.162.

Figures 11.10 and 11.11 show how the axial contact stress varies as the surface radius of a 2.00-in. (50.800-mm)-diameter BK7 lens is changed by successive factors of 10 for convex and concave surface cases, respectively. The preload is held constant [p = 1.0 lb/in. (0.175 N/mm)]. The stress is seen to be independent of the surface radius or its algebraic sign (i.e., convex or concave) for a sharp-corner interface (at the left side of each graph). The greatest changes occur for long-radii toroids on either type of surface. The limits are the tangential interface and the matching radii interface for the convex surface and the concave surface cases, respectively. Once again, the toroids indicated by the circles on each curve (toroid radius = 10R for convex surfaces and 0.5R for concave surfaces) are the recommended minimum sectional radii for the mechanical component. Use of toroids with longer radii than these recommended minimums would, of course, cause the contact stresses to approach even more closely the lower values obtained with tangential or matching radius interfaces for convex and concave surfaces, respectively.

If the surface radius changes from R_i to R_j with all other parameters unchanged, the corresponding contact stress with long-radius toroidal interfaces changes by $(R_i/R_j)^{1/2}$. Hence, for the 10:1 step increases in surface radius depicted in Figs. 11.8 and 11.9, the stress decreases by a factor of $(1/10)^{1/2} = 0.316$ between steps.

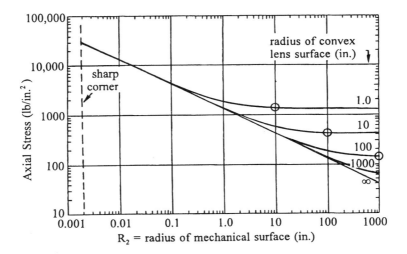

Fig. 11.10 Variation of axial contact stress in a typical preloaded convex lens surface as a function of mechanical interface radius and lens surface radius. (Adapted from Yoder.[6])

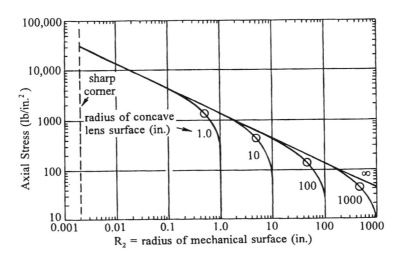

Fig. 11.11 Variation of axial contact stress in a typical preloaded concave lens surface as a function of mechanical interface radius and lens surface radius. (Adapted from Yoder.[6])

11.5 Contact Stress in a Lens Clamped with Spring Clips

11.5.1 Springs with spherical pads

In Sect. 3.5, techniques for axially constraining a lens with multiple spring clips were discussed. Figures 3.19 and 3.20 show typical schematic designs applicable to a rotationally symmetrical lens and a rectangular lens, respectively. The actual interface between the glass surface and the metal surface in each of these designs is at the squared-off end of the spring. This end may be rough with burrs or other defects that present the potential for force, and hence stress, concentration. Even if the metal parts are machined perfectly, they contact the curved glass surface with a sharp edge at points located nominally at the centers of the spring ends. Because of uncertainties in tolerance buildup, the locations and shapes of the interfaces may not be predictable.

It would be preferable to add convex spherical pads to the ends of the springs in somewhat the same manner as cylindrical pads were added to the spring clips holding the prisms in Figs. 7.5, 7.8, and 7.9(b). Then the interfaces will be deterministic, so the stresses at the contacts can be predicted. Within-tolerance machining and assembly errors such as those in the spring deflections or angles would move the contact point only slightly on the curved pad. They would not significantly affect the constraint on the lens.

Models for these interfaces are illustrated in Fig. 11.12. Shown are convex spherical pads contacting: (a) a convex spherical optical surface, (b) a concave optical surface, and (c) a flat optical surface.

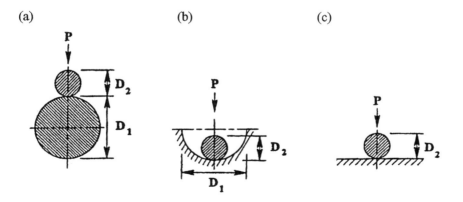

Fig. 11.12 Possible conditions for point contact of elastic bodies. (a) A convex spherical pad touching a convex sphere (lens or mirror). (b) A convex spherical pad touching a concave sphere (lens or mirror). (c) A convex pad touching a flat (lens, mirror, or prism) surface.

Note that in general, either body may be the optic (glass) and the other body the mechanical interface (metal). D_1 and D_2 are then defined as the larger and smaller diameters, respectively. While they are theoretically possible, concave pads are generally not used. In fact, successful designs with point contacts against optical surfaces are rare. The reason for this will be obvious from stress calculation examples using the following equations that were derived from Roark [1].

For all three geometric cases shown in Fig. 11.12, the peak axial contact stress at the center of the contact area is estimated from:

$$S_{C \, SPH} = 0.918 (K_1^2 P_i / K_2^2)^{1/3} \tag{11.9}$$

where:

P_i = preload per spring

$$K_1 = (D_1 + D_2)/(D_1 D_2) \tag{11.5a}$$

$$K_1 = (D_1 - D_2)/(D_1 D_2) \tag{11.5b}$$

$$K_1 = 1/D_1 \tag{11.8}$$

D_1 = twice the radius of the first body
D_2 = twice the radius of the second body

$$K_2 = [(1 - v_G^2)/E_G] + [(1 - v_M^2)/E_M] \tag{11.4}$$

The radius r_C of the circular contact area formed at the interface between a spherical pad and surfaces of different shapes on optical components when those surfaces deform elastically under preload can be calculated from Eq. (11.10). The corresponding area A_C of that circular contact is calculated from Eq. (11.11).

$$r_C = 0.721 (P_i K_2 / K_1)^{1/3} \tag{11.10}$$

$$A_C = \pi r_C^2 \tag{11.11}$$

All terms in these equations are as defined earlier.

Calculations of the peak and average stresses in the glass for the three cases shown in Fig. 11.12 are given in Examples 11.5 through 11.7.

Example 11.5: A convex spherical pad on a cantilevered spring contacting a convex lens surface.
(For design and analysis, use File 41 of the CD-ROM)
Convex spherical pads made of 6061 aluminum and having radii of 1.600 in. (40.640 mm) attached to the ends of three cantilevered springs press directly against the polished convex surface of a 4.310-in. (109.463-mm)-diameter LaSFN30 lens. The total axial preload is 12.500 lb (55.60 N). The radius of curvature of the lens surface is 16.000 in. (406.400 mm). What are (a) the peak and (b) the average stresses in the glass?

From Tables B1 and B12: E_G = 1.80×10^7 lb/in.^{2} (1.24×10^{11} Pa) and υ_G = 0.293
$\qquad\qquad\qquad\qquad\quad$ E_M = 9.9×10^6 lb/in.^{2} (6.82×10^{10} Pa) and υ_M = 0.332

For the lens, D_1 = (2)(16.000) = 32.000 in. (812.800 mm)
For the pad, D_2 = (2)(1.600) = 3.200 in. (81.280 mm)
At each spring, P_i = 12.500/3 = 4.166 lb (18.531 N)

From Eq. (11.5a): K_1 = (32.000 + 3.200)/[(32.000)(3.200)]

$\qquad\qquad\qquad$ = 0.344 in.$^{-1}$ (0.0135 mm^{-1})

From Eq. (11.4), K_2 = [(1 - 0.293^2)/1.80×10^7] + [(1 - 0.332^2)/9.9×10^6]
$\qquad\qquad\qquad$ = 1.407×10^{-7} in.^{2}/ lb (2.041×10^{-11} Pa^{-1})

(a) From Eq. (11.6), $S_{C\ SPH}$ = 0.918[(0.344)^2 (4.166)/(1.407×10^{-7})^2]$^{1/3}$
$\qquad\qquad\qquad\qquad$ = 26,780 lb/in.^{2} (184.6 MPa)

(b) From Eq. (11.10), r_C = 0.721[(4.166)(1.407×10^{-7})/0.344]$^{1/3}$
$\qquad\qquad\qquad\qquad$ = 0.0086 in. (0.219 mm)

From Eq. (11.11), A_C = π(0.0086)^2 = 2.323×10^{-4} in.^{2} (0.150 mm^2)

From Eq. (11.1), S_{AVE} = 4.166/2.323×10^{-4} = 17,934 lb/in.^{2} (123.6 MPa)

These compressive stresses are too great in comparison to our rule-of-thumb tolerance of 50,000 lb/in.^{2} (345 MPa). Possible design modifications that would tend to reduce stress would be to increase the pad radius and/or to increase the number of springs. A pad radius increase by a factor of 100 and doubling the number of springs would reduce the peak stress to 4580 lb/in.^{2} (31.6 MPa) and make the design much better. An even better solution for this sized lens would be to use an optomechanical interface with inherently lower stress such as one with a circular flange or threaded retaining ring and a tangential interface.

Example 11.6: A convex spherical pad on a cantilevered spring contacting a concave lens surface.
(For design and analysis, use File 42 of the CD-ROM)
Repeat Example 11.5 with the lens surface concave instead of convex. The magnitude of the surface radius remains the same. What are (a) the peak and (b) the average stresses in this lens?

From Example 11.5: $D_1 = 32.000$ in. (812.800 mm)
$D_2 = 3.200$ in. (81.280 mm)
$P_i = 4.166$ lb (18.531 N)
$K_2 = 1.407 \times 10^{-7}$ in.$^{-1}$ / lb (2.041×10^{-11} Pa^{-1})

From Eq. (11.5b), $K_1 = (32.000 - 3.200)/(32.000)(3.200)$
$= 0.281$ in.$^{-1}$ (0.011 mm^{-1})

(a) From Eq. (11.6), $S_{C\ SPH} = 0.918[(0.281)^2 (4.166)/(1.407 \times 10^{-7})^2]^{1/3}$
$= 23,400$ lb/in.^{2} (161.3 MPa)

(b) From Eq. (11.10), $r_C = 0.721[(4.166)(1.407 \times 10^{-7})/0.281]^{1/3}$
$= 0.0092$ in. (0.234 mm)

From Eq. (11.11), $A_C = \pi(0.0092)^2 = 2.659 \times 10^{-4}$ in.^{2} (0.172 mm^2)

From Eq. (11.1, $S_{AVE} = 4.166/2.659 \times 10^{-4} = 15,668$ lb/in.^{2} (108.0 MPa)

The peak stress is about 13% smaller than the design with a convex lens surface, but once again, this is not a good design. The changes suggested in Example 11.5 would make it better.

Example No. 11.7: Convex spherical pad on a cantilevered spring pressing against a flat lens surface.
(For design and analysis, use File 43 of the CD-ROM)
Repeat Example 11.5 with the lens surface flat instead of convex. All other parameters remain the same. What are (a) the peak and (b) the average stresses in the lens?

From Example 11.5: $D_2 = 3.200$ in. (81.280 mm)
$P_i = 4.166$ lb (18.531 N)
$K_2 = 1.407 \times 10^{-7}$ in.$^{-1}$ /lb (2.041×10^{-11} Pa^{-1})

From Eq. (11.8), $K_1 = 1/3.200 = 0.312$ in.$^{-1}$ (0.012 mm^{-1})

(a) By Eq. (11.6), $S_{C\,SPH} = 0.918[(0.312)^2 (4.166)/(1.407\times10^{-7})^2]^{1/3}$
$$= 25{,}093 \text{ lb/in.}^2 \text{ (173.0 MPa)}$$

(b) From Eq. (11.10), $r_C = 0.721[(4.166)(1.407\times10^{-7})/0.312]^{1/3}$
$$= 0.0089 \text{ in. (0.226 mm)}$$

From Eq. (11.11), $A_C = \pi(0.0089)^2 = 2.488\times10^{-4} \text{ in.}^2 \text{ (0.160 mm}^2)$

From Eq. (11.1, $S_{AVE} = 4.166/2.488\times10^{-4} = 16{,}744 \text{ lb/in.}^2 \text{ (115.4 MPa)}$

The peak stress is larger than would be desired, so this design is not satisfactory. The changes suggested in Example 11.5 would make it better. If it is carefully made to be parallel to the lens surface, a flat pad could be used. The stresses would then be significantly reduced.

If we divide Eq. (11.10) by Eq. (11.1) using Eqs. (11.12) and (11.11) to determine A_C, we find that all the variables cancel and the ratio of $S_{C\,SPH}$ to S_{AVG} is 1.50 for all spherical pad interface designs. The ratios of calculated stress values in Examples 11.5 through 11.7 correspond closely to this number.

11.5.2 Springs with cylindrical pads

As an alternative to the use of spherical pads between a spring and the optical surface of a lens as described in Sect. 11.5.1, we could provide convex cylindrical pads as the optomechanical interface. Typically, such a pad would be oriented crosswise on the end of the spring and its axial length would equal the width b of the spring. Alternatively, the cylindrical axis could be oriented parallel to the cantilevered length of the spring. A cylindrical pad cannot be used with a concave lens surface. Point contact between the cylinder and the convex spherical lens would occur under light axial loading. With greater preload, the elastic bodies would deform and contact would occur over a small area. From the viewpoint of contact stress, of a cylindrical pad over a spherical one is slight when the lens surface is convex. This advantage increases when the lens surface becomes flat, so the primary use of the cylindrical pad is to provide preload against the outer edges of the faces of plano optical surfaces or against flat or step bevels on curved lens surfaces.

The contact stress in a cylindrical pad interface with a flat optical surface is quantified by Eq. (11.2) with $K_1 = 1/D_2$ as given by Eq. (11.8). The D_2 used in the latter equation is now twice the radius R_{CYL} of the pad. Example 11.8 illustrates this case.

For a constant preload, the stress in a lens with localized point or short line contacts as provided by spherical or cylindrical pads will always be larger than that caused by the annular line contact from a tangential or toroidal interface on a threaded retainer or circular flange. This is due to the larger contact regions with the latter interfaces. From a stress viewpoint, annular contacts would be preferred.

Example 11.8: Cylindrical pad on a cantilevered spring pressing against a flat lens surface.
(For design and analysis, use File 44 of the CD-ROM)
Repeat Example 11.7 with a cylindrical pad of sectional radius R_{CYL} of 1.600 in. (40.640 mm). Assume that the pad length equals the width b of the spring, which is 0.125 in. (3.175 mm). What is now the stress in the glass?

From Example 11.7: D_2 = 3.200 in. (81.280 mm)
P_i = 4.166 lb (18.531 N)
K_2 = 1.407×10^{-7} in.$^{-1}$ (2.041×10^{-11} Pa^{-1})

From Eq. (11.8): K_1 = 1/3.200 = 0.312 in^{-1} (0.012 mm^{-1})

The linear preload p_i = P_i/b = 4.166/0.125 = 33.328 lb/in. (3.765 N/m)

From Eq. (11.2):
$S_{C\ CYL}$ = $0.798[(0.312)(33.328)/1.407 \times 10^{-7})]^{1/2}$ = 6866 lb/in.^{2} (47.3 MPa)

This contact stress is only about one-fourth that produced with the same preload by a spherical pad contact per Example 11.7. If the pad were made longer and/or its sectional radius increased, the stress advantage of the cylindrical pad version over the spherical pad version would be even greater.

11.6 Contact Stress in Small Clamped Mirrors

Figure 11.13 shows three typical interfaces between mechanical parts and small mirrors. In each case, the mirror is clamped in place, with the preload applied by retainers or springs. Figure 11.13(a) features a sharp corner interface on the convex spherical surface of the mirror. The stress in the mirror that is due to the preload would be estimated in the same manner as described in Sect. 11.3.1 for a lens with that type of interface. One would expect this stress to be relatively large. The stress at the retainer on the flat back surface of the mirror in this mounting configuration would be low because of the large area of contact.

Figure 11.13(b) shows two interfaces on a small Mangin mirror. The left interface is a toroidal mechanical surface contacting a flat bevel on the edge of the aperture of the mirror's concave surface. The stress in the mirror that is due to the preload at that interface would be estimated in the same manner as described in Sect. 11.3.2 for a lens with a tangent interface. There K_1 is 0.5 divided by the radius of the toroid.

The convex surface of the mirror in Fig. 11.13(b) has a tangential mechanical

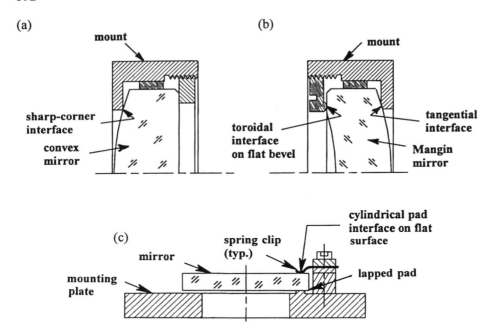

Fig. 11.13 Typical optomechanical interfaces on small mirrors.

interface. The stress in the glass there would also be estimated using the method described in Sect. 11.3.2. Here, K_1 would be 0.5 divided by the radius of the optical surface. Although the preload is the same at both surfaces, the stresses at the bevel and at the convex surface would be somewhat different because the radii contacting the flat surface and the cone are in general different.

Figure 11.13(c) shows a flat mirror preloaded by one of several springs. The convex cylindrical surface of the spring touches a flat glass surface, so the stress there is estimated as indicated in Sect. 11.5.2 for a lens surface contacted in the same manner. Assuming intimate contact between the flat surfaces at the pads opposite the spring contacts, we can estimate the average stress over those contact areas using Eq. (11.1). The same equation can be used to estimate the average stress at the annular interface between the retainer and flat surface of the mirror in Fig. 11.13(a).

The stress in a convex or concave mirror contacted on its optical surface by a toroidal mechanical interface would be estimated by the method described in Sect. 11.3.3 for a lens.

11.7 Contact Stress in Clamped Prisms

11.7.1 Contact stress with curved interfaces

The preferred design concepts for spring-to-prism and locating-pin interfaces described in Sect. 7.1 involve flat (extended area), cylindrical (line), or spherical (point) contacts. From a stress-buildup viewpoint, the larger the area, the less the stress. As mentioned earlier, the flat interface is subject to degeneration into line contact if tolerances are not closely held, so its potential stress advantage may not be achieved. By choosing the contact radius on spring-loaded pads carefully, the stress with a given preload and either a cylindrical or spherical interface can be significantly reduced from that which would occur at a sharp-corner interface for the same preload. The curved interface also offers the advantage that the tilt of the spring end as the spring deflects will not change the nature of the contact or appreciably affect the free length, L, of the spring. This feature is illustrated in Fig. 7.12.

If the mechanical contact interface with a flat prism surface is cylindrical, the geometry of Fig. 11.14 applies. Because $K_1 = 1/D_2 = 0.5/R_{CYL}$ in this case, Eq. (11.2) can

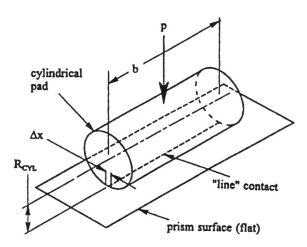

Fig. 11.14 Geometric model of a cylindrical pad interface on a flat prism surface.

be rewritten in the following form and used to estimate the stress, $S_{C\ CYL}$ in the prism. Equation 11.12 results.

$$S_{C\ CYL} = 0.564 [p_i/(R_{CYL} K_2)]^{1/2} \tag{11.12}$$

where:

        p = linear preload = P_i/b
        P_i = total preload per spring = P/N

N = number of springs
b = length of cylindrical contact
R_{CYL} = cylindrical radius of the surface contacting the prism

$$K_2 = [(1 - v_G^2)/E_G] + [(1 - v_M^2)/E_M] \qquad (11.4)$$

v_G and E_G are Poisson's ratio and Young's modulus for the glass (prism)
v_M and E_M are Poisson's ratio and Young's modulus for the metal (pad)

The prism and the pad are assumed to be elastic in this analysis, so the force that presses them together causes each material to deform slightly along the line of contact. The deformed region is a rectangle of size b by Δx (see Fig. 11.14). Equation (11.13) is used to calculate Δx.

$$\Delta x = 2.263 (p_i R_{CYL} K_2)^{1/2} \qquad (11.13)$$

If we divide the contact preload per spring by the contact area for that spring, we obtain the average stress in the contact region as indicated in Eq. (11.14). All terms in Eqs. (11.13) and (11.14) are as defined earlier.

$$S_{AVG} = P_i/(b\Delta x) \qquad (11.14)$$

The value of $S_{C\ CYL}$ derived from Eq. (11.12) is the peak stress along the line parallel to b at the center of the rectangular contact area. It can be shown analytically by dividing Eq. (11.12) by Eq. (11.14) that the peak stress is always 1.277 times the average stress.

Example 11.9: Contact stress in a prism with a spring-loaded cylindrical pad interface.
(For design and analysis, use File 45 of the CD-ROM)
Assume that a preload of 4.167 lb (18.535 N) is applied by a cylindrical pad to a "line" contact of length b = 0.637 in. (16.180 mm) at the top of a BK7 prism. Let the spring and integral pad be made of titanium. Assume in turn that the radius of the pad is 0.1, 1, and 10 in. Calculate $S_{C\ CYL}$ and $S_{C\ AVG}$ for each case. What conclusions can be drawn from these calculations?

R_{CYL}	given	(in.)	0.1	1.0	10
v_G	Table B1		0.208	0.208	0.208
E_G	Table B1	(lb/in.²)	$1.17{\times}10^7$	$1.17{\times}10^7$	$1.17{\times}10^7$
v_M	Table B12		0.310	0.310	0.310
E_M	Table B12	(lb/in.²)	$1.65{\times}10^7$	$1.65{\times}10^7$	$1.65{\times}10^7$
K_2	Eq. (11.4)	(in.²/lb)	$1.366{\times}10^{-7}$	$1.366{\times}10^{-7}$	$1.366{\times}10^{-7}$

P_i	given	(lb)	4.167	4.167	4.167
p_i	P_i/b	(lb/in.)	6.5411	6.5411	6.5411
$S_{C\,CYL}$	Eq. (11.13)	(lb/in.^{2})	12,344	3904	1234
Δx	Eq. (11.14)	(in.)	6.764×10^{-4}	2.139×10^{-3}	6.764×10^{-3}
S_{AVG}	Eq. (11.15)	(lb/in.^{2})	9672	3058	967
$S_{C\,CYL}/S_{AVG}$			1.276	1.276	1.276

Conclusions: (1) longer R_{CYL} give lower stresses, (2) stresses shown here do not pose any damage problems, and (3) the ratio of $S_{C\,CYL}$ to S_{AVG} is as indicated in the text.

Note that the spring deflection required to produce the specified preload is not affected by a change in pad radius.

Examination of Eq. (11.12) shows that a change in R_{CYL} from one value to another would change $S_{C\,CYL}$ by $[(R_{CYL})_2/(R_{CYL})_1]^{1/2}$. The changes in Example 11.9 were by factors of 10, so we would expect the corresponding changes in $S_{C\,CYL}$ to be by factors of $10^{1/2} = 3.162$. This is the case.

We might extrapolate the cylindrical pad dimensional changes of Example 11.9 in the direction of reducing the cylindrical radius further. For $R_{CYL} = 0.002$ in. (0.051 mm) corresponding to a burnished sharp edge, S_{CYL} would increase to 87,650 lb/in.^{2} (604.3 MPa), which would greatly exceed the rule-of-thumb compression tolerance of 50,000 lb/in.^{2}. Hence, "line" contact such as might occur at the machined end of a flat spring that does not have a pad (see Fig. 11.15) could be dangerous because the radius of the sharp metal edge is extremely small. This interface configuration should be avoided.

The analytical technique for estimating stress at cylindrical pad interfaces can be used to estimate the stress produced when a prism is spring loaded against cylindrical pins provided in mounts as locating references. Typical designs are shown in Figs. 7.2, 7.3, and 7.5. An example of such a calculation is given in Sect. 13.27.

If the curved mechanical pad interface with the flat prism surface were to be changed to a spherical contour and all other design features remained constant, Equation 11.9 could be used to estimate the peak contact stress in the glass region surrounding the "point" contact. The radius, r_C, of the elastically deformed circular contact region and the area of that region are given by Eqs. (11.10) and (11.11). The average stress in the contact area could then be estimated using Equation 11.1. The ratio of peak stress to average stress can be shown to be 1.50. Example 11.10 illustrates these calculations.

It can be shown that changing R_{SPH} by some factor, f_R, changes $S_{C\,SPH}$ by $f_R^{-3/2}$ so if the factor is 10 as in Example 11.10, we would expect the $S_{C\,SPH}$ changes to be $10^{2/3}$ or 4.64. This is borne out approximately by the calculations in the example.

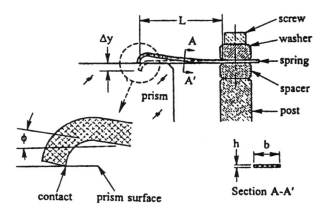

Fig. 11.15 Possible interface of a flat spring end with a prism surface. Excessive stress may well be generated in the glass.

Example 11.10: Contact stress in a prism with a spring-loaded spherical pad interface.
(For design and analysis, use File 46 of the CD-ROM)

Repeat Example 11.9 assuming spherical interfaces with R_{SPH} = 0.1, 1.0, and 10.0 in. What conclusions can be drawn?

R_{SPH}	given	(in.)	0.1	1.0	10.0
υ_G	Table B1		0.208	0.208	0.208
E_G	Table B1	(lb/in.^{2})	1.17×10^7	1.17×10^7	1.17×10^7
υ_M	Table B12		0.310	0.310	0.310
E_M	Table B12	(lb/in.^{2})	1.65×10^7	1.65×10^7	1.65×10^7
K_1	Eq. (11.8)	(in.$^{-1}$)	5.0000	0.5000	0.0500
K_2	Eq. (11.4)	(in.^{2}/lb)	1.366×10^{-7}	1.366×10^{-7}	1.366×10^{-7}
P_i	given	(lb)	4.1667	4.1667	4.1667
$S_{C\ SPH}$	Eq. (11.9)	(lb/in.^{2})	162,456	35,048	7552
r_C	Eq. (11.10)	(in.)	0.0035	0.0075	0.0162
S_{AVG}	Eq. (11.11)	(lb/in.^{2})	108,270	23,579	5054
$S_{C\ SPH}/S_{AVG}$			1.500	1.486	1.494

Conclusions: We see that (1) a longer R_{SPH} gives lower stresses; (2) these contact stresses do not pose severe glass damage problems for a R_{SPH} greater than a few inches; and (3) the ratio of $S_{C\ SPH}$ to S_{AVG} for each case is as indicated in the text.

11.7.2 Contact stress at flat prism locating pads

In many prism mounting designs, the edge dimensions d_p of each locating pad touching the surface of the prism opposite the spring clip interfaces are set to equal the width b of the spring. Typically, each pad is circular. In such designs, the localized contact stress, S_{PAD}, is estimated from Eq. (11.15). This stress should be compared with the rule-of-thumb glass compressive tolerance of 50,000 lb/in.^{2} to determine what safety factor exists in the design.

$$S_{PAD} = 4P_i/(\pi b^2) \hspace{4cm} (11.15)$$

This equation can easily be adjusted to accommodate other pad shapes.

Example 11.11: Contact stress in a prism at a locating pad.
(For design and analysis, use File 47 of the CD-ROM)
Let the spring forces in Example 11.10 be applied normally to three coplanar circular flat areas of diameter = 0.637 in. (16.180 mm) at the base of the prism. Using data from that example, calculate the average stress, S_{PAD} , in the prism.

From Example 11.10: P_i = 4.1667 lb
$\hspace{3.5cm}$ b = 0.637 in.

From Eq. (11.15), $\hspace{0.5cm} S_{PAD}$ = (4)(4.1667)/[$(\pi)(0.637)^2$] = 13.1 lb/in.^{2} (90,300 Pa).

As might be expected, this stress is negligible.

11.8 Tensile Stress in the Single-Sided Bonded Interface

A prism bonded on one side must depend upon the tensile and shear strength of the adhesive joint for integrity of the bond. If it is bonded on two opposite sides, significantly greater reliability exists because an opposing force is felt at the second interface whenever the prism tries to pull away from the first interface. We consider here a means for estimating the stress in the bonding joint under acceleration or shock loading that tends to separate the optical component from the mechanical one in a design typified by Figs. 7.17 through 7.20.

Equation (7.9) gave the minimum bond area Q_{MIN} for a prism with weight W to withstand an acceleration a_G with a safety factor f_S if the adhesive joint has a strength J. Rewriting that equation in terms of the actual area rather than the minimum value, we obtain

$$Q = W a_G f_S / J \qquad\qquad\qquad [7.9(a)]$$

In a simple prism such as a cube, right angle, Porro or penta prism, having no roof or other nonsymmetrical feature and in which the bond covers the entire base area Q of the prism polyhedron, $W = $ (base area)(height)(density) $= Qh\rho$. Usually the prism optical aperture is round and, to a close approximation, the prism edge dimension A equals the aperture diameter. Hence $h = A$ and $W = QA\rho$. Substituting this in Equation 7.9(a) we obtain

$$a_G = J / (A\rho f_S) \qquad\qquad\qquad (11.16)$$

In a more complex prism design such as an Amici, a roof penta, or any other prism having a bonding area Q not equal to the prism base area, the volume of the prism must be determined before we can calculate W. In those cases,

$$a_G = JQ / (V\rho f_S) \qquad\qquad\qquad (11.17)$$

For any given bonded prism assembly, the adequacy of the bond under the expected worst-case acceleration should be confirmed experimentally.

Example 11.12: Stress in a prism and epoxy bond under acceleration.
(For design and analysis, use File 48 of the CD-ROM)
Assume the bonded roof penta prism shown in Fig. 7.17 is subjected to test vibration loads perpendicular to the bonded face equal to 1500 and 4200 times gravity. If the bond has a strength of 2500 lb/in.^{2}, the prism weight is 0.25 lb, and the bond area Q is 0.785 in.^{2}, what is the safety factor for the joint under these loads?

(a) At 1500 × gravity loading: $a_G = 1500 = (2500)(0.785)/[(0.25)(f_S)]$ so $f_S = 5.23$

(b) At 4200× gravity loading: $a_G = 4200 = (2500)(0.785)/[(0.25)(f_S)]$ so $f_S = 1.87$

In part (b), the safety factor is too small so we might expect that the joint may fail under the indicated level of shock or vibration even if that joint is "well-made."

11.9 Bending Stresses in Circular Aperture Clamped Optics

11.9.1 Causes of bending

If, a lens, window, or small circular mirror is clamped axially by a retainer or flange and the annular areas of contact between the mount and the optic's surfaces are not directly opposite (i.e., at the same height from the axis on both sides), a bending moment is created within the optic by the applied axial preload. This moment tends to deform the optic so that one surface becomes more convex and the other surface becomes more concave as illustrated schematically in Fig. 11.16. Deformation of the optical surface(s) may adversely affect the performance of the component. The same effect occurs in noncircular optics.

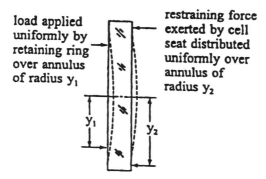

Fig. 11.16 Geometry allowing the estimation of bending moments from axial preloads applied at different heights on opposite sides of a plane parallel plate. (Adapted from Bayar.[10])

When bent, the surface that becomes more convex is placed in tension, while the other surface is compressed. Since glass-type materials break much more easily in tension than in compression (especially if the surface is scratched or has subsurface damage) catastrophic failure may occur if the bending effect is large. The "rule-of-thumb" tolerance for tensile stress given earlier [1000 lb/in.^{2} (68.9 MPa)] applies.

11.9.2 Bending stress in the optical component

Bayar[10] indicated that an analytical model based upon a thin plane parallel plate (as in Fig. 11.16) that uses an equation from Roark[1] applies also to simple lenses. We here extend the analogy to include circular windows and small circular, unperforated mirrors. The degree of approximation depends, in part, on the curvature of the surfaces. Greater curvature decreases the accuracy of the calculation.

The tensile stress in a surface made more convex by bending is given approximately by:

(11.18)

$$S_T = K_6 K_7 / t_E^2$$

where:

P = total axial preload (including an acceleration component as appropriate)

$$K_6 = 3P/(2\pi m) \tag{11.19}$$

$$K_7 = 0.5(m-1) + (m+1)\ln\frac{y_2}{y_1} - (m-1)\frac{y_1^2}{2y_2^2} \tag{11.20}$$

P = total axial preload (including an acceleration component as appropriate)
m = 1/Poisson's ratio υ_G for the glass
t_E = edge or axial thickness of the optic (whichever is the smaller)
y_1 = smaller contact height
y_2 = larger contact height

We should compare the stress from this equation with the tension survival tolerance of 1000 lb/in.² (6.9 MPa). To decrease the probability of breakage from this cause, the contact heights should be made as equal as possible. Increasing the optic's thickness also tends to reduce this danger.

Example 11.13: Bending (tensile) stress in a mirror.
(For design and analysis, use File 49 of the CD-ROM)
A 20.0-in. (50.8-cm)-diameter plane parallel solid fused silica mirror with a diameter-to-thickness ratio of 10:1 is contacted by a toroidal shoulder at $y_1 = 9.50$ in. (24.13 cm) on one side and by a toroidal clamping flange at $y_2 = 9.88$ in. (25.09 cm) on the opposite side. Assume that the total applied preload is 2000 lb (8.90×10^3 N) at low temperature. What tensile stress is created in the bent mirror?

From Table B8a, $\upsilon_G = 0.17$ so m = $1/\upsilon_G$ = 5.882
                t_E = 20.0/10 = 2.000 in. (5.080 cm)

From Eq. (11.19), K_6 = (3)(2000)/[(2π)(5.882)] = 162.348 lb

From Eq. (11.20), K_7 = [(0.5)(5.882 - 1)] + [(5.882 + 1)ln(9.88/9.50)]
                        - {(5.882 - 1)(9.50²)/[(2)(9.88²)]} = 0.454

From Eq. (11.18), S_T = (162.348)(0.454)/(2.00²) = 294.824 lb/in.² (2.03 MPa).

This is well under the survival tolerance for glass-type materials, so the danger of damage is quite low.

11.9.3 Change in surface sag of a bent optic

The following equation for the change in sagittal depth at the center of a plate such as that shown in Fig. 11.16 that is due to the bending moment exerted by the unsymmetrical mounting interface was derived from Roark[1] :

$$\Delta_{SAG} = K_8 K_9 / t_E^3 \tag{11.21}$$

$$K_8 = 3P(m^2 - 1)/(2\pi E_G m^2) \tag{11.22}$$

$$K_9 = \frac{(3m + 1)y_2^2 - (m - 1)y_1^2}{2(m + 1)} - y_1^2(\ln\frac{y_2}{y_1} + 1) \tag{11.23}$$

where all terms are as defined earlier.

To see if this sag is acceptable, it can be compared with the tolerance for surface deformation (such as $\lambda/2$ or $\lambda/20$) corresponding to the required system performance level of the system and the location of the optic in that system.

Example 11.14: Change in sag of a reflecting surface caused by a bending moment.
(For design and analysis, use File 50 of the CD-ROM)
Calculate the change in sag of the mirror described in Example 11.13. Express the change in waves of red light ($\lambda = 0.633$ nm).

From Table B8a, $E_G = 1.06\times10^7$ lb/in.^{2} (7.3$\times$10^4 MPa)
From Ex. 11.13, $\upsilon_G = 0.17$ so m = $1/\upsilon_G$ = 5.882
                    $t_E = 2.000$ in. (5.080 cm)
                    $P = 2000$ lb (8.90$\times$10^3 N)
From Eq. (11.22),
  $K_8 = (3)(2000)(5.882^2 - 1)/[(2\pi)(1.06\times10^7)(5.882^2)] = 8.748\times10^{-5}$ in.^{2}

From Eq. (11.23),
  K_9 = {[(3)(5.882) + 1][9.88^2] - [(5.882 - 1)(9.50^2)]}/[(2)(5.882 + 1)]
              - {9.50^2 [ln(9.88/9.50) + 1]}
     = 6.437 in.^{2}

From Eq. (11.21), $\Delta_{SAG} = (8.748\times10^{-5})(6.437)/(2.000^3)$
                    $= 7.040\times10^{-5}$ in. (1.788$\times$10^{-3} mm) = 2.8 λ_{RED}

This mirror mounting design is probably unsatisfactory from the bending viewpoint for any practical application even though the stress level (from Example 11.13) is quite low. The design could be improved by making y_1 and y_2 more equal.

References

1. Roark, R.J., *Formulas for Stress and Strain*, 3rd ed., McGraw-Hill, New York, 1954. See also Young, W.C., *Roark's Formulas for Stress & Strain*, 6th ed., McGraw-Hill, New York, 1989.

2. Vukobratovich, D., "Optomechanical Systems Design," Chapt. 3 in *The Infrared & Electro-Optical Systems Handbook,* Vol. 4, ERIM, Ann Arbor and SPIE, Bellingham, 1993.

3. Shand, E.B., *Glass Engineering Handbook,* 2nd ed., McGraw-Hill, New York, 1958.

4. Sawyer, K.A., "Contact stresses and their optical effects in biconvex optical elements," S*PIE Proceedings* Vol. 2542, 58, 1995.

5. Delgado, R. F., and Hallinan, M., "Mounting of optical elements," *Opt. Eng.*, 14, S-11, 1975. Reprinted in *SPIE Milestone Series* Vol. 770, 173, 1988.

6. Yoder, P. R., Jr., *Opto-Mechanical Systems Design,* 2nd ed., Marcel Dekker, New York, 1993.

7. Yoder, P.R., Jr., "Optical Mounts: Lenses, Windows, Small Mirrors, and Prisms," Chapt. 6 in *Handbook of Optomechanical Engineering*, CRC Press, Boca Raton, 1997.

8. Yoder, P. R., Jr., "Lens mounting techniques," *SPIE Proceedings* Vol. 389, 2, 1983.

9. Yoder, P. R., Jr., "Axial stresses with toroidal lens-to-mount interfaces," *SPIE Proceedings* Vol. 1533, 2, 1991.

10. Bayar, M., "Lens barrel optomechanical design principles," *Opt. Eng.* Vol. 20, 181, 1981.

CHAPTER 12
Effects of Temperature Changes on Optical Component Mountings

Many things happen in an optical assembly when the temperature changes. Changes occur in optical surface radii, air spaces and lens thicknesses, the refractive indices of optical materials, the refractive index of the surrounding air, and the physical dimensions of structural members. Each of these effects will tend to defocus and misalign the system. Axial and/or radial temperature gradients may also appear. These may cause optics to decenter, tilt, or develop pointing errors, optical surfaces to become distorted, and materials to become less homogeneous in their optical and mechanical properties. Gradients are most significant in systems involving refractive optics. Dimensional changes of optical and mechanical parts forming assemblies usually cause changes in clamping forces (preloads); these changes affect contact stresses. Although these problems may be serious if they are not attended to, most can be eliminated or drastically reduced in magnitude by careful optomechanical design. In this chapter, we point out some of the most common temperature-related problems and indicate typical means for solving them. Included are techniques for athermalizing reflecting, refracting, and catadioptric systems and the effects of temperature changes on axial preload (increasing contact stress at lower temperatures). We consider optical component misalignment caused by loss of contact with the mount at higher temperatures. Radial stress buildup at lower temperatures and shear stress in bonded joints caused by temperature changes are also discussed.

12.1 Athermalization Techniques

Athermalization is the process of stabilizing an instrument's optical performance by designing the optics, mounts, and structures to compensate for temperature changes. We limit our considerations to axial defocus effects that can be approached passively by choices of materials and dimensions.

12.1.1 Reflective systems

All reflective systems offer an advantage over systems that include refractive optics if all optical and mechanical components are made from the same material. An example is shown in Fig. 10.56. This is a schematic section view through the infrared astronomical satellite (IRAS) telescope.[1,2] All structural and optical components of the telescope are beryllium. The flexure mounting for the 24-in. (609.6-cm)-diameter primary mirror is discussed in Sect. 10.3.2. Since all parts of the telescope have the same CTE, changes from room temperature to cryogenic temperature in space will change all component and spacing dimensions equally. Temperature changes do not affect focus or image quality. The same athermal characteristics are offered by the all-aluminum telescope shown in Fig. 9.37.[3]

In the more general configuration for simple reflective systems such as the Cassegrainian or Gregorian telescope with two mirrors separated by an axial distance, the mirrors are made or ULE or Zerodur with low CTEs, and the structure is made of a higher CTE material such as aluminum. A different situation exists in a telescope with glass, aluminum, or beryllium mirrors and an Invar or low-expansion composite structure. In one case, an increase in temperature would cause the focus to move inward while in the other case, this change would move the focus outward. If the mirrors and structure all have different CTEs, more flexibility is available and an athermal design is theoretically possible, especially if the structure is made of different lengths of different materials.

In many cases, however, materials are chosen for reasons other than thermal ones (such as manufacturability, cost, and density) so other means must be employed to reduce the effects of temperature changes. A common means is active control of the location(s) of one or more mirrors by which the temperature distribution within the system is measured and motor-driven mechanisms are used to drive the mirror separation and/or final image distance to optimum values. A better, but more complex, means would be to sense focus or quality of the image and actively servocontrol mirror location(s) to optimize performance. Both techniques require an expenditure of energy that may not be easily available.

The 12.5-in. (31.1-cm)-aperture Cassegrain telescope of the geostationary operational environmental satellite (GOES) uses "metering rods" to passively control the axial air space between the two mirrors. As shown in Fig. 12.1, six Invar tubes connect the cell holding the primary mirror to the spider supporting the secondary mirror. The

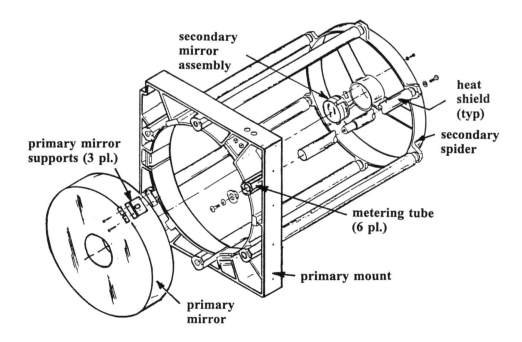

Fig. 12.1 Diagram of the passively athermalized structure of the GOES telescope. (Adapted from Hookman.[4])

primary mount and the secondary spider are made of aluminum. The mount for the secondary mirror is described in Sect. 13.28. The instrument design is axially athermal because the lengths of the dissimilar structural metals have been chosen so that the axial separation between the mirrors remains constant when the temperature ranges from 1°C (34°F) to 54°C (129°F) as the satellite orbits through the Earth's shadow. [4,5]

The way this is accomplished is shown schematically in Fig. 12.2. The materials involved have low or high CTEs, as indicated by the legend. The mirrors are located at the points indicated in the drawing. The plus and minus signs indicate how an increase in temperature affects the central air space between these mirrors. The direction of an individual change is determined by which end of the component is attached to its neighboring components. The algebraic summation of contributions, each consisting of individual component length times CTE times temperature change, for the various structural members defines the mirror separation. The material for one spacer in the secondary mount is selected at assembly to accommodate minor variations in component parameters. The net result is that the air space remains fixed throughout the temperature excursion.

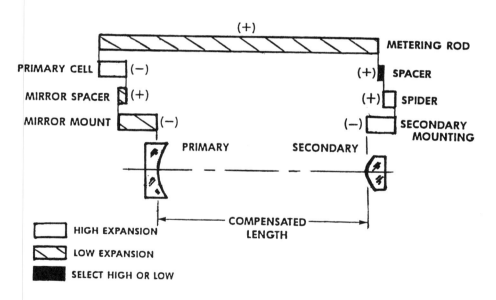

Fig. 12.2 Schematic diagram of the passive thermal compensation mechanism (metering structure) used to stabilize the axial spacing between the GOES telescope primary and secondary mirrors. (Adapted from Zurmehly and Hookman.[5])

To help regulate temperature, aluminum heat shields painted black on the outside surfaces to maximize thermal emissivity and gold plated on the inside surfaces to minimize emissivity are placed over the major mechanical components, including the metering tubes. These shields are not structural members so they do not enter directly into the temperature compensation mechanism described earlier.

12.1.2 Refracting systems

Refractive and catadioptric systems pose more complex athermalization problems because of refractive index variations as well as dimensional variations within transmissive materials when temperature changes. Structures also change dimensions. Along with the CTEs of all materials, key parameters are the optical material's refractive index n_G and the rate of change of that index with temperature. Unless the surrounding medium is a vacuum, the variation with temperature of the refractive index of that medium (usually air) must be considered. To separate these refractive variations, the absolute index for glass $n_{G\ ABS}$ is obtained from the $n_{G\ REL}$ value relative to air (as listed in glass catalogs) at a given temperature and wavelength using the following equation:

$$n_{G\ ABS} = (n_{G\ REL})(n_{AIR}) \tag{12.1}$$

where the air index at 15°C is calculated from Edlen's equation [6]:

$$(n_{AIR\ 15} - 1) \times 10^8 = 6432.8 + \frac{2949810}{146 - (1/\lambda)^2} + \frac{25540}{41 - (1/\lambda)^2} \tag{12.2}$$

and λ is in micrometers.

The index of air varies with temperature at the following rate derived from Penndorf's equation for n_{AIR} [7]:

$$dn_{AIR}/dT = (-0.003861)(n_{AIR\ 15} - 1)/(1 + 0.00366\,T)^2 \tag{12.3}$$

where T is expressed in °C.

At 20°C, dn_{AIR}/dT and $(n_{AIR} - 1)$ have the values at selected wavelengths shown in Table 12.1.

Table 12.1 Values for dn_{AIR}/dT and $(n_{AIR} - 1)$ at various wavelengths

Wavelength (nm)	dn_{AIR}/dT	$(n_{AIR} - 1)$
400	-9.478×10^{-7}	2.780×10^{-4}
550	-9.313×10^{-7}	2.732×10^{-4}
700	-9.245×10^{-7}	2.712×10^{-4}
850	-9.211×10^{-7}	2.701×10^{-4}
1000	-9.190×10^{-7}	2.696×10^{-4}

Jamieson has defined the following expression for the change in focal length of a thin single-element lens with a change in temperature[8] :

$$\Delta f = -\delta_G f \Delta T \qquad (12.4)$$

where:

$\quad f$ = lens focal length in air at a given wavelength and temperature

$\quad \delta_G$ = lens coefficient of thermal defocus given by:

$$\delta_G = [\beta_G / (n_G - 1)] - \alpha_G \qquad (12.5)$$

$$\beta_G = dn_G / dT \qquad (12.6)$$

Equation (12.4) has the same basic form as the temperature variation of a length L of a material with a CTE of α, which is $\Delta L = \alpha L \Delta T$. The parameter δ_G depends only on physical properties and wavelength. It is referred to by some authors as the "thermo-optic coefficient" for the glass. The value of α_G is positive for all refracting materials, and the values of δ_G range from -3.2×10^{-5} to 2.2×10^{-5}. Those glasses with small δ_G values are those for which the increase in focal length, owing to rising temperature and the resultant expansion of surface radii, is nearly balanced by a corresponding decrease because of a reduced index of refraction. The δ_G values for optical plastics and infrared materials are more extreme than those of optical glasses. Table B17 lists the δ_G for 185 Schott glasses, 14 infrared crystals, 4 plastics, and 4 index-matching liquids. [8]

If we mount a thin singlet lens having a positive value for δ_G and focal length f in a simple barrel made of a material (such as a metal) with the CTE = α_M and length L = f as shown in Fig. 12.3, a change in temperature $+\Delta T$ will lengthen the barrel by $\alpha_M L \Delta T = f \Delta T$. At the same time, the lens focal length will lengthen by $\delta_G f \Delta T$. If the materials were to be chosen so $\alpha_M = \delta_G$, the system would be athermal and the image would remain at the end of the barrel at all temperatures. If $\alpha_M \neq \delta_G$, temperature changes will cause defocus. Choosing materials for this system that have nearly the same CTEs does not necessarily make them athermal.

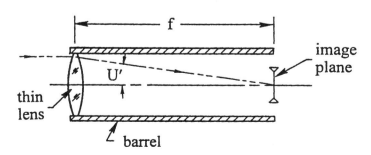

Fig. 12.3 Schematic of a thermally uncompensated single thin lens and mount.

The defocus that occurs in a simple uncompensated thin-lens system is illustrated by Example 12.1.

Example 12.1: Defocus of a thermally uncompensated thin lens mounting. (For design and analysis, use File 51 of the CD-ROM)

Assume a thin BK7 lens with f = 100 mm (3.937 in.) is mounted as in Fig. 12.3 in (a) a 6061 aluminum or (b) a 416 stainless steel barrel. Let the temperature change by +20° C (+36° F). What is the defocus in each case?

From Table B12, $\alpha_{Al} = 23.6 \times 10^{-6}/°C$ $(13.1 \times 10^{-6}/°F$
                      $\alpha_{CRES} = 9.9 \times 10^{-6}/°C$ $(5.5 \times 10^{-6}/°F)$

Then,
$$\Delta L_{AL} = (23.6 \times 10^{-6})(100)(20) = 0.0472 \text{ mm } (0.0019 \text{ in.})$$
$$\Delta L_{CRES} = (8.5 \times 10^{-6})(100)(20) = 0.0198 \text{ mm } (0.0008 \text{ in.}).$$

From Table B17, δ_G for BK7 glass = $- 2.41 \times 10^{-6}/°F$ $(- 4.33 \times 10^{-6}/°C)$

Then, from Eq. (12.4),
$$\Delta f = - (- 4.33 \times 10^{-6})(100)(20) = 0.0087 \text{ mm } (0.0003 \text{ in.}).$$

Hence, defocus$_{AL}$ = 0.0472 - 0.0087 = 0.0385 mm (0.0015 in.)
       defocus$_{CRES}$ = 0.0198 - 0.0087 = 0.0111 mm (0.0004 in.)

The advantage of the lower CTE of the steel material in this application is apparent.

Assuming isothermal conditions, Jamieson[10] explained how to determine the values for δ_G and the change in focal length Δf of a thin doublet and a thin achromatic doublet. His equation for δ_G for the thin doublet case is

$$\delta_{G \text{ DBLT}} = (f/f_1)(\delta_{G1}) + (f/f_2)(\delta_{G2}) \tag{12.7}$$

where f is the focal length of the doublet, f_1 and f_2 are the focal lengths of the elements, and δ_{G1} and δ_{G2} are the coefficients of thermal defocus of the elements. Once δ_G is known, Δf can be calculated for each case from Eq. (12.4).

Jamieson's equation for δ_G for the thin achromatic doublet case is:

$$\delta_{G \text{ ACH DBLT}} = (v_{G1}\delta_{G1} - v_{G2}\delta_{G2})/(v_{G1} - v_{G2}) \tag{12.8}$$

where v_{G1} and v_{G2} are the Abbe numbers for the elements and the other terms are as previously defined.

One means for athermalizing thick lens systems is to design the lenses for the required image quality and through proper choice of glasses, as independent of temperature as possible when properly focused. We then design a mount from multiple materials combining different CTEs so as to make the change in length of the mount equal the change in focal length (or more generally, of image distance). Structures based on the design principles of Fig. 12.4 can create positive or negative changes in overall length from specific lengths of different materials such as Invar, aluminum, titanium, steel, composites (typically graphite epoxy), or plastics (such as Teflon, nylon, or Delrin). The use of a plastic may not always be a wise choice because of its potentially inadequate stability and hysteresis.

Vukobratovich gave equations (here slightly rewritten) for the design of these dual-material structures to thermally compensate an optical system with a coefficient of thermal defocus δ_G, CTEs α_1 and α_2, and focal length f. [11] These equations are

$$\delta_G f = \alpha_1 L_1 + \alpha_2 L_2 \tag{12.9}$$

$$L_1 = f - L_2 \tag{12.10}$$

$$L_2 = (f)(\alpha_1 - \delta_G)/(\alpha_1 - \alpha_2) \tag{12.11}$$

where the geometric parameters are as defined in Fig. 12.4.

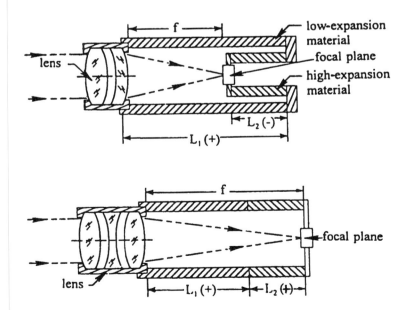

Fig. 12.4 Schematics of dual-material mountings that athermalize the focus of lenses. (a) Reentrant case, (b) series case. (Adapted from Vukobratovich.[11])

Example 12.2: Athermalized thin lens doublet mounting.
(For design and analysis, use File 52 of the CD-ROM)
Consider a closely air-spaced thin lens doublet with characteristics as follows:
f_1 = 60 mm (2.362 in.), BK7 glass, f_2 = - 150 mm (5.905 in.), SF2 glass, and separation d = 0. The effective focal length f of the combination = $f_1 f_2 /(f_1 + f_2 - d)$ = 100 mm (3.937 in.). Let us mount this lens pair in a barrel of the reentrant type shown in Fig. 12.4(a) made of Invar 36 and 6061 aluminum with α_1 = 1.26×10^{-6}/°C and α_2 = 23.6×10^{-6}/°C respectively. What are the appropriate lengths L_1 and L_2 ?

From Table B17, δ_{G1} (BK7) = - 4.33×10^{-6} /°C and δ_{G2} (SF2) = - 3.33×10^{-6} /°C.

From Eq. (12.7),
δ_G = (100/60)(- 4.33×10^{-6}) + (100/- 150)(- 3.33×10^{-6}) = - 4.997×10^{-6} /°C

From Eq. (12.11), L_2 = (100)(1.26×10^{-6} + 4.997×10^{-6})/(1.26×10^{-6} - 23.6×10^{-6})
                              = - 28.008 mm (- 1.103 in.)

From Eq. (12.10), L_1 = 100 - (- 28.008) = 128.008 mm (5.040 in.)

The changes in the two tube lengths, the net changes in the barrel length, and the change in the lens's focal length for a 20°C temperature change are

ΔL_1 = $\alpha_1 L_1 \Delta T$ = (1.26×10^{-6})(128.008)(20) = 0.0032 mm (0.0001 in.)
ΔL_2 = $\alpha_2 L_2 \Delta T$ = (23.6×10^{-6})(- 28.008)(20) = - 0.0132 mm (- 0.0005 in.)
Total change in barrel length = ΔL = $\Delta L_1 + \Delta L_2$ = - 0.0100 mm (- 0.0004 in.)
Δf = $\delta_G f \Delta T$ = (- 4.997×10^{-6})(100)(20)   = - 0.0100 mm (-0.0004 in.)

Since $\Delta L = \Delta f$, the image is at the proper location after the temperature change and the design is athermal.

Modern lens design programs, such as Code V,[12] are capable of athermalization with little intervention by the designer. The programs include thermal modeling features and stored thermal-mechanical properties of a variety of commonly used optical and mechanical materials (including mirror materials). The nominal design typically is known at a specific design temperature such as 20°C. The athermalization design process generally involves (1) calculation of the refractive index of air at the desired extreme high and low temperatures, (2) conversion of the catalog values for refractive indices relative to air into absolute values by multiplying them by the air index, (3) calculation of the absolute glass refractive indices at the extreme temperatures using the dn/dT values from the manufacturer's data, (4) calculation of the surface radii at the extreme temperatures using the known CTEs of the optical materials, (5) calculation of the air spaces and component thicknesses at the extreme temperatures using the known CTEs of the mechanical and optical materials, (6) evaluation of the system's performance at the extreme temperatures and at the best focus locations for those temperatures, (7) design of the mechanical structure and mechanisms as needed to adjust component spacings and/or bring the image to the proper location at each extreme temperature, and, finally, (8) assessment of the system's performance at the extreme temperatures and with the mechanical compensation means having adjusted axial spacings. Presumably if the optomechanical design is proper, the performance degradation that is due to the specified temperature changes will be acceptable.

To illustrate a simple application of this design process, we summarize here an analysis by Friedman[13] in which a mechanical means was devised to correct the final image distance of a 24-in. (60.96-cm)-focal length, f/5 aerial camera lens to optimize performance over the range 20°C to 60 °C. Figure 12.5 shows the lens schematic. It was specified that the temperature of the camera would be stabilized at each temperature considered. The specification required that the performance not be degraded by more than 10% over the full temperature range.

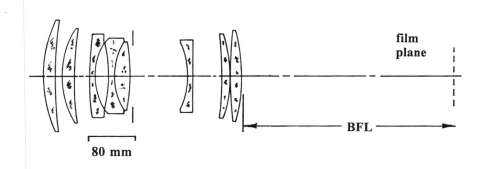

Fig. 12.5 Optical schematic diagram of a 24-in. (60.96-cm)-focal length, f/3.5 aerial camera lens. (Adapted from Friedman.[13])

Friedman's analysis indicated that the back focal length (BFL) of the lens increased monotonically from 365.646 mm at 20°C to 365.947 mm at 60°C for a change of 0.303 mm. To ensure proper performance at all temperatures between these extremes, it would be necessary to utilize a passive mechanical compensation means for adjusting the film location. A bimetallic mechanical design of the additive type shown in Fig. 12.4(b) was created using two different types of aluminum (6061 and 2024) and type 416 stainless steel as the materials. The configuration is shown schematically in Fig. 12.6. The dimensions t_{Al} and t_{CRES} were determined as follows:

From the geometry of Fig. 12.6,

$$(\alpha_{Al\ 6061} t_{Al} + \alpha_{CRES} t_{CRES} - \alpha_{Al\ 2024} t_{Al\ 2024} - \alpha_L t_L)(\Delta T) = \Delta_{BFL}$$

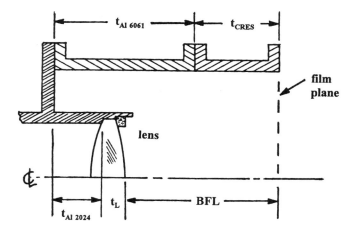

Fig. 12.6 Mechanical schematic of the athermalizing structure for the 24 in (60.96 cm) focal length, f/3.5 aerial camera lens. (Adapted from Friedman[13])

where:

$$\alpha_{Al\ 6061} = 23.6 \times 10^{-6}\,/^{\circ}C \quad \alpha_{Al\ 2024} = 23.2 \times 10^{-6}\,/^{\circ}C\ * \quad \alpha_{CRES} = 9.9 \times 10^{-6}\,/^{\circ}C$$
$$\alpha_L = 6.3 \times 10^{-6}\,/^{\circ}C \quad t_{Al\ 2024} = 154.102\ mm \quad t_L = 15.252\ mm$$
$$\Delta T = 40^{\circ}C \quad \Delta_{BFL} = 0.303\ mm.$$

Substituting into the last equation, we find that

$$236\,t_{Al\ 6061} + 99\,t_{CRES} = 112{,}462.54$$

The following geometric relationship also exists in Fig. 12.6:

$$t_{Al\ 6061} + t_{CRES} = t_{Al\ 2024} + t_L = 535.000$$

Solving the last two equations simultaneously, Friedman obtained $t_{Al\ 6061} = 434.289$ mm and $t_{CRES} = 100.711$ mm. These dimensions were used in the camera's mechanical design.

An evaluation of the system's performance at its best focus and at the lowest and highest temperatures predicted that the polychromatic optical transfer function (OTF) as a function of spatial frequency in the image in line pairs per millimeter (lp/mm) with a minus-blue filter would be as indicated in Figs. 12.7 and 12.8. The response of a particular film type (Panatomic-X, type 136) is also indicated in each figure. The intersections of the latter curve with the OTF curves for different points in the image (on-

---

* Note: This value differs slightly from that given in Table B12 for the material.

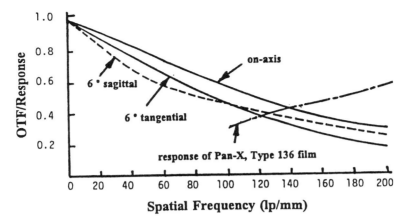

Fig. 12.7 Polychromatic OTF for a 24-in. (60.96-cm)-focal length, f/3.5 aerial camera lens at 20 °C. (Adapted from Friedman.[13])

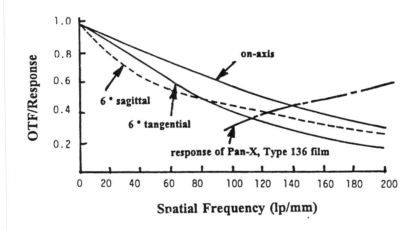

Fig. 12.8 Polychromatic OTF for the camera lens in Fig. 12.7 at 60 °C. (Adapted from Friedman.[13])

axis, 6° off-axis radial and 6° off-axis tangential) represent the "resolution capability" of the lens and film system at the respective temperatures. These resolution predictions are summarized in Table 12.2. During the design, the first six steps given earlier were taken. The results indicate that the design meets the specification over the temperature range. The system therefore is considered athermal.

Table 12.2 Resolution capability of the 24-in. focal length lens and film system[13]

Half-field angle	Resolution (lp/mm)		Percent
	At 20°C	At 60°C	change
On-axis	140	140	0
6° Sagittal	126	123	-2
6° Tangential	122	113	-9

Comprehensive summaries of passive and active mechanisms that have been used to varying degrees of success in providing component motions for athermalization purposes were given by Povey[14] and by Rogers.[15] Zoom lenses that require the movement of components to achieve focal length changes can also incorporate thermal compensation of image quality and focus as small adjustments in the locations of those components in response to temperature changes. See, for example, Parr-Burman and Madgwick[16] and Fischer and Kampe.[17]

12.2 Effects of Temperature Gradients

When all points within an optical instrument are not at the same temperature, the optics and the structure probably have temperature gradients. These may be axial or radial; both types can coexist within the same component. Gradients may result from changes in ambient conditions, movement of the instrument from one temperature environment to another, varying heat load from the sun or more local heat sources, etc. Figure 12.9 schematically illustrates how natural convection of heat generated within an instrument (here a horizontal gas laser) can affect structural dimensions differentially and cause beam pointing errors. These are caused by induced rotation of the laser cavity end mirrors. The problem can be solved equalizing the temperature through appropriate circulation of cooling air.[18]

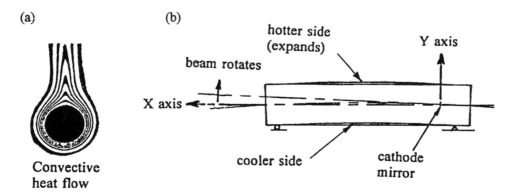

Fig. 12.9 Effect of natural heat convection on beam direction in a gas laser with inadequate temperature gradient control. (Adapted from Hatheway.[18])

If an optical instrument is held in a constant temperature environment for a long time (a process called "soaking"), the temperatures tend to equalize and gradients reduce in severity and may disappear entirely. A special situation exists for long-wavelength infrared sensors that must have their optical components and detectors actively cooled to cryogenic temperatures in order to maximize the signal-to-noise ratio. Uniformity of temperature throughout the instrument is virtually impossible in such cases.

Experience and many experiments with military, industrial, and consumer optical equipment indicate that a moderate-sized instrument may need several hours at constant temperature to stabilize. Other devices are intentionally exposed to rapidly changing temperatures as part of their intended application. One such example is a germanium lens assembly that must survive thermal shock and perform to specification after being cooled from room temperature to 120 K in 5 min. This assembly is described in Sect. 13.1. A more gentle, but also more common instance, is a camera moved from a warm house to the frigid outside world in winter. Proper operation of the camera's mechanisms and full optical performance may not occur in the more severe environment for a long time, if ever. Similar problems may occur when the camera is returned to the warm environment.

Typically, small and moderate sized mirrors are cooled (or heated) by conduction through their mounts or by heat transfer devices attached to their back surfaces. Windows and large mirrors may be temperature stabilized by flowing conditioned air across their surfaces (see Figs. 5.9 and 10.33 for examples). Mirrors used in high-energy laser applications frequently are temperature controlled by flowing cooled fluid through heat-exchange channels within their substrates. The temperatures of lenses, windows, filters, and domes usually must be controlled by heat flow through their mounts around the peripheries of their apertures (see Fig. 5.14). This tends to introduce radial gradients. Prisms typically are temperature stabilized by conduction through mounting surfaces so these optics may have nonsymmetrical temperature gradients.

12.2.1 Radial temperature gradients

A generic radial gradient in a refracting optic is illustrated in Fig. 12.10. Here a simple biconvex lens in air is subjected to a radial gradient in which the glass near the rim is warmer than that near the axis by an amount ΔT. The temperature, lens thickness, and refractive index of the axial region remain essentially constant at T_A, t_A, and n_A, while those parameters at the the rim increase as indicated to $T_A + \Delta T$, $t_A + \Delta t$, and $n_A + \Delta n$. To thin lens approximation (hence neglecting temperature gradients along the axis), the optical path difference (OPD) between the arbitrary ray shown passing between the points A and B compared with the corresponding ray along the axis is approximated by the expression OPD = $(n - 1 + \Delta n)(t + \Delta t) - (n - 1)(t)$. Since $\Delta n = \beta_G \Delta T$ and $\Delta t = \alpha_G t \Delta T$, we obtain:

$$OPD = [(n - 1)(\alpha) + \beta]t_A \Delta T \qquad (12.12)$$

which can be rewritten as:

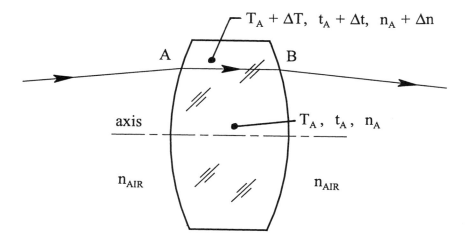

Fig. 12.10 Illustration of a radial temperature gradient in a simple lens.

$$\text{OPD} = (n - 1)(\gamma \, t_A \, \Delta T) \tag{12.13}$$

where, according to Jamieson,[8]

$$\gamma = \alpha + [\beta / (n - 1)] \tag{12.14}$$

The parameter γ_G is a thermo-optical coefficient for the glass that describes its sensitivity to spatial temperature variations. Jamieson[8] indicated that γ_G for most optical glasses lies between $5 \times 10^{-6}/^\circ C$ and $25 \times 10^{-6}/^\circ C$. Exceptions are fluor crown (FK) and phosphate crown (PK) glasses from Schott and Ohara, and some glasses (ATF) from Hoya. Table B17 gives γ_G values for a variety of refractive materials. A few glasses with small or negative values are available. These reduce the sensitivity of lens systems to temperature gradients. Optical plastics and some infrared-transmitting materials (notably germanium) have larger values of γ_G than glasses. The thermal conductivities and heat capacities of plastics are low, so these materials tend to be quite sensitive to spatial temperature gradients. Germanium has a higher conductivity and heat capacity, so lenses made from that material may not suffer as much when the temperature is not uniform. Combinations of materials with high and low γ_G tend to reduce gradient sensitivity. The liquids listed in Table B17 are sometimes used to fill the "air spaces" between lenses to make the system more athermal.[8, 19] To illustrate the use of Eqs. (12.13) and (12.14), consider Example 12.3.

The thin lens approximations made with Eq. (12.13) are not sufficiently accurate for design purposes. They are helpful in making general choices of optical materials or

---

Example 12.3: Estimation of effects of radial gradients in typical thin lenses. (For design and analysis, use File 53 of the CD-ROM)

Thin lenses made of (a) BK7 glass, (b) SF11 glass, and (c) germanium are all 3.500 mm (0.137 in.) thick and have radial temperature gradients causing the rim to be 2 °C hotter than at the axis. What OPDs are created in each case? Assume $\lambda = 0.546$ µm for the glass lenses and 10.6 µm for the Ge lens. Let $n_{\lambda\ BK7} = 1.5187$, $n_{\lambda\ SF11} = 1.7919$, and $n_{\lambda\ Ge} = 4.0000$.

From Table B17, $\gamma_{G\ BK7} = 9.87 \times 10^{-6}\ /°C$
$\gamma_{\lambda\ SF11} = 20.21 \times 10^{-6}\ /°C$
$\gamma_{\lambda\ Ge} = 136.3 \times 10^{-6}\ /°C$

From Eq. (12.13):

(a) OPD $= (0.5187)(3.500)(9.87 \times 10^{-6})(2) = 3.58 \times 10^{-5}$ mm $= 0.07\ \lambda$ @ 0.546 µm

(b) OPD $= (0.7919)(3.500)(20.21 \times 10^{-6})(2) = 1.12 \times 10^{-4}$ mm $= 0.20\ \lambda$ @ 0.546 µm

(c) OPD $= (3.0000)(3.500)(136.3 \times 10^{-6})(2) = 2.86 \times 10^{-3}$ mm $= 0.27\ \lambda$ @ 10.6 µm

These OPDs are large enough to be of concern in high-performance applications.

---

estimating the significance of anticipated temperature gradients. Detailed design requires that ray traces be conducted using realistic input temperature distributions to determine the index and thickness values as functions of zonal locations within the lens apertures and their effects upon lens performance.

Since there is no refraction, given radial temperature gradients will affect reflecting optical components by changing the radii of optical surfaces and surface sagittal depths as functions of height from the axis. Lens design programs handle these changes by considering the surfaces to be aspheric. The resulting effects upon the image are easily determined using such programs.

12.2.2 Axial temperature gradients

An axial temperature gradient can be created in an optical component such as a window, lens, or prism by absorption of an incident heat flux, such as solar or laser radiation. That gradient will cause changes in bending of the optic. Barnes gave a classic treatment of thermal effects on space optics.[20] With uniform axial irradiation, a plane parallel window becomes a shallow, concentric meniscus. Its mean radius of curvature R is given by $1/R = \alpha q/k$, where α is the linear thermal expansion coefficient, q the heat flux per unit area, and k the material's thermal conductivity. If the thickness t is small compared to R, the optical power P of this bowed window is given by:

$$P = 1/f = [(n - 1)/n][tq/k]^2 \tag{12.15}$$

Using this equation, Barnes[20] showed that for an optical system at 300 K in low Earth orbit, the axial thermal gradient in a 2.5-cm (1.0-in.)-thick crown glass window caused by the approximately 15% of solar radiation absorbed is negligible for apertures smaller than 2.9 m (9.5 ft) since the focal shift introduced would be smaller than the Rayleigh $\lambda/4$ tolerance. This critical aperture varies inversely as the square root of the window thickness for a given heat flux absorbed.

Temperature gradients introduced through the edge mounting for a window or corrector plate introduce differences in optical path length at various radii. This is due to changes in mechanical thickness of the material and changes in the refractive index of the material. In general, stresses are built up in the glass and birefringence is introduced. These effects are small.

To illustrate the use of the analytical tools discussed in his paper, Barnes[20] gave an example of an edge-insulated, single-glazed, nominally plane parallel crown glass window 3.0 cm (1.2 in.) thick and 61 cm (24 in.) in aperture. When used in an Earth-oriented satellite at 960 km (600 mi) altitude, this window was found to become a shallow negative lens and to have an optical path difference distribution of zero at the axis and at a zonal radius of 0.9, but a zonal aberration peaking at a zonal radius of 0.6 to 0.7 equivalent to approximately 0.5 wave p-v at visible wavelengths during operation. If used in an f/5 optical system of 55 cm (21.7 in.) aperture, this deformation would cause the system focus to shift about 42 µm; this is nearly twice the Rayleigh quarter-wave tolerance for this system. The zonal aberration would reduce the system's performance even if it were to be refocused. Barnes concluded that the use of a window with an aperture significantly (about 25%) larger than that of the optical system would reduce the error to a much more tolerable magnitude without resorting to complex on-board thermal controls. Reducing the window thickness or decreasing the thermal coupling between the mount and the window by increasing the degree of thermal insulation provided would tend to reduce the effects of such a radial thermal gradient.

12.3 Change in Axial Preload Caused by a Temperature Change

Invariably, lens and mount materials have dissimilar CTEs, so temperature changes of $\pm\Delta T$ cause changes in total axial preload P. Equation (12.18) quantifies this relationship.[21]

$$\Delta P = K_3 \Delta T \tag{12.16}$$

where K_3 is the rate of change of preload with temperature for the design. This factor is sometimes called the design's "temperature sensitivity factor." As shown in Appendix D, K_3 for a single-element lens clamped axially in a simple mount is approximately

$$K_3 = \frac{-E_G A_G E_M A_M (\alpha_M - \alpha_G)}{E_G A_G + 2E_M A_M} \tag{12.17}$$

where:

E_G, E_M = Young's modulus for the glass and metal, respectively
α_M, α_G = CTEs for the glass and metal, respectively
A_G, A_M = cross-sectional areas of the stressed regions in the lens and mount, respectively.

The geometric parameters are shown in Figs. 12.11 and 12.12. Equations (12.18) through (12.20) define A_M and A_G for the mount and lens areas, respectively.

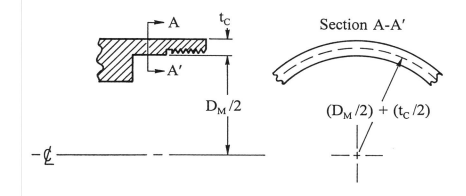

Fig. 12.11 Geometric relationships used to approximate the cross-sectional area of the stressed region within a lens mounting. (From Yoder.[21])

$$A_M = 2\pi t_C [(D_M/2) + (t_C/2)] \tag{12.18}$$

where:

D_G = OD of the lens
D_M = ID of the mount at the lens rim
t_C = radial thickness of the mount wall adjacent to the lens rim

For the lens, either of the following two cases can apply. If $(2y_C + t_E) < D_G$, the stressed region (the diamond-shaped region in Fig. 12.12) lies within the lens rim.

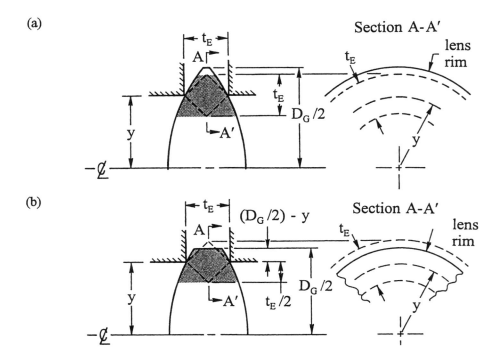

Fig. 12.12 Geometric relationships used to determine cross-sectional area of the stressed region within a lens (a) when completely within the lens rim and (b) when truncated by the rim. (From Yoder.[21])

$$A_G = 2\pi y_C t_E \qquad\qquad\qquad (12.19a)$$

where t_E is the edge thickness of the lens at the contact height y_C. If $(2y_C + t_E) \geq D_G$, the stressed region is truncated by the lens rim and

$$A_G = (\pi/4)(D_G - t_E + 2y_C)(D_G + t_E - 2y_C) \qquad (12.19b)$$

We illustrate the use of these equations with Example 12.4.

Example 12.4: Calculating K_3 for a single lens mounting. (For design and analysis, use File 54 of the CD-ROM)
Assume that the lens shown in Fig. 3.40 is made of SK15 glass and that it is mounted in (a) a 6061 aluminum cell or (b) a 6Al4V titanium cell. Calculate K_3

for each case. The material properties are

$$E_G = 1.22 \times 10^7 \text{ lb/in.}^2 \ (8.41 \times 10^{10} \text{ Pa}) \text{ and } \upsilon_G = 0.275$$
$$\alpha_G = 3.80 \times 10^{-6} / °F \ (6.84 \times 10^{-6} /°C)$$
$$E_{M \ Al} = 9.90 \times 10^6 \text{ lb/in.}^2 \ (6.83 \times 10^{10} \text{ Pa}) \text{ and } \upsilon_{M \ Al} = 0.332$$
$$\alpha_{M \ Al} = 1.31 \times 10^{-5} / °F \ (2.36 \times 10^{-5} /°C)$$
$$E_{M \ Ti} = 1.65 \times 10^7 \text{ lb/in.}^2 \ (1.14 \times 10^{11} \text{Pa}) \text{ and } \upsilon_{M \ Ti} = 0.310$$
$$\alpha_{M \ Ti} = 4.90 \times 10^{-6} / °F \ (8.80 \times 10^{-6} /°C)$$

The pertinent dimensions are

y_C = 3.1020 in. (78.7908 mm)	t_E = 0.2590 in. (6.5786 mm)
D_G = 6.5350 in. (165.9890 mm)	t_C = 0.1960 in. (4.9784 mm)
D_M = 6.5358 in. (166.0093 mm)	

Here $(2y_C + t_E) = (2)(3.102) + 0.259 = 6.463$ in. (164.160 mm), which is smaller than D_G, so the stressed region lies within the lens rim. By Eq. (12.19a),
$$A_G = (2\pi)(3.1020)(0.2590) = 5.0480 \text{ in.}^2 \ (3256.7833 \text{ mm}^2).$$

By Eq. (12.18), $A_M = (2\pi)(0.1960)[(6.5358/2) + (0.1960/2)]$
$$= 4.1451 \text{ in.}^2 \ (2674.2659 \text{ mm}^2)$$

(a) Applying Eq. (12.17) for the aluminum cell:

$$K_{3 \ Al} = \frac{-(1.22 \times 10^7)(5.0480)(9.9 \times 10^6)(4.1451)(1.31 \times 10^{-5} - 3.80 \times 10^{-6})}{(1.22 \times 10^7)(5.0480) + (2)(9.9 \times 10^6)(4.1451)}$$

$$= -163.6 \text{ lb/°F} \ (-1309.9 \text{ N/°C})$$

(b) Applying Eq. (12.17) for the titanium cell:

$$K_{3 \ Ti} = \frac{-(1.22 \times 10^7)(5.0480)(1.65 \times 10^7)(4.1451)(4.90 \times 10^{-6} - 3.80 \times 10^{-6})}{(1.22 \times 10^7)(5.0480) + (2)(1.65 \times 10^7)(4.1451)}$$

$$= -23.3 \text{ lb/°F} \ (-187.0 \text{ N/°C}).$$

With materials having close CTEs (such as SK15 and Ti), the effect of a change in temperature on preload is smaller than if these CTEs differ significantly (such as SK15 and Al). Since contact stress depends on preload, that stress will be more constant with a temperature change with the former combination than with the latter combination. The advantage of similar CTEs wherever they are possible, is apparent.

12.4 Change in Lens Axial Clearance at Increased Temperature

If α_M exceeds α_G (as is usually the case), the metal in the mount will expand more than the glass component for a given temperature increase ΔT. Any axial preload existing at assembly temperature T_A [typically 20°C (68°F)] will then be reduced. If the temperature rises sufficiently, that preload will disappear, and if the lens is not otherwise constrained (as by an elastomeric sealant), it will be free to move within the mount in response to any externally applied forces. In virtually all applications, small changes in position and orientation of the lens within axial and radial gaps created by differential expansion are allowable. Ideally, the mount should maintain contact with the lens to some elevated temperature T_C, defined so that a further temperature increase in the specified maximum survival temperature will not cause the axial gap between the mount and lens to exceed the design tolerance for this parameter.

The axial gap developed between the cell and the lens as temperature rises above T_C can be approximated as:

$$\text{Gap}_A = (\alpha_M - \alpha_G)(t_E)(T_{MAX} - T_C) \tag{12.21}$$

where all terms are as defined earlier.

If Gap_A is equated to the maximum tolerable positive error in axial air space (commonly termed "despace") for the lens, a unique value for T_C of a given design can be calculated. Knowing the rate of change of preload with temperature, K_3, the required preload at assembly on a lens can be adjusted so that it is just reduced to zero at T_C. Defining the temperature change from T_A to T_C as $-\Delta T$, Eq. (12.18) can then be used to estimate the required assembly preload.[21]

Example 12.5: Calculation of T_C based on allowable lens despace. (For design and analysis, use File 55 of the CD-ROM)

Let us assume that an axial movement at a maximum temperature of 160°F (71.1°C) of only 0.0002 in. (0.0051 mm) of a BaK50 lens assembled in a 6061 aluminum mount can be tolerated. The edge thickness of the lens is 0.500 in. (12.7 mm) and assembly takes place at 68°F (20°C). Calculate T_C and verify that the despace tolerance at maximum temperature will be met.

From Tables B1 and B12, $\alpha_G = 2.1\times10^{-6}$ /°F (3.8×10^{-6} /°C)
$\alpha_M = 1.31\times10^{-5}$ /°F (2.36×10^{-5} /°C)

From Eq. (12.21): $\text{Gap}_A = 0.0002 = (1.31\times10^{-5} - 2.1\times10^{-6})(0.5)(160 - T_C)$.

Hence, T_C = 160 - {0.0002/[(11.0×10^{-6})(0.500)]} = 160 - 36.4 = 123.6°F (50.9°C).

This is the temperature at which the mount loses contact with the lens. The further temperature rise to T_{MAX} is 160 - 123.6 = 36.4°F (20.2°C). The corresponding increase in gap is (1.31×10^{-5} - 2.1×10^{-6})(0.5)(36.4) = 0.0002 in. (0.0051 mm).

These calculations show that the design is capable of meeting the specified despace tolerance at T_{MAX}.

12.5 Providing Residual Preload on a Lens at Maximum Temperature

High accelerations (vibration or shock) applied to the lens assembly when clearance exists between the lens and the mounting surfaces may cause damage to the lens from surface-to-surface impacts. Such damage (called "fretting") of glass surfaces under sustained vibrational loading has been reported by Lecuyer[22] and has been experienced by others as well. To minimize this possibility, some lens assemblies are designed to have sufficient residual preload at T_{MAX} to hold the lens firmly against the mechanical interface under the maximum expected acceleration. As indicated by Eq. (3.18), the preload needed to constrain a lens of weight W under acceleration a_G is simply W times a_G and is expressed in pounds. In the SI system, this preload (in newtons) is 9.807Wa_G where W is in kilograms.

Note that in order for this amount of preload to exist at T_{MAX}, the preload to be provided at assembly would be the sum of this value plus the preload change that is due to the temperature change from assembly temperature T_A to temperature $T_C = T_{MAX}$.

Example 12.6: Lens assembly preload required to maintain specified preload at T_{MAX}.
(For design and analysis, use File 56 of the CD-ROM)
Consider a large lens weighing 9.05 lb (4.105 kg) that is to just remain in contact with its mount at a maximum temperature of 160°F (71.1°C) under 250 G acceleration in the axial direction. Assume its K_3 = -30.427 lb/°F (-243.6 N/°C) and assembly takes place at 68°F (28°C). What preload is needed at assembly?

The temperature change ΔT is 160 - 68 = 92°F (51.1°C).

The preload dissipated from T_A to T_{MAX} = (-30.427)(-92)
= 2799.28 lb (1.245×10^4 N).

The additional preload needed to overcome acceleration is $(9.05)(250) = 2262.5$ lb

$(1.01 \times 10^4$ N$)$. The total preload needed at assembly is then $2799.28 + 2262.5 = 5061.8$ lb $(2.25 \times 10^4$ N$)$.

12.6 Contact Stress in a Lens at Low Temperature

In designs where α_M exceeds α_G, the magnitude of the axial preload is increased whenever the temperature drops below temperature T_C. The total preload at any low temperature T can be estimated from Eq. (12.18) by setting ΔT equal to $(T - T_C)$, multiplying by K_3, and adding the assembly preload.

The axial contact stress created by that preload can then be calculated with the aid of Eqs. (11.3) and (11.2). When T equals the specified minimum survival temperature T_{MIN}, the stress should not exceed the rule-of-thumb tolerance on compressive stress in the glass as defined in Sect. 11.1. If these approximation methods indicate a potential problem, calculation of the stress by more exact means (such as finite-element analysis) and estimation of the probability of failure by statistical means are advisable.

> **Example 12.7: Estimating preload on a lens at T_{MIN}.**
> **(For design and analysis, use File 57 of the CD-ROM)**
> Assume that the lens preloaded at assembly as in Example 12.6 is cooled to -40°F (-40°C). What is then the total preload?
>
> The temperature change from T_A to T_{MIN} is -[68 - (-40)] = -108°F (-60°C)
> The preload increase from T_A to T_{MIN} = (-30.427)(-108) = 3286.1 lb (1.46×10⁴ N)
> The total preload at T_{MIN} is then 5062.78 + 3286.1 = 8348.9 lb (3.71×10⁴ N)

> **Example 12.8: Estimated stress in a heavily preloaded lens at T_{MIN}.**
> **(For design and analysis, use File 58 of the CD-ROM)**
> Assume that the lens from Example 12.6 is biconvex with equal radii of 26.926 in. (68.392 cm) and made of BK7 glass. Let the mounting interfaces on both sides be tangential, with contact at $y_C = 3.000$ in. (76.200 mm). If the preload at T_{MIN} is the worst case total value as calculated in Example 12.7, what is the contact stress in the glass?

From Eq. (11.8), $K_{1\,TAN} = 0.5/R = 0.5/26.926 = 0.0186$ in.$^{-1}$ (7.311×10^{-4} mm^{-1})

From Table B1 and Fig. 11.2,
$$K_2 = 8.144 \times 10^{-8} + 8.99 \times 10^{-8} = 1.713 \times 10^{-7} \text{ in.}^2/\text{lb} \; (2.485 \times 10^{-5} \text{ MPa}^{-1})$$

From Eq. 11.3, $p = 8348.9/[(2\pi)(3.000)] = 442.928$ lb/in. (7.757×10^4 N/m)

From Eq. (11.2), $S_C = 0.798[(0.0186)(442.928)/1.713 \times 10^{-7}]^{1/2}$
$$= 5534 \text{ lb/in.}^2 \; (38.2 \text{ MPa})$$

Although the axial force is quite large, the stress is not threatening to the safety of the lens. This is largely due to the redeeming nature of the tangential mount.

12.7 Stress in Multiple-Lens Assemblies

The above theory treated stress in single-element lenses at a temperature different from that at assembly. This theory can be extended to include multiple-lens designs such as cemented doublets and those with spacers or equivalent cell shoulders between separated lenses.[23] The applicable equations and procedures for progressively more complex designs are summarized in the following sections.

12.7.1 Cemented doublet lens

Figure 12.13 shows a typical cemented doublet clamped between a cell shoulder and a threaded retainer. For simplicity, the contact heights are assumed to be the same at both interfaces. The stressed region in the glass is the annulus of radial width $(t_{E1} + t_{E2})$ indicated by the dashed diamond. Equation (12.19) or (12.20), as appropriate, is used to calculate A_G as if the lens were a homogeneous single element. Equation (12.18) is used to determine A_M. These areas, the pertinent component dimensions, and their material properties can then be substituted into Eq. (12.22) (derived in Appendix D) to determine the temperature sensitivity factor K_3. All terms in this equation have been defined previously and have appropriate subscripts to designate the first or second element.

$$K_3 = \frac{-(\alpha_M - \alpha_{G1})(t_{E1}) - (\alpha_M - \alpha_{G2})(t_{E2})}{\dfrac{2t_{E1}}{E_{G1}A_G} + \dfrac{2t_{E2}}{E_{G2}A_G} + \dfrac{(t_{E1} + t_{E2})}{E_M A_M}} \tag{12.22}$$

Given the preload at assembly, the new total and linear preloads at any temperature can be calculated using Eqs. (12.16) and (11.3). These preloads are the same at both the first and third surfaces of the lens. The applicable value of K_2 at each of

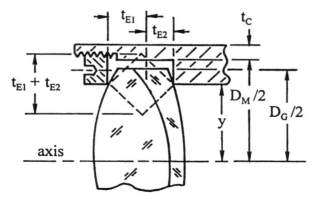

Fig. 12.13 Schematic of a typical cemented doublet lens clamped between a mount's shoulder and a retainer. (From Yoder.[23])

these surfaces can be estimated by Eq. (11.4), using the material properties at that interface. Finally, knowing the type of interface and surface radius at each interface, the value for K_1 can be calculated using the proper form of Eq. (11.5) and the contact stress S_C at that surface can be estimated through use of Eq. (11.2). In general, the stresses at the two surfaces may differ if the glasses have different elastic and/or thermal properties, which determine K_2. The interface types and surface radii may also differ, thereby affecting K_1.

Example 12.9: Contact stresses for a cemented doublet lens. (For design and analysis, use File 59 of the CD-ROM)

The pertinent design parameters for a doublet mounted as in Fig. 12.13 are tabulated below. The lens-to-cell interfaces at R_1 and R_3 are tangential. Assuming a total preload at assembly ($T_A = 68°F$) of $P_A = 44$ lb, estimate the axial contact stress at each interface (a) at assembly and (b) at -80°F.

Parameter	Units	Cell	Lens #1	Lens #2
Material		6061 Al	K5	SF2
D_M, $(D_G)_i$	in.	1.104	1.100	1.100
E_M, $(E_G)_i$	lb/in.^{2}	9.9×10^6	1.03×10^7	7.98×10^6
υ_M, $(\upsilon_G)_i$		0.332	0.227	0.231
α_M, $(\alpha_G)_i$	ppm/°F	1.31×10^{-5}	4.6×10^{-6}	4.7×10^{-6}
K_M, $(K_G)_i$	in.^{2}/lb	8.99×10^{-8}	9.211×0^{-8}	1.187×10^{-7}

t_C, $(t_A)_i$	in.	0.094	0.524	0.187
$(y_C)_i = (y_C)_{i+1}$	in.		0.517	0.517
R_1	in.		2.174	
Sag_1 [Eq. (4.1)]	in.		0.129	
R_2	in.		-2.174	
Sag_2 [Eq. (4.1)]	in.		-0.129	
R_3	in.			-1.730
Sag_3 [Eq. (4.1)]	in.			-0.036
$(t_E)_i$	in.		0.266	0.280
$t_{E\ DBLT}$	in.		0.546	
P_A	lb	44	44	44
$2y_i + t_E$	in.		1.580(> D_G ∴ truncated)	
A_G [Eq. (12.22)] in.²			0.763	
A_M [Eq. (12.18)] in.²		0.354		
K_3 [Eq. (12.22)] lb/°F			-14.621	
$K_{1\ TAN}$ [Eq. (11.8)] in.$^{-1}$			0.230	0.134
$K_2 = K_M + K_G$ in.²/lb			1.82×10^{-7}	2.08×10^{-7}
(a) At $T_A = 68°$ F				
p = $P_{MAX}/(2\pi y_C)$ lb/in.				13.545
S_C lb/in.²			3302	2355
(b) At $T_{MIN} = -80°$ F				
$\Delta T = T_{MIN} - T_A$ °F			-148	
$\Delta P = (K_3)(\Delta T)$ lb			2163.9	
$P_{TOTAL} = P_{MAX} + \Delta P$ lb			2207.9	
p = $P_{TOTAL}/(2\pi y_C)$ lb/in.			679.67	
S_C [Eq. (11.2)] lb/in.²			23,387	16,698

We note that the stresses at R_1 and R_3 are unequal at each temperature and greater at the low temperature. These differences result from the differences in glass properties and radii. The stress at T_{MIN} is tolerable for survival, but large enough to introduce birefringence in the glasses.

If the temperature rises sufficiently to dissipate assembly preload (i.e., to T_C), an axial gap between the doublet and the mount develops for any additional temperature increases in accordance with the following equation:

$$\Delta x = [(\alpha_M - \alpha_{G1})(t_{E1}) + (\alpha_M - \alpha_{G2})(t_{E2})]\Delta T \qquad (12.23)$$

where all terms are as previously defined.

Example 12.10: Axial gap at T_{MAX} for a cemented doublet lens. (For design and analysis, use File 60 of the CD-ROM)
Consider again the cemented doublet of Example 12.9. Find T_C and the axial gap created at $T_{MAX} = 160°F$.

From the prior example, $T_A = 68°F$, $K_3 = -14.621$ lb/°F and $P_A = 44$ lb. This assembly preload dissipates when the temperature rises by $44/14.621 = 3.0°$ to 71.0 °F. The ΔT to T_{MAX} is then $160 - 71.0 = 89.0°F$.

By Eq. (12.23):
$$\Delta x = [(1.31\times10^{-5} - 4.6\times10^{-6})(0.266) + (1.31\times10^{-5} - 4.7\times10^{-6})(0.280)][89.0]$$
$$= (4.613\times10^{-6})(89.0) = 0.0004 \text{ in.}$$

This maximum gap is probably smaller than the tolerance for the axial position of the lens. If so, it would be considered acceptable.

12.7.2 Air-spaced doublet lens

Figure 12.14 shows a simple mounting for an air-spaced doublet consisting of two unequal diameter elements with differing edge thicknesses. The spacer material is not necessarily the same as that of the cell. The glasses may also be different. The contact heights at both surfaces of a given lens are assumed to be equal and the cell wall thickness is assumed to be constant at the lenses. With equal contact heights at both lenses, a cylindrical spacer with parallel OD and ID can be used. This is not the case in the figure, so the spacer has a cylindrical OD and a tapered ID. The assembly preload P_A is the same at all lens surfaces.

The following equations give K_3 (derived in a manner similar to that explained in Appendix D) and the axial gap Δx for temperature increases above T_C, at which temperature the preload imposed at assembly decreases to zero:

$$K_3 = \frac{-(\alpha_M - \alpha_{G1})(t_{E1}) - (\alpha_M - \alpha_S)(t_S) - (\alpha_M - \alpha_{G2})(t_{E2})}{\dfrac{2t_{E1}}{E_{G1}A_{G1}} + \dfrac{t_S}{E_S A_S} + \dfrac{2t_{E2}}{E_{G2}A_{G2}} + \dfrac{(t_{E1} + t_S + t_{E2})}{E_M A_M}} \quad (12.24)$$

$$\Delta x = [(\alpha_M - \alpha_{G1})(t_{E1}) + (\alpha_M - \alpha_S)(t_S) + (\alpha_M - \alpha_{G2})(t_{E2})]\Delta T \quad (12.25)$$

where all terms are as defined earlier.

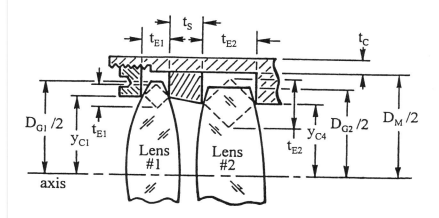

Fig. 12.14 Schematic of two singlet lenses air spaced by a spacer and clamped between a mounting shoulder and a retainer. (From Yoder.[23])

Sectional views of two types of simple lens spacers are shown in Fig. 12.15. Both are solid cylinders fitting closely in the ID of the lens cell (not shown). The version shown in Fig. 12.15(a) is cylindrical while that in Fig. 12.15(b) has a tapered ID to accommodate different heights of contact with the lenses. It also shows tangential interfaces. Equations (12.26) through (12.31) allow the annular area A_S to be calculated for each of these spacers.

For spacer version 12.15(a)

$$w_S = (D_M/2) - y_C \qquad\qquad (12.26)$$

For spacer version 12.15(b), the wall thickness of the tapered spacer is taken as its average annular thickness. This is calculated with the help of the following equations:

$$\Delta y_i = [(D_G)_i/2] - (y_C)_i \qquad\qquad (12.27)$$

$$y'_i = (y_C)_i - \Delta y_i \qquad\qquad (12.28)$$

$$w_S = (D_M/2) - [(y'_1 + y'_2)/2] \qquad\qquad (12.29)$$

In both cases:

(a)

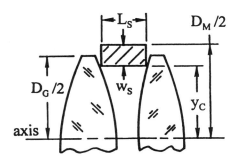

(b)

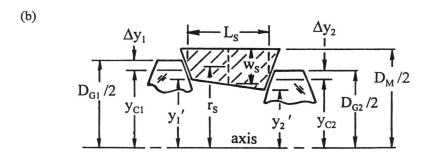

Fig. 12.15 Schematics of typical lens spacers. (a) Cylindrical type with sharp-corner interfaces. (b) Tapered type with tangential interfaces. (From Yoder.[23])

$$r_s = (D_M/2) - (w_s/2) \tag{12.30}$$

$$A_s = 2\pi r_s w_s \tag{12.31}$$

By following the same sequence of calculations as described for the cemented doublet, the contact stresses at the four air/glass interfaces can be estimated (see Example 12.11).

Example 12.11: Contact stress at T_{MIN} for an air-spaced doublet lens. (For design and analysis, use File 61 of the CD-ROM)

A lens assembly like that shown in Fig. 12.14 has tangential interfaces. The pertinent design parameters are tabulated below. Each lens is equiconvex. Assuming a preload P_A at assembly (68°F) of 100 lb, estimate the axial stress at each lens surface at -80°F.

Parameter/Eqn.	Units	Cell	Lens #1	Spacer	Lens #2
Material		Ti	SF2	Ti	BK7
D_M , D_G	in.	4.342	4.336	4.342	4.086
E_i	lb/in.^{2}	1.65×10^7	7.98×10^6	1.65×10^7	1.17×10^7
υ_i		0.340	0.237	0.340	0.208
α_i	ppm/°F	4.9×10^{-6}	4.7×10^{-6}	4.9×10^{-6}	3.9×10^{-6}
K_M , $(K_G)_i$	in.^{2}/lb	5.36×10^{-8}	1.187×10^{-7}	5.36×10^{-8}	8.14×10^{-8}
t_C , L_S	in.	0.100		1.181	
$(t_E)_i$	in.		0.286	1.181	0.509
y_{C1} , y_{C2}	in.		2.014		1.889
R_1 , R_3	in.		7.600		5.391
$P_A = Wa_G$	lb	100	100	100	100
$2y_C + t_E$	in.		4.314		4.287
			($<D_G$)		($>D_G$)
A_{G1} [Eq. (12.22)]	in.^{2}		3.619		
A_{G2} [Eq. (12.23)]	in.^{2}				4.720
Δy_i [Eq. (12.27)	in.		0.154		0.154
y'_i [Eq. (12.28)]	in.		1.860		1.735
w_S [Eq. (12.26)]	in.			0.373	
r_S [Eq. (12.30)]	in.			1.984	
A_M [Eq. (12.18)]	in.^{2}	1.396			
A_S [Eq. (12.31)]	in.^{2}			4.657	
K_3 [Eq. (12.22)]	lb/°F		-4.061		
$K_{1 TAN}$ [Eq. (11.8)]	in.$^{-1}$		0.066		0.093
$K_2 = K_M + (K_G)_i$	in.^{2}/lb		1.722×10^{-7}		1.354×10^{-7}
$\Delta T = T_{MIN} - T_A$	°F	-148			
$\Delta P = K_3 \Delta T$	lb	601			
$P_{TOTAL} = P_{MAX} + \Delta P$	lb		701		701
$p = P_{TOTAL} /(2\pi y_C)$	lb/in.		55.396		59.062
S_C [Eq. (11.2)]	lb/in.^{2}		3677		5083

Because of symmetry, the stresses at R_1 and R_2 are the same as are those at R_3 and R_4. These stresses should cause no damage at T_{MIN}.

12.7.3 General case of the multiple-component lenses

Equation (12.34) allows the factor K3 of a general multiple-component lens design to be defined from terms previously discussed. This equation has in its numerator the sum of negative terms representing the axial thicknesses of each lens element and of the spacer(s) at the applicable heights of contact multiplied by the pertinent differences in CTEs for those parts relative to the CTE of the mount. In the denominator is found the sum of reciprocals of the spring constants for each part of the subassembly. Some terms in the denominator represent parts in compression while others represent parts in tension.

$$K_3 = \frac{-\sum_1^n (\alpha_M - \alpha_i) t_i}{\sum_1^n C_i^{-1}} \tag{12.32}$$

where C_i for a lens is $(E_G A_G / 2 t_E)$ and C_i for a spacer is $(E_M A_M / t_S)$. The factor of 2 in the lens case results from a simplifying approximation that the "effective" area of the annular stressed region in the lens is the average of zero at the lens surface and t_E at the center of the lens.

The general form of the equation for the change in axial gap Δx between the lens and mount after losing contact at T_C is

$$\tag{12.33}$$
$$\Delta x = Gap_A = \sum_1^n (\alpha_M - \alpha_i) t_i \Delta T$$

By applying the general guidelines used in formulating Eqs. (12.32) and (12.33), appropriate equations for analyzing quite complex multiple-component designs can be assembled. The procedure explained earlier can then be used to determine the axial contact stress for those designs at any temperature.

12.8 Radial Stresses in Rim-Mounted, Circular-Aperture Optics

We know that changes in temperature cause differential expansion or contraction of circular lenses, windows, filters, and mirrors with respect to mounting materials in both the axial and radial directions. In the following discussion of the effects of changes in radial dimensions, we assume rotational symmetry of the optics and of the pertinent portions of the mount, a small clearance between the optic OD and the ID of the mount (or of hard radial locating pads, if used), that all components are at a uniform temperature, that the CTEs of the optical materials (glass, ceramic, metal, or composite) and of the mount (usually metal) are α_G and α_M, respectively, and that temperature changes are $\pm \Delta T$.

The CTE of the mount usually exceeds that of the optic mounted in it; a prime exception would be if Invar were used in the mount and a higher CTE material such as Pyrex were used in a mirror. In the usual case, a drop in temperature will cause the mount to contract radially toward the optic's rim. Any radial clearance between these components will decrease in size and if the temperature falls far enough, the ID of the mount will contact the OD of the optic. Further temperature decreases will then cause radial force to be exerted upon the rim of the optic. This force compresses (i.e., strains) the optic radially and creates radially directed stress. To the degree of approximation applied here, the strain and stress are axially symmetrical. If the stress is large enough, the performance of the optic will be adversely affected. Extremely large stresses may cause failure of the optic and/or plastic deformation of the mount.

Temperature increases will, of course, cause the mount to expand away from the optic, thereby increasing any existing radial clearance or creating such a clearance. Significant increases in radial clearance may allow the optic to shift under external forces such as shock or vibration; alignment may then be affected.

12.8.1 Radial stress in an optic at low temperature

The magnitude of the radial stress, S_R, in the optic for a given temperature drop, ΔT, can be estimated as:

$$S_R = -K_4 K_5 \Delta T \tag{12.34}$$

where:

$$K_4 = \frac{(\alpha_M - \alpha_G)}{(1/E_G) + [D_G/(2E_M t_C)]} \tag{12.35}$$

$$K_5 = 1 + \frac{2\Delta r}{D_G \Delta T(\alpha_M - \alpha_G)} \tag{12.36}$$

D_G = optic OD
t_C = mount wall thickness outside the rim of the optic
Δr = radial clearance

Note that ΔT is negative for a temperature decrease. Also, $0 < K_5 < 1$. If Δr exceeds $[D_G \Delta T(\alpha_M - \alpha_G)/2]$, the optic will not be constrained by the mount ID and radial stress will not develop within the temperature range ΔT as a result of rim contact.

Example 12.12: Estimation of radial stress in a lens.
(For design and analysis, use File 62 of the CD-ROM)

A SF2 lens of diameter 2.384 in. (60.554 mm) is mounted in a 416 CRES cell machined to provide 0.0002 in. (5.08×10^{-3} mm) of radial clearance for assembly at 68°F (20°C). The cell wall thickness is 0.125 in. (3.175 mm). What radial stress is developed in the lens at $T_{MIN} = -80°F (-62°C)$?

From Tables B1 and B12:

$E_G = 7.98 \times 10^6$ lb/in.² (5.50×10^4 MPa), $\alpha_G = 4.7 \times 10^{-6}$ /°F (8.4×10^{-6} /°C)

$E_M = 2.9 \times 10^7$ lb/in.² (2.15×10^5 MPa), $\alpha_M = 5.5 \times 10^{-6}$ /°F (9.9×10^{-6} /°C)

$\Delta T = -80 - 68 = -148°F (-82.2°C)$

From Eqs. (12.35) and (12.36),

$$K_4 = \frac{(5.5 \times 10^{-6} - 4.7 \times 10^{-6})}{(1/7.98 \times 10^6) + \{2.384/[(2)(2.9 \times 10^7)(0.125)]\}} = 1.762 \text{ in.}^2/°F$$

$$K_5 = 1 + \frac{(2)(0.0002)}{(2.384)(-148)(5.5 \times 10^{-6} - 4.7 \times 10^{-6})} = -0.417$$

From Eq. (12.34), $S_R = -(1.76)(-0.417)(-148) = -108.6$ lb/in² (- 0.75 MPa)

This negative radial stress at low temperature results from the fact that the CTE difference is insufficient to cause lens rim-to-cell ID contact at T_{MIN}. No radial stress is developed. This condition occurs whenever K_5 is negative.

Example 12.13: Estimation of radial stress in a radially constrained mirror.
(For design and analysis, use File 63 of the CD-ROM)

A mirror made of Ohara E6 glass with a diameter of 20.000 in. (50.800 cm) is mounted in a 6061 aluminum cell machined to provide 0.0002 in. (5.08 µm) of radial clearance for assembly at 68°F (20°C). The cell wall thickness is 0.25 in. (5.080 mm) at the mirror rim. What radial stress is developed in the mirror at $T_{MIN} = -80°F (-62°C)$?

From Tables B8a and B12:

$E_G = 8.5 \times 10^6$ lb/in.^{2} (5.86×10^{10} Pa), $\alpha_G = 1.5 \times 10^{-6}$ /°F (2.7×10^{-6} /°C)

$E_M = 9.9 \times 10^6$ lb/in.^{2} (6.82×10^{10} Pa), $\alpha_M = 13.1 \times 10^{-6}$/°F ($23.6 \times 10^{-6}$ /°C)

$\Delta T = -80 - 68 = -148$°F ($-82.2$°C)

From Eqs. (12.35) and (12.36),

$$K_4 = \frac{(13.1 \times 10^{-6} - 1.5 \times 10^{-6})}{(1/8.5 \times 10^6) + \{20/[(2)(9.9 \times 10^6)(0.25)]\}} = 2.79 \text{ lb/in.}^2 \text{ /°F}$$

$$K_5 = 1 + \frac{(2)(0.0002)}{(20)(-148)(13.1 \times 10^{-6} - 1.5 \times 10^{-6})} = 0.988$$

From Eq. (12.34), $S_R = -(2.79)(0.988)(-148) = 408$ lb/in^2 (2.81 MPa)

This stress would create no threat of damage to the mirror.

12.8.2 Tangential (hoop) stress in the mount wall

Another consequence of differential contraction of the mount relative to the rim contact optic is that stress is built up within the mount in accordance with the following equation:

$$S_M = S_R D_G/(2t_C) \tag{12.37}$$

where all terms are as defined earlier.

With this expression, we can determine if the mount is strong enough to withstand the force exerted upon the optic without exceeding its elastic limit. If the yield strength of the mount material exceeds S_M, a safety factor exists. Examples 12.14 and 12.15 illustrate typical cases.

Example 12.14: Tangential (hoop) stress in a lens cell wall. (For design and analysis, use File 64 of the CD-ROM)
Estimate the stress in the lens cell wall for Example 12.12.

From Example, 12.12, S_R = - 108.6 lb/in.^{2} The fact that this is a negative quantity indicates that there is no radial stress in the glass at low temperature. There can then be no hoop stress in the cell wall at that temperature.

Example 12.15: Tangential (hoop) stress in a mirror cell wall. (For design and analysis, use File 65 of the CD-ROM)
Estimate the stress in the lens cell wall for Example 12.13.

From Example, 12.13, S_R = 408 lb/in.^{2}

By Eq. (12.37), S_M = (408)(20.000)/[(2)(0.250)] = 16,320 lb/in.^{2} (112.53 MPa)

From Table B12, we find that the yield strength of the 6061 aluminum lies between 8000 and 40,000 lb/in.^{2}. The wall might fail (i.e., distort). We should either make the wall thicker or substitute a stronger material for the mount (such as CRES). Note that the stress in the mirror should be recomputed if such a change is made.

12.9 Growth of Radial Clearance at Increased Temperatures

The increase, ΔGap_R, in nominal radial clearance, Gap_R , between an optic and its mount that is due to a temperature increase of ΔT from that at assembly can be estimated by:

$$\Delta Gap_R = (\alpha_M - \alpha_G)(D_G \Delta T/2) \tag{12.38}$$

where all terms are as previously defined.

If there is no axial constraint (as might happen at high temperature), whatever total radial clearance Gap_R exists between the optic OD and mount ID allows the optic to roll (i.e., tilt about a transverse axis) until its rim touches the mount ID at diametrically opposite points of the edge thickness t_A. This roll angle can be estimated by the equation:

$$Roll = \arctan(2 Gap_R/t_E) \tag{12.39}$$

Example 12.16: Growth in radial clearance around a mirror at high temperature.
(For design and analysis, use File 66 of the CD-ROM)
What increase in radial clearance exists in the mirror assembly described in Example 12.13 at $T_{MAX} = 160°$ F (71.1°C)? The radial clearance at assembly is 0.0002 in. ($5.08×10^{-3}$ mm).

$\Delta T = 160 - 68 = 92°$ F (33.3°C).

By Eq. (12.38): $\Delta Gap_R = (13.1×10^{-6} - 1.5×10^{-6})(20)(92)/2)$
$= 0.0107$ in. (0.2711 mm).

The nominal radial gap at T_{MAX} is then $0.0002 + 0.0107 = 0.0109$ in. (0.028 mm).

Example 12.17: Roll (tilt) of a mirror within nominal expanded radial clearance at high temperature.
(For design and analysis, use File 67 of the CD-ROM)
What is the maximum roll that the mirror of the preceding example can experience under vibration at maximum survival temperature, T_{MAX}? Assume that the mirror has an edge thickness t_E of 1.875 in. (47.625 mm).

The expanded radial gap around the mirror is 0.0109 in. (0.028 mm)

By Eq. (12.39), Roll $= \arctan (2)(0.0109)/1.875 = 0.666°$

12.10 Thermally Induced Stresses in Bonded Optics

In Sects. 7.3 and 9.2, we considered techniques for bonding prisms and mirrors to mounts. There are three major sources of stress in the bonded joints between such optics and their mounts. These are shrinkage of the adhesive during curing, acceleration in a direction that tends to pull the optic from the mount, and differential expansion and contraction at high and low temperatures. We consider each of these factors briefly.

Shrinkage during curing typically amounts to a few percent of each dimension of the adhesive layer and may persist throughout the life of the device. Assuming that the material adheres well to both the optic and mount surfaces throughout the contact area, the adhesive layer and the bonded surfaces of the optic and mount are somewhat stressed.

This stress is usually small, but will tend to bend the optic. If the optic is too thin, this may change the figures of optical surfaces suffciently to degrade performance. Corrective actions include making sure that the optic thickness is as large as reasonably possible, choosing an adhesive with minimal curing shrinkage, and minimizing the lateral dimensions of the bond. Using optical materials with high stiffness (i.e., large Young's modulus) also will help in the case of mirrors.

Acceleration directed normal to the bond joint and in a direction that places the joint in tension can cause sufficient force to break something. As explained earlier for prisms, the strength of the adhesive joint often is greater than the tensile strength of the optical material, so fracture of the latter can occur under high tensile stress. The worst situation would be when this happens at an extreme temperature so differential contraction or expansion of the materials and the effect of acceleration act together.

Thermal effects in bonded joints that are due to a mismatch of glass and metal CTEs have their greatest impacts at extreme temperatures. They also tend to bend the optic, but are temporary and usually reversible. In the common case with $\alpha_e >> \alpha_M > \alpha_G$, differential contraction in the three components with changes in temperature introduces stress in all components. Fracture of bonded optical parts has on occasion been attributed to high shear forces exerted in the joint by temperature-induced dimensional changes. Finite-element analysis methods can be used to predict thermally induced stress in the optic caused by this effect, but they are beyond the scope of this book.

Vukobratovich[24] presented an analytical method, based on work by Chen and Nelson,[25] for estimating the shear stress developed in a bonded joint as a result of differential dimensional changes at temperatures other than that at assembly. The pertinent equations are as follows:

$$S_S = (\alpha_M - \alpha_G)(\Delta T)(S_e)[\tanh(\beta L)]/(\beta t_e) \tag{12.40}$$

$$S_e = E_e/[(2)(1 + \nu_e)] \tag{3.46}$$

$$\beta = [(\frac{S_e}{t_e})(\frac{1}{E_M t_M} + \frac{1}{E_G t_G})]^{1/2} \tag{12.41}$$

where:

S_S = shear stress in the joint
α_M, α_G = CTEs of the metal and glass, respectively
ΔT = temperature change from assembly temperature
S_e = shear modulus of the adhesive

tanh = hyperbolic tangent function
L   = width of the bond
t_e = thickness of the adhesive layer
E_M, E_G = Young's modulus of the metal and glass, respectively
υ_e = Poisson's ratio for the adhesive
t_M, t_G = thickness of the metal and glass, respectively

Example 12.18 illustrates the use of these equations for a practical case.

Example 12.18: Stress in a bonded prism caused by differential thermal expansion.
(For design and analysis, use File 68 of the CD-ROM)

The cube-shaped prism shown in Fig. 7.19 is made of fused silica and is bonded to a titanium base with 3M 2216 epoxy. The face width of the prism is 1.378 in. The base is 1.051 in. thick. The bond is circular, 0.004 in. thick, and has a diameter L of 1.378 in. (a) Assuming that the stress in the prism equals the shear stress in the adhesive, what is that stress as a result of a temperature change ΔT of -90°F? (b) Let the large bond be replaced by three equal areas of 0.250 in. width. What would be the stress in each of these bonded areas at -90°F?

From Tables B1, B12, and B14

$\alpha_M = 4.90 \times 10^{-6}$ /°F $\alpha_G = 0.32 \times 10^{-6}$ /°F

$E_M = 16.5 \times 10^6$ lb/in.² $E_G = 10.6 \times 10^6$ lb/in.² $E_e = 1.00 \times 10^5$ lb/in.²

$\upsilon_M = 0.31$ $\upsilon_G = 0.17$ $\upsilon_e = 0.43$ (see Ref. 26)

From Eq. (3.46), $S_e = 1.0 \times 10^5 / [(2)(1 + 0.43)] = 3.50 \times 10^4$ lb/in.²

From Eq. (12.41)

$$\beta = \left\{ \left(\frac{3.50 \times 10^4}{0.004} \right) \left[\frac{1}{(16.5 \times 10^6)(1.051)} + \frac{1}{(10.6 \times 10^6)(1.378)} \right] \right\}^{1/2} = 1.050 \text{ in.}^{-1}$$

(a) From Eq. (12.40) with $\beta L = (1.050)(1.378) = 1.447$

$$S_S = (4.90 \times 10^{-6} - 0.32 \times 10^{-6})(-90)(3.50 \times 10^4)(\tanh 1.447)/[(1.050)(0.004)]$$
$$= -3074 \text{ lb/in.}^2$$

This stress significantly exceeds the rule of thumb tolerance for tensile stress in glass established earlier, so breakage of the prism may be expected at the specified low temperature. As indicated in the discussion of Fig. 7.19, this actually happened.

(b) From Eq. (12.40) with $\beta L = (1.050)(0.250) = 0.262$

$$S_S = (4.90 \times 10^{-6} - 0.32 \times 10^{-6})(-90)(3.50 \times 10^4)(\tanh 0.262)/[(1.050)(0.004)]$$

$$= -880 \text{ lb/in.}^2$$

The stress at low temperature now is reduced to a value that is much more acceptable. We may expect the prism to survive if the bonded surface is free of defects. As indicated in the discussion of Fig. 7.19, this actually was the case.

References

1. Schreibman, M., and Young, P., "Design of Infrared Astronomical Satellite (IRAS) primary mirror mounts," *SPIE Proceedings* Vol. 250, 50, 1980.

2. Young, P., and Schreibman, M., "Alignment design for a cryogenic telescope," *SPIE Proceedings* Vol. 251, 171, 1980.

3. Erickson, D.J., Johnston, R.A., and Hull, A.B., "Optimization of the opto-mechanical interface employing diamond machining in a concurrent engineering environment," *SPIE Critical Review* Vol. CR43, 329, 1992.

4. Hookman, R., "Design of the GOES telescope secondary mirror mounting," *SPIE Proceedings* Vol. 1167, 368, 1989.

5. Zurmehly, G.E., and Hookman, R., "Thermal/optical test setup for the Geostationary Operational Environmental Satellite Telescope," *SPIE Proceedings* Vol. 1167, 360, 1989.

6. Edlen, B., "The Dispersion of Standard Air," *J. Opt. Soc. Am.*, Vol. 43, 339, 1953.

7. Penndorf, R., "Tables of the Refractive Index for Standard Air and the Rayleigh Scattering Coefficient for the Spectral Region between 0.2 and 20 μ and their Application to Atmospheric Optics", *J. Opt. Soc. Am.*, Vol. 47, 176, 1957.

8. Jamieson, T.H., "Athermalization of optical instruments from the optomechanical viewpoint," *SPIE Proceedings* Vol. CR43, 131, 1992.

9. Smith W.J., *Modern Optical Engineering*, McGraw-Hill, New York, 2000.

10. Jamieson, T.H., "Thermal effects in optical systems," *Opt. Eng.* Vol. 20, 156, 1981.

11. Vukobratovich, D., "Optomechanical Systems Design," Chapt. 3 in *The Infrared & Electro-Optical Systems Handbook*, Vol. 4, ERIM, Ann Arbor and SPIE, Bellingham, 1993.

12. Code V is a product of Optical Research Associates, Pasadena, CA.

13. Friedman, I., "Thermo-optical analysis of two long-focal-length aerial reconnaissance lenses," *Opt. Eng.* Vol. 20, 161, 1981.

14. Povey, V., "Athermalization techniques in infrared systems," *SPIE Proceedings* Vol. 655, 142, 1986.

15. Rogers, P.J., "Athermalized FLIR optics," *SPIE Proceedings* Vol. 1354, 742, 1990.

16. Parr-Burman, P.M., and Madgwick, P., "A high-performance athermalized dual field of view I.R. telescope," *SPIE Proceedings* Vol. 1013, 92, 1988.

17. Fischer, R.E., and Kampe, T.U., "Actively controlled 5:1 afocal zoom attachment for common module FLIR," *SPIE Proceedings* Vol. 1690, 137, 1992.

18. Hatheway, A.E., "Thermo-elastic stability of an argon ion laser cavity," *SPIE Proceedings* Vol. 4198, 141, 2001.

19. Andersen, T.B., "Multiple-temperature lens design optimization," SPIE Proceedings Vol. 2000, 2, 1993.

20. Barnes, W.P., Jr., "Some effects of aerospace thermal environments on high-acuity optical systems," *Appl. Opt.* Vol. 5, 701, 1966.

21. Yoder, P.R., Jr., "Advanced considerations of the lens-to-mount interface," *SPIE Proceedings* Vol. CR43, 305, 1992.

22. Lecuyer, J.G., "Maintaining optical integrity in a high-shock environment," *SPIE Proceedings* Vol. 250, 45, 1980.

23. Yoder, P.R., Jr., "Estimation of mounting-induced axial contact stresses in multi-element lens assemblies," *SPIE Proceedings* Vol. 2263, 332, 1994.

24. Vukobratovich, D., "Introduction to Optomechanical Design," *SPIE Short Course Notes SC014*, SPIE Press, Bellingham, 2001.

25. Chen, W.T. and Nelson, C.W., "Thermal stress in bonded joints," *J. Res. Develop.*, Vol. 23, 179, 1979.

26. Private communication from D. Vukobratovich, 2001.

CHAPTER 13
Hardware Examples

In this chapter are found descriptions and illustrations of thirty examples of optical hardware involving, in sequence, mountings for simple and complex lenses, catadioptric systems, and prisms, as well as mirrors and gratings. Concepts and designs described earlier in this book are frequently revisited here. Many of these examples are described in more detail and in context with their applications in other publications. References are provided so the reader can explore those resources for items of particular interest.

13.1 Lens Assembly Designed to Resist Thermal Shock

Stubbs and Hsu[1] described an infrared sensor assembly that was designed to cool from room temperature to <120 K (ΔT > - 150°C) within 5 min. The assembly contained a 26-mm (1.02-in.)-aperture, meniscus-shaped germanium lens element cooled by conduction of heat through its annular interfaces with a multicomponent brazed mount. Figure 13.1 shows a sectional view through the assembly. The mount was made of molybdenum TZM to closely match the CTE of the germanium (CTE_{Mo} = 5.5×10^{-6}/K, CTE_{Ge} = 4.9×10^{-6}/K). Heat flow out of the lens was maximized by establishing intimate

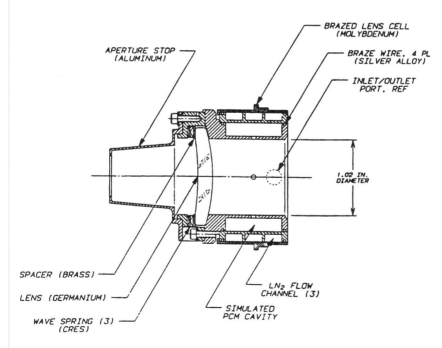

Fig. 13.1 Sectional schematic diagram of a lens assembly designed for rapid cooling by conduction through its rim. (From Stubbs and Hsu.[1])

444 MOUNTING OPTICAL COMPONENTS IN OPTICAL INSTRUMENTS

contact between a flat bevel on the front (concave) lens surface and a brass spacer, and between the spherical rear (convex) lens surface and a matching concave spherical mechanical interface. The latter surface was ground and polished using optical test plates made to match the radius of the lens when at 120 K within two fringes at a 3.39-μm wavelength. The assembly preload of 55 lb (245 N) was provided by three stainless steel wave spring washers in series with a bolted-on, flange-type retainer. The authors indicated that the room-temperature axial preload was 113 lb/in.[2] (0.78 MPa), so the contact area probably was about 0.5 in.[2] (322 mm[2]). With such large surface contacts, stress within the lens from the preload would be minimal.

A flow channel was machined into the housing's outer cylindrical surface and a cylindical plenum cover was brazed over the exposed channel. Fill and vent tubes were then brazed radially onto the cover. The flow channel, labled "simulated PCM cavity" in Fig. 13.1, is a chamber reserved for a phase-change material to be used to stabilize the temperature of the assembly for about 25 min. during operation after cooldown with liquid nitrogen flow through the three channels. Coolant lines were epoxied to the radial tubes using Epibond epoxy type 1210A/9615-10 supplied by CIBA-Geigy Furane Aerospace Products. Figure 13.2 is an exploded view of the assembly showing the optical and mechanical components more clearly.

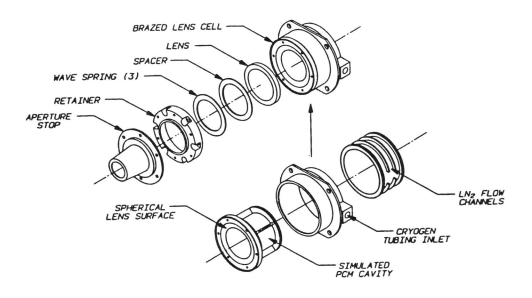

Fig. 13.2 Exploded view of the lens assembly. (From Stubbs and Hsu.[1])

Interferometric tests of a model of the lens assembly indicated that the lens would survive the imposed thermal shock and not be excessively distorted by the compressive forces during operation. Laboratory tests of thermal behavior of the assembly showed that temperatures measured as a function of time after cryogen flow was initiated followed predictions reasonably well and that stabilization at about 100 K appeared to be achieved well within the desired 25-min. time period.

13.2 Infrared Sensor Lens Assembly

The optomechanical configuration of a 69-mm focal length, f/0.87 objective assembly designed for use in an infrared radiation sensor is illustrated in Fig. 13.3. The singlet lens was silicon, while the first element of the cemented doublet was silicon and the second sapphire. The doublet was cemented with AO-805 adhesive (which is no longer available). Wedge angles of the flat bevels on the concave faces of the lenses were held to 10 arcsec for the singlet and 30 arcsec for the doublet to ensure good centration to the axis.

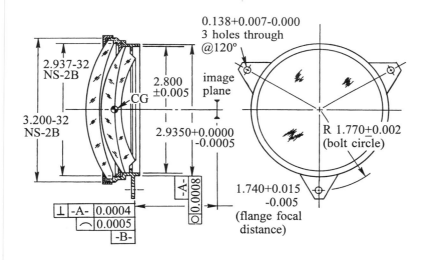

Fig. 13.3 Sectional and frontal views of a triplet infrared sensor assembly. Dimensions are given in inches. (Courtesy of Hughes Danbury Optical Systems, Danbury, CT.)

The cell was made of Invar 36 and was stabilized after rough machining by repeated cycling between - 320° F and room temperature. The registering OD (-A-) and flange ear mounting interface surfaces (-B-) were closely toleranced for diameter and perpendicularity to the optical axis, respectively, to ensure precise alignment with related components of the sensor system.

The lenses were lathe assembled with maximum 0.0002 in. clearances into the cell and constrained axially by threaded 303 CRES retainers. Prior to tightening the retainers, the lenses were differentially rotated about the axis to maximize symmetry of the axial image and to minimize decentration of that image relative to the OD (-A-).

13.3 Cemented Doublet Binocular Objective Assembly

Figure 13.4 shows a sectional view through one objective of the 7×50 M17A1 military binocular designed in the early 1940s and built in large quantity for military use during World War II. It is in many ways similar to designs used in binoculars today. The 7.598-in. focal length, 1.969-in. (50-mm)-aperture (f/3.86) doublet, made of glass types 511635 and 617366, had an OD of 2.048 + 0 - 0.004 in., an axial thickness of 0.571 ± 0.020 in., and a nominal edge thickness of 0.406 in. The lens rim had maximum

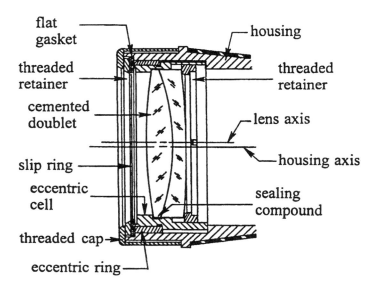

Fig. 13.4 Sectional view of the objective lens mounting in a military binocular of World War II vintage. (Adapted from a U.S. Army drawing.)

protective bevels of 0.020 in. face width at 45°. This doublet was mounted with burnished sharp-corner interfaces in an aluminum cell with stepped ODs machined eccentrically with respect to the centerline of its ID. This cell was inserted into an aluminum ring that had a hole machined eccentrically with respect to its OD. The latter ring was mounted into a recess machined into a cast aluminum telescope housing assembly forming one half of the binocular. The outer edges of the lens cell, eccentric ring, and housing were sealed by a

0.035-in.-thick flat rubber gasket. An axial preload to hold the lens into its cell was provided by a threaded aluminum retainer, while the entire assembly, including the gasket, a thin aluminum slip ring, and a threaded retainer, was covered by a threaded cap. The thin annular slip ring served to prevent torsional distortion of the gasket as the retainer was tightened.

During assembly, the axis of the lens was adjusted laterally by differential rotation of the eccentric parts to align the lines of sight of the individual telescopes parallel to each other and to the hinge of the instrument within specified vertical and horizontal angular tolerances. Concentric tubular tools were used to rotate the eccentrics. No means was provided for axial (focus) adjustment of the objective, the doublet being bottomed against the shoulder in the cell and the cell being bottomed against the shoulder in the body. Static seals were provided between the doublet and the cell and between the slip ring and the cell by sealing compound (originally 3M polysulfide type EC-801) inserted into a shallow annular groove in the cell ID next to the lens rim and into a similar groove in the cell ID at the inner edge of the slip ring.

13.4 Modular Binocular Objective Assembly

The objective module of the 7×50 M19 military binocular (see Trsar et al[2]) shown in Figs. 4.27 and 4.31 is shown in Fig. 13.5. This optical subsystem has an air-spaced triplet of telephoto design with a focal length of 6.012 in. and an aperture of 1.969 in. (50 mm) (f/3.05). The triplet was made of types 517647 (first two elements) and 689309 glasses. The lens diameters were 2.067 in., 1.909 in., and 1.457 in., respectively. Each OD was held to tolerances of + 0, - 0.001 in.

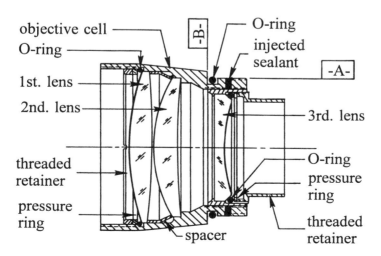

Fig. 13.5 Sectional view of the modular objective assembly for the M19 binocular. (Adapted from Trsar et al[2] .)

The objective housing was wrought aluminum. The crown lenses were mounted directly into the housing with an intermediate tapered spacer. A threaded retainer provided axial preload on these elements through an O-ring that sealed the outermost lens to the housing. A thin annular pressure ring protected the O-ring from distortion as the retainer was tightened. The flint lens was mounted into a focusable cell that threaded into the housing. This cell was sealed to the housing after adjustment by an injected elastomeric sealant. This axial adjustment served to tune the focal length of the triplet. The flint element was sealed into its cell with an O-ring compressed axially through a thin pressure ring by a retainer that also served as a light baffle. The entire objective assembly was sealed to the binocular housing by an O-ring compressed radially during assembly.

After all parts of the objective were assembled, but before its mounting interfaces were machined, the module was sealed, purged, evacuated, and backfilled with dry nitrogen. Centration of the objective to the system optical axis and focus was accomplished by machining the registration OD and shoulder of the module (surfaces -A- and -B-, respectively, of Fig. 13.5) as well as the mating surfaces in the body to close tolerances using sophisticated optical alignment techniques to position the modules in holding and transfer fixtures. The cell (still in its fixture) was precision machined on a numerically controlled lathe. The concentricity of surface -A- to the objective's optical axis was held to $\pm$ 0.010 mm, while the tolerance on flange focal distance was $\pm$ 0.038 mm.

13.5 Air Spaced Triplet Telescope Objective Assembly

A triplet objective assembly used in a high-performance military telescope under severe shock and vibration conditions is shown in Fig. 13.6.[3] The three singlets had identical ODs and fit closely [nominally a 0.006-mm (0.0002-in.) radial clearance] into the ID of a 316 CRES barrel. The lenses were inserted from the right side so the plano front surface of the first element rested against a flat shoulder within the barrel. The first spacer was a thin "washer" cut from a 0.066 $\pm$ 0.005-mm (0.0026 $\pm$ 0.0002-in.)-thick CRES sheet. Under axial preload, this spacer conformed to a "best fit" with the adjacent spherical lens surfaces that had almost identical radii. The second spacer was also 316 CRES; it had tangential interfaces for the contacted lens surfaces. The third singlet had a precision flat bevel that mated with a threaded retainer also made of 316 CRES. This bevel was aligned to the opposite surface of the lens within a 10-μm (0.0004-in.) edge thickness runout tolerance. All metal parts were black passivated.

The three lenses were made of SF4, SK16, and SSK4 glasses, respectively. All had wedge tolerances of 10 arcsec. At assembly, the residual wedges of the lenses were phased (or clocked) by rotation about the axis for maximum symmetry of the on-axis aerial image observed through a microscope. The focal length of the optical assembly was 185.8 $\pm$ 0.7 mm at a 550-nm wavelength and its aperture was 56.64 mm, so it functioned at f/3.28.

The CTEs of the three glasses were 8.0×10^{-6} /°C, 6.3×10^{-6} /°C, and 6.12×10^{-6} /°C,

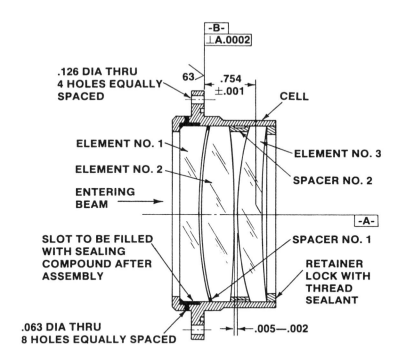

Fig. 13.6 Sectional view of an air-spaced triplet telescope objective assembly. Dimensions are given in inches. (From Yoder.[3])

respectively. That of the barrel was 8.9×10^{-6} /°C. The worst-case radial stress exerted at -80° F (-62° C) on the lens with maximum CTE difference relative to the barrel was estimated as 1551 lb/in.[2] (10.7 MPa). The corresponding tensile stress exerted on the barrel wall was estimated as 14,790 lb/in.[2] (102.0 MPa). The latter stress is about 37% of the metal yield strength of 40,000 lb/in.[2] (276.0 MPa).

13.6 Commercial Mid-IR Lenses

Figure 13.7 is a photograph of a set of four f/2.3 lens assemblies produced by Janos Technologies, Inc. for use with standard commercial infrared cameras in a variety of applications. They are designed to operate to near the diffraction limit in the 3- to 5-μm spectral region and have optical and mechanical characteristics shown in Table 13.1.

Typical construction is indicated by the sectional view through one of the assemblies shown in Fig. 13.8. The following description is adapted from information provided by Palmer and Murray.[4]

The mechanical parts are 6061T6 aluminum and the lenses are silicon and

Table 13.1 Characteristics of f/2.3 commercial mid-IR lenses

Focal length (mm)	Field of View (deg)	Length (mm)	Diameter (mm)	Weight (oz)
13	± 38.9	46.8	57.1	< 8
25	± 22.8	46.8	57.1	< 8
50	± 11.8	46.8	61.9	< 7.5
100	± 6.0	107.6	117.3	< 31

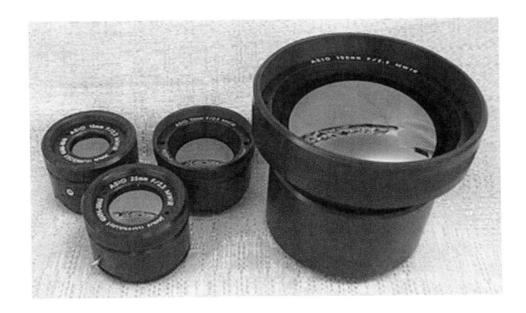

Fig. 13.7 Photograph of four f/2.3 commercial lens assemblies with focal lengths of 13 to 100 mm designed for the mid-infrared region. (Courtesy of Janos Technology, Inc., Townshend, VT.)

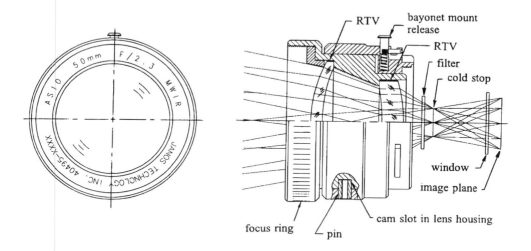

Fig. 13.8 Section view through one of the lenses shown in Fig. 13.7. (Courtesy of Janos Technology, Inc., Townshend, VT.)

germanium. The filter, cold stop, window, and detector array are contained in a separate dewar furnished by the user. Each lens is held in place with RTV Type 655 sealant manufactured by GE. During assembly, the applicable areas of the cell and the rims of each lens are primed with GE primer SS4155 to facilitate adhesion. Special care is exercised in applying the primer to the lenses since it can damage the polished surfaces if they are accidentally contacted. The lenses are then installed with their flat bevels contacting the shoulders provided in the cell and shimmed to center them within $\pm$ 30 μm relative to the mount axis. Once aligned, the RTV is applied with a fluid dispensing system and cured according to the manufacturer's directions. A retaining ring is then installed. It does not apply significant preload to the lens, but serves as a convenient location for lens identification information.

Each lens is focused by rotating the knurled ring at the front. This rotates the lens housing within the fixed mount body and drives the lenses axially by virtue of a helical cam slot in the lens cell that engages a brass pin fixed in the body. The object space range is from infinity to 50, 150, 425, and 1750 mm respectively for the 13, 25, 50, and 100 mm EFL types. Focus is clamped with a soft-tip setscrew (not shown). Each lens attaches to the camera through a bayonet mechanism. The spring-loaded pin shown at top is used to unlock that mechanism.

13.7 Motorized Dual Field-of-View Lens Assembly

The optomechanical layout of a dual focal length f/2.3 lens assembly developed by Janos Technology, Inc. for use with a 3- to 5-μm infrared camera and described by Palmer and Murray[4] is shown in Fig. 13.9. This lens system has focal lengths of 50 and 250 mm and is nearly diffraction limited at both settings. Switching from one EFL (or field size) to the other is accomplished by sliding a cell containing two lenses axially inside the assembly. Focus is established at either setting by an axial movement of another cell containing one lens. A dc motor drives the focal length switching mechanism while a stepper motor is used to drive the focus adjustment. Each mechanism contains a spur gear that rotates a ring gear on a cylindrical cam. Helical slots in the cams engage pins affixed to the lens cell and to the focus cell and drive those cells axially as the cams rotate. The pins also engage slots in the fixed portion of the housing to prevent rotation of the lenses, thereby maintaining constant boresight alignment. Sliding surfaces are hard anodized and have 16 microinch surfaces, but are not lubricated. The radial clearance is typically $\pm$ 12 μm.

Figure 13.10 is a photograph of the exterior of the assembly. It is 321.3 mm long and generally cylindrical in configuration. The maximum lateral dimensions are 126.8 mm high and 133.0 mm wide. The assembly weighs 3.75 kg. The interface with the camera is a bayonet mount. A spring-loaded pin allows that mechanism to be released.

The main housing of the assembly is 6061-T6 aluminum; the lenses are silicon and germanium. The larger lenses are constrained by a threaded retaining ring and located by seating them against shoulders. The spacer between these lenses also provides the seat for the outermost lens. The remaining lenses are held in place by GE RTV-655 seals around their rims in much the same manner as the lenses described in Sect. 13.6 for other infrared lenses made by this same manufacturer.

13.8 All-Plastic Projection Lens Assembly

Figure 4.26 shows a group of all-plastic lens assemblies produced by Corning Precision Lens, Inc. and used primarily for projection television purposes. One of these lenses is shown in Fig. 13.11. It is labeled as a Delta 20 design and consists of an air-spaced triplet mounted in a plastic cell that can be moved axially to focus by rotating the cell within a fixed housing. The dimensions of this assembly are 104.5 $\pm$ 3.5 mm (4.11 $\pm$ 0.14 in.) long, including focus motion, and 117 mm (4.61 in.) diameter, not including the mounting flanges. The weight of the lens assembly shown is approximately 1.5 lb (680 g). Its focal length is 89.7 mm (3.50 in.) and it is designed to operate at a fixed aperture of f/1.2 with a nominal magnification of 9.3×.

The internal optomechanical construction of the lens cell in this assembly is

453

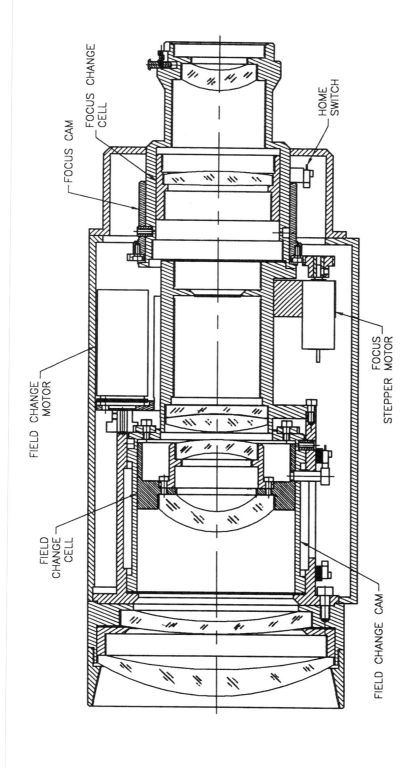

FOCUS CHANGE

FOCUS CHANGE
CELL

FOCUS CAM

HOME
SWITCH

FIELD CHANGE
MOTOR

FOCUS
STEPPER MOTOR

FIELD
CHANGE
CELL

FIELD CHANGE CAM

Fig. 13.9 Section view of a dual field-of-view mid-IR objective lens. (Courtesy of Janos Technology, Inc., Townshend, VT.)

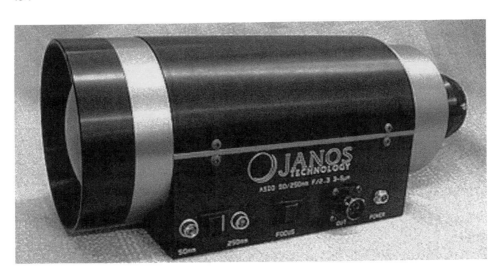

Fig. 13.10 Photograph of the dual field-of-view lens assembly depicted in Fig. 13.9. (Courtesy of Janos Technology, Inc., Townshend, VT.)

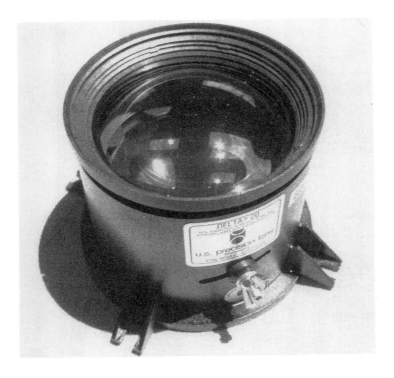

Fig. 13.11 Photograph of an all-plastic television projection lens assembly manufactured by U.S. Precision Lens, Inc., Cincinnati, OH (now Corning Precision Lens, Inc.).

patterned along the lines described by Betinsky and Welham[5] for earlier designs. Figure 13.12 illustrates the concept.[6] The lenses are mounted within a longitudinally split plastic cell molded as two symmetrical halves in what is called a "clamshell mounting." Two types of internal features capture and hold the lenses in position when the halves are

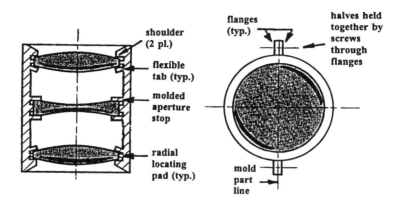

Fig. 13.12 Schematic side and end views of the clamshell lens mounting. Adapted from a publication by U.S. Precision Lens, Inc., Cincinnati, OH.[6])

(a)   (b)

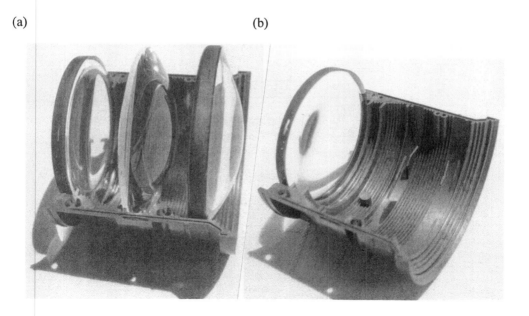

Fig. 13.13 Photographs of the interior of the lens assembly from Fig. 13.11, (a) with half of the cell removed and (b) with two of the three lenses removed. Lens mounting features and stray light-reducing grooves can be seen.

joined and fastened together. Radially, they are constrained by localized pads and axially, they are constrained by narrow tabs projecting inward radially on both sides of the lens. The pads and tabs are sufficiently flexible to allow for slight differences in lens OD and pad ID and lens edge thickness resulting from the production molding process. The halves of the cell are, in the present design, attached by four self-tapping screws. Figure 13.13 is a photograph of the interior of one half of the lens cell with two of the lenses removed. Some of the radial pads, axial tabs, and stray light-suppressing grooves are clearly visible. The holes for the clamshell assembly screws can also be seen.

The assembled lens cell fits snugly into the ID of the outer housing and is focused by sliding axially when rotated. Two screws pass through a helical cam slot molded into the housing wall and are threaded into the wall of the lens cell at diametrically-opposite points. Wing nuts on one or both of these screws allow the adjustment to be clamped after focusing. The housing is designed to be attached to the external supporting structure by screws passing through the mounting ears visible in Fig. 13.11.

13.9 Microscope Objective Assembly

Many lenses (and sometimes mirrors) used in microscope objectives are extremely sensitive to decentration and/or tilt because of their short focal lengths and short radii. Some axial air spaces also are critical to achieving maximum performance when the item is assembled and adjusted. Referring to Fig. 13.14, we summarize here an explanation from Benford[7] of these processes as they apply to a typical refracting type of objective.

The two doublets and the hemispherical front lens are first burnished in their cells in the manner described in Sect. 3.2. After cleaning, these subassemblies are inserted along with a first spacer (of nominal length) into the ID of the main barrel. The first two cells fit snugly into this ID, while the third cell has significant radial clearance. A temporary version of the sleeve labeled "parfocality adjustment" is screwed onto the barrel to provide an axial reference for the stack of lens cells. A second spacer is installed on top of the third cell and held temporarily with the threaded parfocality lock nut. The quality of the aerial image of an artificial star (an axial point object located in the object plane) is examined under high magnification and the first spacer (located between the first two cells) is selected from a stockpile of spacers with slightly different lengths by successive approximations for minimum spherical aberration of the image.

The temporary version of the parfocality adjustment sleeve in place at this time provides access to three radially oriented centering screws that bear against the sides of the third lens cell. The lateral location of the third lens cell is adjusted by turning these screws while observing the axial image until that image appears symmetrical. After this adjustment is completed and the screws tightened firmly, the temporary sleeve is replaced with a permanent version (without access holes) and tightened to hold the setting.

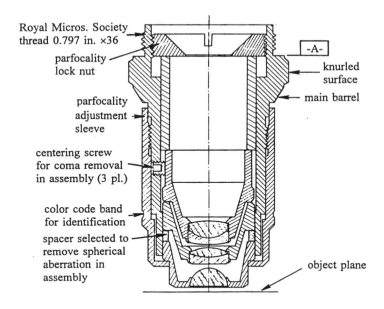

Royal Micros. Society
thread 0.797 in. ×36

parfocality
lock nut

-A-

knurled
surface

main barrel

parfocality
adjustment
sleeve

centering screw
for coma removal
in assembly (3 pl.)

color code band
for identification

spacer selected to
remove spherical
aberration in
assembly

object plane

Fig. 13.14 Construction of a typical microscope objective. (Adapted from Benford.[7])

The flange focal distance of the objective is then adjusted by turning the parfocality adjustment sleeve until the image is located at the standard distance from shoulder -A- on the main barrel. All lenses adjusted in this manner are "parfocalized," i.e., they have a common distance from flange to image. The parfocality lock nut is then tightened. The assembly process is then complete and the lens undergoes final inspection to confirm performance.

13.10 A Simple Focusing Eyepiece Assembly

Figure 13.15 shows a focusing eyepiece from a World War II vintage 7×50 military binocular. The eyepiece itself consists of two lens components: a singlet field lens and a cemented doublet eye lens. These lenses are mounted in an aluminum cell. The lens cell has an external coarse thread that engages a mating internal thread in a fixed tube that is part of the cover assembly. The cover assembly is attached with screws to the rear surface of the binocular housing and sealed to the housing with a flat rubber gasket.

The eye lens registers against the shoulder at the right end of the barrel. A tapered spacer locates the field lens with respect to the eye lens. These coaxial parts are clamped together (i.e., preloaded) by the threaded retainer at left. The eye lens is sealed to the barrel with a polysulfide-type sealing compound. The field lens is not sealed into

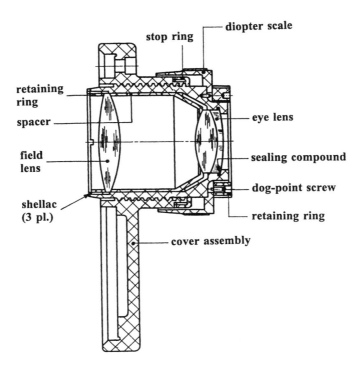

Fig. 13.15 Sectional view through a simple focusing eyepiece for a military binocular. (Adapted from a U.S. Army drawing.)

the cell since it is inside the instrument. Three dabs of shellac placed on the threads of the retaining ring help to secure that part. More suitable thread-locking compounds and sealants are available today.

The entire eyepiece turns on its thread to adjust its focus position for the individual requirements of the user. Wedge and/or decentration defects built into the eyepiece by manufacturing errors cause deviation errors of the eyepiece's optical axis when it is turned to focus the image. This affects parallelism of the lines of sight of the two telescopes of the binocular, especially since both eyepieces are focused independently. The focus threads are prevented from disengaging by a stop ring that threads onto the end of the tubular portion of the cover assembly.

A focus scale calibrated in 0.25 diopter steps is marked on a cylindrical external surface of the knurled focus ring. This ring is held in position on the lens barrel by the clamping action of another ring threaded on the eye end of the lens barrel. Calibration of the diopter scale is adjusted by slipping the focus ring to the proper zero setting before the threaded ring is tightened. The latter ring is fixed in position by a set screw. A phenolic eye guard (not shown) is threaded onto the eye end of the eyepiece to provide a surface that can be rested against the cheek or brow to steady the binocular. More sophisticated rubber eye guards are used on some versions of the binocular. These are usually shaped to fit close to the contour of the face to exclude stray light and enhance night vision.

The focus motion threads of this type eyepiece usually are lapped together during manufacture so they turn freely and smoothly. They then are lubricated with viscous grease that enhanced the feel of the focus motion and resisted penetration of moisture, dirt, and other contaminants into the instrument. The focus mechanism is frequently found to be difficult to turn at the lowest operating temperatures because the grease becomes too stiff.

13.11 Collimator Assembly Designed for High Shock Loading

Figure 13.16 shows a sectional view of a collimating lens assembly designed as part of a military flight motion simulator. This assembly was developed by Janos Technology, Inc. to project an infrared target into a forward-looking infrared system during vibration testing of the FLIR. The collimator has two air-spaced lens groups: the front group is a doublet with an average diameter of 9 in. (22.9 cm), while the rear group is a triplet with an average diameter of about 1.5 in. (3.8 cm). The lenses are made from silicon and germanium, so the optical system would operate in the 3-μm to 5-μm spectral band. The overall dimensions of the assembly are shown as 24.179 in. (61.41 cm) long and 12.43 in. (31.57 cm) diameter at the largest end (neglecting the larger mounting flange). It weighs approximately 80 lb (356 kg).

According to Palmer and Murray,[4] because of the high cost of the larger lenses, the end user of the assembly desired to ensure that those optics would survive without damage a failure on the part of the simulator system that caused severe impact. Rather than designing the entire assembly to withstand the shock, it was designed so that the mechanical supports for the costly components would fail at a load of $a_G = 30$, and those components would be constrained in a safe manner, even under much higher shock loads. The lenses would then not be damaged; they could be salvaged and reused.

It was determined that the severe impact would occur only in a direction transverse to the axis of the assembly. To make the assembly mechanically stiff under under bending forces, the main housing was made of 6061-T6 aluminum and configured with a unique cross-section over most of its length. This construction may be seen in Fig. 13.17, which is a photograph showing the exterior of the assembly. Between the lens groups that occupy the cylindrical portions of the housing, the structure is that of a "paddle wheel" with six ribs of full external diameter supporting conformal wall portions

460

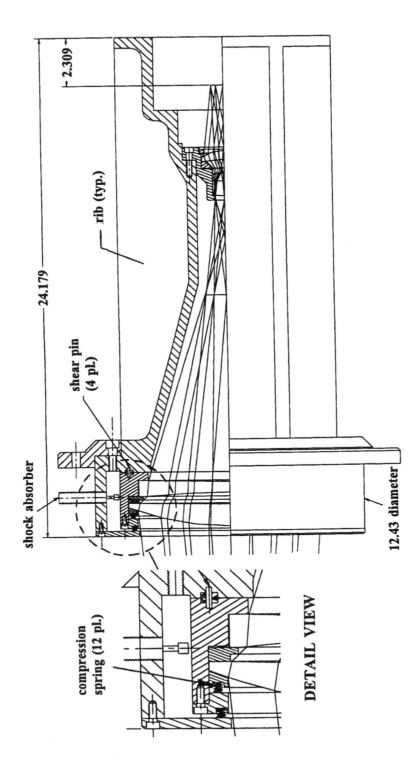

Fig. 13.16 Sectional view of a collimating lens assembly designed to withstand high shock loading. Dimensions are in inches. (Courtesy of Janos Technology, Inc., Townshend, VT.)

(a)

(b)

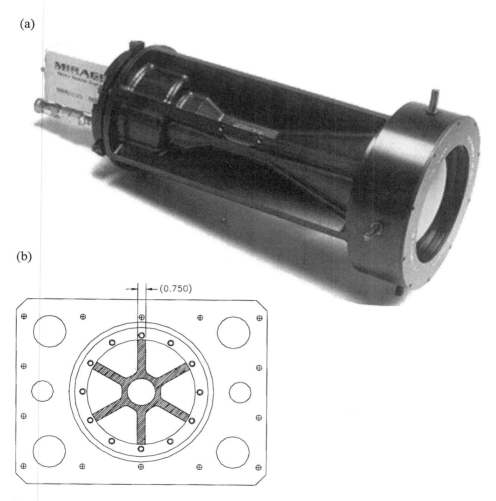

Fig. 13.17 (a) Photograph of the collimator assembly of Fig. 13.16 without the mounting flange. (b) Section view through the midpoint of the assembly. (Courtesy of Janos Technology, Inc, Townshend, VT.)

that enclose the internal light beam emerging from the smaller lenses and expanding to fill the apertures of the larger lenses. These ribs enhance assembly stiffness while minimizing weight. Internal grooves machined into the walls reduce stray light reflections that could degrade image contrast.

The cell for the large lenses was designed with a retaining flange that presses multiple axially oriented compression springs against a pressure ring contacting the first lens. The preload so introduced presses a spacer against the second lens, which in turn registers against a shoulder. The cell is constrained radially in the housing by three axially oriented aluminum shear pins that engage stainless steel inserts pressed into the lens cell and the housing. Without these pins, the cell would be able to slide laterally within clearances provided all around the rim of the cell. At assembly, the pins locate the cell and its lenses radially. The cell is pressed firmly against a shoulder in the housing by additional axially oriented compression springs that bear against the outermost flange.

The pins are designed to shear under the prescribed shock load, allowing the cell to move. This cell motion is dampened by shock absorbers oriented radially at four points around the periphery of the assembly. Three of these are shown in the photograph and one is indicated in the section view. The shock absorbers are nonlinear; they become stiffer under higher accelerations.

13.12 Elastomeric-Supported Camera Lens Assembly

Figure 13.18 shows an aerial camera objective with a focal length of 66 in. (1.67 m) and a fixed relative aperture of f/8. It was decribed by Bayar.[8] Four singlets and one

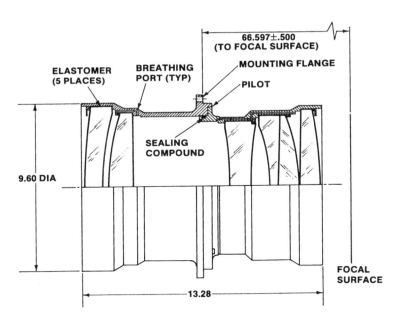

Fig. 13.18 Aerial camera lens with elastomerically mounted lenses. Dimensions are given in inches. (From Bayar.[8])

doublet were mounted separately within annular rings of RTV elastomer in the general manner discussed in Sect. 4.3. For added protection against lens motion within the barrel, each lens was constrained axially against a shoulder by a threaded retainer. The lens barrel was made in two parts that piloted together at a flange. These barrel halves were joined with bolts (not shown) after the lenses were installed.

The front half of the objective was assembled with the barrel mounted with its axis vertical on a rotary table and adjusted until the lens seats and pilot diameter all had minimum mechanical runout as the table and barrel were rotated slowly. The innermost lens was installed and centered to the rotational axis within allowed tolerances using mechanical and/or optical error-detecting means, such as those described in Sect. 3.10. The retainer was snugged down against that lens and a gap between the lens rim and the barrel ID was filled with RTV compound through several radially directed holes (not shown) by means of a hypodermic syringe. The outermost lens was then inserted, aligned to the rotary axis, clamped in place, and "potted" in place. The same procedure was used to assemble and align the rear half of the objective. Once the sealant had cured, the barrel halves were joined to each other and sealed with RTV sealing compound.

The thickness of each annular layer was customized to make the lens mounting athermal radially using Eq. (3.43). This minimized the generation of radial stress within the lenses at low temperatures. Note that in this design, the elastomer was completely surrounded by metal and glass, so the RTV had inadequate space to expand into when the temperature increased. The RTV was then compressed and some radial force undoubtedly was exerted upon the lens rim under some conditions.

An important feature of this assembly and of many others that are evacuated and backfilled with dry gas such as helium or nitrogen after sealing was the set of breathing ports (holes) bored through the housing wall to interconnect all cavities between lenses. Typical ports are shown in Fig. 13.18. In some other designs the same breathing-access function is provided by grinding one or more narrow grooves parallel to the axis through the rim of each of the lenses outside the clear aperture, but inside the IDs of the shoulders and retainers.

13.13 Projection Lens Assembly

Figure 13.19 is a sectional view through a 90-mm (3.54-in.) focal length, f/2 objective assembly designed for motion picture projection. Only single-element lenses are used here since the assembly is typically subjected to very high temperatures during operation and cemented components might be damaged. Large physical apertures are used in the lenses so that geometric vignetting is minimized and illumination remains high at the corners of the format. The MTF at 50 lp/mm is specified as over 70% on-axis, with the average radial and tangential MTF falling only to about 30% at the extreme corners of the image. The field curvature of the design is compatible with the natural cylindrical curvature of the film as it passes through the film gate and helps to maintain image sharpness at the horizontal edges of that image. For the intended application of this lens, an iris is not needed; the lens operates at a fixed relative aperture.

As may be seen from the figure, mechanical construction of the assembly is conventional. All metal parts are anodized aluminum alloy. The barrel is made in two

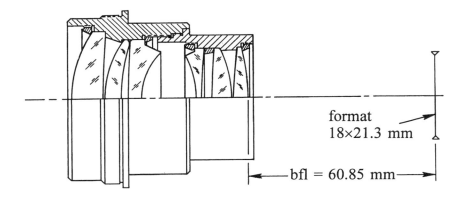

format
18×21.3 mm

bfl = 60.85 mm

Fig. 13.19 A 90-mm focal length, f/2 projection lens assembly. (Courtesy of Schneider Corporation, Hauppauge, NY.)

parts joined at the center by a piloted and threaded interface. Starting at the larger diameter end, the first lens is seated against a shoulder in the barrel and held by a threaded retainer. The second and third lenses are inserted from the right side of this barrel and clamped together without a spacer and against a shoulder in the barrel by a threaded retainer. In this case, the retainer bears against a flat bevel formed at the base of a step ground into the lens rim. The sixth (outermost) lens in the smaller end of the assembly is held against a shoulder by a threaded retainer. The fourth and fifth lenses are held against a shoulder in series with an intermediate spacer of conventional design by another retainer, which also fits into a step on the rim of the fourth lens.

13.14 Astrographic Telescope Objective Assembly

A rugged, yet relatively lightweight large lens assembly is shown in Fig. 13.20. This is a five-element, 81.102-in. (2.06-m) focal length, f/10 objective lens developed at the Optical Sciences Center of the University of Arizona, for astrographic use by the U.S. Naval Observatory.[9] It features individual lens elements and a filter bonded into subcells with annular layers of Dow Corning type 93-500 elastomer on the order of 0.2 in. (5 mm) thick. The cells are installed with interference fits into a barrel and further constrained axially with threaded retainers. Two spacers are also used. All metal parts are 6Al-4V titanium to minimize weight and to provide a close CTE match to the glasses. The overall weight of the assembly is about 44.6 kg (98.3 lb), 21.9 kg (48.4 lb) of which is in the glass. The lens barrel and its component parts are shown in Fig. 13.21.

Each cell was made with a shoulder at one side to provide a reference for

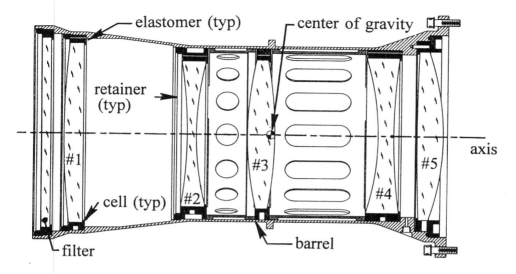

Fig. 13.20 Optomechanical configuration of an 81.102-in. (2.06-m) focal length, f/10 astrographic objective. (Adapted from Vukobratovich et al. [9])

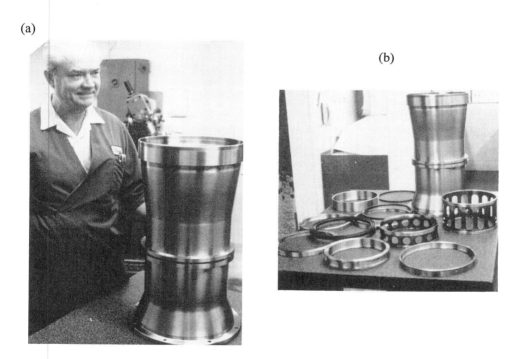

(a)

(b)

Fig. 13.21 Mechanical parts of the astrographic telescope objective, (a) Main titanium barrel; (b) barrel, six cells (solid rings), two spacers (slotted rings), and three retainers. (Courtesy of D. Vukobratovich, Univ. of Arizona, Tucson, AZ.)

squaring on the lens, as indicated schematically in Fig. 13.22(a). The construction technique allowed the lenses to be accurately centered in their subcells. The elastomer was then added and cured. The optomechanical subassemblies were then pressed in place in the barrel so as to rest against axially locating shoulders.

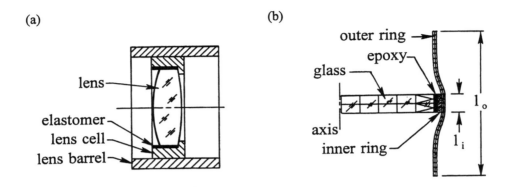

Fig. 13.22 (a) Concept for elastomeric mounting, (b) FEA model used to confirm radial stress calculations. (Adapted from Valente and Richard. [10])

Valente and Richard[10] described how to determine the radial stress introduced into the lens. Using a finite-element analysis technique, those authors verified that essentially the same result would be obtained by their equations and by FEA. Figure 13.22(b) illustrates the model used. Once the radial stress in the glass is known, the stress birefringence can be estimated from the stress optic coefficient of the refractive material and the optical path length in the glass.

As discussed in Sect. 3.7, Eq. (3.45) can be used to calculate the self-weight radial deflection of a lens element such as those in this assembly that results from elastic deformation of the elastomer.[10] Using that equation and assuming 0.2-in.-thick elastomer layers, it can be shown that the worst-case self-weight decentration of the five lenses in this assembly is only 0.0002 in. (5.1 µm), which is considerably smaller than the corresponding centration tolerance of 0.001 in. (25.4 µm).

13.15 Solid Catadioptric Lens Assembly

The optical system of a "solid" catadioptric lens (see Fig. 13.23) was designed as a compact, durable, environmentally stable, long-focal length objective for 35-mm single-reflex camera use.[11] Essentially, it fills the space between the primary and the secondary mirrors of a Cassegrain objective with useful glass. Image quality is maximized while the optical surfaces are closely coupled for mechanical stability. The relatively wide rims of the larger components provide long contacts with the IDs of the lens barrel.

Owing to the telephoto effect of the mirrors, the overall system length is considerably shorter than the focal length.

Several versions of this lens have been manufactured; the one shown here has a focal length of 1200 mm (47.244 in.), a relative aperture of f/11.8 at infinity focus, and covers a 24 × 36-mm format (semifield = ±1.03°). The fifth through tenth elements serve as field lenses for aberration correction and lengthen the focal length in the manner of a Barlow lens.* The system does not have an iris, so variations in lighting conditions are compensated for by exposure variations or by filtering. The filter located following the last lens is easily interchanged for this purpose.

The mechanical construction of the assembly is illustrated in Fig. 13.24. All metal parts are aluminum. The mounting flange mounts to a tripod and the camera attaches to the adapter (shown here without detail). The larger optics are mounted in a barrel with the primary resting against an internal shoulder; the two lenses and primary are secured by a single retainer. The Barlow/field lenses are mounted in a cell that attaches to a threaded central hole in the rear plate portion of the main housing. The focus ring drives the lens barrel on a 14-start Acme thread to focus the lens as close as 23 ft (7 m) with convenient rotation of the focus ring of about one-third turn. Glass-to-metal interfaces are the sharp-corner type. Tolerances were controlled so the lenses and the primary could be installed without lathe assembly.[13]

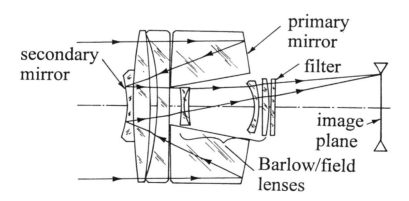

Fig. 13.23 Optical schematic for a 1200-mm (47.244-in.) focal length, f/11.8 solid catadioptric lens assembly. (Adapted from Yoder.[13])

---

* The Barlow lens is defined as a "lens system used in telescopes, in which one or more strongly negatively powered lens elements are used to increase the effective focal length and thereby increase the magnification." (Ref. 12, p. 219)

468

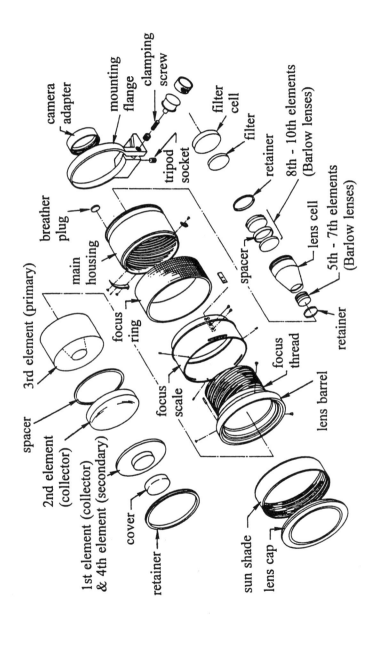

camera
adapter

mounting
flange

clamping
screw

filter
cell

filter

retainer

8th - 10th elements
(Barlow lenses)

tripod
socket

breather
plug

main
housing

spacer

lens cell

5th - 7th elements
(Barlow lenses)

retainer

3rd element (primary)

focus
ring

focus
thread

spacer

2nd element
(collector)

focus
scale

1st element (collector)
& 4th element (secondary)

lens barrel

cover

retainer

sun shade

lens cap

Fig. 13.24 Exploded view of the "solid" catadioptric lens assembly shown in Fig. 13.23. (Adapted from Yoder.[13])

13.16 All-Aluminum Catadioptric Lens Assembly

Figure 13.25 is a photograph of a 557-mm (21.9-in.) focal length, f/2.3 catadioptric lens built by Janos Technology, Inc. The lens, which is designed to operate in the 8- to 12-μm spectral region, is shown mounted on a tripod. The rectangular object at the rear of the assembly is an infrared camera.

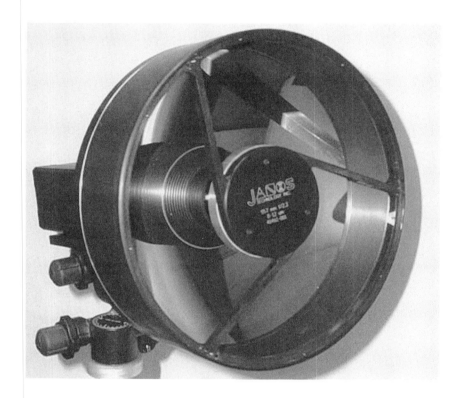

Fig. 13.25 Photograph of a 557-mm (21.93-in.) focal length, f/2.3 catadioptric lens assembly with aluminum mirrors and structure. (Courtesy of Janos Technology, Inc., Townshend, VT.)

Figure 13.26 shows front and sectional side views of the lens. The mirrors and mechanical parts are constructed of 6061-T6 aluminum, while the field lenses are germanium. All optical surfaces and the optomechanical interfaces of this assembly are single-point diamond turned for highest alignment accuracy. Pockets are milled into the back of the primary mirror to reduce weight. The reflecting surfaces are coated with silicon monoxide to protect them during cleaning. Their reflectivities are greater than 98% in the 8-14 μm spectral range and the surfaces are adequately smooth for the application.

470

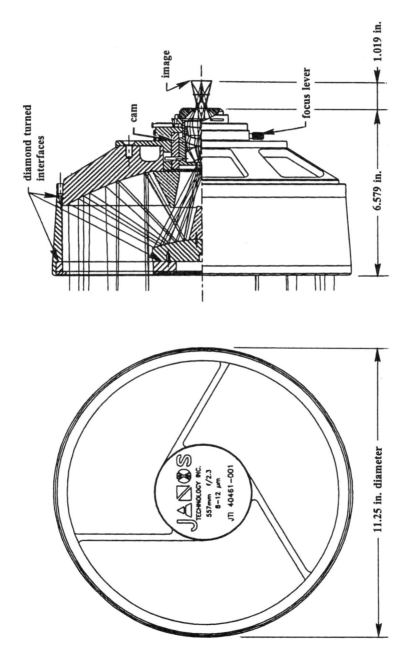

Fig. 13.26 Front and side sectional views of the catadioptric lens assembly from the preceding figure. (Courtesy of Janos Technology, Inc., Townshend, VT.)

No adjustments for axial locations or optical component tilts are needed. Centering of the secondary mirror is accomplished in an interferometer (before installing the refractive components). Wave-front error is measured in the same test setup to ensure that the mirrors are not distorted. The lenses are held in place with RTV655. Internal baffles suppress stray light. The lens assembly is focused for various object distances by manual actuation of a helical cam that drives the lenses axially.

13.17 Catadioptric Star-Mapping Objective Assembly

A catadioptric lens assembly developed for use as a star field-mapping sensor in a spacecraft attitude-monitoring application[14] is illustrated schematically in Fig. 13.27. Figure 13.28 is a photograph of the assembly. This lens has a focal length of 10.0 in. (25.4 cm), a relative aperture of f/1.5, a field of view of ±2.8°, and a charge transfer device as detector. The image quality of the basic Cassegrain telescope formed by spherical primary and secondary mirrors was optimized for the application by two full-aperture refractive correctors (with one aspheric surface) and an air-spaced doublet field lens.[15] The secondary mirror was coated onto the second surface of the second large lens. The image plane was located approximately 1.4 in. (36 mm) beyond the last vertex of the field group to provide space for a thermoelectrically cooled detector array and its adjacent heat sink structure.

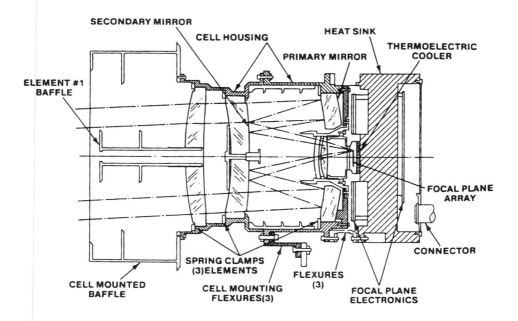

Fig. 13.27 Sectional schematic view of the star-mapper lens assembly. (Adapted from Yoder.[13])

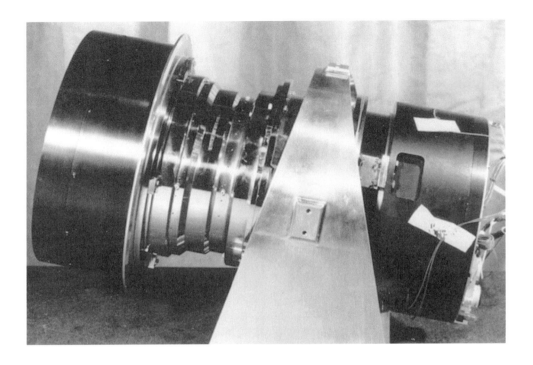

Fig. 13.28 Photograph of the star-mapper lens assembly. (From Cassidy.[14])

Invar was used as the material for the main barrel to minimize the effects of thermal expansion. This barrel was flexure mounted to the aluminum structure of the spacecraft so temperature changes would not affect image quality or alignment between the sensor and the spacecraft attitude control system. The meniscus-shaped, first-surface primary was edge clamped with spring clips against three spherical seats ground into the rear mounting plate attached to the main lens barrel and secured by RTV60 locally injected at six places around the mirror rim as shown in Fig. 13.29. Note that the axial preload was applied at a different height from the axis than the support provided by the seats. The tensile stress developed in the mirror as a result of this mismatch in contact heights was not sufficient to threaten the survivability of the mirror[13] and the surface deformation under operational conditions did not significantly affect performance.

The two larger lenses were provided with flat bevels accurately aligned to the opposite spherical surface. Those lenses were held in place by individual cantilevered flat spring clips. The centering of these lenses was adjusted by radially directed screws passing through the barrel wall and bearing against the lens rims. After alignment, RTV60 elastomer was injected through several radially directed holes into the space between the lens rims and the barrel ID. After curing of the elastomer, the alignment screws were removed and their holes plugged with elastomer.[13]

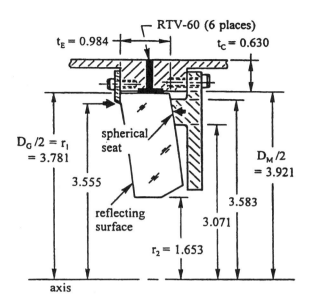

Fig. 13.29 Schematic diagram of the mounting for the spherical meniscus primary mirror used in the star-mapper lens assembly. Dimensions are given in inches.

The field lenses were lathe assembled in their cell as explained in Sect. 4.3. The axial location of this subassembly was adjusted by custom grinding a spacer (not shown) located between the cell flange and the rear housing. Once aligned, that subassembly was pinned in place. The focal plane array, heat sink, thermoelectric cooler, and local electronics were mounted on the lens assembly with flexures as indicated in Fig. 13.27. The axial position of the array was adjusted by customizing the thickness of spacers located at each flexure attachment point.

13.18 Long Focal-Length Catadioptric Objective Assembly

A simple catadioptric assembly is shown in section in Figs. 13.30 and 13.31. This lens had a focal length of 150 in. (3.8 m) and operated at f/10. It was intended for use with a 70-mm-format motion picture camera to photograph missiles during launch. It was designed to be mounted on an antiaircraft gun-type mount to provide the required azimuth and elevation motions for tracking the target. The figures show, respectively, the front and rear (camera) portions of the assembly.[13]

The system was of Cassegrain form with two full-aperture correcting lenses located near the primary mirror's center of curvature and an air-spaced triplet field lens group near the image plane to correct off-axis aberrations. The lens had a flat ±0.6° field.

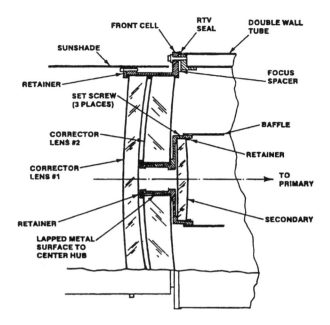

Fig. 13.30 Sectional view of the front portion of a 150-in (3.8-m) focal length, f/10 catadioptric lens assembly. (From Yoder.[13])

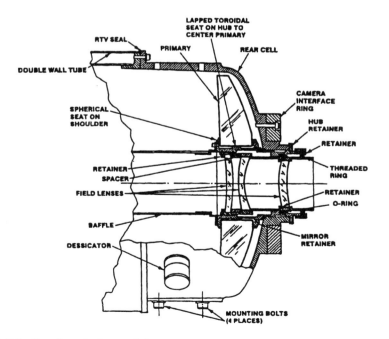

Fig. 13.31 Sectional view of the rear (camera) portion of the catadioptric lens assembly. (From Yoder[13])

The mechanical construction of the lens assembly had a front aluminum cell holding the corrector lenses and secondary mirror and a rear housing holding the primary mirror and field lenses, respectively. The rear housing was an aluminum casting that attached to the gun mount and supported the camera. The front housing was supported from the rear housing through a dual-walled aluminum tube with internal thermal insulation. A tubular lens shade projected forward from the front aperture. The assembly was painted white to reflect sunlight.

In the front cell, the two lenses were clamped by a flange retainer against an internal shoulder with a spacer for separation. The glass-to-metal interfaces at the lens rims were padded locally with single or multiple layers of 0.001-in. (0.025-mm)-thick Mylar tape [See Fig. 13.32(a)]. The required thicknesses of the tape shims were determined by supporting the housing with its axis vertical on a precision rotary table and measuring the runout as the table was slowly rotated. Once centered adequately and shimmed, the retainer was installed and tightened to hold the alignment. The secondary mirror was then mounted in its cell, which had previously been attached through a perforation at the center of the second lens. The interface for this cell to the lens and that for the mirror to the cell were shimmed with Mylar [See Fig. 13.32(b)]. Three setscrews were used to center the secondary mirror to the rotation axis of the table and hence to the lens axis.

In the rear housing, the primary mirror was hub mounted and clamped between a spherically lapped flange shoulder and a threaded retainer. A convex toroidal seat on the cylindrical hub was lapped to match the ID of the primary mirror's central perforation to center that mirror. The hub was in turn axially clamped within the rear housing by another threaded retainer. With the exception of the hub-to-mirror interface, all contacts between the optics and the mount were padded with Mylar shims as shown in Fig. 13.33.

The large-aperture portion of the assembly was focused by inserting metal shims of varying thickness between the tube and the front housing until the central air space was correct and the corrector lenses were squared to the axis. The lateral adjustment was made by successive approximations using motions of the front housing relative to the end of the tube assembly in slightly oversize holes for attachment bolts. After alignment (as measured by viewing an artificial star image under magnification) is accepted, the shims are replaced by custom-ground permanent spacers.

The field lens assembly was lathe assembled as described in Sect. 4.3 and installed in the hub of the rear housing. Axial location was measured mechanically and adjusted to the design value by rotating the threaded ring located at the rear end of the hub. The camera interface was then installed and adjusted for the proper back focus distance using photographic tests to measure residual errors during the process.

An alternative design for the primary mirror and field lens optic-to-mount interfaces is shown in Fig. 13.34. A similar optomechanical interface design could be used to advantage in mounting the optics (corrector lenses and secondary mirror) in the front portion of the assembly. In both cases, no Mylar shims would be used; the mounts are configured with tangential, toroidal, or flat surfaces as now known to be appropriate for direct contacts on the optical surfaces and discussed in Chapter 3. Mounting stresses would then be acceptable throughout the assembly without use of the Mylar padding.

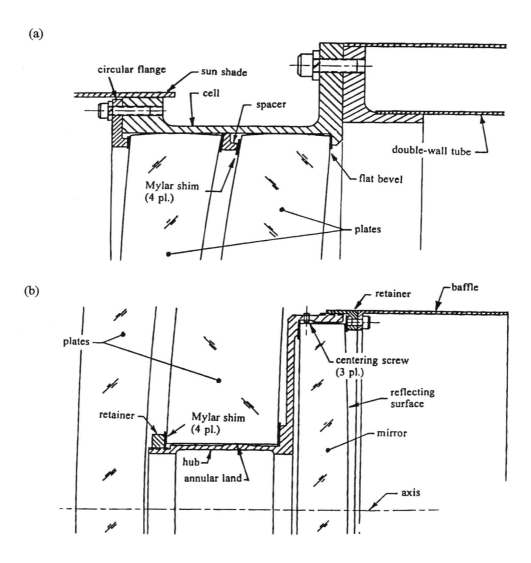

Fig. 13.32 Use of multiple Mylar shims to pad the glass-to-metal interfaces in the front subassembly of the 150-in. (3.8-m) focal length f/10 catadioptric lens (a) at the large lens rims and (b) in the secondary mirror mounting.

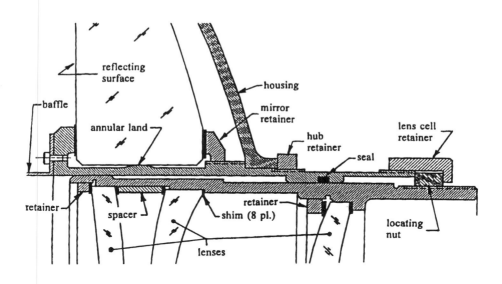

Fig. 13.33 Use of multiple Mylar shims to pad the glass-to-metal interfaces at the primary mirror and field lenses in the rear subassembly of the 150-in. catadioptric lens.

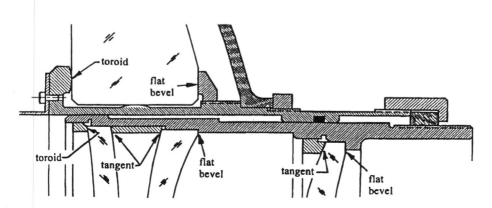

Fig. 13.34 An alternative design for the optic-to-mount interfaces at the primary mirror and field lenses in the 150-in. catadioptric lens.

13.19 A 72-in. (1.8-m) Effective Focal Length f/4 Aerial Camera Objective

Many high-performance photographic objectives with large apertures have been developed for high-altitude aerial reconnaissance purposes. Figure 13.35 shows one such lens that had an aperture of 18-in. (45.7-cm) and a focal length of 72 in. (1.8 m) so it operated at f/4. It was designed optomechanically to function to the diffraction limit in sunlight with a minus-blue filter at an altitude of 100,000 ft (91 km) over a

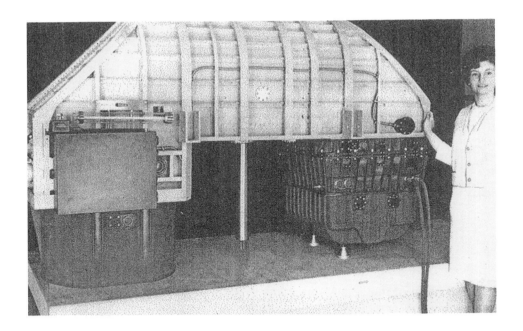

Fig. 13.35 Photograph of an 18-in. (45.72-cm)-aperture, high-acuity aerial reconnaissance camera. (From Yoder.[13])

temperature range of -65 to 130° F (-54 to 54° C).[13] The film magazine is the black subassembly shown below the woman's right hand in the photograph. The optical layout of this assembly is shown in Fig. 13.36. It is of the Petzval type and has three air-spaced triplets, two with approximately the same OD (18.75 in.) and the third having an OD of 17.96 in. The U-shaped configuration provides space for a stabilizing mount (not shown) under the center portion of the assembly.

Figure 13.37 shows the tolerances needed to achieve the performance required from this lens system. It is not simple to mount lenses of these diameters to tight tolerances on centration [typically ± 0.0005 in. (± 12.7 μm)] and in stress-free condition over the specified temperature range. Scott described the mounting for the central triplet subassembly used in this objective.[16] Figure 13.38 shows a sectional view through that subassembly. The positive elements are BaLF6 glass (CTE = 6.7×10^{-6} /°C), while the central negative element is KzFS4 glass (CTE = 4.5×10^{-6} /°C). The cell material was chosen to match as closely as possible the CTE of the BaLF6 glass. This material is A70 titanium (CTE 8.1×10^{-6} /°C). It was machined from a forged cylinder.

At assembly, radially oriented aluminum plugs, nominally 1 in. (25.4 mm) long, were inserted against the rim of the center lens at 120° intervals around that rim. The

479

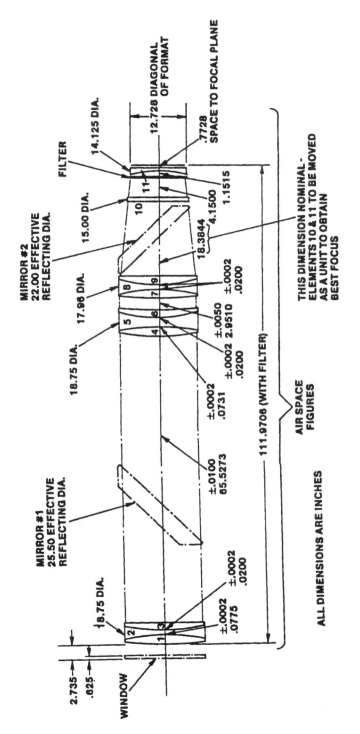

Fig. 13.36 Optical schematic of the large aerial camera lens shown in Fig. 13.35. (From Yoder.[13])

480

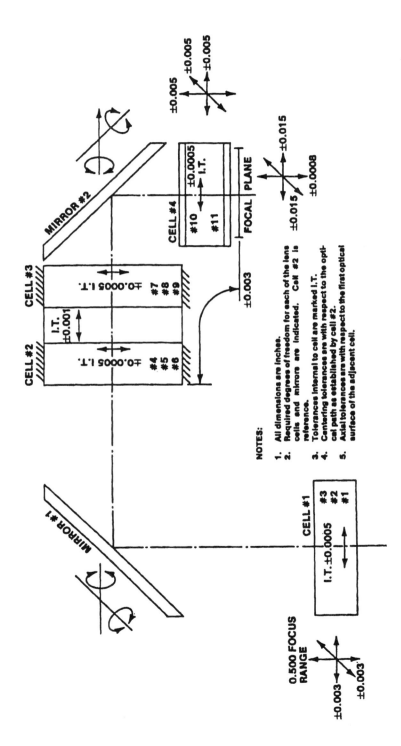

Fig. 13.37 Tolerances on locations and alignment of the lenses, lens cells, mirrors, and image plane for the lens of Fig. 13.35. (From Yoder.[13])

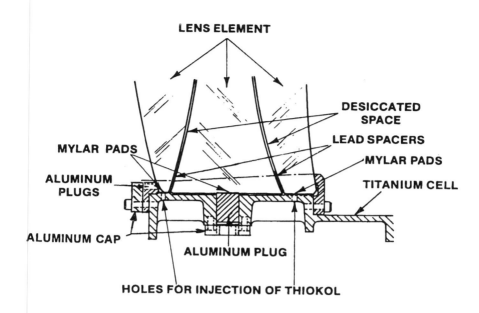

Fig. 13.38 Technique for radially athermalizing the large lenses in the 72-in. (1.8-m) focal length, f/4 aerial camera objective. (Adapted from Scott. [16] **)**

caps over the ends of the plugs were bottomed against the cell wall. Mylar shims were placed between the lens rims and the adjacent metal to pad the interfaces.

This combination of materials of various dimensions served to athermalize the mount in the radial direction. Aluminum plugs also were used to athermalize the subassembly in the axial direction. These plugs were lapped until the right-hand surface of the third lens was pushed against the hard-mounted flange at that end of the assembly and caps over the plug ends were bottomed against the outer surface of the left flange retainer. After assembly, the rims of the positive lenses were sealed to the barrel ID with a polysulfide-type sealant (probably 3M EC-801) to maintain a desiccated environment within the assembly after purging with dry nitrogen.[16]

The method of mounting the lens cells in the housing had to be rigid, compact, lightweight, temperature-stable, and in the case of the front and rear cells, axially adjustable for focus. In the final design, each large cell was supported on three tangent arms, each of which was approximately 0.13 in. (3.3 mm) thick by 3.0 in. (76.2 mm) wide. In the case of the smaller (rear) lens cell, the arms were 1.5 in. (38.1 mm) wide. Their thicknesses were the same as the other arms. One end of each arm was bolted and pinned directly to its cell. In the case of the second and third cells, the fixed ends of the arms were attached to fittings on the structure. In the case of the first and fourth cells, the arms were attached to the structure through adjustable eccentric bolts.[13]

The structure chosen for this assembly was of the semimonocoque type. Here annular aluminum bulkheads were spaced at intervals along the lens axis and tied together by longitudinal stringers in much the same fashion as aircraft fuselages are built. An aluminum skin was attached by rivets to the bulkheads and the stringers for stiffness. The skin was located internally to these latter members to provide space for thermal insulation and a protective cover on the outside. Figure 13.35 shows the assembly before the insulation and cover were added.

To establish the proper focus of the image at the film plane, four adjustable hardened pads were built into the surface of the last lens cell facing the image. Four fixed pads were provided on the film magazine side of the interface. Iterative photographic tests and adjustments of the lens cell pads during final alignment ensured that focus was correct.[13]

13.20 Passively Stabilized 10:1 Zoom Lens Assembly

The Bistovar 15- to 150-mm (0.59- to 5.90-in.) focal length, f/2.8 zoom lens assembly shown in Fig. 13.39 measures about 172 mm (6.77 in.) in length and 155 mm (4.53 in.) in diameter. At the camera end of the housing (item 26) is a standard C-mount interface for a videocamera with an 11.0-mm (0.433-in.) format diagonal. The lens has fixed (infinity) focus; its focal length and relative aperture are electrically variable over a 10:1 range. The relative aperture varies from f/2.8 to f/16. In prototype form, the lens assembly weighs approximately 1600 g (3.57 lb).

The optical system contains, in sequence, a four-element passive stabilization system with ± 5° dynamic range at the entrance aperture, a seven-element 5:1 zoom system, a five-element, dual-position 2:1 zoom system, and a Schott GG475 (minus-blue) filter. The average polychromatic MTF performance over the zoom range at 20 lp/mm on-axis and at 0.9 field is 69% and 25% respectively, including diffraction effects.

Movements of the two zoom lens groups (items 109 and 100, and item 101) in the 5:1 system are synchronized by a motor-driven cylindrical cam (Item 44) carrying slots custom machined for the specific set of lenses used in that assembly. A third moving-lens group (items 102, 110, and 105) moves axially under the control of a separate slot in the same cam so as to switch the 2:1 system whenever the main zoom system reaches its limits. Lenses 108, 97, and 106 remain stationary.

Two air-spaced doublets each consisting of a planoconcave and a planoconvex element, make up the stabilization subsystem. The curved surfaces of each doublet are closely adjacent. The positive singlets (items 92 and 94) are attached to a lightweight tubular structure (item 23) that pivots on ball bearings about either of two orthogonal gimbal axes. A counterweight (item 27) at the camera end of this tube balances the lenses.

483

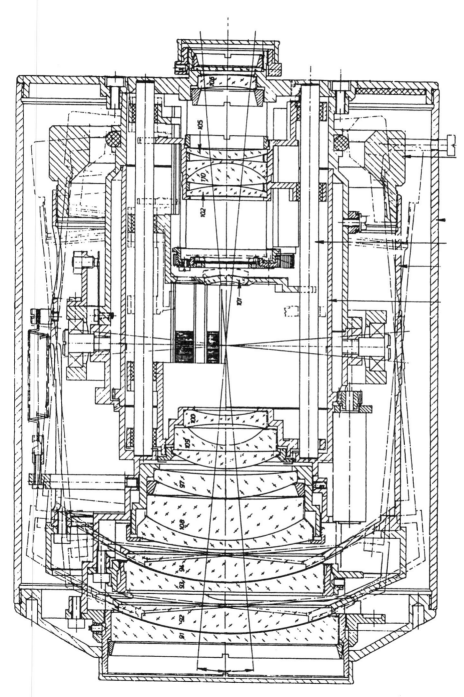

Fig. 13.39 Optomechanical configuration of a stabilized 10:1 zoom lens assembly. (Courtesy of K.M. Bystricky, Bista Research, Inc., Tragöss, Austria.)

Most of the lenses used in this assembly are conventionally mounted in aluminum alloy cells and held in place by threaded retainers. A few glass-to-metal interfaces are spherical, but the majority are of the sharp-corner type. The beveled edge of one lens (item 100) directly contacts a flat bevel on the adjacent doublet (item 109). The pivoted lenses (items 92 and 94) and one fixed lens (item 101) are secured in place with adhesive (Ciba-Geigy Araldite 1118 epoxy) since there is no room for retainers.

13.21 Camera Assembly for the DEIMOS Spectrograph

According to Mast et al.,[17] DIEMOS is a large, multiobject spectrograph with an imaging mode that is part of the Keck 2 telescope on Mauna Kea in Hawaii. It is capable of measuring spectra in the 0.39- to 1.1-μm range of as many as 100 objects simultaneously. The field of view of the system is 16.7 arcmin (equivalent slit length), which produces a 730-mm image at the focus of the telescope. The detector used is a 2×4 mosaic of eight charge-coupled devices (CCDs), each with 2048×4096 pixels at 15 μm per pixel.[18] A series of gratings with 600 to 1200 lines per millimeter provide the necessary dispersion.

The optical system is diagrammed in Fig. 13.40. It has five lens groups with nine lenses. Its EFL is 381 mm, so the plate scale is 125 μm per arcsec in object space. The system includes three aspheric surfaces and the materials indicated in the figure. The combinations of CTEs and the fragility of the three CaF$_2$ lenses posed especially complex mounting problems. Part of the solution was to fill the spaces between the doublets (groups 1 and 4) with optical coupling fluid. The thicknesses of these cavities were small and created with plastic shims. The cavities had to be vented to bladders to accommodate

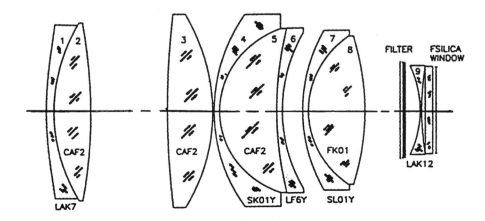

Fig. 13.40 Optical system for the DEIMOS spectrograph camera. (Adapted from Mast et al.[17])

the specified survival temperature excursion (-20° C to 30° C). Experiments reported by Hilyard et al. formed the basis for choice of Cargille LL1074 fluid, ether-based polyethylene film for the bladders, Viton VO763-60 or VO834-70 for O-ring fluid constraints, and Mylar for the shims.[19] These materials proved to be compatible with each other and with the glasses, the CaF_2, and the mounting materials. The bladders were heat sealed to eliminate the need for adhesives.

The optomechanical layout of the camera optics is shown in Fig. 13.41. The barrel contains several 303 CRES segments with spacers to establish the required air spaces between lens groups. The lenses are mounted in ring-shaped CRES cells. The field flattener (lens 9) and the fused silica window shown in Fig. 13.40 are part of the detector assembly, which is mounted in a separate vacuum vessel. The filter shown in Fig. 13.40 is contained in a separately mounted filter wheel. A shutter (not shown) is located in the path near the filter.

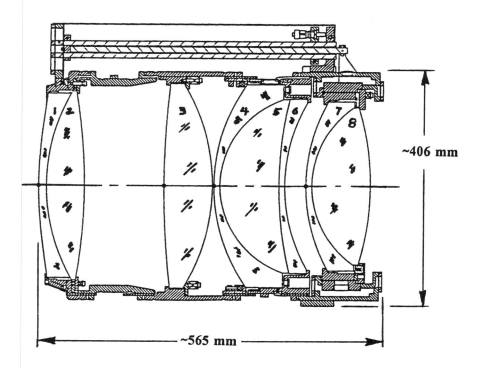

Fig. 13.41 Optomechanical schematic of the DEIMOS camera assembly. (Adapted from Mast et al.[17])

The CaF_2 lenses in groups 1 and 2 are mounted in annular RTV rings inside thin aluminum rings which are, in turn, inside 303 CRES cells. The cells have a slight interference fit (~75 μm) over the rings to compress the crystalline material at all temperatures. This prevents the material going into tension at the lowest expected temperature since that could cause fractures along intercrystalline boundaries. The mathematical basis for this design is explained by Mast et al.[17] The stress in the lenses at assembly (~20°C) is 1.3×10^5 Pa. This decreases to an acceptable 4×10^4 Pa at -20°C.

An error analysis and tolerance budget study conducted by Optical Research Associates indicated that the lens groups should be tilted by no more than 50 arcseconds, decentered by no more than 75 µm, and despaced by no more than 150 µm (all 2σ values). It was known that the aspheric curves on three lenses could be decentered with respect to the mechanical axes by as much as 350 µm. To achieve proper performance in spite of these errors and the residual errors in centration elsewhere in the system during assembly, lens group 4 was designed to be transversely adjustable. Four flexures were built into the mount for this lens group. Two orthogonal adjusting screws and preload springs were provided to make the adjustment. The transverse motion possible is about 500 µm in any direction. Since the flexures can develop high stress points, the cell for this group is 17-4SH CRES.

Lenses within each multiple-lens group are held axially between Mylar shims on flat pads machined locally into shoulders in the lens cells and a spring-loaded Delrin retaining ring. The outer lenses of each multiple-lens group are sealed to adjacent metal parts with GE-560 RTV elastomer. These seals support the lenses radially and serve as dams to constrain the fluid. In most cases, thicknesses of the annular elastomer layers were chosen to render radially athermal designs as developed by Mast et al.[19] The exception is the final doublet (group 4), which has a thicker layer to better match a different steel (tType 17-4SH) used in the cell.

In order to provide a constant scale factor in the dispersed image throughout the operating temperature range of -4°C to 6°C, it was found necessary to move lens group 4 axially as a function of temperature. This was achieved by attaching the lens cell to a bimetallic compensator consisting of a Delrin tube concentric with an Invar rod as indicated in Fig. 13.41. The cell is mounted on flexures to allow this axial motion. The resultant CTE of the compensator is 0.036 mm/°C.

13.22 Nine Cameras for the Earth-Observing System, Multiangle Imaging Spectro-Radiometer

The Multiangle imaging spectro-radiometer (MISR) is a NASA space payload orbiting aboard the EOS-TERRA spacecraft. According to Ford et al.,[21] it employs nine cameras to collect data in four spectral bands within the 0.440- to 0.880-µm range at nine different angles along the flight path. Each observed point on Earth is scanned by each camera and the data compared for similarities and differences. The science goals are to monitor global atmospheric particulates, cloud movements, and vegetative changes during a nominal 6-year mission. Critical design requirements include an operational temperature range of 0° to 10°C, surviving temperature extremes of -40° to -80°C, withstanding launch, and maintaining adequate light transmission in the Earth's polar radiation environment.

   To reduce costs, four lens designs are used in the nine cameras. The innermost three systems are identical (designated type A) while the remaining designs (designated types B, C, and D) are located in pairs symmetrically disposed relative to the nadir. Focal lengths increase in the sequence from the nadir outward. Figure 13.42 shows the four lens designs. Their characteristics are listed in the figure caption. Glass types for all the designs are as indicated in the figure for design type D. Unmarked elements are filters. The detectors are at right in each design. Note that the image sizes are essentially constant.

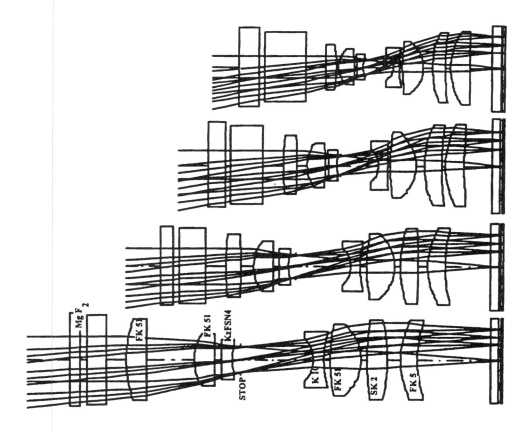

Fig. 13.42 Optical schematics for the four MISR lens designs. Characteristics are, from top to bottom, type A, EFL = 59.3 mm, field = ±14.9°, length = 111 mm; type B, EFL = 73.4 mm, field = ±12.1°, length = 124 mm; type C, EFL = 95.3 mm, field = ±9.4°, length = 144 mm; and type D, EFL = 123.8 mm, field = ±7.3°, length = 181 mm. (From Ford et al. [21])

Figure 13.43 shows a sectional view through lens design D. This is representative of all four designs. The main housing is aluminum, with walls about 6.3 mm (0.25 in.) thick to minimize radiation penetration in orbit. To control clamping force changes with temperature, spacers made of Vespel SP1 were used under each retaining ring. This material has a CTE larger than that of aluminum. The thickness of each spacer was computed to compensate for the difference in CTEs for the housing, the spacer, and the lens. This rendered the preload essentially constant with temperature at that achieved with about 5 oz-in. (0.035 N-m) of torque on each threaded retainer. This preload was found experimentally to be adequate under the specified vibration/shock loading.

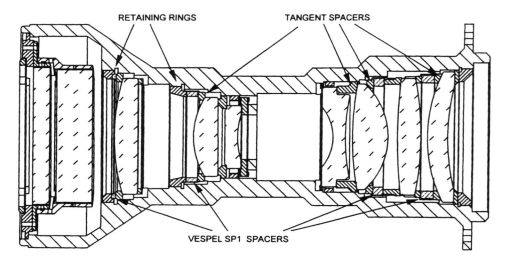

Fig. 13.43 Sectional view through MISR lens type D. (From Ford et al. [21])

The optomechanical interfaces between the spacers and all lenses with convex surfaces are tangents to minimize contact stress. The radial force from the axial preload acting at each tangent interface with a convex surface was found to adequately center those lenses. The assemblies were vibrated gently after the retainers were tightened to help seat the lenses with minimal axial separations. This condition corresponds to the maximum possible degree of centration with the existing frictional conditions. The retainers were then retorqued to the specified value.

Lenses with concave surfaces were centered mechanically to the IDs of the housing at each lens location using annular spacers made of Vespel SP1 and configured as indicated in Fig. 13.44. The IDs and ODs of the spacers were machined for close sliding fits in the housing and to the lens ODs, then milled locally to create flexures that would spring load the lenses radially. This creates rim contact interfaces without the radial stress problems that would occur with hard mounting under the expected temperature changes.

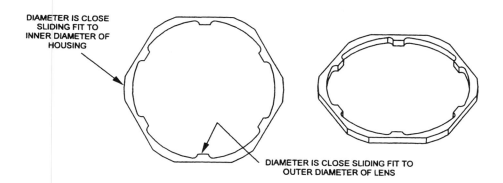

DIAMETER IS CLOSE SLIDING FIT TO INNER DIAMETER OF HOUSING

DIAMETER IS CLOSE SLIDING FIT TO OUTER DIAMETER OF LENS

Fig. 13.44 Vespel SP1 centering spacer ring design for MISR lenses with concave surfaces. (From Ford et al. [21])

Analysis of the lens designs indicated that temperature compensation would be required to keep them in focus over the specified operational temperature range. A passive approach was chosen in which the detector is moved as a function of temperature to keep it at or near the optimum location of the image formed by each lens. It was found that complete compensation at all temperatures could not be achieved for all four types of lenses with identical optomechanical designs, but the performance degradation resulting from the use of one compromise design was deemed acceptable.

Figure 13.45 shows the adopted compensator design. One of these assemblies is attached to the end of each lens housing as indicated in Fig. 13.46. Optimization of the detector location relative to the image is achieved in this design with a set of concentric tubes made of different materials connected at alternate ends so their length variations with temperature add and subtract as a more complex version of the reentrant compensator configuration of Fig. 12.4(a). In this case, however, the materials used in the components tending to reduce the total length with increasing temperature are made of a low CTE material (Invar and fiberglass), while those tending to increase that length are made of a high CTE material (aluminum and magnesium). The result is to create a compensator with minimal overall length, but effective expansion and contraction characteristics adequately matching the BFL changes of the four lens designs.

The detectors are cooled with thermal electric coolers to -10°C. They are thermally insulated from the surrounding structure. Details of the final design of the mechanical and temperature control systems that minimize thermal gradients in the lens assemblies are given in the paper by Ford et al.[21] Tests that confirmed the achievement of required performance in the laboratory also are summarized in that paper.

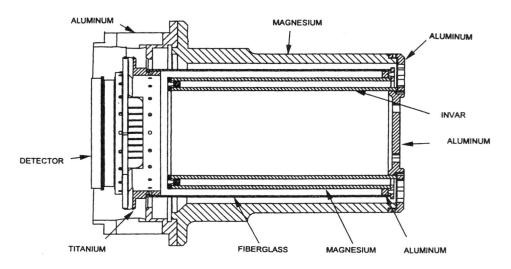

Fig. 13.45 Schematic of the temperature compensator used with each MISR lens assembly. (From Ford et al. [21])

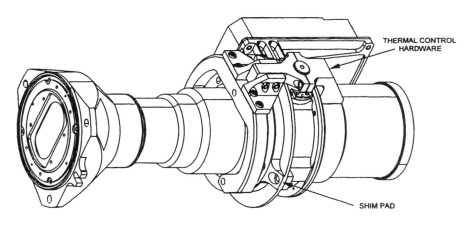

Fig. 13.46 Schematic of one assembled MISR camera. (From Ford et al. [21])

13.23 Bonded Porro Prism Erecting System for a Binocular

The optomechanical layout of the U.S. Army's 7×50 M19 binocular, developed in the 1950s as a replacement for the modified commercial binoculars used in World War II and the Korean conflict is shown in Fig. 4.31. This binocular was a totally new design featuring significantly reduced weight and size, improved optical performance, large-quantity producibility, and improved reliability and maintainability compared with all prior designs. These advantages were achieved by making the device modular, with only five optomechanical parts, all of which were interchangeable in any reasonably clean location without adjustment and without special tools.[2,22] These modules are shown in Fig. 4.27. Because the success of modular construction in other applications depends largely on the detailed optomechanical design, the availability of optically based tooling, and special care exercised during manufacture, we describe here in considerable detail how the prealigned Porro prism image-erecting system was assembled and incorporated into the body housing.

A drawing and photographs of the Porro prism cluster are shown in Figs. 13.47 and 13.48. The prisms were made of high-index (type 649338) glass to ensure total internal reflection and were tapered to have minimal volume and weight without vignetting.

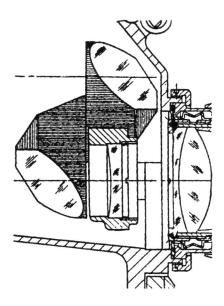

Fig. 13.47 Section of the optomechanical layout of the M19 binocular (from Fig. 4.31) showing the erecting prism assembly, its mounting bracket, and the lens/reticle mounting. (Adapted from a U.S. Army drawing.)

The first step in assembly was to bond one Porro prism to a die-cast aluminum bracket with adhesive per MIL-A-4866 (such as Summers Milbond) in a fixture built to exacting tolerances and carefully maintained throughout use. After that bond was cured, the prism and bracket subassembly was mounted in a second precision fixture. Ultraviolet-curing optical cement (Norland 61) was applied to the appropriate portion of the prism's hypotenuse surface. The second prism was positioned with respect to the first prism so that the input and output axes were parallel (pointing) and displaced by the proper

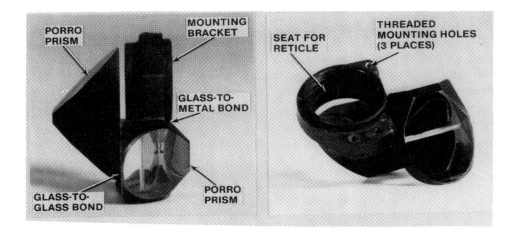

Fig. 13.48 Photographs of the M19 bonded Porro prism subassembly. (From Yoder. [13]**)**

distance. In addition, that prism was rotated in the interface plane to correct rotation (tilt) of the image around the optical axis. A video camera and monitor were used to display to the operator the pointing and tilt relationships for the prism assembly. The operator first adjusted the free prism laterally until the image of a reticle projected through the system was positioned within a prescribed rectangular tolerance envelope on the monitor screen. Then, while the image was maintained inside this rectangle, the prism was rotated slightly to align tilt reference indicators also displayed on the monitor screen. Once adjusted, the prism was clamped in position in the fixture. Curing of the cement took place under a bank of ultraviolet lamps adjacent to the setting station. Multiple setting and curing fixtures were necessary to support the required production rate. After curing, the same optical alignment apparatus was used as a test device to ensure that the desired prism setting was retained through the curing process.

Both housings started out as identical thin-walled, vinyl-clad aluminum investment castings; they were machined differently to form their unique left and right shapes. The wall thickness was nominally 1.524 mm. Over this, a 0.38 mm thick coating of soft vinyl was applied prior to machining of the critical mounting seats for the eyepiece, the prism assembly, and the objective. The locations of the eyepiece and prism assembly seats were established mechanically during the machining process. Normally, with a rigid, stable part, these would not have presented unusual problems despite the very demanding tolerances required. However, the structural flexibility of the thin-walled housing was a serious handicap. In addition, owing to the soft vinyl, it was not possible to reliably locate the housings from any of the vinyl-clad surfaces or to clamp on them without causing cosmetic damage. Elaborate fixtures relying upon a few previously machined surfaces that were not vinyl clad had to be developed before acceptable production yields and rates could be attained.

Machining of the housing with the prism assembly installed was the critical step in obtaining the module precision required to permit interchangeability. Horizontal and vertical collimation requirements (divergence and dipvergence, respectively) for the monocular's optical axis with respect to the hinge pin centerline were such that the bore for the objective had to be properly located radially within 0.0127 mm and the requirement for perpendicularity between the objective seat and the optical axis was 0.0051 mm measured across the objective seat. In addition, the objective seat had to be located axially to obtain the proper flange focal distance. To obtain these accuracies, it was necessary to use optical alignment techniques to position the housing for machining.

Initially, the housing was mounted directly on a computer numerically controlled lathe, with a hollow lathe spindle that permited passage of a light beam for monitoring alignment optically. Alignment in place proved to be very difficult and time-consuming. This resulted in inefficient use of the machine tool. Only a fraction of its available time was actually being used for machining; most of the time was devoted to aligning the housing. This was unacceptable for high-volume production, so this approach was abandoned.

The production approach that was finally developed was to hold the housing in a transferable setting and machining fixture. The housing was positioned using optical alignment instrumentation and locked in place on the fixture at an offline setting station. Then the fixture was transferred to the spindle of a CNC multitool lathe for final machining. Multiple transferable fixtures were provided so that setting and machining could proceed in parallel.

The fixture and the optical alignment technique used at the setting station are shown schematically in Fig. 13.49. The fixture base was designed to mate precisely with the lathe spindle so that the fixture centerline was coincident with the rotational axis of the spindle during machining. In this way the mounting seat for the objective could be machined concentric with the fixture centerline. Atop the fixture base was a sliding plate that could be translated laterally. This plate carried a post simulating a binocular hinge pin. The post centerline was always parallel to the fixture centerline.

An optical system in the setting station (not shown in Fig. 13.49) provided an image of a target at infinity along the input optical axis, which was coincident with the fixture axis. A master objective was mounted at a fixed location in the setting station and centered on this axis. This objective formed an image of the target at an image plane inside the housing. This image was then viewed through a master eyepiece (temporarily attached to the housing) by a videocamera, with the output being displayed on a video monitor. The proper flange focus position for machining the objective lens seat in the housing was obtained by moving the housing vertically along the hinge post until the best

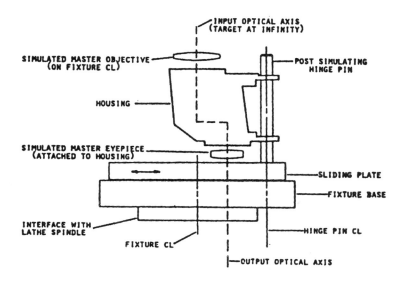

Fig. 13.49 Schematic of prism-adjusting and holding fixture used to machine the M19 body housing with a prealigned prism installed. (From Trsar et al.[2])

focus was obtained on the video monitor. The housing was then clamped to the post and sliding plate. Axial positioning of the housing on the fixture now was completed, but lateral adjustment to obtain collimation was still needed.

The collimation requirements for the monocular were that the output optical axis be parallel to the hinge pin centerline within ± 5 arcmin in the dipvergence plane (normal to the plane of Fig. 13.49) and be diverging by 5 to 17 arcmin in the plane of the figure. Since the hinge pin and fixture centerlines were parallel, the collimation requirement was referenced to the fixture centerline. After focus adjustment, the housing and sliding plate assembly were adjusted laterally (in two directions) with respect to the fixture base and the master objective until the required collimation conditions were achieved. This was indicated by a predetermined positioning of the target image on the video monitor. The sliding plate was then locked to the fixture base and the assembly transferred to the CNC lathe for machining of the objective mounting seat.

A similar procedure was used to orient the housing for machining the eyepiece interface. The result was a body housing with a prealigned prism assembly that would mate properly with any objective module and any eyepiece module to form one half of the binocular instrument. The left and right housing assemblies also were properly aligned to fit together at the hinge without adjustment.

13.24 Large Flexure-Mounted Mirror Assembly

Large prisms frequently pose difficult mounting problems, not only because of their weight and size, but also because large separations of mounting supports may cause significant thermal expansion problems from the dissimilarities in the CTEs of the optical and mechanical materials. For example, the three-component prism shown in Figs. 13.50 and 13.51 is 6 in. (15.2 cm) wide and 7.3 in. (18.5 cm) long. The prisms are made of Zerodur (CTE ~ zero); they are mounted at three points on a cast-aluminum base structure (CTE ≈ 12 ppm/°F). The mounting points are separated by as much as 4 in. Over this distance, differential expansion for a temperature change of 40°F is about 2×10^{-3} in. (0.051 mm). Forces are then exerted on the prism, and its high-precision reflecting surfaces can be distorted. To accommodate temperature changes with different CTEs without optical effects, flexures were used to attach the prism to the structure. The basic principle of the flexure mount is explained in Section 7.4 in conjunction with Fig. 7.29.

The prism shown in Figs. 13.50 and 13.51(a) consists of a triplet of first-surface mirrors fashioned as a right-angle reflector and a mirror version of an Amici prism. Each mirror is inclined at 45° to the optical axis of a microlithography mask projection system

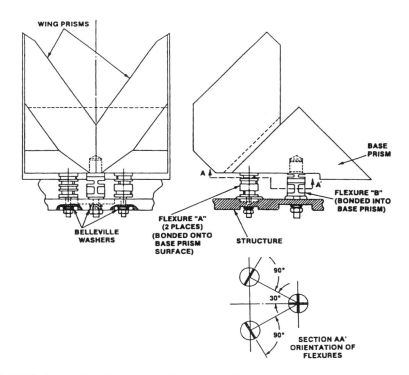

Fig. 13.50 Schematic of a large prism assembly attached to structure through flexure posts. (Courtesy of SVG Lithography Systems, Wilton, CT.)

(a)

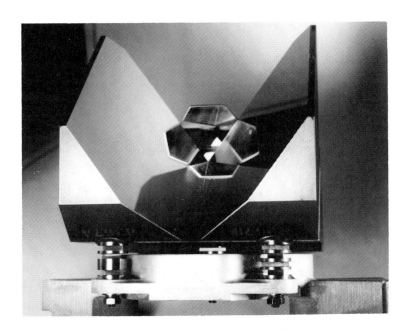

(b)

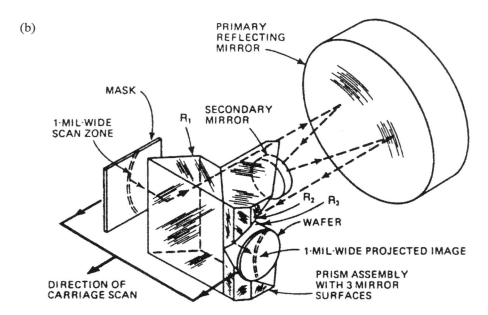

Fig. 13.51 (a) Photograph of the prism assembly of Fig. 13.50; (b) Schematic of the optical system for the microlithography mask projection system using this prism assembly. (Courtesy of SVG Lithography Systems, Wilton, CT.)

of the type shown in Fig. 13.51(b). The beam from a light condenser (not shown) passes through the mask within the narrow arc indicated in the figure and reflects from one face (R_1) of the base prism to a 1:1 magnification imaging system. The beam then reflects from both surfaces (R_2 and R_3) of the wing prisms to form an image of the illuminated portion of the mask on the silicon wafer. The mask and wafer are attached to a carriage that scans in the direction shown to expose the entire information-carrying area of the mask on a corresponding area on the wafer.

The wing prisms are optically contacted to one face of the right-angle base prism that is in turn mounted on the system's structure by the three flexures attached to the hypotenuse of the base prism. The multiple flexure blades are 0.020 in. thick and 0.120 in. long; they are machined into 0.750-in.-diameter Invar posts. Post "B" has a torsion flexure and a universal joint; it is bonded with 3M 2216 epoxy into a hole in the base prism. The other two posts are bonded to the lower surface of the base prism. One of these posts has one universal joint and a single flexure blade that is compliant in the direction toward post "B." The third post has two universal joints. The sectional view AA' of Fig. 13.50 shows the locations of the posts at the corners of a nearly equilateral triangle and the orientations of some flexure blades. Each post has a threaded section at the bottom that passes through holes in the base plate and is secured with nuts acting through stacks of Belleville washers to preload the threads and provide the axial compliance required for the anticipated temperature changes.[13]

13.25 Mounting for Large Dispersing Prisms in an Echellette Spectrograph/Imager

As described by Sheinis et al.,[23] the Echellette spectrograph and imager (ESI) developed for use at the Cassegrain focus of the Keck II 10-m telescope employs two large (approx. 25 kg each) prisms for cross dispersion. In order to maintain optical stability in the operational modes, these prisms must maintain a fixed angle relative to the nominal spectrograph optical axis under a variety of flexural and thermal loads. These include gravity- and thermally induced motions of the optical elements, stress-induced deformations of the optical surfaces, and thermally induced changes in the refractive index of the materials making up the components. The major components of the ESI are shown in Fig. 13.52. The ESI has three scientific modes: medium-resolution echellette mode, low-resolution prismatic mode, and imaging mode. To switch from one mode to another, one prism must be moved out of the beam as shown in Fig. 13.53. That prism is mounted on a single-axis stage. A mirror is moved into the beam to switch to the direct imaging mode. The spectrograph optical system is described by Epps and Miller[24] and by Sutin.[25]

The design philosophy for the ESI is characterized by the use of determinate structures or space frames wherever possible. A determinate structure is one that constrains the six degrees of freedom of a solid body by six structural elements or struts connected to the outside world at six points or nodes. Up to three pairs of the nodes may

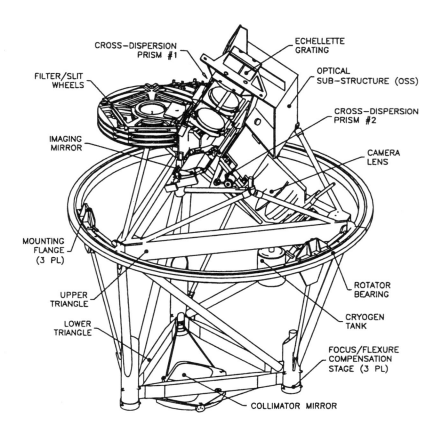

Fig. 13.52 Major components of the Echellette spectrograph and imager developed for use with the Keck II telescope. (From Sheinis et al.[23])

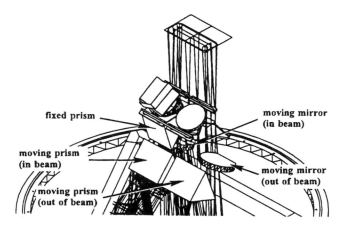

Fig. 13.53 Another view of the ESI showing the dispersing prisms. (From Sutin.[25])

be degenerate. Struts are used in compression and tension only. Thus, deflections of the struts are linear with length, as opposed to struts or plates used in bending where the deflections are proportional to the third power of the part length. Other examples can be found in the description by Radovan et al.[26] of the active collimator used for tilt correction of the ESI and in the description by Bigelow and Nelson[27] of the space frame that provides the backbone for the entire instrument. The desirable features of this type of mounting occur because no moments can be imparted at the strut connections. This has the advantage that distortions of one structural member will introduce displacements without inducing stresses in a second member (i.e., an optical component) mounted on the first member. The challenge to the designer is to create a design that allows only motions of each component and of combined groups of optics so that the combined set of errors is smaller than the tolerances prescribed by the error budget. To do this, the mechanical designer must work very closely with the optical designer to establish the predicted performance of the system prior to actual construction.

In the ESI, the cross-dispersing prisms are in collimated light; therefore, to a first order, small translations of the prisms will produce pupil motion only and no corresponding image motion. Tilts of the prisms will produce combinations of the following: image motion, change of the cross-dispersion direction, change in the amount of cross-dispersion, change in the anamorphic magnification factor, and increased distortion. Therefore the most important stability criterion for the prisms is control of tip and tilt, with almost no requirement for displacement stability. The sensitivities for ESI are $\pm$ 0.013, $\pm$ 0.0045, and $\pm$ 0.014 arcsec of image motion for $\pm$ 1 arcsec of prism tilt about the X-, Y-, and Z-axes, respectively. The desired spectrograph performance is $\pm$ 0.06 arcsec of image motion without flexure control and $\pm$ 0.03 arcsec of image motion with flexure control for a 2-hr integration. For a reasonable choice of the allowable percentage of the total error allotted to the prism motion, these sensitivities give a requirement of less than $\pm$ 1.0, $\pm$ 2.0, and $\pm$ 1.0 arcsec rotation about the X-, Y-, and Z-axes. The normal operating temperature range for the Keck instruments is 2 $\pm$ 4°C, and the total range seen at the summit of Mauna Kea is -15 to 20°C. The instrument must maintain all the above translational and rotational specifications over the entire working temperature range. Therefore the prism mounts need to be designed to be athermal with respect to tilts over this working temperature range and must keep stresses below the acceptable limits over the complete temperature range of the site as well as extremes experienced during shipping.

In addition, attention must be paid to the stresses induced in the prisms. Not only is the potential for fracture of the bond joint or of the glass a cause for concern, but stress induced in the glass will induce a corresponding local change in the index of refraction of the glass, causing a possible wave-front distortion. To ensure against glass breakage, the calculated stress should be limited to 2% of the yield stress of the glass at the bond joint under normal operation. This would also apply to loads occuring during shipping, in earthquakes, with drive errors, and during collisions of the telescope with other objects in the dome (e.g., cranes). Equally important requirements of the mounting design are (1) minimization of measurable hysteresis, which limits the accuracy of the open-loop flexure control system; (2) the ability to make a one-time alignment adjustment of the prism tilts over a 30 arcmin range during the initial assembly; and (3) the ability to remove the prisms for recoating, with a repeatable alignment position upon reassembly.

The ESI design approach held the optics with determinate space frames and interconnected optical assemblies with space frames. However, it was found that it was easier to build the central structure on which all of the optical elements and assemblies (except the collimator mirror) were mounted to a plate as an optical substructure (OSS). It turned out that this was adequate for the task. The prisms were attached to the OSS through six struts. The actual attachment to the prism consisted of two parts: a pad that was permanently bonded to the prism and a mating, detachable part that was permanently attached to the ends of the struts. This allowed the prism to be readily and repeatably installed and removed from its determinate support system.

The fixed and movable prism mounting designs are shown in Figs. 13.54 and 13.55, respectively. Joined pairs of struts are connected to each prism in one point on each of the three nonilluminated faces via a bonded tantalum pad. The CTE of tantalum (6.5 $\times 10^{-6}$ /°C) closely matches that of the BK7 prisms (7.1$\times 10^{-6}$ /°C). The struts attach either directly to the OSS (in the case of the fixed prism) or to the translation stage (in the case of the movable prism), which in turn is bolted to the OSS. The largest refracting faces of the fixed and movable prisms measure 36.0 by 22.8 cm and 30.6 by 28.9 cm, respectively. The glass path is long (>80 cm), so it was necessary for the refractive index to be

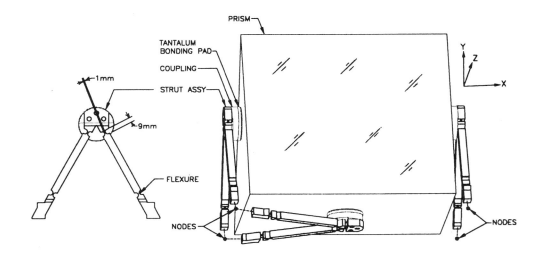

Fig. 13.54 Sketch of the fixed prism assembly showing its six-strut mounting configuration. (From Sheinis et al.[23])

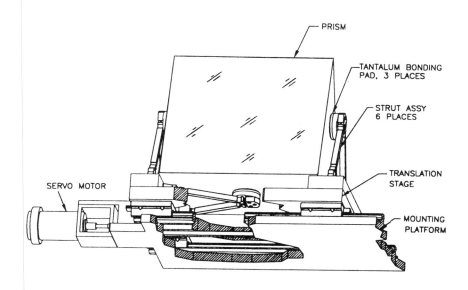

Fig. 13.55 Sketch of the movable prism assembly showing its six-strut mounting configuration and translation stage. (From Sheinis et al.[23])

unusually uniform throughout the prisms. These were made of Ohara BSL7Y glass having a measured index homogeneity better than $\pm\ 2\times10^{-6}$. This achievement is believed to represent the state of the art for prisms of this size.

Each pair of struts was milled from a single piece of ground steel stock. Since each strut should constrain only one degree of freedom of the prism, crossed flexures were cut into each end of each strut to remove four degrees of freedom (one rotational and one translational per flexure pair). The fifth degree of freedom, axial rotation, is removed by the low torsional stiffness of the strut and flexure combination.

Flexure thicknesses and lengths were designed to impart less stress than the self-weight loading of the prism into the prism pad connection and to be below the flexure material's elastic limit over the full range of adjustment, while keeping the strut as stiff as possible. Pad areas were chosen to give a self-weight-induced stress of 125,000 Pa. If we consider the tensile strength of glass to be 7 MPa,[27] this gives a safety factor of 50. The glass-to-metal bond adhesive was Hysol 9313 and the thickness was chosen to be the same (0.25 mm) as that developed by Iraninejad et al.[28] during development of the bonded connections for the Keck primary segments. To confirm these choices, extensive stress testing over various temperature ranges was performed for BK7-to-tantalum and BK7-to-steel bonds. Several samples of BK7 were fabricated with the same surface finish as specified on the prisms. These were bonded to tantalum and steel pads mechanically similar to the actual bonding pads for the prism mounts. These assemblies were subjected to tensile and shear loads up to 10 times the expected loading in the instrument. The test jigs were then cycled 20 to 30 times through the expected temperature excursion range on the Mauna Kea summit. None failed. The joints were then examined for stress birefringence under crossed polarizers. The level of wave-front error was calculated to be less than the limit prescribed by the error budget in the case of the tantalum pad, but not for the steel pad. The tantalum material was then designated for use in the bonding pads. Note that the CTE difference between tantalum and BK7 is 0.6×10^{-6} /°C, whereas the best match to BK7 reported elsewhere[13] uses 6Al-4V titanium with a CTE difference of 1.7×10^{-6} /°C.

13.26 Mountings for Prisms in an Articulated Telescope

Conventionally, the main weapon of an armored vehicle (tank) is operated by a gunner who has two optical intruments to acquire and fire at hostile targets. The primary fire control sight is usually a periscope protruding through the turret ceiling while the secondary sight usually is a telescope protruding through the front of the turret alongside and attached by linkages to the weapon. The key design features of a typical embodiment of the latter type of instrument are discussed here. The specific telescope considered is of the articulated form, i.e., it is hinged near its midsection so the front end can swing in elevation with the gun, while the rear section is essentially fixed in place so the gunner has access to the eyepiece without significantly moving his head.

Figure 13.56 shows the optical system schematically. It has a fixed magnification of 8-power and a field of view of about 8°. The exit pupil diameter is about 5 mm, so the entrance pupil diameter is about 40 mm. The telescope housing diameter throughout its length is generally about 2.5 in.; the prism housings naturally are somewhat larger. Widely separated relay lenses erect the image and transfer the image from the objective focus to the eyepiece focus. Two prism assemblies are shown in the figure. The first contains three prisms, two 90° prisms and a Porro prism, that function within the mechanical hinge and keep the image erect at all gun elevation angles. The second prism assembly with two 90° prisms offsets the axis vertically and turns that axis 20° in a horizontal plane to bring the eyepiece to a convenient location near the gunner's eye. The balance of this section deals with the articulated joint and the mounting arrangement for the prisms in it.

The articulated joint mechanism is shown in Fig. 13.57. The first right-angle prism of the articulated joint is mounted in "Housing, 90° Prism" (see Fig. 13.58). The prism is bonded to a bracket that is attached with two screws and two pins to a plate that is in turn attached with four screws to the housing. After assembly and alignment, a cover is installed over the screws and sealed in place. Surface "W" of that housing attaches to the exit end of the reticle housing.

The second right-angle prism is mounted in "Housing, Erector" as indicated in Fig. 13.59. It also is bonded to a bracket that is attached with two screws and two pins

503

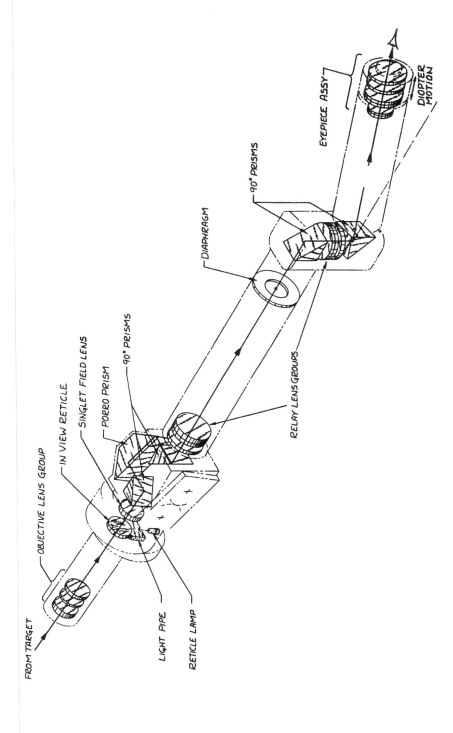

Fig. 13.56 Optical schematic of an articulated telescope. (Courtesy of the U.S. Army.)

504

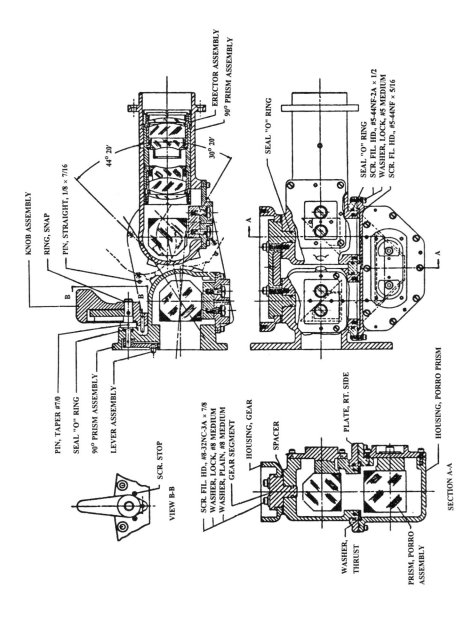

Fig. 13.57 The articulated joint mechanism for the telescope of Fig. 13.56. (Courtesy of the U.S. Army.)

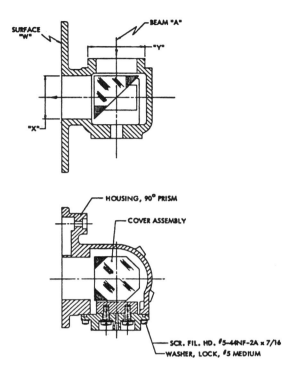

Fig. 13.58 First right-angle prism assembly. (Courtesy of the U.S.Army.)

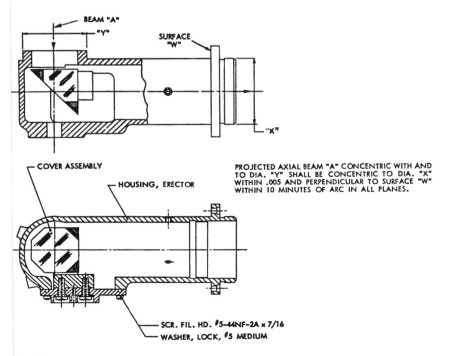

PROJECTED AXIAL BEAM "A" CONCENTRIC WITH AND TO DIA. "Y" SHALL BE CONCENTRIC TO DIA. "X" WITHIN .005 AND PERPENDICULAR TO SURFACE "W" WITHIN 10 MINUTES OF ARC IN ALL PLANES.

Fig. 13.59 Second right-angle prism assembly. (Courtesy of the U.S.Army.)

to a plate that is screwed fast to the housing. The note in this figure indicates the alignment requirements for the prism. Surface "W" mentioned there is shown in Fig. 13.58. After alignment, a cover is sealed over the screws.

As shown in Fig. 13.57, the Porro prism is contained within a separate housing and, together with a gear housing on the opposite side of the telescope, forms the mechanical link between the telescope's front and rear portions. The action of the gear train keeps the prism oriented angularly midway between the front and rear portions of the telescope. This angular relationship maintains the erect image. The housing for the Porro prism is made of hardened stainless steel since it acts as a bearing for the angular motion. The rotary joints in the assembly are sealed with lubricated O-rings that seat in grooves in the mating parts. The prism is bonded to a bracket that is attached to a cover by two screws riding in two slots. After installation of the bonded prism assembly in the housing, the prism is slid in the slots to adjust the optical path through the assembly; the screws are then secured and the plate pinned in place. A protective cover is then installed.

13.27 Semikinematic Design for Constraining a Penta Prism with Springs

In Sect. 7.1, a concept for semikinematically mounting a penta prism is described. The prism is constrained in one direction by clamping it with three cantilevered spring clips against three coplanar pads on a baseplate. In the orthogonal direction, it is spring loaded with a single straddling spring against three locating pins pressed into the baseplate. For the convenience of the reader, Fig. 7.5 showing the mounting configuration is reproduced here as Fig. 13.60. Note that all six degrees of freedom are uniquely constrained. This minimizes bending moments that might distort the optical surfaces.

13.27.1 Constraint perpendicular to the plane of reflection

Figure 13.61 shows one of the three cantilevered spring clips pressing against the top of the prism to preload it against a pad directly below on the baseplate. The interface with the prism is a cylinder of radius R_{CYL}. The following example illustrates analysis of a typical design.

Example 13.1: Analysis of the interface between a cylindrical pad on a cantilevered spring and a prism surface.
(For design and analysis, use File 69 of the CD-ROM)

A BK7 penta prism with A = 1.250 in. (31.750 mm) is constrained perpendicular to its pentagonal faces by three cantilevered beryllium copper springs of width b = 0.250 in. (6.350 mm), thickness t = 0.011 in. (0.279 mm), and free length L = 0.375 in. (9.525 mm). A total preload sufficient to withstand acceleration a_G = 12 is

(a)

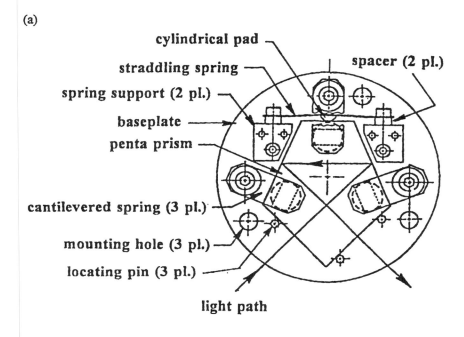

cylindrical pad

straddling spring

spring support (2 pl.)

baseplate

penta prism

spacer (2 pl.)

cantilevered spring (3 pl.)

mounting hole (3 pl.)

locating pin (3 pl.)

light path

(b)

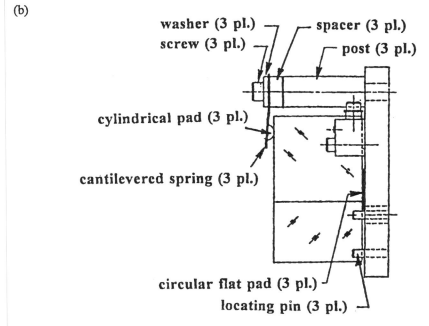

washer (3 pl.)

screw (3 pl.)

spacer (3 pl.)

post (3 pl.)

cylindrical pad (3 pl.)

cantilevered spring (3 pl.)

circular flat pad (3 pl.)

locating pin (3 pl.)

Fig. 13.60 Repeat of Fig. 7.5, semikinematic mounting for a penta prism. (a) Plan view, (b) side view.

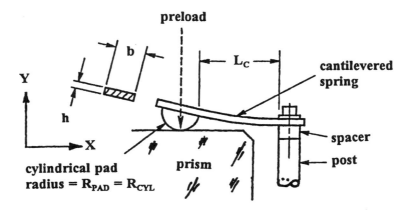

Fig. 13.61 Configuration of one of the cantilevered springs with cylindrical pads applying preload to the prism of Fig. 13.60.

required. Integral cylindrical pads of radius $R_{CYL} = 0.250$ in. (6.350 mm) and length equal to b on each spring touch the prism surface. (a) What spring deflection is required? (b) What is the bending stress developed in the spring and what is its safety factor? (c) What is the contact stress in the prism?

From Fig. 6.17, $V = 1.5A^3 = (1.5)(1.250)^3 = 2.930$ in.^{3} (48.014 cm^3)
From Table B1, $\rho = 0.091$ lb/in.^{3} so $W = (2.930)(0.091) = 0.267$ lb (0.121 kg)
From Eq. (7.1), $P_i = Wa_G/N = (0.267)(12)/3 = 1.068$ lb (4.744 N)
The linear preload = $p_i = P_i/b$
$$= (1.068)/0.250 = 4.272 \text{ lb/in. } (0.7481 \text{ N/mm})$$
From Table B12, S_Y for BeCu = 155,000 lb/in.^{2} (1.069×10^3 MPa)
$$E_M = 18.50 \times 10^6 \text{ lb/in. } (1.27 \times 10^5 \text{ MPa}) \text{ and } \upsilon_M = 0.35$$

(a) From Eq. (3.28):
Δ = spring deflection = $(1 - 0.35^2)(4)(1.068)(0.375^3)/(18.5 \times 10^6)(0.250)(0.011^3)$
$$= 0.032 \text{ in. } (0.816 \text{ mm})$$

(b) From Eq. (3.29):
S_B = spring stress = $(6)(1.068)(0.375)/(0.250)(0.011^2)$
$$= 79,438 \text{ lb/in.}^2 (547.7 \text{ MPa})$$

$f_S = S_Y/S_B = 155,000/79,438 = 1.95$

(c) From Table B1: $K_G = 8.177 \times 10^{-8}$ in.^{2}/lb

From Eq. (11.4): $K_M = (1 - 0.35^2)/18.5 \times 10^6 = 4.743 \times 10^{-8}$ in.^{2}/lb

Hence, $K_2 = 1.29 \times 10^{-7}$ lb/in.^{2}

From Eq. (11.12):

$S_{C\ CYL} = 0.564[p_i/(K_2 R_{CYL})]^{1/2} = 0.564\{4.272/[(1.29 \times 10^{-7})(0.250)]\}^{1/2}$

$= 6491$ lb/in.^{2} (44.7 MPa)

Since glass can withstand compressive stress of about 50,000 lb/in.^{2}, this is not a problem. The safety factor for the spring is satisfactory, as is the spring deflection.

13.27.2 Constraint in the plane of reflection

Figure 13.60(a) shows a straddling leaf spring holding the prism horizontally against three cylindrical locating pins pressed into the baseplate. The mechanical interface with the prism surface is at a cylindrical pad of radius R_{CYL} located at the center of the spring. In the following example, we continue our analysis of the design.

Example 13.2: Analysis of the interface between a cylindrical pad on a straddling spring and a prism surface.
(For design and analysis, use File 70 of the CD-ROM)

The prism is as described in the last example. The straddling spring is BeCu and has the following dimensions: b = 0.250 in. (6.350 mm), t = 0.014 in. (0.356 mm), and L = 1.040 in. (26.416 mm). The cylindrical pad radius is 0.250 in. (6.350 mm). The pad presses against the end of the prism as shown in Fig. 13.60. Find (a) the spring deflection, (b) the stress in the spring and its f_S, and (c) the worst case stress in the prism?

From Example 13.1 for BeCu: $S_Y = 155,000$ lb/in.^{2} (1.069×10^3 MPa)

$E_M = 18.5 \times 10^6$ lb/in. (1.27×10^5 Pa), $\upsilon_M = 0.35$

$W = 0.267$ lb (0.121 kg), $a_G = 12$

From Eq. (7.1), $P_i = Wa_G/N = (0.267)(12)/1 = 3.204$ lb (14.252 Pa)

$p_i = P_i/b = (3.204)/0.250 = 12.816$ lb/in. (2244.41 N/m)

(a) From Eq. (7.7):

$\Delta y = $ deflection $= (0.0625)(1 - 0.35^2)(3.204)(1.040^3)/(18.5 \times 10^6)(0.250)(0.014^3)$

$= 0.016$ in. (0.406 mm)

(b) From Eq. (7.8): $S_B = $ spring stress $= 0.75 P_i L/bt^2$

$= (0.75)(3.204)(1.040)/[(0.250)(0.014^2)] = 51,002$ lb/in.^{2} (351.7 MPa)

$f_S = S_Y / S_B = 155,000/51,002 = 3.0$

(c) From Example 13.1: $K_2 = 1.29 \times 10^{-7}$ lb/in.^{2}

From Eq. (11.12): $S_{C\ CYL} = 0.564[p_i /(R_{CYL})(K_2)]^{1/2}$
$= (0.564)\{12.816/[(0.250)(1.29 \times 10^{-7})]\}^{1/2} = 11{,}243$ lb/in.^{2} (77.5 MPa)

All results of this analysis seem to be acceptable.

The total preload P_i is applied normal to the base of the prism as illustrated in Fig. 13.62 and has components P_x directed toward the single pin 1 at the prism's

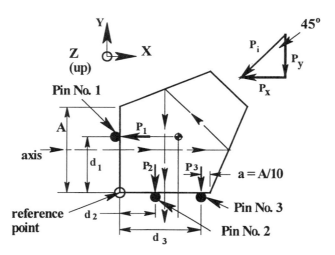

Fig. 13.62 Applied preload and locations of pin constraints for the penta prism analyzed in Examples 13.1 through 13.3.

entrance face and P_y directed toward pins 2 and 3 on the exit face. From the geometry of the design, the force components on the pins are

$$P_1 = P_x = P_i \sin 45° \qquad\qquad (13.1)$$

$$P_2 + P_3 = P_y = P_i \cos 45° \qquad\qquad (13.2)$$

A third equation results from the requirement that the clockwise and counterclockwise moments about an axis through any point in the plane of Fig. 13.62 and normal to that plane balance each other. If we (arbitrarily) choose the apex of the prism as the reference point, then

$$P_1 d_1 = P_2 d_2 + P_3 d_3 \qquad (13.3)$$

Combining these three equations, we obtain

$$(13.4)$$
$$P_2 = P_i (d_1 \sin\theta - d_3 \cos\theta)/(d_2 - d_3)$$

$$(13.5)$$
$$P_3 = P_i \cos\theta - P_2$$

Note that static instability would result if the preload force at any locating pin goes to zero.

One possible constraint configuration with pin contact length $h_P = A/10$ would locate the pins as indicated in Fig. 13.62 with respect to the center of gravity of the prism. This would minimize overturning moments under shock or vibration in the X-Y plane. This would not, however, reduce moments in the Y-Z or X-Z planes because the pins and the straddling spring are not in the same Z plane as the CG. Since it is not convenient to locate the constraints in the plane containing the CG, we must rely on the cantilevered springs to withstand moments in the Y-Z and X-Z planes.

At this point in the development of the design, we should examine the possibility of beam obscuration. To do so, we must make certain assumptions about the prism and mounting geometry. The results we obtain apply only to this geometry, but the analytical procedure can easily be adapted to other geometries.

Figure 13.63(a) shows the shadows of pins protruding a distance $A/10$ above the bottom face of the prism at the entrance and exit faces. The center of pin 3 is $A/10$ from the nearest prism corner. The projected location of the CG at 0.648A from a refracting face is indicated in each view. The entrance and exit clear apertures (CA) of the prism are assumed to have diameters of 0.9A; they are indicated by the dashed circles. Obviously, some vignetting of the transmitted beam occurs at pins 1 and 2.

Locations for pins 1 and 2 that just eliminate vignetting with $h_P = A/10$ are shown in Fig. 13.63(b). Here the corners of the pin shadows are tangent to the CA. From the geometry of the figure, we determine that the pins are now located as follows:

(a)

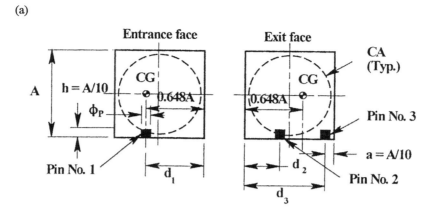

(b)

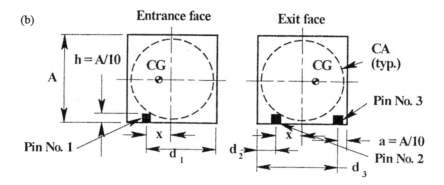

Fig. 13.63 Vignetting effects caused by the pins (a) if aligned to the prism CG and (b) with pins 1 and 2 moved outboard to be tangent to the clear aperture.

$$x = [(0.5\,CA)^2 - (0.5A - h_P)^2]^{1/2} \qquad (13.6)$$

$$d_1 = 0.5A + x + 0.5\phi_P \qquad (13.7)$$

$$d_2 = 0.5A - x - 0.5\phi_P \qquad (13.8)$$

$$d_3 = A - a \qquad (13.9)$$

where h_P = contact length of the pin on the prism and ϕ_P = pin diameter.

Setting $\theta = 45°$ in Eqs. (13.1 through 13.3), we obtain:

$$P_1 = 0.707P_i \tag{13.10}$$

$$P_2 = 0.707(d_1 - d_3)P_i/(d_2 - d_3) \tag{13.9}$$

$$P_3 = 0.707P_i - P_2 \tag{13.12}$$

Knowing the magnitudes of the preloads at all pins, we can now determine the stress in the prism at each pin interface. If we assume all the pins to be the same, it is necessary only to find the stress at pin 1 because it has the greatest preload and hence represents a worst case for damage. This is illustrated in the following example.

Example 13.3: Estimation of worst-case stress in a penta prism at a locating pin. (For design and analysis, use Files 71.1 & 71.2 of the CD-ROM)

The prism considered in Examples 13.1 and 13.2 is located horizontally by pins made of type 416 stainless steel with diameters ϕ_P = 0.125 in. (3.175 mm). The preload P_i is 3.204 lb (14.252 N) as calculated in Example 13.2. Pin 1 of Fig. 13.62 has the greatest component of this preload. Line contact occurs along a length of h_P = 0.125 in. (3.175 mm) on this cylindrical pin. (a) What stress develops in the glass under this preload?

From Table B12 and Ex. 13.1, E_M = 29.0×10⁶ lb/in.² (2.0×10⁵ MPa), υ_M = 0.283
$K_M = (1 - 0.283^2)/29.0 \times 10^6 = 3.172 \times 10^{-8}$ in.²/lb $K_G = 8.177 \times 10^{-8}$ in.²/lb
Hence, $K_2 = K_M + K_G = 1.135 \times 10^{-7}$ in.²/lb
From Eq. (13.8), $P_1 = 0.707P_i = (0.707)(3.204) = 2.265$ lb (10.076 N)
The linear preload is $p_i = P_i/h_P = 2.265/0.125 = 18.120$ lb/in. (3173.28 N/m)
From Eq. (11.12),
$$S_{C\ CYL} = 0.564[p_i/(K_2 R_{CYL})]^{1/2} = 0.564\{18.120/[(1.135 \times 10^{-7})(0.0625)]\}^{1/2}$$
$$= 28{,}505\ \text{lb/in.}^2\ (196.5\ \text{MPa}) \quad \text{This stress is excessive.}$$

(b) Assume that the clear aperture of the prism is 0.9A = 1.125 in. (28.575 in.) and a = A/10 = 0.125 in. (3.175 mm). Lengthen all the pins to 0.250 in. (6.350 mm) and move pins 1 and 2 outboard to be tangent to the clear aperture. Where are the pins and what are the stresses in the prism at the contacts?

From Eq. (13.4),

$x_1 = x_2 = \{[(0.5)(1.1250)]^2 - [(0.5)(1.250) - 0.250)^2]\}^{1/2} = 0.419$ in. (10.649 mm)

From Eqs. (13.7 through (13.12),

$d_1 = (0.5)(1.250) + (0.5)(0.125) + 0.419 = 1.106$ in. (28.105 mm)

$d_2 = (0.5)(1.250) - (0.5)(0.125) - 0.419 = 0.143$ in. (3.645 mm)

$d_3 = 1.250 - 0.125 = 1.125$ in. (28.575 mm)

$P_1 = (0.707)(3.204) = 2.265$ lb (10.078 N)

$P_2 = (0.707)(1.106 - 1.125)(3.204)/(0.143 - 1.125) = 0.044$ lb (0.195 N)

$P_3 = (0.707)(3.204) - 0.044 = 2.221$ lb (9.880 N)

The linear preloads are

$p_1 = 2.265/0.250 = 9.060$ lb/in. (1586.641 N/m)

$p_2 = 0.044/0.250 = 0.176$ lb/in. (0.031 N/mm)

$p_3 = 2.221/0.250 = 8.884$ lb.in. (1.556 N/mm)

From Eq. (11.12),

At pin 1, $S_{C\ CYL} = 0.564\{9.060/[(1.135\times10^{-7})(0.0625)]\}^{1/2}$
$= 20,156$ lb/in.^{2} (138.97 MPa)

At pin 2, $S_{C\ CYL} = 0.564\{0.176/[(1.135\times10^{-7})(0.0625)]\}^{1/2}$
$= 2809.3$ lb/in.^{2} (19.4 MPa)

At pin 3, $S_{C\ CYL} = 0.564\{8.884/[(1.135\times10^{-7})(0.0625)]\}^{1/2}$
$= 19,959.3$ lb/in.^{2} (137.6 MPa)

These stresses should be acceptable from a damage viewpoint.

13.28 The mounting for the Geostationary Operational Environmental Satellite Telescope Secondary Mirror

The configuration of the Cassegrainian telescope used in NASA's Geostationary Operational Environmental Satellite (GOES) is shown in Fig. 13.64. The aperture of the primary mirror is 12.25 in. (31.1 cm), while that of the secondary mirror is 1.53 in. (3.9 cm). The mounting of the latter mirror as described by Hookman[29] is considered here.

The ULE secondary mirror is mounted in an Invar cell as shown in the sectional view of Fig. 13.64. It is supported radially and axially by pads of RTV566 and registered against three 0.002-in. (0.05-μm)-thick Mylar pads equally spaced around the periphery of the mirror's aperture. The pads are bonded in place with epoxy to ensure that they do not move. The radial RTV pads are 0.200 in. (5.1 mm) in diameter and 0.01 in. (0.25 mm) thick, while the axial pads have the same diameters and are 0.025 in. (0.64 mm) thick. The Invar retaining ring is held by three screws to the end of the cell as shown in the exploded view of Fig. 13.65. When bottomed against the cell, the cured axial RTV pads are compressed 0.002 in. (0.05 mm) to preload the subassembly nominally by about 2.15 lb (9.6 N). The radial pads are centered axially at the neutral plane of the mirror.

To minimize temperature effects caused by a mismatch of CTEs of the Invar mirror cell and the aluminum mounting, the cell is supported on the ends of three flexure blades machined integrally into the mounting shown in Fig. 13.65. The mount is 6061-T6 aluminum. The flexure blades are 0.5 in (12.7 mm) long, 0.32 in. (8.1 mm) wide, and 0.020 in. (0.5 mm) thick. Temperature changes do not disturb the radial location or tilt of the mirror. Tests of the spider-mounted secondary mirror indicated that the natural frequency of the assembly was 830 Hz. This safely avoided strong driving frequencies of the applicable environment.

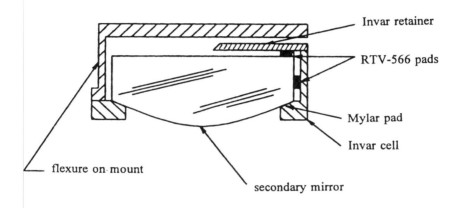

Fig. 13.64 Partial sectional view of the GOES secondary mirror mount. (Adapted from Hookman.[29])

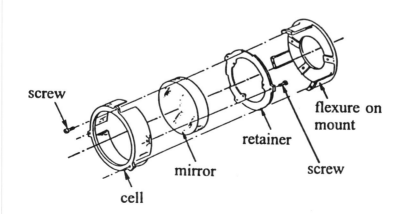

Fig. 13.65 Exploded view of the GOES secondary mirror mount. (From Hookman.[29])

13.29 Mounting for the Far Ultraviolet Spectroscopic Explorer Spectrograph Gratings

The Far Ultraviolet Spectroscopic Explorer (FUSE) is a NASA-sponsored, low earth-orbiting astrophysical observatory designed to provide high spectral resolution observations across a 905 to 1195 Å spectral band. Figure 13.66 schematically shows the optical arrangement of the spectrograph.[30] Light is collected by four off-axis parabolic telescope mirrors (not shown) and focused onto four slit mirrors that act both as movable entrance slits for the spectrometer and as mirrors that direct the visible star field to fine error sensors (also not shown). The diverging light passing through the slits is diffracted and reimaged by four holographic grating mount assemblies (GMAs). The spectra are

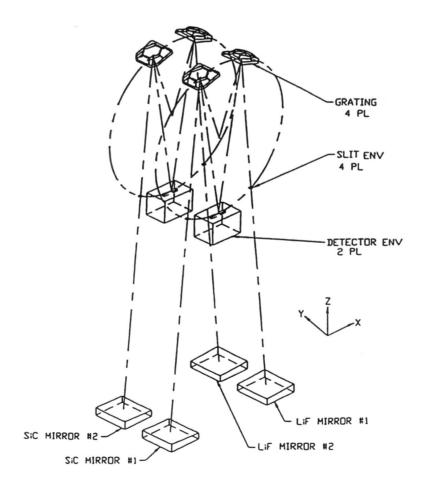

Fig. 13.66 Optical configuration of the FUSE spectrograph. (From Shipley et al.[30])

collected on two microchannel plate detectors. The orbital temperature operating range is 15° to 25°C while the survival range is -10° to 40°C. During an observation, the temperature will be stabilized within 1°C.

The four gratings are identical in size (266 by 275 by 68.1 mm). They are made of Corning 7940 fused silica, class 0, grade F. This material was chosen for its low CTE and availability to accommodate the process of adding holographic gratings. The weight of each blank is reduced by machining the rib pattern shown in Fig. 13.67 in its back surface. Two corners are removed to accommodate an anticipated envelope interference. Strength and fracture control requirements dictate that the blank be acid etched after ruled surfaces are coated with LiF or SiC to optimize performance in these bands.

The Invar mounting brackets are bonded in place with Hysol EA9396 epoxy. Tests of bonded samples showed that the bond strength consistently was >4000 lb/in.^{2}, with some samples exceeding 5000 lb/in.^{2}. This bond strength is more than adequate for the application.

Calculations of fracture probability using Gaussian and Weibull statistical methods were inconclusive.[31] The fact that the nonoptical surfaces of the gratings were not polished contributes significantly to this problem. In order to ensure success, a conservative mechanical interface design was employed; this was thoroughly evaluated by finite-element means throughout the design evolution. One major improvement was to add the flex pivots shown in Fig. 13.68 to allow compliance in the directions

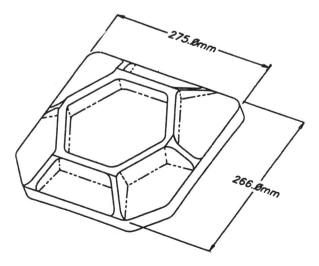

Fig. 13.67 View of the back side of the grating blank showing its machined rib structure. (From Shipley et al.[30])

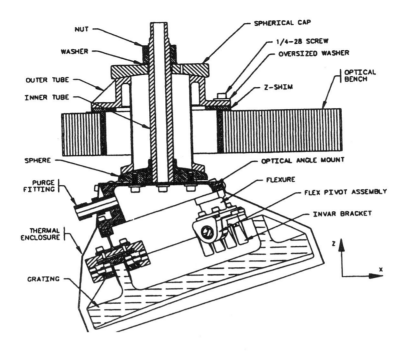

Fig. 13.68 Sectional view of the grating mount assembly showing its adjustment provisions. (From Shipley et al.[30])

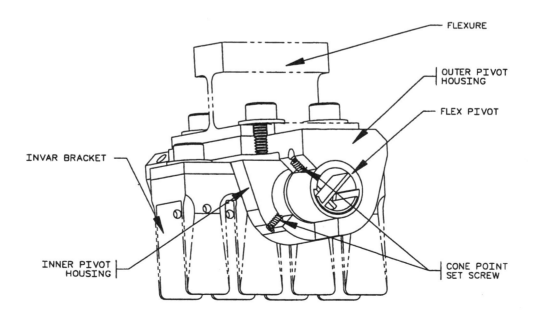

Fig. 13.69 Detail view of the flex pivot feature in the grating mount design. (From Shipley et al.[31])

perpendicular to the radial flexures. The radial flexure blades were reduced in length to accommodate this addition while maintaining the height of the mechanism.

Figure 13.69 shows details of the flex pivot installation. Each pivot consists of outer and inner pivot housings, two 0.625-in.-diameter welded cantilever flex pivots, and eight cone point setscrews. The location of each pivot is maintained by the setscrews, which are driven into shallow conical divots machined at two places in each cantilevered end of the flexure. Rigorous vibration testing of prototype and flight model grating mounts confirmed the success of the design.

The wedge-shaped optical angle mounting seen in Fig. 13.68 between the radial flexures and the bottom of the outer tubular central structure serves to orient the grating at the proper angle relative to the coordinate system of the device. A spacer (shim) is used between the outer tube and the optical bench for axial adjustment. The outer tube interfaces with spherical seats at top and bottom. This allows fine adjustment of the angular orientation by external motorized screws in an alignment fixture. This adjustment is clamped by torquing the nut at the top of the assembly. Optical cubes attached to the backs of the gratings are used with theodolites as the metrology means during alignment.

Titanium was used extensively in the grating mount because of its high strength and relatively low CTE. All titanium parts except the flexures are Tiodized [32] to reduce friction between mating surfaces during alignment and to facilitate cleaning at assembly. The convex sphere and the spherical washer of Fig. 13.68 are made of type 17-4-PH stainless steel, the nut is type 303 stainless steel, and the Z-shim is a type 400 stainless steel.

13.30 The Mounting Configuration for the Very Large Telescope Secondary Mirror

The European Southern Observatory (ESO) very large telescope (VLT) consists of an array of four 8-m (26.25-ft)-diameter telescopes that can operate together (i.e., coupled) or independently. If coupled, the light-gathering power is equivalent to a 16-m (52.50-ft)-diameter single-aperture telescope. Optical performance is monitored and optimized by adjusting 150 axial and 64 lateral hydraulic supports on the primary mirrors[33] and focusing, centering, and tilt/chopping stages on the secondary mirrors.

Each secondary mirror is a convex aspheric, 1.2 m (47.24 in.) in diameter and 130 mm (5.12 in.) thick. A sectional view though one mirror is shown in Fig. 13.70. The mirrors are made of hot isostatic pressed I220H beryllium. They are lightweighted by machining pockets into the back surface, plated with electroless nickel plated (front and back surfaces), and polished. The mirror mounts were integrated with the substrates before polishing. The mirrors were thermal cycled at various points during manufacture to minimize residual stresses. Its weight is 42.3 kg (93.2 lb). The mirror is supported from

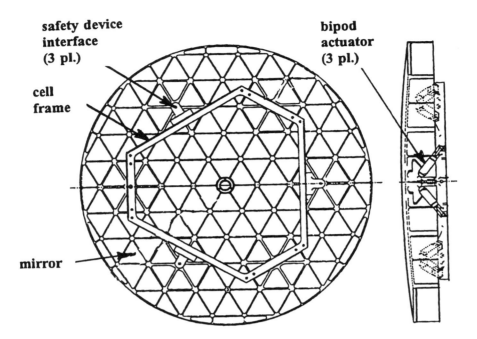

safety device
interface
(3 pl.)

bipod
actuator
(3 pl.)

cell
frame

mirror

Fig. 13.70 The configuration of the VLT secondary mirror substrate. (Adapted from Cayrel. [33])

a truncated triangular frame by six actuators in bipod configuration. Attachment is at the neutral plane of the substrate.[34] The frame is in turn attached to the armature of the secondary mirror chopping assembly and thence to the other mechanisms in the overall optomechanical system.

The following mechanisms depicted in Fig. 13.71 and described by Cayrel[33] provide the motions required of the mirror during alignment and operation:

• Focusing stage: moves the inner tube and all components mounted on it (including the secondary mirror) axially with respect to the fixed central tube in a stepwise fashion during operation and to switch the telescope mode from Nasmyth to Cassegrain focus. Roller bearings between the two tubes allow precise motion with minimal backlash.

• Centering stage: moves the vertex of the secondary mirror with axially separated drivers that provide transverse motions radially or angularly, depending upon the sense of the independent motions. This stage also compensates for gravity effects as the telescope axis is moved in elevation.

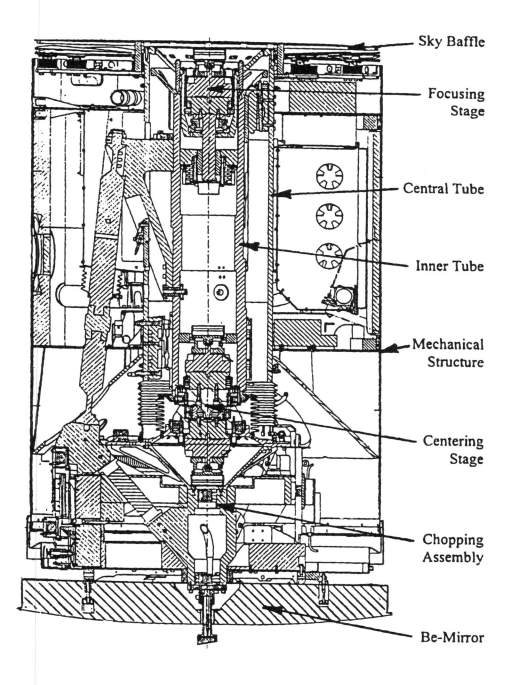

Fig. 13.71 Optomechanical configuration of the VLT secondary mirror unit. (Adapted from Barho et al.[35])

• Chopping stage: tilts the secondary mirror continuously to compensate for telescope tracking errors and in a preprogrammed stepwise oscillatory motion to switch the telescope line of sight between the sky background and the star image.

The secondary mirror assembly's thermal environment is stabilized by several heater pads operating under thermister control. The temperature of various electronic heat sources is stabilized with liquid and fan cooling as needed. Radiation cooling of the mirror's rear surface is compensated for with a nearby electric heater pad.

References

1. Stubbs, D.M., and Hsu, I.C., "Rapid cooled lens cell," *SPIE Proceedings* Vol. 1533, 36, 1991.

2. Trsar, W.J., Benjamin, R.J., and Casper, J.F., "Production engineering and implementation of a modular military binocular," *Opt. Eng.* Vol. 20, 201, 1981.

3. Yoder, P. R., Jr., "Lens mounting techniques," *SPIE Proceedings* Vol. 389, 2, 1983.

4. Private communication from T.A. Palmer and D.A. Murray, Janos Technology, Inc., Townshend, VT.

5. Betensky, E.I., and Welham, B.H., "Optical design and evaluation of large aspherical-surface plastic lenses," *SPIE Proceedings* Vol. 193, 78, 1979.

6. U.S. Precision Lens, Inc., *The Handbook of Plastic Optics*, 2nd ed., Cincinnati, OH, 1983.

7. Benford, J.R., "Microscope Objectives," Chapt. 4 in *Applied Optics and Optical Engineering*, Vol. III, Academic Press, New York, 1965.

8. Bayar, M., "Lens barrel optomechanical design principles," *Opt. Eng.,* Vol. 20, 181, 1981.

9. Vukobratovich, D., Valente, T.M., Shannon, R.R., Hooker, R.A., and Sumner, R.E., "Design and fabrication of an astrographic astrograph," *SPIE Proceedings* Vol. 1752, 245, 1992.

10. Valente, T.M., and Richard, R.M., "Interference fit equations for lens cell design using elastomeric lens mountings," in *Opt. Eng.* Vol. 33, 1223, 1994.

11. *Dictionary of Science and Technology*, C. Morris, ed., Academic Press, San Diego, 1992.

12. Rayces, J.L., Foster, F., and Casas, R.E., "Catadioptric System," U.S. Patent No. 3,547,525, 1970.

13. Yoder, P.R., Jr., *Opto-Mechanical Systems Design,* 2nd ed., Marcel Dekker, New York, 1993.

14. Cassidy, L.W., "Advanced Stellar Sensors - A New Generation," in *Digest of Papers, AIAA/SPIE/OSA Symposium, Technology for Space Astrophysics Conference: The Next 30 Years*, 164, American Institute of Aeronautics and Astronautics, Reston, VA, 1982.

15. Bystricky, K.M., and Yoder, P.R., Jr., "Catadioptric lens with aberrations balanced with an aspheric surface," *Appl. Opt.* Vol. 24, 1206, 1983.

16. Scott, R. M., "Optical Engineering," *Appl. Opt.* Vol. 1, 387, 1962.

17. Mast, T., Faber, S.M., Wallace, V., Lewis, J., and Hilyard, D., "DEIMOS camera assembly," *SPIE Proceedings* Vol. 3786, 499, 1999.

18. Mast, T., Brown, W., Gilmore, K., and Pfister, T., "DEIMOS detector mosaic assembly," *SPIE Proceedings* Vol.3786, 493, 1999.

19. Hilyard, D.F., Laopodis, G.K., and Faber, S.M., "Chemical reactivity testing of optical fluids and materials in the DEIMOS Spectrographic Camera for the Keck II Telescope," *SPIE Proceedings* Vol. 3786, 482, 1999.

20. Mast, T., Choi, P.I., Cowley, D., Faber, S.M., James, E., and Shambrook, A., "Elastomeric lens mounts," *SPIE Proceedings* Vol. 3355, 144, 1998.

21. Ford, V.G., White, M.L., Hochberg, E, and McGown, J., "Optomechanical design of nine cameras for the Earth Observing System Multi-Angle Imaging Spectro-Radiometer, TERRA Platform," *SPIE Proceedings* Vol. 3786, 264, 1999.

22. Yoder, P.R., Jr., "Two new lightweight military binoculars," *J. Opt. Soc. Am.* Vol. 50, 491, 1960.

23. Sheinis, A.I., Nelson, J.E., and Radovan, M.V., "Large prism mounting to minimize rotation in Cassegrain instruments," *SPIE Proceedings* Vol. 3355, 59, 1998.

24. Epps, H.W., and Miller, J.S., "Echellette spectrograph and imager (ESI) for Keck Observatory," *SPIE Proceedings* Vol. 3355, 48, 1998.

25. Sutin, B.M., "What an optical designer can do for you AFTER you get the design," *SPIE Proceedings* Vol. 3355, 134, 1998.

26. Radovan, M.V., Nelson, J.E., Bigelow, B.C., and Sheinis, A.I., "Design of a collimator support to provide flexure control on Cassegrain instruments," *SPIE Proceedings* Vol. 3355, 1998.

27. Bigelow, B.C. and Nelson, J.E., "Determinate space-frame structure for the Keck II Echellete Spectrograph and Imager (ESI)," *SPIE Proceedings* Vol. 3355, 164, 1998.

28. Iraninejad, B., Lubliner, J., Mast, T., and Nelson, J., "Mirror deformations due to thermal expansion of inserts bonded to glass," *SPIE Proceedings* Vol. 748, 206, 1987.

29. Hookman, R., "Design of the GOES telescope secondary mirror mounting," *SPIE Proceedings* Vol. 1167, 368, 1989.

30. Shipley, A., Green, J.C., and Andrews, J.P., "The design and mounting of the gratings for the Far Ultraviolet Spectroscopic Explorer," *SPIE Proceedings* Vol. 2542, 185, 1995.

31. Shipley, A., Green, J., Andrews, J., Wilkinson, E., and Osterman, S., "Final flight grating mount design for the Far Ultraviolet Spectroscopic Explorer," *SPIE Proceedings* Vol. 3132, 98, 1997.

32. *Tiodize Process Literature*, Tiodize Co., Inc., Huntington Beach, CA.

33. Cayrel, M., "VLT beryllium secondary mirror No. 1 - performance review," *SPIE Proceedings* Vol. 3352, 721, 1998.

34. Hovsepian, T., Michelin, J-M., Stanghellini, S., "Design and tests of the VLT M1 mirror passive and active supporting system," *SPIE Proceedings* Vol. 3352, 424, 1998.

35. Barho, R., Stanghellini, S., and Jander, G., "VLT secondary mirror unit performance and test results," *SPIE Proceedings* Vol.3352, 675, 1998.

APPENDIX A
Unit Conversion Factors

To facilitate conversion from U.S. Customary System (USC) units to metric or System International (SI) units, we list here the standard factors for changing the units commonly used in measuring selected physical parameters mentioned in this text. This involves multiplying the value in USC units by the factor listed. Conversion in the reverse direction requires division by the same factor.

To change **length** in
> feet (ft) to meters (m), multiply by 0.3048.
> inches (in.) to millimeters (mm), multiply by 25.4.
> inches (in.) to nanometers (nm), multiply by 2.54×10^7.

To change **weight** in
> pounds (lb) to kilograms (kg), multiply by 0.4536.
> ounces (oz) to grams (g), multiply by 28.3495.

To change **force** in
> pounds (lb) to newtons (N), multiply by 4.4482.
> kilograms (kg) to newtons, multiply by 9.8066.

To change **linear force** in
> lb/in. to N/mm, multiply by 0.1751.

To change **pressure, stress, or units for Young's modulus** in
> lb/in.^{2} (psi) to N/m^2, multiply by 6894.757.
> lb/in.^{2} (psi) to megapascals (MPa), multiply by 6.8947×10^{-3}.
> lb/in.^{2} (psi) to N/mm^2, multiply by 6.895×10^{-3}.
> atmospheres to MPa, multiply by 0.1103.
> atmospheres to lb/in.^{2}, multiply by 14.7.

To change **torque** or **bending moment** in
> lb-in. to N-m, multiply by 0.11298.
> oz-in. to N-m, multiply by 7.0615×10^{-3}.
> lb-ft to N-m, multiply by 1.35582.

To change **volume** in
> in.^{3} to cm^3, multiply by 16.3871.

To change **density** in
> lb/in.^{3} to g/cm^3, multiply by 27.6804.

To change **acceleration** in
> gravitational units (G) to m/sec^2, multiply by 9.80665.
> ft/sec^2 to m/sec^2, multiply by 0.3048.

To change **temperature** in
> degrees F to degrees C, subtract 32 and multiply by 5/9.
> degrees C to degrees F, multiply by 9/5 and add 32.
> degrees C to degrees K, add 273.1.

APPENDIX B
Mechanical Properties of Materials

This appendix provides tables of material properties derived from various sources as noted. Included are:

Table B1 - Selected mechanical properties of 68 selected Schott glasses.

Table B2 - Comparison of 11 lightweight optical glasses (L) with the nearest standard glass types (S).

Table B3 - Selected optical and mechanical characteristics of commonly used optical plastics.

Table B4 - Optomechanical properties of selected alkali halides and alkaline earth halides.

Table B5 - Mechanical properties of selected IR-transmitting glass and other oxides.

Table B6 - Mechanical properties of diamond and selected IR-transmitting semiconductor materials.

Table B7 - Mechanical properties of selected IR-transmitting chalcogenide materials.

Table B8a - Mechanical properties of selected nonmetallic mirror substrate materials.

Table B8b - Mechanical properties of selected metallic and composite mirror substrate materials.

Table B9 - Comparison of material figures of merit especially pertinent to mirror design.

Table B10a - Characteristics of aluminum alloys used in mirrors.

Table B10b - Characteristics of aluminum matrix composites.

Table B10c - Beryllium grades and some of their properties.

Table B10d - Characteristics of major silicon carbide types.

Table B11 - Techniques for machining, finishing, and coating materials for optical applications.

Table B12 - Mechanical properties of selected metals used for mechanical parts in optical instruments.

Table B13 - Typical physical characteristics of optical cements.

Table B14 - Typical characteristics of representative structural adhesives.

Table B15 - Typical physical characteristics of representative elastomeric sealants.

Table B16 - Typical minimum values for fracture strength S_F of infrared window materials.

Table B17 - Coefficient of thermal defocus (δ) and thermo-optical coefficient (γ) for selected optical materials.

Table B1 - Selected mechanical properties of 68 selected Schott glasses* (Page 1 of 4)

Rank	Glass name	Glass type	Young's modulus (E_G) (lb/in.^{2})	(Pa)	Poisson's ratio (υ_G)	$K_G = (1-\upsilon_G^2)/E_G$ (in^2/lb)	(1/Pa)	Thermal expansion coefficient (α_G) (1/°F)	(1/°C)	Density (ρ) (lb/in^3)	(g/cm^3)
1	K10	501564	9.57e+06	6.60e+10	0.192 a	1.006e-07	1.459e-11	3.6e-06	6.5e-06	0.091	2.52
2	ZKN7	508612	1.03e+07	7.10e+10	0.214	9.266e-08	1.344e-11	2.5e-06	4.5e-06	0.090	2.49
3	BK1	510635	1.07e+07	7.40e+10	0.210	8.906e-08	1.292e-11	4.3e-06	7.7e-06	0.089 a	2.46 a
4	K7	511604	1.00e+07	6.90e+10	0.218	9.518e-08	1.380e-11	4.7e-06	8.4e-06	0.091	2.53
5	KF3	515547	9.57e+06	6.60e+10	0.216	9.959e-08	1.444e-11	4.5e-06	8.1e-06	0.092	2.56
6	BK7	517642	1.17e+07	8.10e+10	0.208	8.177e-08	1.181e-11	3.9e-06	7.1e-06	0.091	2.51
7	UBK7	517643	1.17e+07	8.10e+10	0.212	8.129e-08	1.179e-11	3.9e-06	7.0e-06	0.091	2.51
8	BaLKN3	518602	1.04e+07	7.20e+10	0.212	9.146e-08	1.326e-11	4.4e-06	7.9e-06	0.094	2.61
9	PK2	518651	1.22e+07	8.40e+10	0.209	7.850e-08	1.138e-11	3.8e-06	6.9e-06	0.091	2.51
10	PK50	521697	9.57e+06	6.60e+10	0.235	9.870e-08	1.431e-11	4.9e-06	8.8e-06	0.094	2.59
11	K5	522595	1.03e+07	7.10e+10	0.227	9.211e-08	1.336e-11	4.6e-06	8.2e-06	0.094	2.59
12	KF9	523515	9.72e+06	6.70e+10	0.202	9.871e-08	1.432e-11	3.8e-06	6.8e-06	0.098	2.71
13	LLF6	532488	9.14e+06	6.30e+10	0.205	1.048e-07	1.521e-11	4.2e-06	7.5e-06	0.102	2.81
14	BaK2	540597	1.03e+07	7.10e+10	0.233	9.184e-08	1.332e-11	4.4e-06	8.0e-06	0.103	2.86
15	LLF1	548458	8.70e+06	6.00e+10	0.210	1.098e-07	1.593e-11	4.5e-06	8.1e-06	0.106	2.94
16	KzFN1	551496	8.85e+06	6.10e+10	0.224	1.074e-07	1.557e-11	3.9e-06	7.1e-06	0.098	2.71
17	PSK3	552635	1.22e+07	8.40e+10	0.226	7.789e-08	1.130e-11	3.4e-06	6.2e-06	0.105	2.91

* Ranked in order of increasing value of refractive index, n_d

Table B1 - Selected mechanical properties of 68 selected Schott glasses (Page 2 of 4)

Rank	Glass name	Glass type	Young's modulus (E_G) (lb/in.^{2})	(Pa)	Poisson's ratio (ν_G)	$K_G = (1-\nu_G{}^2)/E_G$ (in.^{2}/lb)	(1/Pa)	Thermal expansion coefficient (α_G) (1/°F)	(1/°C)	Density (ρ) (lb/in.^{3})	(g/cm^3)
18	BaK5	557587	1.04e+07	7.20e+10	0.241	9.020e-08	1.308e-11	4.3e-06	7.8e-06	0.109	3.02
19	SK11	564608	1.15e+07	7.90e+10	0.239	8.229e-08	1.194e-11	3.6e-06	6.5e-06	0.111	3.08
20	BaK50	568580	1.17e+07	8.10e+10	0.259	7.941e-08	1.152e-11	2.1e-06 a	3.7e-06 a	0.106	2.93
21	BaK1	573575	1.07e+07	7.40e+10	0.253	8.721e-08	1.265e-11	4.2e-06	7.6e-06	0.115	3.19
22	LF7	575415	8.56e+06	5.90e+10	0.217	1.114e-07	1.615e-11	4.4e-06	7.9e-06	0.116	3.20
23	LF4	578416	8.70e+06	6.00e+10	0.219	1.094e-07	1.587e-11	4.5e-06	8.1e-06	0.116	3.21
24	BaLF4	580537	1.10e+07	7.60e+10	0.244	8.532e-08	1.237e-11	3.6e-06	6.4e-06	0.115	3.17
25	LF5	581409	8.56e+06	5.90e+10	0.226	1.109e-07	1.608e-11	5.1e-06	9.1e-06	0.116	3.22
26	BaF3	583465	9.28e+06	6.40e+10	0.261	1.004e-07	1.456e-11	4.3e-06	7.8e-06	0.118	3.28
27	SK5	589613	1.22e+07	8.40e+10	0.256	7.670e-08	1.112e-11	3.1e-06	5.5e-06	0.119	3.30
28	F3	596392	8.41e+06	5.80e+10	0.224	1.129e-07	1.638e-11	4.4e-06	8.0e-06	0.128	3.55
29	F14	601382	8.41e+06	5.80e+10	0.218	1.132e-07	1.642e-11	4.4e-06	7.9e-06	0.124	3.44
30	F5	603380	8.41e+06	5.80e+10	0.220	1.131e-07	1.641e-11	4.4e-06	8.0e-06	0.125	3.47
31	BaF4	606439	9.57e+06	6.60e+10	0.247	9.809e-08	1.423e-11	4.4e-06	7.9e-06	0.126	3.50
32	SK2	607567	1.13e+07	7.80e+10	0.263	8.228e-08	1.193e-11	3.3e-06	6.0e-06	0.128	3.55
33	F4	617366	7.98e+06 a	5.50e+10 a	0.225	1.190e-07 a	1.726e-11 a	4.6e-06	8.3e-06	0.129	3.58
34	SSKN8	618498	1.20e+07	8.30e+10	0.256	7.763e-08	1.126e-11	3.9e-06	7.1e-06	0.120	3.33
35	F2	620364	8.41e+06	5.80e+10	0.225	1.129e-07	1.637e-11	4.6e-06	8.2e-06	0.130	3.61
36	FN11	621362	1.22e+07	8.40e+10	0.230	7.774e-08	1.128e-11	4.2e-06	7.5e-06	0.096	2.66

Table B1 - Selected mechanical properties of 68 selected Schott glasses (Page 3 of 4)

Rank	Glass name	Glass type	Young's modulus (E_G) (lb/in.²)	(Pa)	Poisson's ratio (ν_G)	$K_G = (1-\nu_G{}^2)/E_G$ (in²/lb)	(1/Pa)	Thermal expansion coefficient (α_G) (1/°F)	(1/°C)	Density (ρ) (lb/in³)	(g/cm³)
37	BaF8	624470	1.06e+07	7.30e+10	0.260	8.806e-08	1.277e-11	3.9e-06	7.0e-06	0.133	3.67
38	F7	625356	7.98e+06 a	5.50e+10 a	0.239	1.182e-07	1.714e-11	5.4e-06 a	9.8e-06 a	0.131	3.62
39	F1	626357	8.12e+06	5.60e+10	0.229	1.167e-07	1.692e-11	4.8e-06	8.7e-06	0.132	3.65
40	BaSF1	626390	8.99e+06	6.20e+10	0.242	1.047e-07	1.518e-11	4.7e-06	8.5e-06	0.132	3.66
41	F6	636353	8.27e+06	5.70e+10	0.231	1.145e-07	1.661e-11	4.7e-06	8.5e-06	0.136	3.76
42	SF12	648338	8.70e+06	6.00e+10	0.228	1.089e-07	1.580e-11	4.3e-06	7.8e-06	0.135	3.74
43	SF2	648339	7.98e+06 a	5.50e+10 a	0.231	1.187e-07	1.721e-11	4.7e-06	8.4e-06	0.139	3.86
44	LaKN22	651559	1.31e+07	9.00e+10	0.268	7.111e-08	1.031e-11	3.7e-06	6.6e-06	0.135	3.73
45	BaSF2	664358	9.57e+06	6.60e+10	0.245	9.820e-08	1.424e-11	4.6e-06	8.2e-06	0.141	3.90
46	SF19	667330	8.41e+06	5.80e+10	0.228	1.127e-07	1.635e-11	4.3e-06	7.7e-06	0.145	4.02
47	SF5	673322	8.12e+06	5.60e+10	0.233	1.164e-07	1.689e-11	4.6e-06	8.2e-06	0.147	4.07
48	LaF20	682482	1.36e+07	9.40e+10	0.273	6.788e-08	9.845e-12	4.1e-06	7.4e-06	0.140	3.87
49	BaF50	683445	1.35e+07	9.30e+10	0.266	6.889e-08	9.992e-12	4.6e-06	8.3e-06	0.137	3.80
50	SF8	689312	8.12e+06	5.60e+10	0.233	1.164e-07	1.689e-11	4.6e-06	8.2e-06	0.152	4.22
51	SF15	699301	8.70e+06	6.00e+10	0.235	1.086e-07	1.575e-11	4.4e-06	7.9e-06	0.147	4.06
52	SFN64	706303	1.35e+07	9.30e+10	0.250	6.950e-08	1.008e-11	4.7e-06	8.5e-06	0.108	3.00
53	SF1	717295	8.27e+06	5.70e+10	0.234	1.143e-07	1.658e-11	4.5e-06	8.1e-06	0.161	4.46
54	SF18	722293	8.12e+06	5.60e+10	0.238	1.161e-07	1.685e-11	4.5e-06	8.1e-06	0.162	4.49
55	SF10	728284	9.28e+06	6.40e+10	0.232	1.019e-07	1.478e-11	4.2e-06	7.5e-06	0.155	4.28

Table B1 - Selected mechanical properties of 68 selected Schott glasses (Page 4 of 4)

Rank	Glass name	Glass type	Young's modulus (E_G)		Poisson's ratio (υ_G)	$K_G = (1-\upsilon_G{}^2)/E_G$		Thermal expansion coefficient (α_G)		Density (ρ)	
			(lb/in.²)	(Pa)		(in.²/lb)	(1/Pa)	(1/°F)	(1/°C)	(lb/in.³)	(g/cm³)
56	SF53	728287	8.41e+06	5.80e+10	0.238	1.121e-07	1.626e-11	4.6e-06	8.2e-06	0.161	4.45
57	SF13	741276	9.28e+06	6.40e+10	0.233	1.019e-07	1.478e-11	3.9e-06	7.1e-06	0.158	4.36
58	SF54	741281	8.41e+06	5.80e+10	0.237	1.122e-07	1.627e-11	4.3e-06	7.7e-06	0.165	4.56
59	SF14	762265	9.43e+06	6.50e+10	0.235	1.002e-07	1.454e-11	3.7e-06	6.6e-06	0.164	4.54
60	SF55	762270	8.12e+06	5.60e+10	0.247	1.156e-07	1.677e-11	4.6e-06	8.2e-06	0.171	4.72
61	SF11	785258	9.57e+06	6.60e+10	0.237	9.860e-08	1.430e-11	3.4e-06	6.1e-06	0.171	4.74
62	SFL56	785261	1.32e+07	9.10e+10	0.255	7.084e-08	1.027e-11	4.8e-06	8.7e-06	0.118 b	3.28 b
63	SF56	785261	8.41e+06	5.80e+10	0.242	1.119e-07	1.623e-11	4.4e-06	7.9e-06	0.178	4.92
64	LaSF32	803304	1.64e+07	1.13e+11	0.256	5.702e-08	8.270e-12	4.4e-06	7.9e-06	0.127	3.52
65	LaSFN30	803464	1.80e+07 a	1.24e+11 a	0.293 a	5.083e-08 a	7.372e-12 a	3.4e-06	6.2e-06	0.161	4.46
66	SFL6	805254	1.35e+07	9.30e+10	0.260	6.913e-08	1.003e-11	5.0e-06	9.0e-06	0.122 b	3.37 b
67	SF6	805254	8.12e+06	5.60e+10	0.248	1.155e-07	1.676e-11	4.5e-06	8.1e-06	0.187 a	5.18 a
68	LaSFN9	850322	1.58e+07	1.09e+11	0.286	5.808e-08	8.424e-12	4.1e-06	7.4e-06	0.160	4.44
Ratio (max./min.)			2.25		1.53	2.34		2.57		2.11	

Note: "a" indicates extreme low or high value, "b" indicates lightweight version.

Sources: Glass selection from B.H. Walker, "Select Optical Glasses," in *The Photonics Design and Applications Handbook*, Lauren Publishing, Pittsfield, MA, H-356, 1993. Data (except for K_G) from Schott Optical Glass Catalog, Schott Glass Technologies, Inc., Duryea, PA.

Table B2 - Comparison of 11 lightweight optical glasses (L) with the nearest standard glass types (S)

Glass name	n_d	v_d	Density ρ (g/cm^3)	Weight reduction (%)	Resistance to: acid "SR"	alkali "AR"	Knoop hardness "HK"
(L) FN11	1.62096	36.18	2.66	26	1	1.0	510
(S) F2	1.62004	36.37	3.61		1	2.3	370
(L) SFL4	1.75520	27.21	3.37	30	1.0	1.3	500
(S) SF4	1.75520	27.58	4.79		51	2.3	330
(L) SFL6	1.80518	25.39	3.37	35	2	1	500
(S) SF6	1.80518	25.43	5.18		52	2.3	310
(L) SFL56	1.78470	26.08	3.28	33	2	1.3	530
(S) SF56A	1.78470	26.08	4.92		3	2.2	330
(L) SFL57	1.84666	23.62	3.55	36	1.3	1	510
(S) SF57	1.84666	23.83	5.51		52	2.3	300
(L) SFN64	1.70585	30.30	3.00	26	1-2	1.2	500
(S) SF15	1.69895	30.07	4.06		1	1.2	370
(L) BaSF64A	1.70400	39.38	3.20	19	2	1.2	540
(S) BaSF13	1.69761	38.57	3.97		51	1.2	450
(L) LaSF32	1.80349	30.40	3.52	28	1-2	1.0	560
(S) LaSF8	1.80741	31.61	4.87		52	1.2	420
(L) LaSF36A	1.79712	35.08	3.60	20	3	1.0	570
(S) LaSF33	1.80596	34.24	4.48		51	1.2	440
(L) LaKL12	1.67790	54.93	3.32	19	52	2.2	600
(S) LaKN12	1.67790	55.20	4.10		53	4.2	470
(L) LaKL21	1.64048	59.75	2.97	21	53	4.2	590
(S) LaK21	1.64050	60.10	3.74		53	4.2	460

Source: Schott Optical Glass Catalog, Schott Glass Technologies, Inc., Duryea, PA.

Table B3 - Selected optical and mechanical characteristics of commonly used optical plastics (Page 1 of 2)

Properties*	ASTM** test method	Units	Methyl methacrylate (acrylic)	Polystyrene	Polycarbonate	Methyl methacrylate styrene co-polymer (NAS)	Styrene acrylonitrile (SAN)	Allyl diglycol carbonate (CR39)
Refractive index								
(n_D)	D542		1.492	1.590	1.586	1.564	1.567–1.571	1.504
Abbe value								
(v_D)	D542		57.2	30.8	34.0	35	38	56
$dn/dT(\times 10^{-5})$		(/°C)	-8.5	-12.0	-14.3	-14.0		-14.3
Haze	D1003	(%)	<2	<3	<3	<3	3	3
Deflection temperature $(\times 10^{-5})$	D648-56	(°F)						
3.6° F/min, 264 psi			198	180	280		99–104	
3.6° F/min, 66 psi			214	230	270	212	100	
CTE $(\times 10^{-5})$	D696-44	(°F)	3.6	3.5	3.8	3.6	3.6–3.7	6.3 @25–75°C
Recommended maximum continuous service temperature		(°F)	175	175	240	175	212	

534

Table B3 - Selected optical and mechanical characteristics of commonly used optical plastics (Page 2 of 2)

Properties*	ASTM** test method	Units	Methyl methacrylate (acrylic)	Polystyrene	Polycarbonate	Methyl methacrylate styrene co-polymer (NAS)	Styrene acrylonitrile (SAN)	Allyl diglycol carbonate (CR39)
Water absorption (immersed 24 hr @ 73°F)	D570-63	(%)	0.3	0.2	0.15	0.15	0.2	
Specific gravity (ρ)	D792		1.19	1.06	1.20	1.09		
Hardness (0.25 in. sample)	D785-62		M97	M90	M70	M75		
Thermal conductivity (k)		(cal/sec-cm-°C)	4.96	2.4-3.3	4.65	4.5	2.9	5

Notes: * Material formulation data should be confirmed prior to design and specification.

** American Society for Testing and Materials, West Conshohocken, PA

Sources: From various manufacturer's publications; *The Handbook of Plastic Optics*, 2nd ed., U. S. Precision Lens, Inc., Cincinnati, OH, 1983; and H.D. Wolpert, "Optical Plastics: Properties and Tolerances," in *The Photonic Design and Application Handbook*, Lauren Publishing, Pittsfield, MA, H-321, 1989.

Table B4 - Optomechanical properties of selected alkali halides and alkaline earth halides (Page 1 of 2)

Material name and symbol	Refractive index n @ λ in μm	dn/dT @ λ in μm ($\times 10^{-6}$/°C)	CTE α ($\times 10^{-6}$/°C)	Young's modulus E ($\times 10^{10}$ N/m²)	Poisson's ratio ν	Density ρ (g/cm³)	Knoop hardness (kg/mm²)	$K_G = (1 - \nu_G^2)/E_G$ $\times 10^{-11}$ (Pa⁻¹)
Barium fluoride (BaF₂)	1.463 @ 0.63 1.458 @ 3.8 1.449 @ 5.3 1.396 @ 10.6	-16.0 @0.63 -15.9 @3.4 -14.5 @10.6	6.7 @ 75 K 18.4 @ 300 K	5.32	0.343	4.89	82 (500 g)	1.659
Calcium fluoride (CaF₂)	1.431 @ 0.7 1.420 @ 2.7 1.411 @ 3.8 1.395 @ 5.3	-10.4 @0.66 - 8.1 @3.4	18.9 @300 K	9.6	0.29	3.18	160–178	0.954
Potassium bromide (KBr)	1.555 @ 0.6 1.537 @ 2.7 1.529 @ 8.7 1.515 @ 14	-41.9 @1.15 -41.1 @10.6	25.0 @ 75 K	2.69	0.203	2.75	7 (200 g)	3.564
Potassium chloride (KCl)	1.474 @ 2.7 1.472 @ 3.8 1.469 @ 5.3 1.454 @ 10.6	-36.2 @1.15 -34.8 @10.6	36.5	2.97	0.216	1.98	7.2 (200 g)	3.210

Table B4 - Optomechanical properties of selected alkali halides and alkaline earth halides (Page 2 of 2)

Material name and symbol	Refractive index n @ λ in μm	dn/dT @ λ in μm ($\times 10^{-6}$/°C)	CTE α ($\times 10^{-6}$/°C)	Young's modulus E ($\times 10^{10}$ N/m²)	Poisson's ratio ν	Density ρ (g/cm³)	Knoop hardness (kg/mm²)	$K_G = (1-\nu_G^2)E_G$ $\times 10^{-11}$ (Pa⁻¹)
Lithium fluoride (LiF)	1.394 @ 0.5 1.367 @ 3.0 1.327 @ 5.0	-16.0 @0.46 -16.9 @1.15 -14.5 @3.39	5.5	6.48	0.225	2.63	102–113 (600 g)	1.465
Magnesium fluoride (MgF₂)	1.384 @ 0.4o* 1.356 @ 3.8o* 1.333 @ 5.3o*	+0.88@1.15 +1.19@3.39	14.0(∥) 8.9 (⊥)	16.9	0.269	3.18	415	0.549
Sodium chloride (NaCl)	1.525 @ 2.7 1.522 @ 3.8 1.517 @ 5.3	-36.3 @3.39	39.6	4.01	0.28	2.16	15.2 (200 g)	2.298
Thallium bromo-iodide (KRS5)	2.602 @ 0.6 2.446 @ 1.0 2.369 @ 10.6 2.289 @ 30	-254 @0.6 -240 @1.1 -233 @10.6 -152 @40	58	1.58	0.369	7.37	40.2 (200 g)	5.467

Notes: * Birefringent material, o = ordinary axis.

Sources: P.R. Yoder, Jr., *Opto-Mechanical Systems Design*, 2nd ed., Marcel Dekker, New York, 1993; W.J. Tropf, M.E. Thomas, and T.J. Harris, "Properties of Crystals and Glasses," Chapt. 33 in *OSA Handbook of Optics*, 2nd ed., Vol. II, McGraw-Hill, New York, 1995.

Table B5 - Mechanical properties of selected IR-transmitting glass and other oxides (Page 1 of 3)

Material name and symbol	Refractive index n @ λ in μm	dn/dT @ λ in μm (×10⁻⁶/°C)	CTE α (×10⁻⁶/°C)	Young's modulus E (×10¹⁰ N/m²)	Poisson's ratio υ	Density ρ (g/cm³)	Knoop hardness (kg/mm²)	$K_G=(1-\upsilon_G{}^2)E_G$ ×10⁻¹¹ (Pa⁻¹)
Aluminum oxynitride (ALON)	1.793 @ 0.6 1.66 @ 4.0		5.8	32.2	0.24	3.71	1970	0.293
Calcium alumino-silicate (Schott IRG11)	1.684 @ 0.55 1.608 @ 4.6 1.635 @ 3.3		8.2 @ 293–573 K	10.8	0.284	3.12	608	0.851
Calcium alumino-silicate (Corning 9753)	1.61 @ 0.5 1.57 @ 2.5		6.0 @ 293–573 K	9.86	0.28	2.798	600 (500 g)	0.935
Calcium alumino-silicate (Schott IRGN6)	1.592 @ 0.55 1.562 @ 2.3 1.521 @ 4.3		6.3 @ 293–573 K	10.8	0.284	3.12	608	0.851

Table B5 - Mechanical properties of selected IR-transmitting glass and other oxides (Page 2 of 3)

Material name and symbol	Refractive index n @ λ in μm	dn/dT @ λ in μm (×10^{-6}/°C)	CTE α (×10^{-6}/°C)	Young's modulus E (×10^{10} N/m^2)	Poisson's ratio υ	Density ρ (g/cm^3)	Knoop hardness (kg/mm^2)	$K_G=(1-\upsilon_G{}^2)/E_G$ ×10^{-11} (Pa^{-1})
Fluoride glass (Ohara HTF1)	1.51 @ 1.0 1.49 @ 3.0	-8.19	16.1	6.42	0.28	3.88	311	1.436
Fluoro-phosphate glass (Schott IRG9)	1.488 @ 0.55 1.469 @ 2.3 1.458 @ 3.3		16.1 @ 293–573 K	7.7	0.288	3.63	346 (200 g)	1.191
Germanate (Corning 9754)	1.67 @ 0.5 1.63 @ 2.5 1.61 @ 4.0		6.2 @ 293–573 K	8.41	0.290	3.581	560 (100 g)	1.089
Germanate (Schott IRG2)	1.899 @ 0.55 1.841 @ 2.3		8.8 @ 293–573 K	9.59	0.282	5.00	481 (200 g)	0.960
Lanthanum dense flint (Schott IRG3)	1.851 @ 0.55 1.796 @ 2.3 1.776 @ 3.3		8.1 @ 293–573 K	9.99	0.287	4.47	541 (200 g)	0.918

Table B5 - Mechanical properties of selected IR-transmitting glass and other oxides (Page 3 of 3)

Material name and symbol	Refractive index n @ λ in μm	dn/dT @ λ in μm ($\times 10^{-6}$/°C)	CTE α ($\times 10^{-6}$/°C)	Young's modulus E ($\times 10^{10}$ N/m²)	Poisson's ratio υ	Density ρ (g/cm³)	Knoop hardness (kg/mm²)	$K_G = (1-\upsilon_G^2)/E_G$ $\times 10^{-11}$ (Pa^{-1})
Lead silicate (Schott IRG7)	1.573 @ 0.55 1.534 @ 2.3		9.6 @ 293–573 K	5.97	0.216	3.06	379	1.597
Sapphire* (Al₂O₃)	1.684 @ 3.8 1.586 @ 5.8	13.7	5.6 (∥) 5.0 (⊥)	40.0	0.27	3.97	1370 (1000 g)	0.232
Fused silica (Corning 7940)	1.561 @ 0.193 1.460 @ 0.55 1.433 @ 2.3 1.412 @ 3.3	10–11.2 @ 0.5–2.5 μm	-0.6 @ 73K 0.58 @ 273–473 K	7.3	0.17	2.202	500 (200 g)	1.333

Notes: * Birefringent material.

Sources: Corning, Inc. data sheets; Schottglaswerke data sheets; P.R. Yoder, Jr., *Opto-Mechanical Systems Design*, 2nd ed., Marcel Dekker, New York, 1993; W.J. Tropf, M.E. Thomas, and T.J. Harris, "Properties of Crystals and Glasses," Chapt. 33 in *OSA Handbook of Optics*, 2nd ed., Vol. II, McGraw-Hill, New York, 1995.

Table B6 - Mechanical properties of diamond and selected IR-transmitting semiconductor materials (Page 1 of 2)

Material name and symbol	Refractive index n @ λ in μm	dn/dT @ λ in μm ($\times 10^{-6}$/°C)	CTE α ($\times 10^{-6}$/°C)	Young's modulus E ($\times 10^{10}$ N/m²)	Poisson's ratio υ	Density ρ (g/cm³)	Knoop hardness (kg/mm²)	$K_G = (1 - \upsilon_G^2)E_G$ $\times 10^{-11}$ (Pa^{-1})
Diamond (C)	2.382 @2.5 2.381 @5.0 2.381 @10.6		-0.1 @ 25 K 0.8 @ 293 K 5.8 @ 1600 K	114.3	0.069 (CVD)	3.51	9000	0.094
Indium antimonide (InSb)	3.99 @8.0	4.7	4.9	4.3		5.78	225	
Gallium arsenide (GaAs)	3.1 @10.6	1.5	5.7	8.29	0.31	5.32	721	1.090
Germanium (Ge)	4.055 @2.7 4.026 @3.8 4.015 @5.3 4.00 @10.6	424 @ 250–350 K	2.3 @100 K 5.0 @200 K 6.0 @300 K	10.37	0.278	5.323	800	0.890

Table B6 - Mechanical properties of diamond and selected IR-transmitting semiconductor materials (Page 2 of 2)

Material name and symbol	Refractive index n @ λ in μm	dn/dT @ λ in μm ($\times 10^{-6}/°C$)	CTE α ($\times 10^{-6}/°C$)	Young's modulus E ($\times 10^{10}$ N/m^2)	Poisson's ratio υ	Density ρ (g/cm^3)	Knoop hardness (kg/mm^2)	$K_G=(1-\upsilon_G^2)E_G$ $\times 10^{-11}$ (Pa^{-1})
Silicon (Si)	3.436 @2.7 3.427 @3.8 3.422 @5.3 3.148 @10.6	1.3	2.7–3.1	13.1	0.279	2.329	1150	0.704

Sources: Various manufacturer's data sheets; P.R. Yoder, Jr., *Opto-Mechanical Systems Design*, 2nd ed., Marcel Dekker, New York, 1993; P.M. Amirtharaj and D.G. Seiler, "Optical Properties of Semiconductors," Chapt. 36 in *OSA Handbook of Optics*, 2nd ed., Vol. II, McGraw-Hill, New York, 1995.

Table B7 - Mechanical properties of selected IR-transmitting chalcogenide materials

Material name and symbol	Refractive index n @ λ in μm	dn/dT @ λ in μm ($\times 10^{-6}$/°C)	CTE α ($\times 10^{-6}$/°C)	Young's modulus E ($\times 10^{10}$ N/m²)	Poisson's ratio υ	Density ρ (g/cm³)	Knoop hardness (kg/mm²)	$K_G = (1-\upsilon_G^2)/E_G$ $\times 10^{-11}$ (Pa^{-1})
Arsenic trisulfide (AsS₃)	2.521 @0.8 2.412 @3.8 2.407 @5.0	85 @0.6 17 @ 1.0	26.1	1.58	0.295	3.43	180	5.778
Ge₃₃As₁₂Se₅₅ (AMTIR-1)	2.605 @1.0 2.503 @8.0	101 @1.0 72 @10.0	12.0	2.2	0.266	4.4	170	4.224
Zinc sulfide (ZnS)	2.36 @0.6 2.257 @ 3.0 2.246 @ 5.0 2.192 @10.6	63.5 @0.63 49.8 @1.15 46.3 @10.6	4.6	7.45	0.29	4.08	230	1.229
Zinc selenide (ZnSe)	2.61 @0.6 2.438 @3.0 2.429 @5.0 2.403 @10.6	91.1 @0.63 59.7 @1.15 52.0 @10.6	5.6 @163 K 7.1 @273 K 8.3 @473 K	7.03	0.28	5.27	105	1.311

Sources: P.R. Yoder, Jr., *Opto-Mechanical Systems Design*, 2nd ed., Marcel Dekker, New York, 1993; W.J Tropf, M.E. Thomas, and T.J. Harris, "Properties of Crystals and Glasses," Chapt. 33 in *OSA Handbook of Optics*, 2nd ed., Vol. II, McGraw-Hill, New York, 1995.

Table B8a - Mechanical properties of selected nonmetallic mirror substrate materials (Page 1 of 2)

Material name and symbol	Source	CTE α $\times 10^{-6}$/°C ($\times 10^{-6}$/°F)	Young's modulus E $\times 10^{10}$ Pa ($\times 10^{6}$ lb/in.^{2})	Poisson's ratio ν	Density ρ g/cm^3 (lb/in.^{3})	Specific heat C_P J/kg-K (Btu/lb-°F)	Thermal conductivity k W/m-K (Btu/hr-ft-°F)	Knoop hardness (kg/mm^2)	Best surface smoothness (Å rms)
Duran 50	Schott	3.2 (1.8)	6.17 (8.9)	0.20	2.23 (0.081)	835 (0.20)	1.02 (0.59)		~5
Pyrex 7740	Corning	3.3 (1.86)	6.30 (9.1)	0.2	2.23 (0.081)	1050 (0.25)	1.13 (0.65)		~5
Borosilicate crown E6	Ohara	2.8 (1.5)	5.86 (8.5)	0.195	2.18 (0.079)				
Fused silica	Corning or Heraeus	0.58 (0.32)	7.3 (10.6)	0.17	2.205 (0.080)	741 (0.177)	1.37 (0.8)	500	~5
ULE 7971	Corning	0.015 (0.008)	6.76 (9.8)	0.17	2.205 (0.080)	766 (0.183)	1.31 (0.76)	460	~5
Zerodur	Schott	0 ± 0.05 (0 ± 0.03)	9.06 (13.6)	0.24	2.53 (0.091)	821 (0.196)	1.64 (0.95)	630	~5

Table B8a - Mechanical properties of selected nonmetallic mirror substrate materials (Page 2 of 2)

Material name and symbol	Source	CTE α ×10⁻⁶/°C (×10⁻⁶/°F)	Young's modulus E ×10¹⁰ Pa (×10⁶ lb/in.²)	Poisson's ratio ν	Density ρ g/cm³ (lb/in.³)	Specific heat C_P J/kg-K (Btu/lb-°F)	Thermal conductivity k W/m-K (Btu/hr-ft-°F)	Knoop hardness (kg/mm²)	Best surface smoothness (Å rms)
Zerodur M	Schott	0 ± 0.05 (0 ± 0.03)	8.9 (12.9)	0.25	2.57 (0.093)	810 (0.194)	1.6 (0.92)	540	~5
Cer-Vit C-101*	Owens-Illinois	0 ± 0.03 (0 ± 0.02)	9.18 (13.3)	0.25	2.50 (0.090)	840 (0.20)	1.70 (1.0)	540	~5

Notes: * Obsolete material.

Sources: Various manufacturer's data sheets; W.P. Barnes, Jr., "Optical Materials - Reflective," Chapt. 4 in *Applied Optics and Optical Engineering*, Vol. VII, Academic Press, New York; R.A. Paquin, Materials and Processes for Dimensionally Stable Mirrors, *Short Course Notes*, SPIE Press, Bellingham, 1991.

Table B8b - Mechanical properties of selected metallic and composite mirror substrate materials (Page 1 of 2)

Material name and symbol	CTE α ×10⁻⁶/°C (×10⁻⁶/°F)	Young's modulus E ×10¹⁰ Pa (×106 lb/in.²)	Poisson's ratio υ	Density ρ g/cm³ (lb/in.³)	Specific heat C_p J/kg–K (Btu/lb–°F)	Thermal conductivity k W/m–K (Btu/hr–ft–°F)	Hardness	Best surface smoothness Å rms
Beryllium I-70A	11.3 (6.3)	28.9 (42)	0.08	0.08 (0.067)	1820 (0.436)	194 (112)		60–80*
Aluminum 6061-T6	23.6 (13.1)	6.82 (9.9)	0.332	2.68 (0.100)	960 (0.23)	167 (96)	30–95 Brinell	~200
Copper OFHC**	16.7 (9.3)	11.7 (17)	0.35	8.94 (0.323)	385 (0.092)	392 (226)	40 Rockwell F	40
Molybdenum TZM	5.0 (2.8)	31.8 (46)	0.32	10.2 (0.368)	272 (0.065)	146 (84.5)	200 Vickers	10
Silicon carbide RB-30% Si	2.64 (1.47)	31.0 (45)		2.92 (0.106)	660 (0.16)	158 (91)		
Silicon carbide RB-12% Si	2.68 (1.49)	37.3 (54.1)		3.11 (0.112)	680 (0.16)	147 (85)		

Table B8b - Mechanical properties of selected metallic mirror substrate materials (Page 2 of 2)

Material name and symbol	CTE α $\times 10^{-6}$/°C ($\times 10^{-6}$/°F)	Young's modulus E $\times 10^{10}$ Pa ($\times 10^6$ lb/in.^{2})	Poisson's ratio υ	Density ρ g/cm^3 (lb/in.^{3})	Specific heat C_P J/kg–K (Btu/lb–°F)	Thermal conductivity k W/m–K (Btu/hr–ft–°F)	Hardness	Best surface smoothness Å rms
Silicon carbide CVD	2.4 (1.3)	46.6 (67.6)	0.21	3.21 (0.116)	700 (0.17)	146 (84)	2540 Knoop (500 g)	
SXA metal matrix of 30% SiC$_P$ in 2124 Al***	12.4 (6.9)	11.7 (17)		2.90 (0.105)	770 (0.18)	130 (75)		
Graphite epoxy GY-70/x30	0.02 (0.01)	9.3 (13.5)		1.78 (0.064)		35 (20)		

Notes; * Sputtered; ** Oxygen free, high conductivity; *** With SiC particles of mean size 3.5 µm (0.0014 in.) per Advanced Composite Materials Corp., San Diego.

Sources: Various manufacturer's data sheets; W.P. Barnes, Jr., "Optical materials - Reflective," Chapt. 4 in *Applied Optics and Optical Engineering*, Vol.VII, Academic Press, New York; R.A. Paquin, "Materials and Processes for Dimensionally Stable Mirrors", *Short Course Notes*, SPIE Press, Bellingham, 1991.

547

Table B9 - Comparison of material figures of merit especially pertinent to mirror design (Page 1 of 2)

	Weight and self-weight deflection proportionality factors				Thermal distortion coefficients	
	$(E/\rho)^{1/2}$ Resonant frequency for same geometry	ρ/E Mass or deflection for same geometry*	ρ^3/E Deflection for same mass	$(\rho^3/E)^{1/2}$ Mass for same deflection	α/k Steady state	α/D Transient
Preferred value	large	small	small	small	small	small
Pyrex	5.3	3.53	1.76	0.420	2.92	5.08
Fused silica	5.7	3.04	1.46	0.382	0.36	0.59
ULE	5.5	3.30	1.61	0.401	0.02	0.04
Zerodur	6.0	2.78	1.78	0.422	0.03	0.07
Al 6061	5.0	3.97	2.90	0.538	0.13	0.33
Metal matrix 30% SiC–Al	6.3	2.49	2.11	0.459	0.10	0.22
Be I-70H or I-220H	12.5	0.64	0.22	0.149	0.05	0.20
Cu, OFHC	3.6	7.64	61.1	2.471	0.53	0.14
Invar 36	4.2	5.71	37.0	1.924	0.10	0.38
Super Invar	4.3	5.49	36.3	1.906	0.03	0.12

Table B9 - Comparison of material figures of merit especially pertinent to mirror design (Page 2 of 2)

Preferred value	Weight and self-weight deflection proportionality factors				Thermal distortion coefficients	
	$(E/\rho)^{1/2}$ Resonant frequency for same geometry	ρ/E Mass or deflection for same geometry*	ρ^3/E Deflection for same mass	$(\rho^3/E)^{1/2}$ Mass for same deflection	α/k Steady state	α/D Transient
	large	small	small	small	small	small
Molybdenum	5.6	3.15	32.8	1.812	0.04	0.09
Silicon	7.5	1.78	0.97	0.311	0.02	0.03
SiC: HP alpha	11.9	0.70	0.72	0.268	0.02	0.03
SiC: CVD	12.0	0.69	0.71	0.267	0.02	0.03
SiC: RB–30% Si	10.7	0.88	0.73	0.270	0.01	0.03
CRES: 304	4.9	4.15	26.5	1.629	0.91	3.68
CRES:416	5.2	3.63	22.1	1.486	0.34	1.23
Ti 6Al4V	5.1	3.89	7.63	0.873	1.21	3.03

Note: This parameter is the reciprocal of "specific stiffness" defined on Pg. 14.

Source: R.A. Paquin, "Materials for Optical Systems," Chapt. 3 in *Handbook of Optomechanical Engineering*, CRC Press, Boca Raton, 1997.

Table B10a - Characteristics of aluminum alloys used in mirrors

Alloy Type	Form	Hardenable?	Remarks
1100	Wrought	No	Relatively pure, low strength, can be diamond turned
2014/2024	Wrought	Yes	High strength and ductility, multiphase, must be plated
5086/5486	Wrought	No	Moderate strength when annealed, weldable, available in large plates
6061	Wrought	Yes	Low alloy, all-purpose, reasonably high strength, weldable, can be diamond turned and/or plated, all forms readily available
7075	Wrought	Yes	Highest strength, usually plated, strength more temperature sensitive than other alloys
B201	Cast	Yes	Sand or permanent mold cast, high strength, cqan be diamond turned
A356/357	Cast	Yes	Sand or permanent mold cast, moderate strength, most common, extensive processing for dimensional stability
713/Tenzalloy	Cast	Yes	Sand or permanent mold cast, moderate strength
771/Precedent 71A	Cast	Yes	Sand cast, moderate strength, very stable, expensive casting procedures required, easiest to machine

Source: R.A. Paquin, "Metal Mirrors," Chapt. 4 in *Handbook of Optomechanical Engineering*, CRC Press, Boca Raton, 1997.

Table B10b - Characteristics of aluminum matrix composites

Property	Instrument grade	Optical grade	Structural grade
Matrix alloy	6061-T6	2124-T6	2021-T6
Volume % SiC	40	30	20
SiC form	Particulate	Particulate	Whisker
CTE ($\times 10^{-6}$/K)	10.7	12.4	14.8
Thermal conductivity (W/m–K)	127	123	not available
Young's modulus (MPa)	145	117	127
Density (g/cm^3)	2.91	2.91	2.86

Source: W.R. Mohn, and D. Vukobratovich, "Recent applications of metal matrix composites in precision instruments and optical systems," *Opt. Eng.* Vol. *27*, 90, 1988.

551

Table B10c – Beryllium grades and some of their properties

Property	O-50	I-70-H	I-220-H	I-250	S-200-FH
Maximum beryllium oxide content (%)	0.5	0.7	2.2	2.5	1.5
Grain size (μm)	15	10	8	2.5	1.5
2% offset yield strength (MPa)	172	207	345	544	296
Microyield strength (MPa)	10	21	41	97	34
Elongation (%)	3.0	3.0	2.0	3.0	3.0

Sources: R.A. Paquin, "Metal Mirrors", Chapt. 4 in *Handbook of Optomechanical Engineering*, CRC Press, Boca Raton, 1997; Brush Wellman, Inc., Elmore, OH.

Table B10d - Characteristics of major silicon carbide types

SiC type	Structure/ Composition	Density	Fabrication Process	Properties*	Remarks
Hot pressed	>98% alpha plus others	>98%	Powder pressed in heated dies	High E, ρ, K_{lc}, MOR; lower k	Simple shapes only; size limited
Hot isostatic pressed	>98% alpha/beta plus others	>99%	Hot gas pressure on encapsulated preform	High E, ρ, K_{lc}, MOR; lower k	Complex shapes possible; size limited
Chemically vapor deposited	100% beta	100%	Deposition of hot mandrel	High E, ρ, k; lower K_{lc}, MOR	Thin shell or plate forms; built-up shapes
Reaction bonded	50–92% alpha plus silicon	100%	Cast, prefired, porous preform fired with silicon infiltration	Lower E, ρ, MOR, k; lowest K_{lc}	Complex shapes readily formed; large sizes; properties are silicon content dependent

Notes: * MOR = modulus of rupture, K_{lc} = plane strain fracture toughness.
Source: R.A. Paquin, "Metal Mirrors", Chapt. 4 in *Handbook of Optomechanical Engineering*, CRC Press, Boca Raton, 1997.

Table B11 - Techniques for machining, finishing, and coating materials for optical applications (Page 1 of 3)

Material	Figure Control Method	Surface Finish Control Method	Coatings
Al alloys 6061, 2024 (most common)	SPDT, SPT, CS, CM, EDM, ECM, IM	EN + SPDT + PL Polish with oil distillates + diamond	MgF_2, SiO, SiO_2, AN, AN + Au, ELNiP and most others
Al matrix Al or Al + SiC	HIP, CS, EDM, ECM, GR, PL, IM, (CM, SPT - Diff)	EN + SPDT + PL	MgF_2, SiO, SiO_2, AN, EN + Au
Low silicon Al castings A-201, 520	SPDT, SPT, CS, CM, EDM, ECM, IM	EN + SPDT + PL Polish with oil + diamond	MgF_2, SiO, SiO_2, AN, EN + Au and most others
Al silicon hypereutectic 393.2 Vanasil + lower silicon A-356.0	CS, EDM, CE, IM, SPDT, SPT, GR, CM, CM - easier than composite Al-SiC	EN + SPDT + PL	EN or ELNiP followed by most others
Beryllium alloys	CM, EDM, ECM, EM, GR, HIP not SPDT	EN + SPDT + PL Polish with oil + diamond	None or coat EN

Table B11 - Techniques for machining, finishing, and coating materials for optical applications (Page 2 of 3)

Material	Figure Control Method	Surface Finish Control Method	Coatings
Magnesium alloys	SPDT, SPT, CS, CM, EDM, ECM, IM	GR, PL with oil + diamond	Similar to Al, EN
SiC Sintered, CVD, RB, carbon + Si *	HIP/mandrel + GR, CVD/mandrel + GR molded carbon + reaction with Silane to SiC	GR + PL	Vacuum processes
Silicon	HIP/mandrel, GR, CVD/mandrel	GR + PL	Vacuum processes
Steels Austenitic PH - 17-5, 17-7 Ferritic 416	CM, EDM, ECM, Gr, not SPDT CM, EDM, ECM, GR not SPDT	EN or ELNiP + SPDT + PL	EN, ELNiP, and most others
Titanium alloys	CM, HIP, ECM, EDM, GR not SPDT	PL, IM	EN + most others Cr/Au

Table B11 - Techniques for machining, finishing, and coating materials for optical applications (Page 3 of 3)

Material	Figure Control Method	Surface Finish Control Method	Coatings
Glass, quartz, Low expansion ULE, Zerodur	CS, GR, IM, PL, CE, SL	PL, IM, CMP, GL (laser or flame)	Vacuum processes Cr/Au, Cr, Ti-W, Ti-W/Au, SiO, SiO_2, MgF_2, Ag/Al_2O_3

Notes: AN = anodize, CE = chemical etch, CM = conventional machine, CMP = chemical mechanical polish, CS = cast, CVD = chemical vapor deposit, ECM = electrochemical machine, EDM = electrode discharge mill, ELNiP = electrolytic nickel phosphorus plate (can replace EN), EN = electroless nickel (usually ~11% by weight), GL = glaze, GR = grind, HIP = hot isostatic press, IM = ion mill, PL = polish, SPDT = single-point diamond turn, SPT = precision turn with tool other than diamond, SL = slump casting over mold.
* An interesting new process by POCO Graphite, Inc., Decatur, TX

Source: D. Englehaupt, Center for Applied Optics, University of Alabama in Huntsville, Huntsville, AL, private communication, 2002 (a revision and expansion of information from Chapt. 10 in *Handbook of Optomechanical Engineering*, CRC Press, Boca Raton, 1997).

Table B12 - Mechanical properties of selected metals used for mechanical parts in optical instruments (Pg. 1 of 4)

Material	CTE (α) $\times 10^{-6}/°C$ ($\times 10^{-6}/°F$)	Young's modulus* (E_M) $\times 10^{10}$ Pa ($\times 10^6$ lb/in.^{2})	Yield strength* (S_Y) $\times 10^7$ Pa (10^3 lb/in.^{2})	Poisson's ratio (ν_M)	Density (ρ) g/cm^3 (lb/in.^{3})	Thermal Conductivity* (k) W/m-K (Btu/hr-ft-°F)	Hardness*	$K_M = (1 - \nu_M^2)/E_M$ $\times 10^{-11}$ m^2/N ($\times 10^{-8}$ in.^{2}/lb)
Aluminum 1100	23.6 (13.1)	6.89 (10.0)	3.4–15.2 (5–22)		2.71 (0.098)	218–221 (126–128)	23–44 Brinell	
Aluminum 2024	22.9 (12.7)	7.31 (10.6)	7.6–39.3 (11–57)	0.33	2.77 (0.100)	119–190 (69–110)	47–130 Brinell	1.22 (8.41)
Aluminum 6061	23.6 (13.1)	6.82 (9.9)	5.5–27.6 (8–40)	0.332	2.68 (0.097)	167 (96.5)	30–95 Brinell	1.30 (8.99)
Aluminum 7075	23.4 (13.0)	7.17 (10.4)	10.3–50.3 (15–73)		2.79 (0.101)	142–176 (82–102)	60–150 Brinell	
Aluminum 356	21.4 (11.9)	7.17 (10.4)	17.2–20.7 (25–30)		2.68 (0.097)	150–168 (87–97)	60–70 Brinell	
Beryllium S-200	11.5 (6.4)	27.6–30.3 (40–44)	20.7 (30)		1.85 (0.067)	220 (127)	80–90 Rockwell-B	

Table B12 – Mechanical properties of selected metals used for mechanical parts in optical instruments (Pg. 2 of 4)

Material	CTE (α) $\times 10^{-6}$ /°C ($\times 10^{-6}$ /°F)	Young's modulus* (E_M) $\times 10^{10}$ Pa ($\times 10^6$ lb/in.^{2})	Yield strength* (S_Y) $\times 10^7$ Pa (10^3 lb/in.^{2})	Poisson's ratio (υ_M)	Density (ρ) g/cm^3 (lb/in.^{3})	Thermal Conductivity* (k) W/m-K (Btu/hr-ft-°F)	Hardness*	$K_M = (1 - \upsilon_M{}^2)/E_M$ $\times 10^{-11}$ m^2/N ($\times 10^{-8}$ in.^{2} /lb)
Beryllium I-400	11.5 (6.4)	27.6–30.3 (40–44)	34.5 (50)	0.08	1.85 (0.067)	220 (127)	100 Rockwell-B	1.63 (2.37)
Beryllium I-70A	11.3 (6.3)	28.9 (42)		0.08	1.85 0.067)	194 (112)		1.63 (2.37)
Copper C10100 (OFHC)	16.9 (9.4)	11.7 (17)	6.9–36.5 (10–53)	0.343	8.94 (0.323)	391 (226)	10–60 Rockwell-B	3.56 (5.16)
Copper C17200 (BeCu)	17.8 (9.9)	12.7 (18.5)	107–134 (155–195)	~0.35	8.25 (0.298)	107–130 (62–75)	27–42 Rockwell-C	3.27 (4.74)
Copper 360 (brass)	20.5 (11.4)	9.65 (14.0)	12.4–35.9 (18–52)		8.50 (0.307)	116 (67)	62–80 Rockwell-B	

Table B12 - Mechanical properties of selected metals used for mechanical parts in optical instruments (Pg. 3 of 4)

Material	CTE (α) $\times 10^{-6}$/°C ($\times 10^{-6}$/°F)	Young's modulus* (E_M) $\times 10^{10}$ Pa ($\times 10^6$ lb/in.²)	Yield strength* (S_Y) $\times 10^7$ Pa ($\times 10^3$ lb/in.²)	Poisson's ratio (υ_M)	Density (ρ) g/cm³ (lb/in.³)	Thermal Conductivity* (k) W/m-K (Btu/hr-ft-°F)	Hardness*	$K_M = (1 - \upsilon_M{}^2)/E_M$ $\times 10^{-11}$ m²/N ($\times 10^{-8}$ in.²/lb)
Copper C260	20.0 (11.1)	11.0 (16)	7.6–44.8 (11–65)		8.52 (0.308)	121 (70)	55–93 Rockwell-B	
Invar 36	1.26 (0.7)	14.1 (21.4)	27.6–41.4 (40–60)	0.259	8.05 (0.291)	10.4 (6.0)	160 Brinell	0.663 (4.57)
Super Invar	0.31 (0.17)	14.8 (21.5)	30.3 (44)	0.29	8.13 (0.294)	10.5 (6.1)	160 Brinell	0.629 (4.34)
Magnesium AZ-31B-H24	25.2 (14)	4.48 (6.5)	14.5–25.5 (21–37)	0.35	1.77 (0.064)	97 (56)	73 Brinell	1.95 (13.5)
Magnesium M1A	25.2 (14)	4.48 (6.5)	12.4–17.9 (18–26)		1.77 (0.064)	138 (79.8)	42–54 Brinell	
Steel 1015 (low carbon)	11.9 (6.6)	20.7 (30)	28.3–31.0 (41–45)	0.287	7.75 (0.28)		111–126 Brinell	0.44 (3.05)

Table B12 - Mechanical properties of selected metals used for mechanical parts in optical instruments (Pg. 4 of 4)

Material	CTE (α) $\times10^{-6}$/°C ($\times10^{-6}$/°F)	Young's modulus* (E_M) $\times10^{10}$ Pa ($\times10^{6}$ lb/in.²)	Yield strength* (S_Y) $\times10^{7}$ Pa (10^{3} lb/in.²)	Poisson's ratio (ν_M)	Density (ρ) g/cm³ (lb/in.³)	Thermal Conductivity* (k) W/m-K (Btu/hr-ft-°F)	Hardness*	$K_M = (1 - \nu_M^2)/E_M$ $\times10^{-11}$ m²/N ($\times10^{-8}$ in.²/lb)
Steel 304 (CRES)	14.7 (8.2)	19.3 (28)	51.7–103 (75–150)	0.27	8.0 (0.29)	16.2 (9.4)	83 Rockwell-B 42 Rockwell-C	0.48 (3.31)
Steel 416 (CRES)	9.9 (5.5)	20.0 (29)	27.6–103 (40–150)	0.283	7.8 (0.28)	24.9 (14.4)	82 Rockwell-B 42 Rockwell-C	0.46 (3.17)
Titanium 6Al4V	8.8 (4.9)	11.4 (16.5)	82.7–106 (120–154)	0.34	4.43 (0.16)	7.3 (4.2)	36-39 Rockwell-C	0.79 (5.47)
SXA Metal Matrix (SiC & 2124 Al)	12.4 (6.9)	11.7 (17)			1.78 (0.064)	35 (20)	Variable within sample	

* Range of values pertains to various tempers.

Sources: Adapted from P.R. Yoder, Jr., *Opto-Mechanical Systems Design*, 2nd ed., Marcel Dekker, New York, 1993; R.A. Paquin, "Materials Properties and Fabrication for Stable Optical Systems," *SPIE Short Course Notes* SC219, SPIE Press, Bellingham, 2001.

Table B13 - Typical physical characteristics of optical cements

Refractive index (n) after curing: 1.55 @ 25 °C

Thermal expansion coefficient (α):
  @ 27°C to 100°C $63\times10^{-6}/°C$ ($35\times10^{-6}/°F$)
  @ 100°C to 200°C $56\times10^{-6}/°C$ ($31\times10^{-6}/°F$)

Shear strength: 36 MPa (5200 lb/in.^{2})

Young's modulus   4275 MPa (6.2×10^5 lb/in.^{2})

Water absorption (bulk material)   0.3% after 24 hr @ 25 °C

Shrinkage during curing: Approximately 4%

Viscosity: 275 to 320 cP

Density: 1.22 g/cm^3 (0.044 lb/in.^{3})

Hardness (Shore D):   Approximately 90

Total mass loss in vacuum: 3%

Source: Adapted from P.R. Yoder, Jr., *Opto-Mechanical Systems Design,* 2nd ed., Marcel Dekker, New York, 1993.

Table B14 - Typical characteristics of representative structural adhesives (Page 1 of 4)

Material (Mfr. code)*	Recommended curing time @ °C	Uncured viscosity (cP)	Shear strength MPa (lb/in.^{2}) @ °C	Temperature range of use °C (°F)	CTE (α) $\times 10^{-6}$/°C ($\times 10^{-6}$/°F)	Joint thickness mm (in.)	Young's modulus MPa (lb/in.^{2})	Poisson's ratio
one-part epoxies								
2214 Regular Gray (3M)	60 min @121	thixotropic paste (aluminum filled)	20.7 (3000) @ -55 31.0 (4500) @ 24 31.0 (4500) @ 82 10.3 (1500) @ 121 2.7 (400) @ 177	-53–121 (-67–250)	49 (27) @ 0–80° C		~5170 (~7.5×10^5)	
two-part epoxies								
Milbond 1:1 weight mix ratio (SO)	3 hr @ 71 7 day @ 25		17.7 (2561) @ -50 14.5 (2099) @ 25 6.8 (992) @ 70	-54–70 (-65–158)	62 @ -54–20 72 @ 20–70	0.381+0.025 (0.015+0.001)	592 (85,900) @ -50 °C 158 (23,000) @ 20 °C	
2216 B/A Gray 2:3 volume mix ratio (3M)	30 min @ 93 2 hr @ 66 7 day @ 24	~80,000	13.8 (2000) @ -55 17.2 (2500) @ 24 2.7 (400) @ 82 1.3 (200) @ 121	-55–150 (-67–302)	102 (57) @ 0-40 °C 134 (74) @40–80 °C	0.102+0.025 (0.004+0.001)	~689.5 (~1.0×10^5)	~0.43

Table B14 - Typical characteristics of representative structural adhesives (Page 2 of 4)

Material (Mfr. code)*	Recommended curing time @ °C	Uncured viscosity (cP)	Shear strength MPa (lb/in.²) @ °C	Temperature range of use °C (°F)	CTE (α) $\times10^{-6}$/°C ($\times10^{-6}$/°F)	Joint thickness mm (in.)	Young's modulus MPa (lb/in.²)	Poisson's ratio
2216 B/A Translucent 1:1 volume mix ratio (3M)	60 min @ 93 4 hr @ 66 30 day @ 24	~10,000	20.7 (3000) @ -55 13.8 (2000) @ 24 1.4 (200) @ 82 0.7 (100) @ 121	-55–150 (-67–302)	81 (45) @ -50–0 °C 207 (115) @60–150 °C	0.102±0.025 (0.004±0.001)	~6.9×10⁴ (~10×10⁵)	~0.43
Urethanes								
3532 B/A Brown 1:1 volume mix ratio (3M)	24 hr @ 24	30,000	13.8 (2000) @ -40 13.8 (2000) @ 24 2.1 (300) @ 82			~0.127 (~0.005)		
U-05FL off-white 2:1 volume mix ratio (L)	24 hr @ 25 & 50% RH		5.2 (750) @ 25			0.076–0.229 (0.003–0.009)		

Table B14 - Typical characteristics of representative structural adhesives (Page 3 of 4)

Material (Mfr. code)*	Recommended curing time @ °C	Uncured viscosity (cP)	Shear strength MPa (lb/in.^{2}) @ °C	Temperature range of use °C (°F)	CTE (α) $\times 10^{-6}$/°C ($\times 10^{-6}$/°F)	Joint thickness mm (in.)	Young's modulus MPa (lb/in.^{2})	Poisson's ratio
UV Curing								
349 Single component (L)	UV Cure @100 mW/cm^2 Fix: <8 sec @ ~0 gap Full: 36 sec @ 0.25 gap	~9500	11.0 (1600)	-54 to 130 (-65 to 266)	80 (44)	<0.35 (<0.014)		
OP-30 Single component low stress (DY)	UV cure @ 200 mW/cm^2 10–30 sec	400	5.2 (750)	<150 (<302)	111 (200) @ 125 °C		17.2 (2500)	
OP-60-LS Single component <0.1% cure shrinkage (DY)	UV cure @ <300 mW/cm^2 5–30 sec	80,000	31.7 (4600)	-45 to 180 (-50 to 350)	27 (15) @ <50 °C 66 (37) @ > 50 °C		6900 (1×10^6)	

Table B14 - Typical characteristics of representative structural adhesives (Page 4 of 4)

Material (Mfr. code)*	Recommended curing time @ °C	Uncured viscosity (cP)	Shear strength MPa (lb/in.^{2}) @ °C	Temperature range of use °C (°F)	CTE (α) ×10^{-6}/°C (×10^{-6}/°F)	Joint thickness mm (in.)	Young's modulus MPa (lb/in.^{2})	Poisson's ratio
Cyanoacrylates								
460 (L)	Fix: 1 min @22 Full: 24 hr @22 @ 50% RH	45	11.7 (1700)		80 (44)			

Notes: * Mfr. Code/Website: (3M) = 3M/www.3m.com, (SO) = Summers Optical/www.emsdiasum.com, (DY) = Dymax Corp/www.dymax.com, (L) = Loctite/www.loctite.com.

Source: Various manufacturer's data sheets, P.R. Yoder, Jr., *Opto-Mechanical Systems Design*, *2nd* ed., Marcel Dekker, New York, 1993; D. Vukobratovich, "Introduction to Optomechanical Design", *SPIE Short Course Notes*, SC014, SPIE Press, Bellingham, 2001, D. Vukobratovich, private communication, 2001.

Table B15 - Typical physical characteristics of representative elastomeric sealants (Page 1 of 3)

Material (Mfr. code)*	Suggested curing time @ °C	Uncured viscosity**	Cured hardness (Shore A)	Temperature range of use °C (°F)	Shrinkage % after 3 days @ 25°C	Effluent or mass loss % after hrs @ °C	CTE (α) $\times 10^{-6}$/°C ($\times 10^{-6}$/°F)	Tensile strength MPa (lb/in.^{2})
One-part silicone products								
732 (DC)	24 hr @ 25 & 50% RH (0.125 in. bead)	320 g/min 0.125 in. ID orifice @ 90 lb/in.^{2} air pressure	25	-60 to 177 (-76 to 350) continuous < 204 (400) intermittent		acetic acid		2.2 (325)
RTV112 (GE)	24 hr @ 25 for 3 mm thickness.	200 P	25	<204 (400) continuous <260 (500) intermittent	1.0	acetic acid	270 (150)	2.2 (325)
Two-part silicone products								
93-500 10:1 mix by weight (DC)	7 day @ 77 & 50% RH		40	-65 to 200 (-85 to 392)	nil	0.16 @ 24 hr & 125 & <10^{-6} Torr	300 (167)	

Table B15 - Typical physical characteristics of representative elastomeric sealants (Page 2 of 3)

Material (Mfr. code)*	Suggested curing time @ °C	Uncured viscosity**	Cured hardness (Shore A)	Temperature range of use °C (°F)	Shrinkage % after 3 days @ 25°C	Effluent or mass loss % after hrs @ °C	CTE (α) ×10⁻⁶/°C (×10⁻⁶/°F)	Tensile strength MPa (lb/in.²)
RTV88 200:1 mix by weight*** (GE)	24 hr @ 25 & 50% RH	8800 P	58	-54 to 260 (-65 to 500) continuous <316 (600) intermittent	0.6	alcohol	210 (117)	5.7 (830)
RTV560 200:1 mix by weight (GE)	24 hr @ 25 & 50% RH	300 P	55	-115 to 260 (-175 to 500)	1.0		200 (110)	4.8 (690)
RTV8111 ~33/1 mix by weight*** (GE)	<72 hr @ 25 & 50% RH	99 P	45	-54 to 204 (-65 to 400)	1.0	alcohol	250 (140)	2.4 (350)

Table B15 - Typical physical characteristics of representative elastomeric sealants (Page 3 of 3)

Material (Mfr. code)*	Suggested cure time @ °C	Uncured viscosity**	Cured hardness (Shore A)	Temperature range of use °C (°F)	Shrinkage % after 3 days @ 25°C	Effluent or mass loss % after hrs @ °C	CTE (α) $\times 10^{-6}$/°C ($\times 10^{-6}$/°F)	Tensile strength MPa (lb/in.^{2})
Other products:								
EC801B/A polysulfide (3M)	tack free: <72 hr @ 25 full cure: 1 wk @ 25	heavy liquid	>35-60 (40 Rex)	-54 to 82 (-65 to 180)				

Notes: * Mfr. code/website: (DC) = Dow Corning/www.dowcorning.com, (GE) = General Electric Silicones/www.gesilicones.com; ** Units: g/min = grams per minute extrusion rate; P = poise; cP = centipoise; *** Vacuum deaerate before use.
Source: Various manufacturer's data sheets; P.R. Yoder, P.R., *Opto-Mechanical Systems Design*, 2nd ed., Marcel Dekker, New York, 1993

Table B16 - Typical minimum values for fracture strength f_S of infrared window materials*

Material	f_S (MPa)	f_S (lb/in.^{2})
MgF$_2$ (single crystal)	142	2.05×10^4
MgF$_2$ (polycrystalline)	67	9.71×10^3
Sapphire (single crystal)	300	4.35×10^4
ZnS	100	1.45×10^4
Diamond (CVD)**	100	1.45×10^4
ALON	300	4.35×10^4
Silicon	120	1.74×10^4
CaF$_2$	100	1.45×10^4
Germanium	90	1.30×10^4
Fused silica	60	8.70×10^3
ZnSe	50	7.25×10^3

* Note that these values are approximate. They depend upon the quality of the surface finish, fabrication method, material purity, type of test, and size of the sample.
** Chemical vapor deposited
Source: D.C. Harris, *Materials for Infrared Windows and Domes, Properties and Performance*, SPIE Press, Bellingham, 1999.

Table B17 - Coefficient of thermal defocus and thermo-optical coefficient for 185 Schott glasses, 14 crystals, 4 plastics, and 4 index-matching liquids (Page 1 of 5)

Material	Coeff. of thermal defocus (δ_G) ($\times 10^{-6}$/°C)	Thermo-optical coeff. (γ_G) ($\times 10^{-6}$/°C)	Material	Coeff. of thermal defocus (δ_G) ($\times 10^{-6}$/°C)	Thermo-optical coeff. (γ_G) ($\times 10^{-6}$/°C)	Material	Coeff. of thermal defocus (δ_G) ($\times 10^{-6}$/°C)	Thermo-optical coeff. (γ_G) ($\times 10^{-6}$/°C)
Optical Glasses								
FK3	-11.66	4.74	SK15	-5.89	7.91	F2	-3.82	12.58
FK52	-30.68	-1.88	SK19	-4.14	8.66	F5	-2.48	13.52
PK3	-4.58	9.62	SK52	0.34	12.34	FN11	-3.93	11.07
PK51A	-28.12	-2.72	KF9	-1.42	12.18	BASF1	-5.11	11.89
PSK50	-11.64	5.56	BALF5	-7.27	8.93	BASF10	-5.38	11.82
BK1	-6.54	8.86	BALF50	-8.19	8.41	BASF52	4.51	14.91
BK7	-4.33	9.87	SSK2	-1.51	10.89	BASF56	-2.36	13.84
BALKN3	-5.82	9.98	SSKN8	-4.94	9.26	LAF2	-9.02	7.18
K5	-7.76	8.64	LAKN7	-7.86	6.34	LAF9	3.11	17.51
K11	-2.31	10.49	LAK10	-1.15	10.25	LAF22	-4.24	9.76
ZK5	-6.80	10.60	LAKN13	-11.03	5.77	FK5	-14.89	3.51
BAK2	-6.96	9.04	LAK21	-7.63	5.97	FK54	-30.66	-1.46
BAK6	-4.91	9.69	LAK28	-0.73	10.67	PK50	-11.42	6.18
SK2	-0.67	11.33	LLF6	-3.53	11.47	PSK2	-3.97	8.83
SK6	-0.94	11.46	BAF5	-2.74	11.26	PSK52	-11.55	5.45
SK11	-3.51	9.49	BAF50	-7.17	9.43	BK3	1.81	12.41
			BAF54	-1.96	10.44	BK10	-1.49	10.11
			LF5	-6.75	11.45	K3	-7.08	9.52

Table B17 - Coefficient of thermal defocus and thermo-optical coefficient for 185 Schott glasses, 14 crystals, 4 plastics, and 4 index-matching liquids (Page 2 of 5)

Material	Coeff. of thermal defocus (δ_G) ($\times 10^{-6}$ /°C)	Thermo-optical coeff. (γ_G) ($\times 10^{-6}$/°C)	Material	Coeff. of thermal defocus (δ_G) ($\times 10^{-6}$ /°C)	Thermo-optical coeff. (γ_G) ($\times 10^{-6}$/°C)	Material	Coeff. of thermal defocus (δ_G) ($\times 10^{-6}$ /°C)	Thermo-optical coeff. (γ_G) ($\times 10^{-6}$/°C)
K7	-8.03	9.52	LAKN14	-2.27	8.73	FK51	-29.35	-2.15
K50	-2.18	11.82	LAKL21	-3.28	8.92	PK2	-3.95	9.85
ZKN7	6.07	15.07	LLF1	-5.01	11.19	PK51	-31.82	-5.62
BAK4	-3.00	11.00	BAF3	-4.09	11.51	PSK3	-3.58	8.82
BAK50	8.99	16.39	BAF8	-1.69	12.31	PSK53	-15.37	3.43
SK4	-4.22	8.58	BAF52	-8.00	8.80	BK6	-5.88	9.72
SK9	-0.26	11.74	LF1	-6.45	10.55	BALK1	-10.94	7.26
SK12	-3.54	9.26	LF8	-6.76	10.24	K4	-3.01	11.59
SK16	-5.68	6.92	F3	-2.58	13.42	K10	-1.04	11.96
SK20	-3.38	9.42	F6	-3.79	13.21	K51	5.75	14.35
SK55	-3.05	8.95	F14	-2.36	13.44	BAK1	-5.72	9.48
KF50	-1.63	12.97	BASF5	6.36	22.16	BAK5	-6.73	8.87
BALF6	-2.03	11.37	BASF13	-2.17	12.03	SK1	-1.62	10.58
BALF51	-6.75	9.45	BASF54	-0.06	14.54	SK5	-1.67	9.33
K3	-1.84	11.36	BASF57	-2.21	11.99	SK10	-5.03	8.97
SSK51	-6.86	8.34	LAF3	-7.33	7.87	SK14	-3.60	8.40
LAK8	-1.07	10.13	LAFN10	-0.15	11.25	SKN18	0.18	12.98
LAK11	-7.96	6.44	LAFN23	-9.08	7.12	SK51	-12.69	5.11

Table B17 - Coefficient of thermal defocus and thermo-optical coefficient for 185 Schott glasses, 14 crystals, 4 plastics, and 4 index-matching liquids (Page 3 of 5)

Material	Coeff. of thermal defocus (δ_G) ($\times 10^{-6}$ /°C)	Thermo-optical coeff. (γ_G) ($\times 10^{-6}$ /°C)	Material	Coeff. of thermal defocus (δ_G) ($\times 10^{-6}$ /°C)	Thermo-optical coeff. (γ_G) ($\times 10^{-6}$ /°C)	Material	Coeff. of thermal defocus (δ_G) ($\times 10^{-6}$ /°C)	Thermo-optical coeff. (γ_G) ($\times 10^{-6}$ /°C)
KF3	-3.96	12.24	F15	-3.26	12.94	SF53	0.42	16.82
BALF4	0.26	13.06	BASF6	-3.69	11.11	SF56	-0.10	15.70
BALF8	-6.50	10.10	BASF51	6.32	17.12	SF58	4.09	22.09
SSK1	-1.40	11.20	BASF55	5.63	15.83	SF63	0.82	17.22
SSK4	-3.46	8.74	BASF64	-3.68	10.92	TIF2	-9.87	7.33
SSK52	-3.53	9.87	LAFN7	3.46	14.06	KZFS1	-2.01	7.99
LAK9	-2.89	9.71	LAF21	-1.90	9.90	KZFSN5	2.04	11.04
LAKN12	-9.69	5.51	LAFN24	0.85	11.65	KZFS8	3.30	13.90
LAKN16	1.25	11.85	LAF25	2.79	14.39	LAF26	3.35	14.55
LAK23	-11.19	4.61	LASF3	0.66	11.66	LASFN9	-3.18	11.62
LLF4	-5.73	10.67	LASF13	3.10	15.50	LASFN15	-2.33	10.67
BAF4	-4.04	11.76	LASFN31	-2.64	10.96	LASF32	-4.37	11.43
BAF9	-0.60	12.40	SF2	-3.33	13.47	SF3	0.33	17.13
BAF53	-1.92	11.08	SF5	-2.18	14.22	SF6	3.72	19.92
LF3	-5.07	11.13	SF7	-1.82	13.98	SF9	0.97	17.32
F1	-5.32	12.08	SF11	8.01	20.21	SF12	-1.89	13.71
F4	-4.37	12.23	SF14	5.75	18.95	SF15	-1.15	14.65
F9	-2.20	13.20	SF18	1.02	17.22	SF19	-0.27	15.13

Table B17 - Coefficient of thermal defocus and thermo-optical coefficient for 185 Schott glasses, 14 crystals, 4 plastics, and 4 index-matching liquids (Page 4 of 5)

Material	Coeff. of thermal defocus (δ_G) ($\times 10^{-6}$/°C)	Thermo-optical coeff. (γ_G) ($\times 10^{-6}$/°C)	Material	Coeff. of thermal defocus (δ_G) ($\times 10^{-6}$/°C)	Thermo-optical coeff. (γ_G) ($\times 10^{-6}$/°C)	Material	Coeff. of thermal defocus (δ_G) ($\times 10^{-6}$/°C)	Thermo-optical coeff. (γ_G) ($\times 10^{-6}$/°C)
SF54	1.69	17.09	SF55	0.64	17.04	Infrared Crystals		
SFL56	-8.36	9.04	SF57	4.81	21.41			
SF61	1.62	17.42	SF62	-1.17	15.23	germanium	124.87	136.27
SFN64	-7.30	9.70	TIK1	-17.85	2.75	silicon	61.93	66.93
KZFN1	-3.39	10.81	KZFSN2	-1.54	10.66	ZnSe	34.12	49.32
KZFSN2	1.82	10.82	KZFSN4	1.89	10.89	ZnS	26.17	41.97
KZFS6	-0.96	9.24	KZFSN7	2.61	12.21	CdTe	52.46	61.46
LGSK2	-20.31	3.89				AMTIR1	33.47	59.47
LAFN28	-1.18	10.42				GaAs	58.56	70.36
LASFN30	-2.04	10.36				KRS5	-233.22	-111.22
SF1	0.11	16.31				KCl	-99.25	-27.25
SF4	2.51	18.51				KBr	-106.44	-51.24
SFL6	-9.61	8.39				NaCl	-97.44	-9.44
SF10	1.05	16.05				CsBr	68.84	164.64
SF13	2.96	17.16				CsI	-174.05	-74.05
SF16	-3.01	13.79						
LASF11	-0.14	11.46						
SF50	-8.73	11.47						

Table B17 - Coefficient of thermal defocus and thermo-optical coefficient for 185 Schott glasses, 14 crystals, 4 plastics, and 4 index-matching liquids (Page 5 of 5)

Material	Coeff. of thermal defocus (δ_G) ($\times 10^{-6}$ /°C)	Thermo-optical coeff. (γ_G) ($\times 10^{-6}$ /°C)	Material	Coeff. of thermal defocus (δ_G) ($\times 10^{-6}$ /°C)	Thermo-optical coeff. (γ_G) ($\times 10^{-6}$ /°C)
Plastics			**Liquids**		
Acrylic	-278.4	-154.4	CG305974	-1076.26	1076.26
Polycarbonate	-253.4	-117.4	CG505257	-923.66	-923.66
Polystyrene	-289.7	-189.7	CG710209	-926.27	-926.27
SAN	-246.5	-146.5	CG810184	-1113.27	-1113.27

Source: Adapted from T.H. Jamieson, "Athermalization of optical instruments from the optomechanical standpoint," *SPIE Proceedings* Vol. CR43, 131, 1992.

APPENDIX C
Torque-Preload Relationship for
a Threaded Retaining Ring

The threaded retainer acts as a body moving on an inclined plane. Figure C1 shows the geometry and the forces acting on the body. We follow the general guidelines of Chapter 10 in Boothroyd and Poli [1] to derive the appropriate equations.

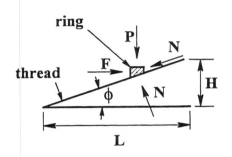

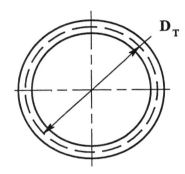

Fig. C1 Side view.   **Fig. C2 End view.**

For horizontal equilibrium, $F - \mu N\cos \phi - N\sin \phi = 0$
Solve for N: $N = F/(\mu\cos \phi + \sin \phi)$

For vertical equilibrium, $P + \mu N\sin \phi - N\cos \phi = 0$
Solve for N: $N = P/(-\mu\sin \phi + \cos \phi)$

Equate equations for N to get: $F = [(P)(\sin \phi + \mu\cos \phi)/(\cos \phi - \mu\sin \phi)]$

Divide by $\cos \phi$ to get: $F = (P)(\tan \phi + \mu)/(1 - \mu\tan \phi)$

Since $\tan \phi = H/L = H/(\pi D_T)$ where H = thread pitch and L = thread circumference, we have: $F = [PH/(\pi D_T)]/[1 - (\mu H/\pi D_T)]$

The torque applied to the retainer is $Q = FD_T/2 = [PD_T/2][(H + \pi\mu D_T)/(\pi D_T - \mu H)]$

We assume that the threads are triangular with a half-angle γ so they wedge together and increase the terms involving friction by $1/\cos \gamma = \sec \gamma$. This factor is 1.155 for a 60° thread.

Hence: $Q = [PD_T /2][(H + (\pi\mu D_T)(1.155))/(\pi D_T - (\mu H)(1.155))]$

Since $H \ll D_T$, we can safely neglect it.

So $Q = [PD_T /2][((\pi\mu D_T)(1.155))/(\pi D_T)] = 1.155\, PD_T\, \mu/2 = 0.577\, PD_T\, \mu.$

But there is another term to consider. This accounts for friction between the end of the retaining ring and the lens and is $Q_L = P\mu_G y_C$. We add this to the first term, approximate y_C as $D_T/2$, and get:

$$Q = 0.577 PD_T\, \mu_M + (P\mu_G D_T /2) = (PD_T)(0.577\mu_M + 0.5\mu_G)$$

Hence: $P = Q/(D_T)(0.577\mu_M + 0.5\mu_G)$ (C1)

Measurements of the angle of inclination for a slowly sliding dry anodized aluminum plate on a dry anodized aluminum inclined plane yield a value for μ_M of about 0.19. Similar measurements for BK7 glass on anodized aluminum yield a μ_G of about 0.15. Substituting these values into Eq. (C1) gives

$$P = 5.42 Q/D_T$$ (C2)

Vukobratovich,[2] Kowalski,[3] and Yoder,[4] state that this equation is usually written as:

$$P = 5 Q/D_T.$$ (C3)

The correlation between Eqs. (C2) and (C2) is within about 8%. It is doubtful if the coefficients of friction are known this accurately in any real situation.

Equations C1 through C3 are applied in Sect. 3.4.1.

References

1. Boothroyd, G., and Poli, C., *Applied Engineering Mechanics*, Marcel Dekker, New York, 1980.
2. Vukobratovich, D., "Optomechanical Design," in *SPIE Short Course Notes*, SPIE Press, Bellingham, 1993.
3. Kowalskie, B.J., "A Users Guide to Designing and Mounting Lenses and Mirrors," *Digest of Papers, OSA Workshop on Optical Fabrication and Testing, North Falmouth, MA*, Optical Society of America, Washington, 98, 1980.
4. Yoder, P.R., Jr., *Opto-Mechanical Systems Design* 2nd ed., Marcel Dekker, New York, 1993.

APPENDIX D
The Lens Temperature Sensitivity Factor K$_3$

D1 Single Lens Element

Consider a simple biconvex lens clamped by a retainer as shown in Fig. D1. It is assumed that the retainer is stiff and firmly attached (by the thread) to the cell. For simplicity, we ignore the slight weakening effect of the undercut and thread in the cell wall. The stressed regions in the metal cell and in the glass lens are modeled as annular rings. Figure D2 shows a section through one side of each ring with dimensions exaggerated. The temperature is T_1 and the coefficients of expansion are as indicated in Fig. D2.

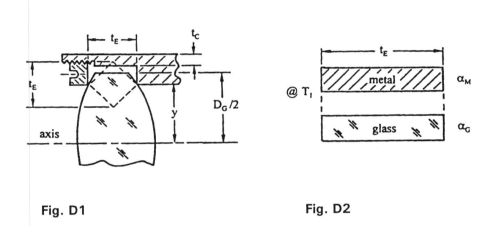

Fig. D1   **Fig. D2**

Assume $\alpha_M > \alpha_G$. At a lower temperature T_2, the metal cell would shrink more than the glass if each were unconstrained (see Fig. D3). Actually, the glass is compressed by the cell and the cell stretches (see Fig. D4). We define the axial strains as ξ_M and ξ_G.

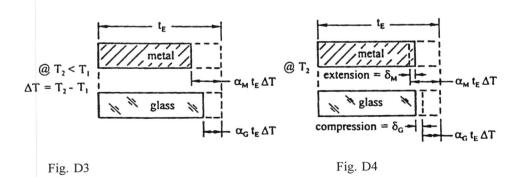

Fig. D3   Fig. D4

577

Then:

New length of the glass $= t_E - \alpha_G t_E \Delta T - \xi_G$

New length of the metal $= t_E - \alpha_M t_E \Delta T + \xi_M$

Equate the new glass length to the new metal length and rearrange:

$$(\alpha_M - \alpha_G) t_E \Delta T = \xi_G + \xi_M \qquad\qquad\qquad\qquad \text{(D1)}$$

The spring constants of the rings are

$$C_G = (E_G A_G)/2t_E \qquad \text{and} \qquad C_M = (E_M A_M)/t_E$$

Note: The factor 2 in the equation for C_G results from a simplifying approximation that the "effective" radial width of the annular stressed region in the lens is the average of zero at the lens surface and t_E at the center of the lens.

The force exerted on both parts is $P = C_G \xi_G = C_M \xi_M$

Then: $\xi_G = P/C_G = 2Pt_E /E_G A_G$ and $\xi_M = P/C_M = Pt_E /E_M A_M$

Substitute these into Eq. (D1):

$$(\alpha_M - \alpha_G) t_E \Delta T = Pt_E [(2/E_G A_G) + (1/E_M A_M)]$$

Cancel the lengths, simplify the fractions and solve for P:

$$P = \frac{E_G A_G E_M A_M (\alpha_M - \alpha_G)\Delta T}{E_G A_G + 2E_M A_M}$$

In Eq. (12.16), this is written as $P = K_3 \Delta T$

so:

$$K_3 = \frac{- E_G A_G E_M A_M (\alpha_M - \alpha_G)}{E_G A_G + 2E_M A_M} \qquad \text{This is Eq. (12.22).}$$

Note: The negative sign was added to the numerator to make P a positive (compressive) force for a negative ΔT.

D2 - Cemented Doublet Lens

Consider a cemented doublet lens clamped as in Sect. D1 by a retainer, (see Fig. D5). Figure D6 is a section through one side of the glass and metal ring elements with the dimensions exaggerated. The temperature is T_1 and the coefficients of expansion are as indicated in Fig. D6.

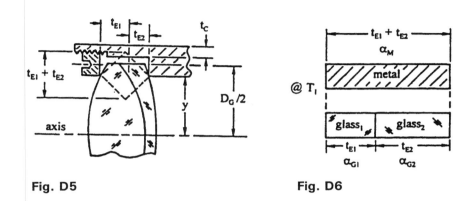

Fig. D5   Fig. D6

We assume α_M > either α_{G1} or α_{G2}. At a lower temperature T_2, the metal cell would shrink more than the glasses if each were unconstrained (see Fig. D7). Actually, the glass is compressed by the cell and the cell stretches (see Fig. D8). We define the axial strains as ξ_M for the cell and ξ_{G1} and ξ_{G2} for the two lens elements.

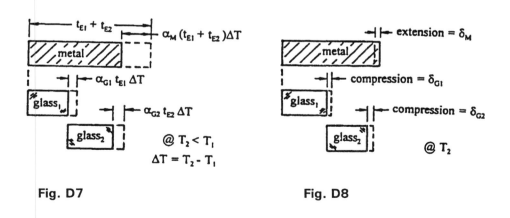

Fig. D7   Fig. D8

Then:

New length of lens 1 $= t_{E1} - \alpha_{G1} t_{E1} \Delta T - \xi_{G1}$

New length of lens 2 $= t_{E2} - \alpha_{G2}\, t_{E2}\, \Delta T - \xi_{G2}$

New length of the cell $= t_{E1} + t_{E2} - \alpha_M\,(t_{E1} + t_{E2})\Delta T + \delta_M$

Equate the total new length of the glass to the new length of the metal and rearrange:

$$(-\alpha_{G1} t_{E1} - \alpha_{G2}\, t_{E2} + \alpha_M\,(t_{E1} + t_{E2}))\,\Delta T = \xi_M + \xi_{G1} + \xi_{G2} \qquad (D2)$$

Define the "spring constants" of the metal and glass rings as:

$$C_{G1} = (E_{G1}\, A_{G1})/2t_{E1}\,, \qquad C_{G2} = (E_{G2}\, A_{G2})/2t_{E2} \quad \text{and} \quad C_M = (E_M\, A_M)/(t_{E1} + t_{E2})$$

Note: The factor of 2 in the equations for C_{G1} and C_{G2} results from a simplifying approximation that the "effective" radial width of the annular stressed region in the lens is the average of zero at the lens surface and t_E at the center of the lens.

The force exerted on all three parts is the same so $P = C_{G1}\, \xi_{G1} = C_{G2}\, \xi_{G2} = C_M\, \xi_M$

Then: $\quad \xi_{G1} = P/C_{G1} = 2Pt_{E1}/E_{G1}\, A_{G1}\,, \qquad \xi_{G2} = P/C_{G2} = 2Pt_{E2}/E_{G2}\, A_{G2}$

and $\quad \xi_M = P/C_M = P(t_{E1} + t_{E2})/E_M\, A_M$

Substitute these into Eq. (D2):

$$[-\alpha_{G1} t_{E1} - \alpha_{G2}\, t_{E2} + \alpha_M\,(t_{E1} + t_{E2})]\,\Delta T$$

$$= (2Pt_{E1}/E_{G1}\, A_{G1}) + (2Pt_{E2}/E_{G2}\, A_{G2}) + [P(t_{E1} + t_{E2})/E_M\, A_M]$$

Solve for P noting that $A_{G1} = A_{G2} = A_G$ from the geometry of the analytical model and express this in the form of Eq. (12.16) as $P = K_3\, \Delta T$.

So:

$$K_3 = \frac{- (\alpha_M - \alpha_{G1})t_{E1} - (\alpha_M - \alpha_{G2})t_{E2}}{\dfrac{2t_{E1}}{E_{G1} A_G} + \dfrac{2t_{E2}}{E_{G2} A_G} + \dfrac{(t_{E1} + t_{E2})}{E_M A_M}}$$

This is Eq. (12.24). Once again the negative sign was added to make P a positive (compressive) force for a negative ΔT.

INDEX

a_G (see acceleration factor)

Abbe erecting system, 169, 171

Abbe version of the Porro prism, 167, 168

Aberration from prisms, 155, 156, 162, 163, 185, 186

Abrasion (see Erosion)

Acceleration factor (a_G), 72, 74, 163, 194, 201, 202, 213, 217, 277, 278, 280, 397, 398, 419, 423, 425, 431, 459, 506, 509

defined, 43

Acrylic (see Polymethylmethacrylate)

Adhesive

properties of, App. B13, B14

optical (see Optical cement)

structural, App. B14

Air bag mirror support, 342, 348-350

Alignment

by lathe assembly, 102-104

of multiple lenses, 104-115

of single lenses, 81-88

Al_2O_3 (see Sapphire)

Allyl diglycol carbonate (CR39)

properties of, App. B3

ALON (see Aluminum oxynitride)

Aluminum (Al)

properties of, App. B9, B10a, B12

Aluminum matrix materials, App. B9, B10b

Aluminum oxynitride (ALON)

properties of, App. B5

American National Standards Institute (ANSI), 42

Amici prism, 165, 166, 206, 207, 212, 398, 495

Amici/penta erecting system, 170, 172

AMTIR ($Ge_{33}AS_{12}Se_{55}$)

properties of, App. B7, B17

ANSI (see American National Standards Institute)

ANSI Publication B1.1-1982, 44, 51, 269

Antireflection (A/R) coating, 141, 142, 144, 230-232

Aperture estimation of, 157-161

Arsenic trisulfide (As_2O_3)

properties of, App. B7

Articulated telescope

prism mounting for, 502-506

As_2O_3 (see Arsenic trisulfide)

Athermalization techniques, 403-414

AXAF (see Chandra telescope)

Axicon, internally reflecting, 179, 180

BaF_2 (see Barium Fluoride)

Barium fluoride (BaF_2)

properties of, App. B4

Bauernfeind 45° prism, 179

Be (see Beryllium)

Beamsplitter prism

design of, 163-165

mounting for, 193-195

Bearing

flexure, 313

spherical, 362

Beryllium (Be)

properties of, App. B10c, B12

Binocular

M17, 446

M19, 447, 491-494

Swarovski, 130, 221, 222

Zeiss, 129

Biocular prism, 181, 182

Birefringence, 29, 30, 372, 418, 427, 466, 502

Bladder (see Air bag mirror support)

Bonding area 163, 213, 214, 217, 277, 398

Brass
    properties of, App. B12
Burnishing lenses into cells, 33, 35, 36, 57, 104, 148, 456

C (see Diamond)
$CaAl_2O_3$ (see Calcium aluminosilicate)
CaF_2 (see Calcium fluoride)
Calcium fluoride (CaF_2)
    properties of, App. B4
Calcium aluminosilicate ($CaAl_2O_3$)
    properties of, App B5
Catadioptric systems, 121-123, 233, 295, 403, 406, 433, 466-477
Cement, optical (see Optical cement)
Centering of lenses (see Decentration)
CeO_2 (see Cerium oxide)
Cerium oxide (CeO_2) (see Radiation-resistant glass)
Chalcogenide materials
    properties of, App. B7
Chandra telescope, 464-466
Coatings
    antireflection, 141, 142, 144, 230-232
    electroless nickel (EN), 260, 262, 263, 519, 553
    reflecting, 14, 83, 175, 177, 179, 209, 227, 230, 275, 469
Coefficient of thermal expansion (CTE, α)
    definition, 10
Coefficient of thermal defocus (δ_G)
    definition, 407
    values for selected optical materials, App. B17
Composites, 11, 14, 15, 259, 329, 404, 409, 432, App. B8d
Conical interface (see Tangential interface)
Contact stress, estimation of
    in lenses, 373-391

in prisms, 392-397, 506-513
in small mirrors, 391, 392
Contamination, 1, 3, 5, 366
Convection heating, 414
Cooled lens assemblies (see Thermal shock)
Copper (Cu)
    properties of, App. B12
Corner-cube prism (see Cube-corner prism)
Corrosion, 1, 3, 5, 15, 16
CR39 (see Allyl diglycol carbonate)
Crash safety, 3
CRES (see Steel, stainless)
Crystals, optical
    properties of, App. B4-7
Cu (see Copper)
Cube-corner prism, 180, 181, 285, 286
Cyanoacrylate adhesive
    properties of, App. B14
Cyclic olefin copolymer, 88

Decentration, 21, 22, 24, 25, 72-74, 76, 94, 104, 126, 277, 291, 403, 446, 456, 458, 466, 486
Delta prism, 177, 178, 210
Density
    definition of, 11
Diamond (C)
    properties of, App. B6
Differential thread, 107, 126-128, 293
Dispersing prism, 2, 183-185, 497-502
Dispersion, 11, 14, 183-186, 484, 497, 499
Dome, optical 3, 29, 30, 135, 151-153, 415
Double-Dove prism, 156, 163, 174-176, 210
Dove prism, 156, 163, 173-175, 210
Drop-in assembly, 93, 101
Duran 50
    properties of, App. B8a

E6 (see Ohara E6 glass)

Echellette spectrograph/imager (ESI), 497-502

Edge-contacted lenses, 99, 100

Elastomer
properties of, App. B15

Environmental testing, 3

Epoxy
properties of, App. B14

Epoxy pinning, 85, 114, 115

Erosion
sand/dust, 7, 141, 151
rain, 7, 141, 142, 151

Expansion, thermal (see Thermal expansion)

Eyepiece,
diopter adjustment, 127, 129
fixed focus, 101
focusing, 30, 106, 127-129
sealing of, 124, 125

Far Ultraviolet Spectroscopic Explorer (FUSE) spectrograph, 515-519

Filter, optical
heated, 147, 150, 415
laminated, 148-150
segmented (mosaic), 149-151

Flexure bearing, 313, 314, 353

Flexure supports
lenses, 76-81, 84, 85
mirrors, 279, 280, 287-294
prisms, 222-224

Fluoride glass (HTF1)
properties of, App. B5

Fluorite (see Calcium fluoride)

Fluorophosphate glass (IRG9)
properties of, App. B5

Flushing (see Purging)

Focus adjustment
eyepiece, 30, 106, 127-129
wedge system, 187-189

Force (see also Preload)

definition of, 10

Fresnel reflection, 110, 192, 229-233

Friction, coefficient of (see Coefficient of friction)

Frit bonding (see Mirror, frit bonded)

Fungus, 1, 3, 7

Fused silica
properties of, App. B5

GaAs (see Gallium arsenide)

Gallium arsenide (GaAs)
properties of, App. B6, B17

$Ge_{33}AS_{12}Se_{55}$ (see AMTIR)

Gemini telescope, 340-343

Geostationary Orbiting Environmental Satellite (GOES) telescope, 404, 405, 514, 515

Germanate (9754)
properties of, App. B5

Germanium (Ge)
properties of, App. B6, B17

Glass,
infrared transmitting, App. B5
lightweight, 14, App. B2
map, 11, 12
optical
properties of, App. B1, B17
radiation resistant, 3, 7, 14

Graphite epoxy
properties of, App. B8b

Gratings, mountings for (see Far Ultraviolet Spectrographic Explorer (FUSE) spectrograph,

Gravitational effects on optics, 6, 43, 72, 73, 121, 194, 199, 216, 217, 237, 246, 248, 283, 296, 300-308, 311, 317-319, 322, 323, 333, 342, 343, 346, 348, 354, 357, 360, 361, 398, 520

Gravity (see Acceleration factor, Self-weight deflection)

Hale telescope, 247, 312, 316-318

Hindle mounting for mirrors, 303-305, 319-322, 324-330

Hoop stress (see Stress, tangential)

Hubble telescope, 311, 350-354, 360-364

Humidity, 5
   typical extremes, 8

Hyperhemisphere (see Dome, optical)

Image displacement
   axial by prism, 155-157
   lateral by tilted plate, 231, 232

Image
   ghost, 166, 227, 229-233, 264
   inverted, 166
   left-handed, 2
   reverted, 2
   right-handed, 2

Indium antimonide (InSb)
   properties of, App. B6

Infrared Astronomical Satellite (IRAS) telescope, 311, 357-360, 403

InSb (see Indium antimonide)

Interface
   cylindrical pad, 203, 205-208, 274, 386, 390, 391, 393-395, 506, 508, 509,
   elastomeric, 29, 33, 66-76, 81, 104, 136, 145, 146, 148, 151-153, 179, 213, 278, 285, 462-464, 466,
   flat bevel, 33, 39-41, 54, 65, 75, 89, 102, 271, 277, 295, 372, 391, 444, 445, 448, 451, 464, 472, 476, 484
   kinematic, 21, 26, 27, 193
   nonkinematic, 29, 193, 208, 277, 278, 343
   rim contact, 22, 433
   semikinematic, 26, 28, 29, 56, 193-198, 200, 275, 300, 343, 506, 507
   sharp-corner, 33, 56-59, 63, 96, 100, 101, 207, 270, 271, 376-381, 383, 384, 393, 430, 446, 467, 484

spherical, 33, 63-65, 76, 380, 381, 383, 444, 472, 475, 484
spherical pad, 208, 277, 386-391, 396
step bevel, 33, 65, 66, 102, 390
surface contact, 23
tangential, 33, 59, 60, 61, 75, 76, 102, 270, 271, 378-381, 383, 384, 388, 390, 391, 424-426, 429, 430, 448, 476
toroidal, 33, 54, 60-65, 76, 85, 108, 270, 271, 380, 381, 383, 384, 390-392, 400, 476

International Standards Organization (ISO), 3

Invar
   properties of, App. B12

IRAS telescope (see Infrared Astronomical Observatory telescope)

IRG 11
   properties of, App. B5

ISO (see International Standards Organization)

KBr (see Potassium bromide)

KCl (see Potassium chloride)

Keck telescope, 319-326, 484, 497, 499, 501

Kinematic mounting (see Interface, kinematic)

Kitt Peak National Observatory telescope, 313-316

KRS5 (see Thallium bromoiodide)

Kuiper (KAO) telescope, 261-263

Lathe assembly technique, 102-104

Left-handed image (see Image, left-handed)

Lens-to-mount interface (see Interface)

LiF (see Lithium fluoride)

Lightweight glasses (see Glass, lightweight)

Lightweighting of mirrors, 236-267
Liquid pinning (see Epoxy pinning)
Lithium fluoride (LiF)
   properties of, App. B4

Magnesium fluoride (MgF_2)
   properties of, App. B4
Magnesium (Mg)
   properties of, App. B12
Metal matrix
   properties of, App. B10b (see also
   SXA)
M e t h y l m e t h a c r o l a t e   (s e e
   Polymethylmethacrylate)
Methylmethacrolate styrene copolymer
   (NAS)
   properties of, App. B3
Mg (see Magnesium)
MgF_2 (see Magnesium fluoride)
Microscope objective
   alignment of, 456, 457
   use of burnished lenses in, 33, 35,
   456
Microyield strength
   definition of, 10
Military specifications, U.S.
   M I L - S T D - 2 1 0   (c l i m a t i c
   information), 3, 7
   M I L - S T D - 8 1 0   (environmental
   testing), 10
   MIL-S-11031 (sealants), 135
Mirror configuration
   built-up, 233, 236, 248-254, 257
   contoured-back, 237-247
   first-surface, 227-229, 277, 279,
   472, 495
   frit-bonded, 248, 252-254
   machined-back, 248, 255-257, 261,
   262
   metal, 121, 248, 261, 262-264, 297-
   300
   penta, 281-284

retroreflector, 285, 286
roof penta, 283, 284
second-surface, 14, 227, 229-233
Mirror
   principal uses for, 2
MMT (see Multiple-Mirror telescope)
Mo (see Molybdenum)
Modulation (optical) transfer function
   of athermalized lens, 412, 513
   with double-Dove prism, 174
Modulus of elasticity (see Young's
   modulus)
Molybdenum lens cell, 443,444
Molybdenum (Mo)
   properties of, App. B12
Mounting techniques
   mirror,
      adaptive, 259, 260
      air bag, 342, 348-350
      bonded, 277-281
      clamped, 269-278
      elastomeric, 285, 286
      flange, 271-273
      flexure, 287-294
      Hindle, 319-330
      multiple-ring, 329, 333, 334
      parallel post, 305-308
      rim support, 264-267, 301-303
      roller chain/strap, 354-357
      spring clip, 273-278
      threaded retaining ring, 269-271
      three point, 301-303
      whiffletree (see Hindle)
   lens
      burnished, 33, 35, 104, 148
      cantilevered spring, 33, 53-56
      elastomeric, 29, 33, 66-75, 104,
         135, 136, 145, 146, 148, 151-
         153
      flange, 33, 43, 48-53, 121, 137-
         139, 145, 150-153 390, 398
      nonsymmetrical, 33, 55, 56

ring, 36-43
spring, 33, 34
threaded retainer, 33, 44-48,
prism,
    cantilevered bonded, 212-217
    clamped, 193-212
    double-sided bonded, 217-223
    elastomeric, 179
    flexure, 222, 224
    kinematic, 193
    nonkinematic, 208-212
    semikinematic, 193-208
MTF [see Modulation (optical) transfer function]
Multiple-lead thread, 128
Multiple-Mirror telescope (MMT), 334-341

NaCl (see Sodium chloride)
NAS (see Methylmethacrylate styrene copolymer)
Nonkinematic (see Mounting type, prism, nonkinematic)

Ohara E6 glass, 336, 434
  properties of, App. B8a
Optical cement
  properties of, App. B13
Optical transfer function (OTF) [see Modulation (optical) transfer function]

Pechan prism (see Prism types, Pechan)
Pellicle, 265, 266
Penta prism (see Prism types, penta)
Periscope relay lens, 97-99
Pinning (see Epoxy pinning)
Plastic doweling, (see Epoxy pinning)
Plastic lenses
  mounting of, 88-91, 116-118
Plastics, optical

properties of, App. B3
Plate, tilted
  beam displacement introduced by, 231, 232
PMMA (see Polymethylmethacrylate)
Poisson's ratio (υ)
  definition of, 11
Poker-chip assembly, 104-108
Polycarbonate
  properties of, App. B3
Polymethylmethacrylate (PMMA)
  properties of, App. B3
Polystyrene
  properties of, App. B3
Porro prism (see Prism types, Porro)
Porro prism erecting system (see Prism types, Porro erecting system)
Potassium chloride (KCl)
  properties of, App. B4, B17
Potassium bromide (KBr)
  properties of, App. B4, B17
Preload,
  definition of, 22
  variation with temperature, 418-421
Pressure, atmospheric, 4, 5
  typical extremes, 8
Pressure differential, effects of, 145-149
Prism types,
  Abbe erecting system, 169-171
  Abbe version of Porro, 167, 168
  Amici, 165-166
  Amici/penta erecting system, 170, 172, 173
  anamorphic, 189-192
  axicon, 179, 180
  Bauernfeind 45°, 179
  beamsplitter (or beamcombiner)
    cube, 163-165
    plate, 275, 276
  biocular, 181, 182
  constant deviation, 167, 169, 170,

183, 281
cube-corner, 180, 181
delta, 177, 178
dispersing, 182-185
Dove, 173, 174
double-Dove, 173-175
focus-adjusting wedge, 187, 189
Pechan, 176, 177
penta, 170, 171
Porro, 166-168
Porro erecting system, 169, 170
retroreflector (see Cube-corner prism)
reversion, 175, 176
rhomboid, 167, 169
right-angle, 163, 164
right-angle/roof penta, 170, 172
Risley wedge, 187, 188
roof penta, 170, 172
Schmidt, 178
sliding wedge, 187, 189
thin wedge, 185, 186
Power spectral density, 9
Prism, mounting for (see Mounting techniques, prism)
Prism tunnel diagram
illustrations of, 157-161
Purging, 31
Pyrex,
properties of, App. B8a, B9

Quartz (see Fused silica)

Radiation, high-energy, 7
Radiation resistant glass, 7
Rain erosion (see Erosion)
Rectangular lens mounting (see Mounting techniques, lens, nonsymmetrical)
Reflection,
law of, 156
total internal (TIR), 161, 162

Refractive index,
absolute, 406
relative, 406
variation with temperature (dn_G/dT, β_G), 407
variation with wavelength (dispersion), 182, 183
Relative humidity (see Humidity)
Reversion prism (see Prism types, reversion)
Rhomboid prism (see Prism types, rhomboid)
Right-angle prism (see Prism types, right-angle)
Right-handed image (see Image, right-handed),
Rim, lens
spherical, 75, 76
crowned, 76
Risley wedge system (see Prism types, Risley wedge)
Roof penta prism (see Prism types, roof penta)
RTV (see Elastomer)

SAN (see Styrene acrylonitrile)
Sapphire (Al_2O_3)
properties of, App. B5
Schmidt prism (see Prism types, Schmidt)
Sealant (see Elastomer)
Sealing
static, 30, 31, 123-125
dynamic, 124
Self-weight deflection
lens decentration due to, 72-74
of vertical-axis mirror, 300-303
of horizontal-axis mirror, 305-308
Semikinematic mounting (see Interface, semikinematic)
Semiconductor material
properties of, App B6

Sharp-corner interface (see Interface, sharp-corner)

Shell, optical, mounting for, 151-153

Shock
mechanical, 5, 6,
  typical extremes, 8
thermal, 443, 445

Si (see Silicon)

SiC (see Silicon carbide)

Silicon (Si)
properties of, App. B6, B17

Silicon carbide
properties of, App. B8b, B9
characteristics of, App. B10d

Single-point diamond turning (SPDT), 16, 97, 121, 131, 261, 262, 299, 300

Snap ring (see Mounting techniques, lens, ring)

Snell's law, 156

Sodium chloride (NaCl)
properties of, App. B4, B17

SOFIA telescope, 326, 329-332

Spacer
configurations of, 93-99
cross-sectional area,
fabrication of, 96-98
length computation, 93, 94

SPDT (see Single-point diamond turning)

Specific stiffness
definition of, 14
typical values for mirror materials, App. B9

Specific heat
definition of, 11

Spectrograph, FUSE (see Far Ultraviolet Spectroscopic Explorer spectrograph)

Spherical-seat mirror mounting (see Interface, spherical)

Spring mounting for lenses (see Mounting techniques, lens, spring)

Steel, stainless
properties of, App. B12

Steel, corrosion resistant (CRES) (see Steel, stainless)

Steel, carbon
properties of, App. B12

Strain
definition of, 10

Stray light baffling, 99, 167, 208, 227, 445, 456, 459, 461, 571

Stress optic coefficient. 30, 372, 466
definition of, 11

Stress
average, 46, 372, 376, 379, 387-389, 392, 394, 395, 397
contact, 59, 60, 63, 65, 135, 270, 271, 371, 373, 376, 377, 379-387, 390-392, 394, 395, 397, 403, 421, 424, 426, 430, 432, 488, 508,
definition of, 10
radial, 403, 432-436, 449, 463, 466, 488
shear, in bonded interface, 438-440
tangential (hoop) in cell wall, 435, 436
tensile in bent optic, 398-400
tolerance for in glass-type materials, 371

Stress birefringence (see Birefringence)

Styrene (see Polystyrene)

Super Invar
properties of, App. B12

SXA metal matrix
properties of, App. B12

Sylvite (see Potassium chloride)

Tangential interface (see Interface, tangential)

Temperature compensation (see athermalization)

Temperature
effect on axial preload, 418-424

588

gradient, effects of, 414-418
typical extremes, 8
Thallium bromoiodide (KRS5)
properties of, App. B4, B17
Thermal diffusivity
definition of, 11
Thermal conductivity
definition of, 10
Thermal expansion coefficient (see Coefficient of thermal expansion)
Thermal shock, 443, 445
Thermo-optic coefficient (see Coefficient of thermal defocus)
Ti (see Titanium)
TIR (see Reflection, total internal)
Titanium (Ti)
properties of, App. B12
Toroidal interface (see Interface, toroidal)
Torque applied to a retainer, 44-48, App. C

UK telescope, 333, 334
ULE
properties of, App. B8a, B9
Unit conversion factors, App. A
Urethane adhesive
properties of, App. B14

Vibration, 1, 3, 5-10
power spectral density, 7, 9, 10
typical extremes, 8

Weight reduction in mirrors (see Lightweighting of mirrors)
Whiffletree mounting (see Hindle mounting)
Window
deformations of
from temperature gradient, 417, 418
from pressure differential, 145-147

elastomeric mounting of, 135, 136,
heated, 141, 150, 151
laminated, 140, 141, 148, 151
vacuum-tight, 137-139

Yield strength (S_Y)
definition of, 10
Young's modulus (E)
definition of, 10

Zerodur
properties of, App. B8a, B9
Zinc sulfide (ZnS)
properties of, App. B7, B17
Zinc selenide (ZnSe)
properties of, App. B7, B17
ZnS (see Zinc sulfide)
ZnSe (see Zinc selenide)
Zoom mechanisms, 126, 130-132, 414, 482, 483

Biographical Sketch of the Author

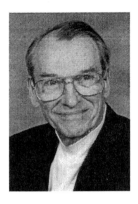 Paul R. Yoder, Jr., retired recently from a career as an independent consultant in optical engineering. For more than 50 years he conducted theoretical and experimental research in optics; designed and analyzed optical instruments; and planned, organized, and managed optical technology and electro-optical system projects ranging from conceptual studies and prototype developments to quantity production of hardware. He has held various technical and engineering management positions with the U.S. Army's Frankford Arsenal, The Perkin-Elmer Corp., and Taunton Technologies, Inc.

Yoder authored or coauthored more than 60 technical papers on optical engineering topics as well as *Opto-Mechanical Systems Design* (Marcel Dekker, New York, 1986 and 2nd ed., 1993); *BASIC-Programme fur die Optik* (Oldenbourg, Munich, 1986); Chapter 37, "Mounting Optical Components," in OSA's *Handbook of Optics* Vol.I (McGraw-Hill, New York, 1994); and Chapter 6 "Optical Mounts" in the *Handbook of Optomechanical Engineering* (CRC Press, Boca Raton). He received his B.S. and M.S. degrees in physics from Juniata College (1947) and The Pennsylvania State University (1950), respectively; he is a Fellow of SPIE, a Fellow of OSA, a member of Sigma Xi; and is listed in *Who's Who in Science and Engineering*. Yoder has served SPIE as a member of the board of directors 1982-1984, 1990-1992 and 1994, and was chairman of the publications committee and member of the executive committee, 1991 and 1994. He also is a founding member of SPIE's Optomechanical/Instrument Working Group. He has served as book reviews editor for *Optical Engineering* and as a topical editor for *Applied Optics*. A frequent organizer and chairman as well as an active participant in SPIE and OSA symposia, he has taught numerous short courses on optical engineering, precision mounting of optical components, principles for mounting optical components, basic optomechanical design, and analysis of the optomechanical interface for SPIE, industry, and U.S. government agencies. He also has taught two nationally broadcast courses for the National Technological University Network and has lectured at the University of Arizona and the National University in Taiwan. He received the Director's Award from SPIE in 1996, the Engineering Excellence Award from OSA in 1997, and the George W. Goddard Award from SPIE in 1999.